Physiotherapy for Respiratory and Cardiac Problems

D1465086

*To John R Plant OBE
whose enthusiasm and interest have always encouraged
development of the Physiotherapy Department at Royal
Brompton Hospital.*

For Churchill Livingstone:

Editorial Director (Nursing and Allied Health): Mary Law
Project Manager: Valerie Burgess
Project Development Editor: Dinah Thom
Design Direction: Judith Wright
Project Controller: Derek Robertson
Copy Editor: Sue Beasley
Indexer: Jill Halliday
Promotion Manager: Hilary Brown

Physiotherapy for Respiratory and Cardiac Problems

Edited by

Jennifer A Pryor MBA MSc FNZSP MCSP
Head of Physiotherapy, Royal Brompton Hospital, London, UK

Barbara A Webber FCSP DSc(Hon)
Formerly Head of Physiotherapy, Royal Brompton Hospital, London, UK

SECOND EDITION

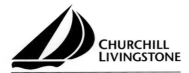
CHURCHILL
LIVINGSTONE

EDINBURGH LONDON NEW YORK PHILADELPHIA SAN FRANCISCO SYDNEY TORONTO 1998

CHURCHILL LIVINGSTONE
A Division of Harcourt Brace and Company Limited

Churchill Livingstone, Robert Stevenson House, 1–3 Baxter's Place, Leith Walk, Edinburgh EH1 3AF, UK

© Longman Group (UK) Limited 1993
© Harcourt Brace and Company Limited 1995

⚏ is a registered trade mark of Harcourt Brace and Company Limited

All rights reserved. No part of this publication may be reproduced, stored in retrieval system, or transmitted in any form or by any means, electronic, mechanical, photocopying, recording or otherwise, without either the prior permission of the publishers (Churchill Livingstone, Robert Stevenson House, 1–3 Baxter's Place, Leith Walk, Edinburgh EH1 3AF), or a licence permitting restricted copying in the United Kingdom issued by the Copyright Licensing Agency Ltd, 90 Tottenham Court Road, London, W1P 9HE.

First edition 1993
Second edition 1998

ISBN 0 443 05841 5

British Library Cataloguing in Publication Data
A catalogue record for this book is available from the British Library.

Library of Congress Cataloging in Publication Data
A catalog record for this book is available from the Library of Congress.

Medical knowledge is constantly changing. As new information becomes available, changes in treatment, procedures, equipment and the use of drugs become necessary. The editors, contributors and the publishers have, as far as it is possible, taken care to ensure that the information given in this text is accurate and up to date. However, readers are strongly advised to confirm that information, especially with regard to drug usage, complies with the latest legislation and standards of practice.

The publisher's policy is to use **paper manufactured from sustainable forests**

Produced by Longman Singapore Publishers (Pte) Ltd.
Printed in Singapore

Contents

Contributors

Stephen J. Barton RGN RMN
Senior Nurse, Respiratory Division, Royal
Brompton Hospital, London, UK

Delva D. Bethune MHSc PT & OT Dip
Associate Professor, School of Rehabilitation
Therapy, Queen's University, Kingston, Ontario,
Canada

Julia Bott MCSP
Consultant Respiratory Physiotherapist,
London, UK

Catherine E. Bray BAppSc(Phty)
Senior Physiotherapist, Cardiopulmonary
Transplant Unit, St Vincent's Hospital,
Sydney, Australia

Wendy Burford RGN BTTA
Director of Nursing, St Ann's Hospice,
Manchester, UK
Formerly Clinical Nurse Specialist, Palliative
Care, Royal Brompton Hospital, London, UK

Conor D. Collins BSc MB MRCPI FRCR
Consultant Radiologist, Christie Hospital,
Manchester, UK
Honorary Lecturer in Radiology, University of
Manchester, UK

Elizabeth Dean PhD PT
Associate Professor, School of Rehabilitation
Medicine, University of British Columbia,
Vancouver, British Columbia, Canada

Elizabeth R. Ellis Grad Dip Phty PhD
Senior Lecturer, School of Physiotherapy,
Faculty of Health Sciences, University of
Sydney, Sydney, Australia

David M. Hansell MD MRCP FRCR
Consultant Radiologist, Royal Brompton
Hospital, Honorary Senior Lecturer, Imperial
College School of Medicine, London, UK

Denise Hills MCSP
Formerly Superintendent Physiotherapist,
Westminster Hospital, London, UK

Diana M. Innocenti FCSP
Formerly Superintendent Physiotherapist, Guy's
Hospital, London, UK

Sue Jenkins PhD GradDipPhys
Senior Lecturer, School of Physiotherapy,
Curtin University of Technology, Perth,
Australia

Mandy Jones MSc MCSP
Senior Physiotherapist, Charing Cross Hospital,
The Hammersmith Hospitals NHS Trust,
London, UK

Helen McBurney PhD BAppSc(Phty)
GradDipPhysio(Cardiothoracic) MAPA
Head, School of Physiotherapy, La Trobe
University, Melbourne, Australia
Physiotherapist (sessional), Box Hill Hospital,
Melbourne, Australia

Debbie McKenzie MCSP
Senior Physiotherapist, Royal Brompton
Hospital, London, UK

Peter G. Middleton MBBS BSc(Med) PhD FRACP
Consultant Physician, Department of
Respiratory Medicine, Westmead Hospital,
Sydney, Australia

Sally Middleton BAppSc(Phty) MSc(Med)
Clinical Research Officer, Institute of
Respiratory Medicine, University of Sydney,
Sydney, Australia

Michael D. L. Morgan MA MD FRCP(UK)
Consultant Physician, Department of
Respiratory Medicine, Glenfield Hospital,
Leicester, UK
Honorary Senior Lecturer, University of
Leicester, UK

Annette Parker MCSP
Superintendent Paediatric Physiotherapist,
Taunton and Somerset Hospital, Taunton, UK

Amanda J. Piper BAppSc Med PhD
Senior Physiotherapist, Centre for Respiratory
Failure and Sleep Disorders, Royal Prince Alfred
Hospital, Sydney, Australia

Helen M. Potter BAppSci(Phty) GradDipManipTher, MSc
Lecturer (Manipulative Therapy), School of
Physiotherapy, Curtin University of
Technology, Perth, Australia

Ammani Prasad MCSP
Respiratory Physiotherapist / Research Assistant,
Cystic Fibrosis Unit, Great Ormond Street
Hospital for Children, London, UK

Jennifer A. Pryor MBA MSc FNZSP MCSP
Head of Physiotherapy, Royal Brompton
Hospital, London, UK

Sarah C. Ridley MCSP
Superintendent Physiotherapist / Medical and
Surgical Specialties, The Royal Infirmary of
Edinburgh, Edinburgh, UK

Julius Sim BA MSc PhD MCSP
Professor, Department of Physiotherapy Studies,
Keele University, Staffordshire, UK

Sally J. Singh PhD BA MCSP
Pulmonary Rehabilitation Coordinator,
Department or Respiratory Medicine, Glenfield
Hospital, Leicester, UK
Honorary Lecturer, University of Leicester,
UK

Beatrice Tucker BAppSc(Phty), PGradDip Physio,
Lecturer, School of Physiotherapy, Curtin
University of Technology, Perth, Australia

John S. Turner MBChB MMed(UCT) FCP(SA)
Physician / Critical Care Specialist, Cape Town,
South Africa

Trudy Ward MCSP GradDipPhys
Therapy Manager, Duke of Cornwall Spinal
Treatment Centre, Salisbury District Hospital,
Salisbury, UK

Fran H. Woodard MCSP
Superintendent Physiotherapist, Charing Cross
Hospital, The Hammersmith Hospitals NHS
Trust, London, UK

Barbara A. Webber FCSP DSc(Hon)
Formerly Head of Physiotherapy, Royal
Brompton Hospital, London, UK

Preface to second edition

During the last five years the term 'evidence based medicine' has had an increasing profile in medicine and 'purchasers' of physiotherapy services are asking for outcomes and evidence that physiotherapy is of benefit in specific patients with specific problems.

We cannot answer all these questions but the database of clinical trials is growing. In assessing the evidence it is important to remember the definition of Sackett et al (1996): 'Evidence based medicine involves integrating individual clinical expertise and the best external evidence available from systematic research'.

In this book we have referenced statements where possible, but there are still many areas of practice which are anecdotal. We must not lose the skills and techniques in these areas if there are indications of patient benefit.

The second edition includes separate and new chapters on surgery and intensive care, and new chapters on non-invasive ventilation and pulmonary rehabilitation. Other chapters have been expanded with sections written by physiotherapy specialists in the field — manual therapy and acupuncture. All the chapters have been updated and new references included.

No text can meet every reader's need but we hope that the material here will lead the reader on to other sources and contacts, and by open exchange of information and ideas we should be able to take the profession forward to benefit our patients.

London 1997

J.A.P
B.A.W

Preface to first edition

This book is intended for physiotherapy students, new graduates and postgraduate physiotherapists with an interest in patients with respiratory and cardiac problems.

Assessment of the patient should reveal the patient's problems. If some or all of these problems can be influenced by physical means, physiotherapy is indicated. Physiotherapy is also indicated when potential problems have been identified and preventative measures should be taken. The role of the physiotherapist as an educator in both the prevention and treatment of problems is another important aspect.

Diagnoses will continue to provide useful medical categories, but treatment can become prescriptive and inappropriate or ineffective if given in response to a diagnosis alone. The pathology behind the problem provides the key as to whether it is a physiotherapy problem or a medical problem.

It is by accurate assessment of the patient that short- and long-term patient goals can be identified and agreed, and an effective treatment plan outlined. Continuous reassessment of the patient and the treatment outcomes will identify the need for continuation or modification of treatment.

This book begins with assessment of the patient and the interpretation of medical investigations. This is followed by a section on mechanical support and cardiopulmonary resuscitation.

An important part of our role is communication, counselling and health education. The skills available to the cardiorespiratory physiotherapist are many and varied. Practical skills have been outlined and referenced where possible. All skills are not yet supported by rigorous clinical studies, but it is important that we continue to use them if outcome measures support their place in clinical practice. In the future measurement tools could validate their use. Research should be an integral part of the practice of physiotherapy.

Patients' problems and their management are outlined in the context of differing pathologies. One pathological process may present as several patient problems. Pneumothorax, for example, appears under the problems of both pain and breathlessness. The characteristic problems of some patient groups and diagnostic categories are then discussed detailing the pathology, medical management, physiotherapy and evaluation of treatment.

This book should be read in conjunction with specialized texts on anatomy, physiology and pathology. Further reading is indicated within each chapter. Throughout the text, for simplicity, the patient is referred to as he/him and the physiotherapist as she/her, but it is not intended to imply that all patients are male or that all physiotherapists are female.

It is hoped that the problem orientated approach to physiotherapy practice will facilitate the learning process for the physiotherapist and improve the quality of the care we provide.

London 1993

B.A.W.
J.A.P.

Acknowledgements

We would like to thank all the authors who have enabled us to bring together expertise from throughout the world. We also thank the many people who so generously shared their experience and knowledge in response to our many questions and read, constructively criticized and contributed to sections of the text: Philippa Carter, Derek Cramer, Mary Dodd, Margaret Hodson, Mandy Jones, Pallav Shah, Peter Wills and Fran Woodard. Milena Potucek and Paul Hyett again took several photographs for us. We are most grateful to all these friends and colleagues.

J.A.P
B.A.W

Investigations, patients' problems and management

1

Assessment

Sally Middleton   Peter G. Middleton

INTRODUCTION

The aim of assessment is to define the patient's problems accurately. It is based on both a subjective and an objective assessment of the patient. Without an accurate assessment it is impossible to develop an appropriate plan of treatment. Equally, a sound theoretical knowledge is required to develop an appropriate treatment plan for those problems which may be improved by physiotherapy. Once treatment has commenced it is important to assess its effectiveness regularly in relation to both the problems and goals.

The system of patient management used in this book is based on the problem oriented medical system (POMS) first described by Weed in 1968. This system has three components:

- Problem oriented medical records (POMR)
- Audit
- Educational programme.

The POMR is now widely used as the method of recording the assessment, management and progress of a patient. It is divided into five sections, as shown in Figure 1.1 and summarized below.

- *Database.* Here personal details, medical history, relevant social history, results of investigations and tests, together with the physiotherapist's assessment of the patient are recorded.
- *Problem list.* This is a concise list of the patient's problems, compiled after the assessment is complete. Problems are not always written in order of priority. The list includes

3

problems both related and unrelated to physiotherapy. The resolution of problems and the appearance of new ones are noted appropriately.

• *Initial plan and goals.* A treatment plan is formulated to address the physiotherapy-related problems, keeping in mind the patient's other problems. Long- and short-term goals are then formulated. Long-term goals are what the patient and the physiotherapist want to finally achieve and should relate to the problems. Short-term goals are the stages by which the long-term goals should be achieved.

• *Progress notes.* These are written to document the patient's progress, especially highlighting any changes. The notes are written in the 'subjective, objective, analysis, plan' (SOAP) format for each problem, and provide an up-to-date summary of the patient's progress.

• *Discharge summary.* This is written when the patient is discharged from treatment or transferred to another institution. It includes presenting problems, treatment given, outcomes of treatment, together with any home programme or follow-up instructions.

DATABASE

The database contains a concise summary of the relevant information about the patient taken from the medical notes, together with the subjective and objective assessment made by the physiotherapist. The format may differ from hospital to hospital, but will contain the same information.

The first part contains the patient's personal details including name, date of birth, address, hospital number, and referring doctor. It may also contain the diagnosis and reason for referral. The second part summarizes the history from the medical notes and the physiotherapy assessment. This is often divided into several sections:

History of presenting condition (HPC) summarizes the patient's current problems, including relevant information from the medical notes.

Previous medical history (PMH) summarizes the entire list of medical and surgical problems that the patient has had in the past. It may be written in disease-specific groupings or as a chronological account.

Drug history (DH) is a list of the patient's current medications (including dosage) taken from the medication charts. Drug allergies should also be noted.

Family history (FH) includes a list of any major

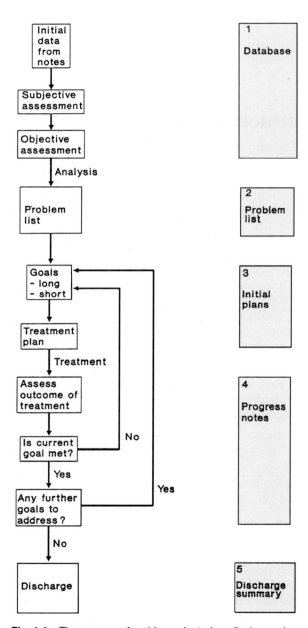

Fig. 1.1 The process of problem oriented medical records.

diseases suffered by members of the immediate family.

Social history (SH) provides a picture of the patient's social situation. It is important to specifically question the patient about the level of support available at home, and to gain an idea of the patient's expected contribution to household duties. The layout of the patient's home should also be ascertained with particular emphasis on stairs. Occupation and hobbies, both past and present, give further information about the patient's lifestyle. Finally, history of smoking and alcohol use should be noted.

Patient examination includes all information collected in the physiotherapist's subjective and objective assessment of the patient.

Test results contain any significant findings as they become available. These may include arterial blood gases, spirometry, blood tests, sputum analysis, chest radiographs, computerized tomography (CT) and any other relevant tests (e.g. hepatitis B positive).

Subjective assessment

Subjective assessment is based on an interview with the patient. It should generally start with open-ended questions – What is the main problem? What troubles you most? – allowing the patient to discuss the problems that are most important to him at that time. Indeed, by asking such questions, previously unmentioned problems may surface. As the interview progresses, questioning may become more focused on those important features that need clarification. There are five main symptoms of respiratory disease:

- Breathlessness (dyspnoea)
- Cough
- Sputum and haemoptysis
- Wheeze
- Chest pain.

With each of these symptoms, enquiries should be made concerning:

- *Duration* – both the absolute time since first recognition of the symptom (months, years) and the duration of the present symptoms (days, weeks)
- *Severity* – in absolute terms and relative to the recent and distant past
- *Pattern* – seasonal or daily variations
- *Associated factors* – including precipitants, relieving factors, and associated symptoms, if any.

Breathlessness

Breathlessness is the subjective awareness of an increased work of breathing. It is the predominant symptom of both cardiac and respiratory disease. It also occurs in anaemia where the oxygen-carrying capacity of the blood is reduced, in neuromuscular disorders where the respiratory muscles are affected, and in metabolic disorders where there is a change in the acid–base equilibrium (see Ch. 3) or metabolic rate (e.g. hyperthyroid disorders). Breathlessness is also found in hyperventilation syndrome where it is due to psychological factors (e.g. anxiety).

The pathophysiological mechanisms causing breathlessness are still the subject of intensive investigation. Many factors are involved, including respiratory muscle length–tension relationships, respiratory muscle fatigue, stimulation of pulmonary stretch receptors, and alterations in central respiratory drive.

The duration and severity of breathlessness is most easily assessed through enquiries about the level of functioning in the recent and distant past. For example, a patient may say that 3 years ago he could walk up five flights of stairs without stopping, but now cannot even manage one flight. Some patients may deny breathlessness as they have (unconsciously) decreased their activity levels so that they do not get breathless. They may only acknowledge breathlessness when it interferes with important activities, e.g. bathing. The physiotherapist should always relate breathlessness to the level of function that the patient can achieve.

Comparison of the severity of breathlessness between patients is difficult because of differences in perception and expectations. To overcome these difficulties, numerous gradings have

Table 1.1 The New York Heart Association classification of breathlessness

Class I	No symptoms with ordinary activity, breathlessness only occurring with severe exertion, e.g. running up hills, fast bicycling, cross-country skiing
Class II	Symptoms with ordinary activity, e.g. walking up stairs, making beds, carrying large amounts of shopping
Class III	Symptoms with mild exertion, e.g. bathing, showering, dressing
Class IV	Symptoms at rest

been proposed. The New York Heart Association grading (1964) shown in Table 1.1, was developed for patients with cardiac disease, but is also applicable to respiratory patients. No scale is universal and it is important that all staff within one institution use the same scale.

Breathlessness is usually worse during exercise and better with rest. The one exception is hyperventilation syndrome where breathlessness may improve with exercise. Two patterns of breathlessness have been given specific names:

- *Orthopnoea* is breathlessness when lying flat.
- *Paroxysmal nocturnal dyspnoea* (*PND*) is breathlessness that wakes the patient at night. In the cardiac patient, lying flat increases venous return from the legs so that blood pools in the lungs, causing breathlessness. A similar pattern may be described in patients with severe asthma, but here the breathlessness is caused by nocturnal bronchoconstriction.

Further insight into a patient's breathlessness may be gained by enquiring about precipitating and relieving factors. Breathlessness associated with exposure to allergens and relieved by bronchodilators is typically found in asthma.

Cough

Coughing is a protective reflex which rids the airways of secretions or foreign bodies. Any stimulation of receptors located in the pharynx, larynx, trachea, or bronchi may induce cough. Cough is a difficult symptom to clarify as most people cough normally every day, yet a repetitive persistent cough is both troublesome and

distressing. Smokers may discount their early morning cough as being 'normal' when in fact it signifies chronic bronchitis.

Important features concerning cough are its effectiveness, and whether it is productive or dry. The severity of cough may range from an occasional disturbance to a continual trouble. A loud, barking cough, which is often termed 'bovine', may signify laryngeal or tracheal disease. Recurrent coughing after eating or drinking is an important symptom of aspiration. A chronic productive cough every day is a fundamental feature of chronic bronchitis and bronchiectasis. Interstitial lung disease is characterized by a persistent, dry cough. Nocturnal cough is an important symptom of asthma in children and young adults, but in older patients it is more commonly due to cardiac failure. Drugs, especially beta-blockers and some other anti-hypertensive agents, can cause a chronic cough. Chronic cough may cause fractured ribs (cough fractures) and hernias. Stress incontinence is a common complication of chronic cough, especially in women. As this subject is often embarrassing to the patient, specific questioning may be required (see page 8).

Postoperatively, the strength and effectiveness of cough is important for the physiotherapist to assess.

Sputum

In a normal adult, approximately 100 ml of tracheobronchial secretions are produced daily and cleared subconsciously. Sputum is the excess tracheobronchial secretions that is cleared from the airways by coughing or huffing. It may contain mucus, cellular debris, microorganisms, blood and foreign particles. Questioning should determine the colour, consistency and quantity of sputum produced each day. This may clarify the diagnosis and the severity of disease (Table 1.2).

A number of grading systems for mucoid–mucopurulent–purulent sputum have been proposed. For example, Miller (1963) suggested:

M1 mucoid with no suspicion of pus
M2 predominantly mucoid, suspicion of pus

Table 1.2 Sputum analysis

	Description	Causes
Saliva	Clear watery fluid	
Mucoid	Opalescent or white	Chronic bronchitis without infection, asthma
Mucopurulent	Slightly discoloured, but not frank pus	Bronchiectasis, cystic fibrosis, pneumonia
Purulent	Thick, viscous: Yellow Dark green/brown Rusty Red currant jelly	 Haemophilus Pseudomonas Pneumococcus, mycoplasma Klebsiella
Frothy	Pink or white	Pulmonary oedema
Haemoptysis	Ranging from blood specks to frank blood, old blood (dark brown)	Infection (tuberculosis, bronchiectasis), infarction, carcinoma, vasculitis, trauma, also coagulation disorders, cardiac disease
Black	Black specks in mucoid secretions	Smoke inhalation (fires, tobacco, heroin), coal dust

P1 1/3 purulent, 2/3 mucoid
P2 2/3 purulent, 1/3 mucoid
P3 > 2/3 purulent.

However, in clinical practice sputum is often classified as mucoid, mucopurulent or purulent, together with an estimation of the volume (1 teaspoon, 1 egg cup, ½ cup, 1 cup).

Sputum 'plugs' are hard rubbery casts in the shape of the bronchial tree which may be produced in asthma, allergic bronchopulmonary aspergillosis (ABPA) and occasionally in bronchiectasis.

Haemoptysis is the presence of blood in the sputum. It may range from slight streaking of the sputum to frank blood. Frank haemoptysis can be life threatening, requiring bronchial artery embolization or surgery. Isolated haemoptysis may be the first sign of bronchogenic carcinoma, even when the chest radiograph is normal. Patients with chronic infective lung disease often suffer from recurrent haemoptyses.

Odour emanating from sputum signifies infection. In general, particularly offensive odours suggest infection with anaerobic organisms (e.g. aspiration pneumonia, lung abscess).

Wheeze

Wheeze is a whistling or musical sound produced by turbulent airflow through narrowed airways. These sounds are generally noted by patients when audible at the mouth. Stridor, the sound of an upper airway obstruction, is often mistakenly called 'wheeze' by patients. Heart failure may also cause wheezing in those patients with significant mucosal oedema. For a full discussion of wheeze see page 18.

Chest pain

Chest pain in respiratory patients usually originates from musculoskeletal, pleural or tracheal inflammation, as the lung parenchyma and small airways contain no pain fibres.

Pleuritic chest pain is caused by inflammation of the parietal pleura, and is usually described as a severe, sharp, stabbing pain which is worse on inspiration. It is not reproduced by palpation.

Tracheitis generally causes a constant burning pain in the centre of the chest, aggravated by breathing.

Musculoskeletal (chest wall) pain may originate from the muscles, bones, joints or nerves of the thoracic cage. It is usually well localized and exacerbated by chest and/or arm movement. Palpation will usually reproduce the pain.

Angina pectoris is a major symptom of cardiac disease. Myocardial ischaemia characteristically causes a dull central retrosternal gripping or band-like sensation which may radiate to either arm, neck or jaw.

Pericarditis may cause pain similar to angina or pleurisy.

A differential diagnosis of chest pain is given in Table 1.3.

Incontinence

Incontinence is a problem which is often aggravated by chronic cough. Coughing and huffing increase intra-abdominal pressure which may precipitate urine leakage. Fear of this may influence compliance with physiotherapy. Thus identification and treatment of incontinence is important. Questions may need to be specific to elicit this symptom: *'When you cough, do you find that you leak some urine?' 'Does this interfere with your physiotherapy?'*.

Other symptoms

Of the other symptoms a patient may report, a number have particular importance.

Table 1.3 Syndromes of chest pain

Condition	Description	Causes
Pulmonary		
Pleurisy	Sharp, stabbing, rapid onset, limits inspiration, well localized, often 'catches' at a certain lung volume, not tender on palpation	Pleural infection or inflammation of the pleura, trauma (haemothorax), malignancy
Pulmonary embolus	Usually has pleuritic pain, with or without severe central pain	Pulmonary infarction
Pneumothorax	Severe central chest discomfort, with or without pleuritic component, severity depends on extent of mediastinal shift	Trauma, spontaneous, lung diseases (e.g., cystic fibrosis, AIDS)
Tumours	May mimic any form of chest pain, depending on site and structures involved	Primary or secondary carcinoma, mesothelioma
Musculoskeletal		
Rib fracture	Localized point tenderness, often sudden onset, increases with inspiration	Trauma, tumour, cough fractures (e.g. in chronic lung diseases, osteoporosis)
Muscular	Superficial, increases on inspiration and some body movements, with or without palpable muscle spasm	Trauma, unaccustomed exercise (excessive coughing during exacerbations of lung disease), accessory muscles may be affected
Costochondritis (Tietze's syndrome)	Localized to one or more costochondral joints, with or without generalized, non-specific chest pain	Viral infection
Neuralgia	Pain or paraesthesia in a dermatomal distribution	Thoracic spine dysfunction, tumour, trauma, herpes zoster (shingles)
Cardiac		
Ischaemic heart disease (angina or infarct)	Dull, central, retrosternal discomfort like a weight or band with or without radiation to the jaw and/or either arm, may be associated with palpitations, nausea, or vomiting	Myocardial ischaemia, onset at rest is more suggestive of infarction
Pericarditis	Often retrosternal, exacerbated by respiration, may mimic cardiac ischaemia or pleurisy, often relieved by sitting	Infection, inflammation, trauma, tumour
Mediastinum		
Dissecting aortic aneurysm	Sudden onset, severe, poorly localized central chest pain	Trauma, atherosclerosis, Marfan's syndrome
Oesophageal	Retrosternal burning discomfort, but can mimic all other pains, worse lying flat or bending forward	Oesophageal reflux, trauma, tumour
Mediastinal shift	Severe, poorly localized central discomfort	Pneumothorax, rapid drainage of a large pleural effusion

Fever (pyrexia) is one of the common features of infection, but low-grade fevers can also occur with malignancy and connective tissue disorders. Equally, infection may occur without fever, especially in immunosuppressed (e.g. chemotherapy) patients or those on corticosteroids. High fevers occurring at night, with associated sweating (night sweats), may be the first indicator of pulmonary tuberculosis.

Headache is an uncommon feature of respiratory disease. Morning headaches in patients with severe respiratory failure may signify nocturnal carbon dioxide retention. Early morning arterial blood gases or nocturnal transcutaneous carbon dioxide monitoring are required for confirmation.

Peripheral oedema in the respiratory patient suggests right heart failure which may be due to cor pulmonale (right ventricular failure secondary to hypoxic pulmonary vasoconstriction). Peripheral oedema may also occur in patients taking high-dose corticosteroids, as a result of salt and water retention.

Functional ability

It is important to assess the patient as a whole, enquiring about his daily activities. If the patient is employed, what does his job *actually* entail? For example, a surveyor may sit behind a desk all day, or he may be climbing 25-storey buildings. The home situation should also be documented, in particular the number of stairs to the front door and within the house. With whom does the patient live? What roles does the patient perform in the home (shopping, housework, cooking)? Finally, questions concerning activities and recreation often reveal areas where significant improvements in quality of life can be made.

Disease awareness

During the interview it is important to ascertain the patient's knowledge of his disease and treatment. The level of compliance with treatment, often difficult to assess initially, may become evident as rapport develops. These issues will influence the goals of treatment.

Objective assessment

Objective assessment is based on examination of the patient, together with the use of tests such as spirometry, arterial blood gases and chest radiographs. Although a full examination of the patient should be available from the medical notes, it is worthwhile to make a thorough examination at all times as the patient's condition may have changed since the last examination, and the physiotherapist may need greater detail of certain aspects than is available from the notes. A good examination will provide an objective baseline for the future measurement of the patient's progress. By developing a standard method of examination, the findings are quickly assimilated, and the physiotherapist remains confident that nothing has been omitted.

General observation

Examination starts by observing the patient from the end of the bed. Is the patient short of breath, sitting on the edge of the bed, distressed? Is he obviously cyanosed? Is he on supplemental oxygen? If so, how much? What is his speech pattern – long fluent paragraphs without discernible pauses for breath, quick sentences, just a few words, or is he too breathless to speak? When he moves around or undresses, does he become distressed? With a little practice, these observations should become second nature and can be noted whilst introducing yourself to the patient.

In the intensive care patient there are a number of further features to be observed. The level of ventilatory support must be ascertained. This includes both the mode of ventilation (e.g. supplemental oxygen, continuous positive airway pressure, intermittent positive pressure ventilation) and the route of ventilation (mask, endotracheal tube, tracheostomy). The level of cardiovascular support should also be noted, including drugs to control blood pressure and cardiac output, pacemakers and other mechanical devices. The patient's level of consciousness should also be noted. Any patient with a decreased level of consciousness is at risk of aspiration and reten-

Table 1.4 The Glasgow Coma Scale

Eye opening	Spontaneous	4
	To speech	3
	To pain	2
	None	1
Best verbal response	Oriented	5
	Confused speech	4
	Inappropriate words	3
	Incomprehensible sounds	2
	None	1
Best motor response	Obeys commands	6
	Localizes to pain	5
	Withdraws (generalized)	4
	Flexion	3
	Extension	2
	No response	1

Maximum total score is 15; minimum total score is 3.

tion of pulmonary secretions. In those patients who are not pharmacologically sedated, the level of consciousness is often measured using the Glasgow Coma Scale (Table 1.4). This gives the patient a score (from 3 to 15) based on his best motor, verbal and eye responses.

The patient's chart should then be examined for recordings of temperature, pulse, blood pressure and respiratory rate. These measurements are usually performed by the nursing staff immediately on admission of the patient and regularly thereafter.

For details of the assessment of the infant and child see page 332.

Body temperature. Body temperature can be measured in a number of ways. Oral temperatures are the most convenient method in adults but should not be performed for at least 15 minutes after smoking or consuming hot or cold food or drink. Aural, axillary and rectal temperature may also be measured.

Body temperature is maintained within the range 36.5–37.5°C. It is lowest in the early morning and highest in the afternoon.

Fever (pyrexia) is the elevation of the body temperature above 37.5°C, and is associated with an increased metabolic rate. For every 0.6°C (1°F) rise in body temperature, there is an approximately 10% increase in oxygen consumption and carbon dioxide production. This places extra demand on the cardiorespiratory system which causes a compensatory increase in heart rate and respiratory rate.

Heart rate. Heart rate is most accurately measured by auscultation at the cardiac apex. The pulse rate is measured by palpating a peripheral artery (radial, femoral or carotid). In most situations, the heart rate and pulse rate are identical; a difference between the two is called the 'pulse deficit'. This indicates that some heart beats have not caused sufficient blood flow to reach the periphery and is commonly found in atrial fibrillation and some other arrhythmias.

The normal adult heart rate is 60–100 beats per minute.

Tachycardia is defined as a heart rate greater than 100 beats/min at rest. It is found with anxiety, exercise, fever, anaemia and hypoxia. It is also common in patients with cardiac disorders. Medications such as bronchodilators and some cardiac drugs may also increase heart rate.

Bradycardia is defined as a heart rate less than 60 beats/min. It may be a normal finding in athletes and may also be caused by some cardiac drugs (especially beta-blockers).

Blood pressure (BP). With every contraction of the heart (systole) the arterial pressure increases, with the peak called the 'systolic' pressure. During the relaxation phase of the heart (diastole), the arterial pressure drops, with the minimum called the 'diastolic' pressure. Blood pressure is usually measured non-invasively by placing a sphygmomanometer cuff around the upper arm, and listening over the brachial artery with a stethoscope. The cuff width should be approximately one-half to two-thirds of the length of the upper arm, otherwise readings may be inaccurate. Cuff inflation to above systolic pressure collapses the artery, blocking flow. With release of the air, the cuff pressure gradually falls to a point just below systolic. At this point, the peak pressure within the artery is greater than the pressure outside the artery, so flow recommences. This turbulent flow is audible through the stethoscope. As the cuff is further deflated the noise continues. When the cuff pressure drops to just below diastolic, the pressure within the artery is greater than that of the cuff throughout the cardiac cycle, so turbulence abates and the noise ceases.

Blood pressure is recorded as systolic/diastolic pressure. Normal adult blood pressure is between 95/60 and 140/90 mmHg.

Hypertension is defined as a blood pressure of greater than 145/95 mmHg, usually due to changes in vascular tone and/or aortic valve disease.

Hypotension is defined as a blood pressure of less than 90/60 mmHg. It is often a normal finding during sleep. Daytime hypotension may be due to heart failure, blood loss or decreased vascular tone.

Postural hypotension is a drop in blood pressure of more than 5 mmHg between lying and sitting or standing, and may be due to decreased circulating blood volume, or loss of vascular tone.

Pulsus paradoxus is the exaggeration of the drop in blood pressure that occurs with inspiration. Normally, during inspiration the negative intrathoracic pressure reduces venous return and drops cardiac output slightly. Exaggeration of this normal response where blood pressure drops by more than 10 mmHg is seen in situations where the intrathoracic pressure swings are greater, as occurs in severe airway obstruction.

Respiratory rate. Respiratory rate should be measured with the patient seated comfortably. The normal adult respiratory rate is approximately 12–16 breaths/min.

Tachypnoea is defined as a respiratory rate greater than 20 breaths/min, and can be seen in any form of lung disease. It may also occur with metabolic acidosis and anxiety.

Bradypnoea is defined as a respiratory rate of less than 10 breaths/min. It is an uncommon finding, and is usually due to central nervous system depression by narcotics or trauma.

Body weight. Weight is often recorded on the observation chart. Respiratory function can be compromised by both obesity and severe malnourishment. As ideal body weight has a large normal range, the body mass index (BMI) has been proposed as an alternative. This is calculated by dividing the weight in kilograms by the square of the height in metres (kg/m^2); the normal range is 20–25 kg/m^2. Patients with values below 20 are underweight, those with values of 25–30 are overweight, and those with values over 30 are classified as obese.

Malnourished patients often exhibit depression of their immune system with increased risk of infection. They also have weaker respiratory muscles which are more likely to fatigue. Obesity causes an increase in residual volume (RV) and a decrease in functional residual capacity (FRC) (Rubinstein et al 1990). Thus tidal breathing occurs close to closing volumes. This is particularly important postoperatively, where the obese are more prone to subsegmental lung collapse.

An accurate daily weight gives a good estimate of fluid volume changes, as any change in weight of more than 250 g/day is usually due to fluid accumulation or loss. Daily weights are commonly used in intensive care, renal and cardiac patients to assess fluid balance.

Other measures. In the intensive care patient there is a plethora of monitoring that can be performed. As well as the parameters listed above, measures of central venous pressure (CVP), pulmonary artery pressure (PAP), and intracranial pressure (ICP) will need to be reviewed as part of the physiotherapy assessment. Some intensive care units now record this information on bedside computer terminals. Further details of intensive care monitoring can be found in Chapters 4 and 5.

Apparatus. At this point the lines and tubes going into and coming out of the patient should be noted. Venous lines provide constant direct access to the bloodstream, and vary widely in site, complexity and function. The simplest cannula in a small peripheral vein, usually in the forearm, is called a 'drip'. It is used for the administration of intravenous (IV) fluids and most IV drugs. At the other end of the spectrum are the multi-lumen lines placed in the subclavian, internal jugular or femoral veins, ending in the venae cavae close to the heart. These central lines allow simultaneous administration of multiple drugs and can be used for central venous pressure monitoring. Central lines can be potentially dangerous, as disconnection of the line can quickly suck air into the central veins, causing an air embolus which may be fatal.

Some patients, especially those in intensive care, may have an arterial line for continuous recording of blood pressure and for repeated sampling of arterial blood. These lines are usually inserted in the radial or brachial artery. If accidentally disconnected, rapid blood loss will occur.

After cardiac surgery, most patients have cardiac pacing wires which exit through the skin overlying the heart. In most cases these wires are not required and are removed routinely before discharge. In the event of clinically significant cardiac arrhythmias, these wires are connected to a pacing box that electrically stimulates the heart. In medical patients, pacemaker wires are introduced through one of the central veins and rest in the apex of the right ventricle. Care must be taken with all pacing wires as dislodgement may be life threatening.

Intercostal drains are placed between two ribs into the pleural space to remove air, fluid or pus which has accumulated. They are also used routinely after cardiothoracic surgery. In general, the tube is attached to a bottle partially filled with sterile water, called an 'underwater seal drain'. The bottle should be positioned at least 0.5 metres below the patient's chest (usually on the floor). Bubbling indicates that air is entering the tube from the pleural space at that time. Frequent observations must be made of the fluid level within the tube which should oscillate or 'swing' with every breath. If the fluid does not swing, the tube is not patent and requires medical attention. In certain situations the bottle may be connected to continuous suction which will dampen the fluid 'swing'. Those patients who are producing large volumes of fluid or pus may be connected to a double bottle system, where the first bottle acts as a reservoir to collect the fluid and the second provides the underwater seal. More recently, fully enclosed disposable plastic systems have been devised. Any patient with a chest drain should have a pair of large forceps available at all times to clamp the tube if any connection becomes loosened.

Postoperatively, drains may be placed at any operation site (e.g. abdomen) to prevent the collection of fluid or blood. These are generally connected to sterile bags. Nasogastric tubes are placed for two reasons: soft, fine-bore tubes are used to facilitate feeding, whilst firm, wider-bore tubes allow aspiration of gastric contents.

The hands. The hands provide a wealth of information. A fine tremor will often be seen in association with high-dose bronchodilators. Warm and sweaty hands with an irregular flapping tremor may be due to acute carbon dioxide retention. Weakness and wasting of the small muscles in the hands may be an early sign of an upper lobe tumour involving the brachial plexus (Pancoast's tumour). Examination of the fingers may show nicotine staining from smoking.

Clubbing is the term used to describe the changes in the fingers and toes as shown in Figure 1.2. The first sign of clubbing is the loss of the angle between the nail bed and the nail itself. Later, the finger pad becomes enlarged. The nail bed may also become 'spongy', but this is a difficult sign to elicit. A summary of the diseases associated with clubbing is given in Table 1.5. The exact cause of clubbing is unknown. It is interesting to note that clubbing in cystic fibrosis patients disappears after heart and lung or lung transplant.

The eyes. The eyes should be examined for pallor (anaemia), plethora (high haemoglobin) or jaundice (yellow colour due to liver or blood disturbances). Drooping of one eyelid with enlargement of that pupil suggests Horner's syndrome where there is a disturbance in the sympathetic nerve supply to that side of the head (sometimes seen in cancer of the lung).

Cyanosis. This is a bluish discolouration of the skin and mucous membranes. Central cyanosis, seen on examination of the tongue and mouth, is caused by hypoxaemia where there is an increase in the amount of haemoglobin not bound to oxygen. The degree of blueness is related to the quantity of unbound haemoglobin. Thus a greater degree of hypoxia is necessary to produce cyanosis in an anaemic patient (low haemoglobin), whilst a patient with polycythaemia (increased haemoglobin) may appear

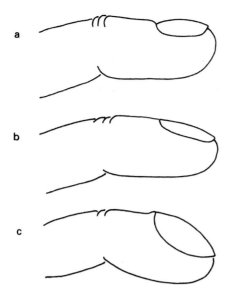

Fig. 1.2 Clubbing: **a** normal; **b** early clubbing; **c** advanced clubbing.

Table 1.5 Causes of clubbing

Lung disease	Infective (bronchiectasis, lung abscess, empyema) Fibrotic Malignant (bronchogenic cancer, mesothelioma)
Cardiac disease	Congenital cyanotic heart disease Bacterial endocarditis
Other	Familial Cirrhosis Gastrointestinal disease (Crohn's disease, ulcerative colitis, coeliac disease)

cyanosed with only a small drop in oxygen levels. Peripheral cyanosis, affecting the toes, fingers and earlobes may also be due to poor peripheral circulation, especially in cold weather.

Jugular venous pressure. On the side of the neck the jugular venous pressure (JVP) is seen as a flickering impulse in the jugular vein. It is normally seen at the base of the neck when the patient is lying back at 45°. The JVP is usually measured in relation to the sternal angle as this point is relatively fixed in relation to the right atrium. A normal JVP at the base of the neck corresponds to a vertical height approximately 3–4 cm above the sternal angle. The JVP is generally expressed as the vertical height (in centimetres) above normal. The JVP provides a quick assessment of the volume of blood in the great vessels entering the heart. Most commonly it is elevated in right heart failure. This may occur in patients with chronic lung disease complicated by cor pulmonale. In contrast, dehydrated patients may only have a visible JVP when lying flat.

Peripheral oedema. This is an important sign of cardiac failure, but may also be found in patients with a low albumin level, impaired venous or lymphatic function, or those on high-dose steroids. When mild it may only affect the ankles, with increasing severity it may progress up the body. In bedbound patients, it is important to check the sacrum.

Observation of the chest

When examining the chest it is important to remember the surface landmarks of the thoracic contents (Fig. 1.3).

Some important points are:

• The oblique fissure, dividing the upper and middle lobes from the lower lobes, runs underneath a line drawn from the spinous process of T2 around the chest to the 6th costochondral junction anteriorly.

• The horizontal fissure on the right, dividing the upper lobe from the middle lobe, runs from the 4th intercostal space at the right sternal edge horizontally to the midaxillary line, where it joins the oblique fissure.

• The diaphragm sits at approximately the 6th rib anteriorly, the 8th rib in the midaxillary line, and the 10th rib posteriorly.

• The trachea bifurcates just below the level of the manubriosternal junction.

• The apical segment of both upper lobes extends 2.5 cm above the clavicles.

Chest shape. The chest should be symmetrical with the ribs, in adults, descending at approximately 45° from the spine. The transverse diameter should be greater than the anteroposterior (AP) diameter. The thoracic spine should have

Anterior

Posterior

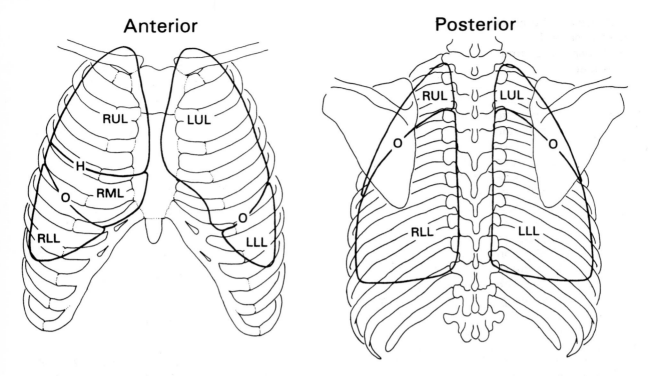

Fig. 1.3 Surface markings of the lungs: H, horizontal fissure; O, oblique fissures; RUL, right upper lobe; LUL, left upper lobe; RML, right middle lobe; LLL, left lower lobe; RLL, right lower lobe.

a slight kyphosis. Important common abnormalities include:

Kyphosis, where the normal flexion of the thoracic spine is increased.

Kyphoscoliosis, which comprises both lateral curvature of the spine with vertebral rotation (scoliosis) and an element of kyphosis. This causes a restrictive lung defect which, when severe, may cause respiratory failure.

Pectus excavatum, or 'funnel' chest, is where part of the sternum is depressed inwards. This rarely causes significant changes in lung function but may be corrected surgically for cosmetic reasons.

Pectus carinatum, or 'pigeon' chest, is where the sternum protrudes anteriorly. This may be present in children with severe asthma and rarely causes significant lung function abnormalities.

Hyperinflation, where the ribs lose their normal 45° angle with the thoracic spine and become almost horizontal. The anteroposterior diameter of the chest increases to almost equal the trans-

verse diameter. This is commonly seen in severe emphysema.

Breathing pattern. Observation of the breathing pattern gives further information concerning the type and severity of respiratory disease.

Normal breathing should be regular with a rate of 12–16 breaths/min, as mentioned previously. Inspiration is active and expiration passive. The approximate ratio of inspiratory to expiratory time (I : E ratio) is 1 : 1.5 to 1 : 2.

Prolonged expiration may be seen in patients with obstructive lung disease, where expiratory airflow is severely limited by dynamic closure of the smaller airways. In severe obstruction the I : E ratio may increase to 1 : 3 or 1 : 4.

Pursed-lip breathing is often seen in patients with severe airways disease. By opposing the lips during expiration the airway pressure inside the chest is maintained, preventing the floppy airways from collapsing. Thus overall airflow is increased.

Apnoea is the absence of breathing for more than 15 seconds.

Hypopnoea is diminished breathing with inadequate ventilation. It may be seen during sleep in patients with lung disease.

Kussmaul's respiration is rapid, deep breathing with a high minute ventilation. It is usually seen in patients with metabolic acidosis.

Cheyne–Stokes respiration refers to irregular breathing with cycles consisting of a few relatively deep breaths, progressively shallower breaths (sometimes to the point of apnoea), and then slowly increasing depth of breaths. This is usually associated with heart failure, severe neurological disturbances, or drugs (e.g. narcotics).

Ataxic breathing consists of haphazard, unco-ordinated deep and shallow breaths. This may be found in patients with cerebellar disease.

Apneustic breathing is characterized by prolonged inspiration, and is usually the result of brain damage.

Chest movement. During normal inspiration, there are symmetrical increases in the anteroposterior, transverse and vertical diameters of the chest. The increase in vertical diameter is achieved by contraction of the diaphragm, causing the abdominal contents to descend. Sternal and rib movements are responsible for the increases in anteroposterior and transverse diameters of the chest. These movements can be divided into two components (Fig. 1.4). When elevated, the anterior ends of the ribs move forward and upwards with anterior movement of the sternum. This increase in anteroposterior diameter is likened to the movement of an old fashioned 'pump handle'. At the same time, rotation of the ribs causes an increase in the transverse diameter, likened to the movement of a 'bucket handle'.

During normal quiet breathing, the diaphragm is the main inspiratory muscle increasing the vertical diameter. There is also an increase in the lower thoracic transverse diameter due to external intercostal muscle contraction. Expiration is passive, caused by the elastic recoil of the lung and chest wall. When breathing is increased, all the accessory inspiratory muscles (sternomastoid, scalenes, trapezii) contract to

Pump handle

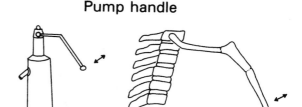

Bucket handle

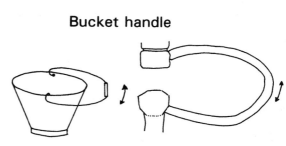

Fig. 1.4   Chest wall movement.

increase the anteroposterior and transverse diameters, and the diaphragm activity increases, thus further increasing the vertical dimensions. Expiration may become active with contraction of the abdominal and internal intercostal muscles.

Intercostal indrawing occurs where the skin between the ribs is drawn inwards during inspiration. It may be seen in patients with severe inspiratory airflow resistance. Larger negative pressures during inspiration suck the soft tissues inwards. This is an important sign of respiratory distress in children, but is less often seen in adults.

Palpation of the chest

Trachea. Firstly, the trachea is palpated to assess its position in relation to the sternal notch. Tracheal deviation indicates underlying mediastinal shift. The trachea may be pulled towards a collapsed or fibrosed upper lobe, or pushed away from a pneumothorax or large pleural effusion.

Chest expansion. This can be assessed by observation, but palpation is more accurate. The patient is instructed to expire slowly to residual volume. At residual volume the examiner's hands are placed spanning the posterolateral segments of both bases, with the thumbs touching in the midline posteriorly, as shown in Figure 1.5. In obese patients, it helps if the skin of the anterior chest wall is slightly retracted by the fingertips. The patient is then instructed to inspire slowly and the movement of both thumbs is observed. Both sides should move equally, with 3–5 cm being the normal displacement.

A similar technique may be used anteriorly, again to measure basal movements. Measurement of apical movement is more difficult. By placing the hand over the upper chest anteriorly, a qualitative comparison of the two sides can be made. In all cases, diminished movement is abnormal.

Paradoxical breathing is where some or all of the chest wall moves inwards on inspiration and outwards on expiration. It can involve anything from a localized area to the entire chest wall. Localized paradox occurs when the integrity of the chest wall is disrupted. Fractures of multiple ribs with two or more breaks in each rib will result in the central section losing the support usually provided by the rest of the thoracic cage. Thus, during inspiration, this loose segment (often called a 'flail segment') is drawn inwards as the rest of the chest wall moves out. In expiration the reverse occurs.

Paradoxical movement of one hemithorax may be remarkably difficult to observe. It may be caused by unilateral diaphragm paralysis. Paradox of the entire chest wall occurs in bilateral diaphragm weakness or paralysis. It is most apparent when the patient is supine.

Paradoxical movement of the lower chest can occur in patients with severe chronic airflow limitation who are extremely hyperinflated. As the dome of the diaphragm cannot descend any further, diaphragm contraction during inspiration pulls the lower ribs inwards. This is called 'Hoover's sign'.

Surgical emphysema. Air in the subcutaneous tissues of the chest, neck or face should also be noted. On palpation there is a characteristic crackling in the skin. This occurs when a pneumomediastinum (air in the mediastinum) has tracked outwards. A chest radiograph must

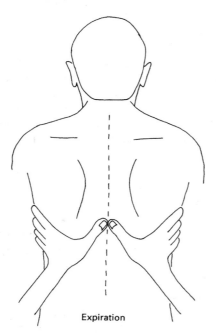 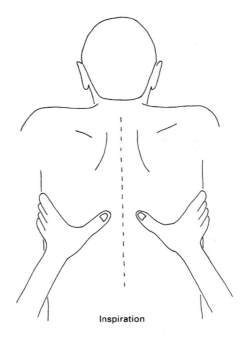

Expiration   Inspiration

Fig. 1.5 Palpation of thoracic expansion.

be performed immediately, as a pneumo-mediastinum may be associated with a pneumothorax.

Vocal fremitus. Vocal fremitus is the measure of speech vibrations transmitted through the chest wall to the examiner's hands. It is measured by asking the patient to repeatedly say '99', whilst the examiner's hands are placed flat on both sides of the chest. The hands are moved from apices to bases, anteriorly and posteriorly, comparing the vibration felt. Vocal fremitus is increased when the lung underneath is relatively solid (consolidated), as this transmits sound better. As sound transmission is decreased through any interface between lung and air or fluid, vocal fremitus is decreased in patients with a pneumothorax or a pleural effusion.

Percussion

Percussion of the chest provides further information that can help in the assessment and localization of lung disease. It is performed by placing the left hand firmly on the chest wall so that the fingers have good contact with the skin. The middle finger of the left hand is struck over the distal interphalangeal joint with the middle finger of the right hand. The right wrist should be relaxed so that the weight of the entire right hand is transmitted through the middle finger. Both sides of the chest from top to bottom should be percussed alternately, paying particular attention to the comparison between sides.

Resonance is generated by the chest wall vibrating over the underlying tissues. Normal resonance is heard over aerated lung, whilst consolidated lung sounds dull, and a pleural effusion sounds 'stony dull'. Increased resonance is heard when the chest wall is free to vibrate over an air-filled space, such as a pneumothorax or bulla. In situations where the chest wall is unable to move freely, as may occur in obese patients, the percussion note may sound dull, even if the underlying lung is normal.

Auscultation

Chest auscultation is the process of listening to and interpreting the sounds produced within the thorax. A stethoscope simplifies auscultation and facilitates localization of any abnormalities. It consists of a diaphragm and bell connected by tubing to two ear-pieces. The diaphragm is generally used for listening to breath sounds, whilst the bell is best for the very low frequencies generated by the heart (especially the third and fourth heart sounds). The diaphragm and bell must be intact for a sound to be heard properly, and the tubing relatively short to minimize absorption of the sound. The ear-pieces, made of plastic or rubber, should fit snugly within the ears, pointing slightly forward in order to maximize sound transmission into the auditory canal.

A teaching stethoscope (Fig. 1.6) is a useful tool to allow both the experienced and inexperienced physiotherapist to hear the same sounds simultaneously (Ellis 1985).

Chest auscultation should ideally be performed in a quiet room, with the chest exposed. The patient is instructed to take deep breaths through an open mouth, as turbulence within the nose can interfere with the breath sounds. There is a wide variation in the intensity of breath sounds depending on chest wall thickness. The terms used are described below.

Breath sounds.

Normal breath sounds are generated by turbulent airflow in the trachea and large airways. These sounds, which can be heard directly over the trachea, comprise high, medium and low frequencies. The higher frequencies are attenuated by normal lung tissue so that breath sounds heard over the periphery are softer and lower pitched. Originally it was thought that the higher-pitched sounds were generated by the bronchi (bronchial breath sounds) and the lower ones by airflow into the alveoli (vesicular breath sounds). It is now known that normal breath sounds (previously called 'vesicular') simply represent filtering of the 'bronchial' breath sounds generated in the large airways. Although technically incorrect, normal breath sounds are still sometimes referred to as 'vesicular' or 'bronchovesicular'. Normal breath sounds are heard all over the chest wall throughout inspiration and for a short period during expiration.

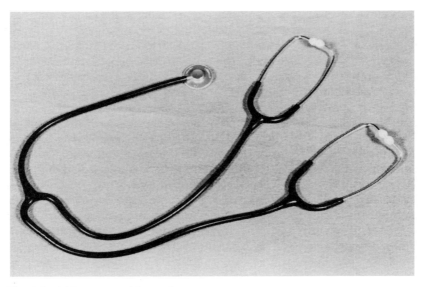

Fig. 1.6 A Littmann teaching stethoscope.

Bronchial breath sounds are the normal tracheal and large airway sounds, transmitted through airless lung which does not attenuate the higher frequencies. Thus, the sounds heard over an area of consolidated lung are similar to those heard over the trachea itself. Bronchial breath sounds are loud and high pitched, with a harsh quality. They are heard equally throughout inspiration and expiration, with a short pause between the two. Thus in all three respects, bronchial breath sounds differ from normal breath sounds which are faint, lower pitched and absent during the latter half of expiration.

If the bronchus supplying an area of consolidated lung is obstructed (e.g. carcinoma, large sputum plug) bronchial breath sounds may not be heard as the obstruction blocks sound transmission.

Diminished sounds occur when there is a reduction in the initial generation of the sound or when there is an increase in sound attenuation. As the breath sounds are generated by flow-related turbulence, reduced flow causes less sound. Thus patients who will not (e.g. due to pain), or cannot (e.g. due to muscle weakness) breathe deeply, will have globally diminished breath sounds. Similarly, diminished breath sounds are heard in some patients with emphysema where the combination of parenchymal destruction and hyperinflation cause greater attenuation of the normal breath sounds.

Locally diminished breath sounds may represent obstruction of a bronchus by tumour or large sputum plugs. Localized accumulation of air or fluid in the pleural space will block sound transmission so that breath sounds are absent.

Added sounds.

Wheezes, previously called 'rhonchi', are musical tones produced by airflow vibrating a narrowed or compressed airway. A fixed, monophonic wheeze is caused by a single obstructed airway, while polyphonic wheezes are due to widespread disease. Any cause of narrowing, for example, bronchospasm, mucosal oedema, sputum or foreign bodies, may cause wheezes. As the airways are normally compressed during expiration, wheezes are first heard at this time. When airway narrowing is more severe, wheezes may also be heard during inspiration. The pitch of the wheeze is directly related to the degree of narrowing, with high-pitched wheezes indicating near total obstruction. However, the volume of the wheeze may be misleading as the moderate asthmatic may have loud wheezes while the very severe asthmatic may have a 'quiet chest' because he is not generating sufficient airflow to cause wheezes.

Low-pitched, localized wheezes are caused by sputum retention and can change or clear after coughing.

Crackles, previously called 'crepitations' or 'râles', are clicking sounds heard during inspiration. They are caused by the opening of previously closed alveoli and small airways during inspiration. Crackles are described as 'early' or 'late', 'fine' or 'coarse', and 'localized' or 'widespread'. Coarse, early inspiratory crackles occur when bronchioles open (often heard in bronchiectasis and bronchitis), whilst fine, late inspiratory crackles occur when alveoli and respiratory bronchioles open (often heard in pulmonary oedema and pulmonary fibrosis). When severe, the late inspiratory crackles of pulmonary oedema and pulmonary fibrosis may become coarser and commence earlier in inspiration.

Localized crackles may occur in dependent alveoli which are gradually closed by compression from the lung above. This early feature of subsegmental lung collapse resolves when the patient breathes deeply or coughs. The crackles of pulmonary oedema are also more marked basally, but only clear transiently after coughing. The differentiation between subsegmental lung collapse and pulmonary oedema may be difficult, and sometimes auscultation will not clarify the situation. Elevation of the jugular venous pressure and peripheral oedema suggest pulmonary oedema, whereas ineffective cough, recent anaesthesia and pyrexia suggest sputum reten-

tion which could lead to subsegmental lu collapse (Table 1.6). Postoperative and intensiv care patients may have a combination of both pulmonary oedema and sputum retention.

Pleural rub is the creaking or rubbing sound which occurs with each breath when the pleural surfaces are roughened by inflammation, infection or neoplasm. Normally the visceral and parietal pleura slide silently. Pleural rubs range from being localized and soft to being loud and generalized, sometimes even palpable. In certain instances, they may be difficult to differentiate from crackles. An important distinguishing feature is that pleural rubs are heard equally during inspiration and expiration, with the sounds often recurring in reverse order during expiration.

Vocal resonance. Vocal resonance is the transmission of voice through the airways and lung tissue to the chest wall where it is heard through a stethoscope. It is usually tested by instructing the patient to say '99' repeatedly (like vocal fremitus which is felt with the hands). As mentioned previously, normal lung attenuates the higher frequencies so that the lower frequencies dominate. Thus, speech normally becomes a low-pitched mumble. Consolidated lung transmits all sounds better, especially the high frequencies, so the transmitted sound is louder and higher pitched. In this situation speech can actually be understood. Whispered speech lacks the lower frequencies and is normally not transmitted to the chest wall. However, over areas of consolidation the whisper is clearly heard and intelligible – this is called 'whispering pectoriloquy'.

Table 1.6 Differentiation between pulmonary oedema and sputum retention

Chest sign	Pulmonary oedema	Sputum retention
Auscultation	Fine crackles, especially at bases, with or without wheezes	Scattered or localized crackles, with or without wheezes, may move with coughing
Sputum	Frothy white or pink	Thicker, more viscid, any colour
Other signs	Elevated JVP Peripheral oedema Increased weight, positive fluid balance History of previous cardiac disease	Pyrexia History of intercurrent chest disease, recent anaesthetic, aspiration, respiratory muscle weakness

ary of chest examination in selected chest problems

	Breath sounds	PN	VF	VR
...tion:				
With open airway	Bronchial	Dull	↑	↑
With blocked airway	↓	Dull	↓	↓
Pneumothorax	↓ or absent	Hyperresonant	↓ or absent	↓ or absent
Pleural effusion	↓ or absent	Stony dull	↓ or absent	↓ or absent

PN, percussion note; VF, vocal fremitus; VR, vocal resonance; ↑, increased; ↓; decreased

As with auscultation of breath sounds, vocal resonance is decreased when the transmission of sound through the lung or from the lung to chest wall is impeded. This occurs with emphysema, pneumothorax, pleural thickening or pleural effusion.

A summary of the chest examination of selected chest problems is given in Table 1.7.

Heart sounds. The normal heart sounds represent the closure of the four heart valves. The first heart sound is caused by closure of the mitral and tricuspid valves, while the second heart sound is due to closure of the aortic and pulmonary valves. A third heart sound indicates cardiac failure in adults, but may be normal in children. It is attributed to vibration of the ventricular walls caused by rapid filling in early diastole. The fourth heart sound is caused by vibration of the ventricular walls in late diastole as the atria contract. It may be heard in heart failure, hypertension and aortic valve disease.

A murmur is the sound generated by turbulent flow through a valve. The murmur of valvular incompetence is caused by back flow across the valve, whilst stenotic valves generate murmurs by turbulent forward flow.

Sputum

At the end of the respiratory examination, it is often worthwhile to instruct the patient to huff to a low lung volume to assess the presence of retained secretions. Any sputum produced should be examined for colour, consistency, and quantity as described on page 6.

Physiotherapy techniques

In those patients who have previously been taught physiotherapy, it is important to ascertain which techniques are used, how well they are performed, and their effectiveness. For example, patients who use huffing to clear retained secretions should have its effectiveness assessed. Suboptimal techniques need to be identified and their correction incorporated in the treatment plan.

Exercise capacity

For a complete assessment of the respiratory system, exercise capacity should also be measured. Depending on the situation, this may vary from a full exercise test for measuring maximum oxygen uptake, to a simple assessment of breathlessness during normal activities. An exercise test provides the best measure of functional limitation, which may differ from that suggested by a patient's lung function. Two of the most common methods used to assess patients with respiratory disease are the 6-minute walking test and the shuttle walking test (for further details, see Ch. 3).

Test results

The final stage of assessment of a respiratory patient involves the use of tests, in particular spirometry, arterial blood gases, and chest radiography. The following is a brief summary of the application of these tests. A full discussion is given in Chapters 2 and 3.

Spirometry

The forced expiratory volume in 1 second (FEV_1), the forced vital capacity (FVC) and peak expiratory flow (PEF) are important measures of ventilatory function. Normal values, based on population studies, depend on age, height, sex and race. Weight is not an important determinant of lung function, except in the markedly obese or malnourished.

Although often expressed as absolute values, lung function should always be compared with the predicted values and with the previous recordings for that patient. For example a 21-year-old, 6-foot-tall male asthmatic changing his spirometry (FEV_1/FVC) from 4.0/5.0 litres to 1.5/3.0 litres should cause concern, while a normal 81-year-old, 5-foot female may never manage to blow more than 1.3/1.8 litres!

Arterial blood gases

Arterial blood gases (ABGs) provide an accurate measure of oxygen uptake and carbon dioxide removal by the respiratory system as a whole. The arterial blood is usually sampled from the radial artery at the wrist. Rarely, arterialized capillary samples may be taken from the earlobe. Arterial blood gases are best used as a measure of steady state gas exchange; thus it is imperative that the patient is resting quietly with a constant inspired oxygen level (FiO_2) and mode of ventilation for at least 30 minutes prior to sampling. When analysing the results, consideration must be given to all these factors.

Normal values for arterial blood gases are:

pH	7.35–7.45
PaO_2	10.7–13.3 kPa (80–100 mmHg)
$PaCO_2$	4.7–6.0 kPa (35–45 mmHg)
HCO_3^-	22–26 mmol/l
Base excess	−2 to +2

Chest radiographs

Chest radiographs are an important aid to physical examination as they provide a clear picture of the extent and severity of disease at that time. In some instances, chest radiographs may show more extensive disease than e[x] others they may underestima[te] present. Comparison with prev[ious] provides an excellent measure ....nt or deterioration over time, and an objective assessment of the response to treatment. However, the chest radiograph may sometimes lag 1–2 days behind the clinical findings.

PROBLEM LIST

The second part of the problem oriented medical record (POMR) is the problem list (see Fig. 1.1). The information in the database, together with the subjective and objective assessment are then analysed as a whole, and integrated with the physiotherapist's knowledge of disease processes.

The problem list is then compiled. It consists of a simple, functional and specific list of the patient's problems at that time, not always listed in order of priority. Each problem is numbered and dated at the time of assessment. The problem list should not only include those problems that may improve with physiotherapy (e.g. breathlessness on exertion), but should also include other relevant problems that may have a bearing on the treatment chosen (e.g. anaemia). The problem list should not be a list of signs and symptoms, as this would provide the wrong emphasis for treatment. In the past, disease-based treatment tended to result in standardized treatment, ignoring the patient's individual problems. This meant that all chronic airflow limitation patients were given treatment for increased sputum production. All intubated patients also received standard treatment, irrespective of the presence or absence of excess secretions and the patient's ability to clear them. The best system is one that is individualized to each patient.

Problems once resolved should be signed off and dated. Any subsequent problems are added and dated appropriately.

INITIAL PLANS

For each of the problems listed, long- and short-term goals are formulated. These should be specific, measurable, achievable, realistic and med (SMART). A treatment plan is then devised for each of these goals. This process must be performed, where possible, in consultation with the patient. The importance of involving the patient himself cannot be overstressed, as cooperation is fundamental to nearly all physiotherapy treatment.

Long-term goals are generally directed at returning the patient to his maximum functional capacity. Specifically, goals may be simplified to functions that are important to the patient, e.g. to be able to walk home from the shops carrying one bag of shopping. When setting goals for an inpatient, consideration must be given to his discharge. If the home situation includes two flights of stairs to the bedroom then the goal of exercise ability should reflect this. If physiotherapy is to be continued at home after discharge, one of the goals must be to teach the patient or a relative how to perform the treatment effectively.

Short-term goals are the steps taken to achieve the long-term goals. In general these are small, simple activities that are more easily achieved. All goals, both short- and long-term, should state expected outcomes and time frames. The goals, especially the short-term goals, should be reviewed regularly as some patients may improve faster than others. If goals are not met within the agreed time frame, then revision is necessary. The time frame may have been too short, the goal inappropriate, or other problems need attention before this goal can be met.

The treatment plan includes the specifics of treatment, together with its frequency and equipment requirements. Patient education must not be omitted from the treatment plan as it is an important component of physiotherapy.

A summary, as a reminder of the key points of assessment, is given in Box 1.1.

PROGRESS NOTES

These are written on a daily basis using the 'subjective, objective, analysis, plan' (SOAP) format:

- **S**ubjective – what the patient, doctors or nurses report
- **O**bjective – any change in physical

> **Box 1.1** Key points of assessment
>
> **Database**
> - Medical records
>
> **Subjective assessment**
> - Breathlessness, cough, sputum, wheeze, chest pain
> - Duration, severity, pattern, associations
> - Functional ability, disease awareness
>
> **Objective assessment**
> - General observation from end of bed
> - Chest – observation, palpation, percussion, auscultation
> - Sputum
> - Physiotherapy techniques, exercise capacity
>
> **Test results**
> - Spirometry
> - Arterial blood gases
> - Chest radiographs
>
> **Problem list → Treatment plan**

examination or test, e.g. auscultation, chest radiograph
- **A**nalysis – the physiotherapist's professional opinion of the subjective and objective findings
- **P**lan – including changes in treatment and any further action.

Entries are made for each problem, signed and dated. If there have been no changes, nothing further needs to be written.

Progress notes may also include a graph or flow chart. Graphs are particularly useful in displaying the change in a parameter with time, for example an asthmatic's peak expiratory flow rates. Flow chart displays are useful if multiple factors are changing over a period of time, as may occur in the intensive care patient.

Outcomes. The short- and long-term goals provide a basis for evaluating the effectiveness of treatment in relation to the various problems. One of the best indicators of outcome is the change in objective findings after treatment. Although changes that occur immediately after a single treatment are related to physiotherapy intervention alone, changes over longer periods of time reflect treatment by the entire health team. Chest auscultation before and after a treatment may provide a simple indication of the effectiveness of that treatment. Similarly, the chest radiograph can demonstrate the effectiveness of physiotherapy treatment by showing diminution in the area of collapsed/consolidated lung. On a long-term basis, changes in lung function or exercise tolerance provide the most valuable measures of treatment outcome.

The analysis of outcome is then compared with that expected (i.e. the goals). If there are discrepancies between the actual and expected outcomes then the plan (P) documents the changes to the goals and/or treatment, as required.

DISCHARGE SUMMARY

Upon discharge or transfer elsewhere, a summary should be written of the patient's initial problems, treatment and outcomes. Instruction for home programmes and any other relevant information should also be included. Discharge summaries are helpful to other physiotherapists who may treat the patient in the future. The summary should always contain adequate information for future audit and studies of patient care.

AUDIT

'Audit' refers to the systematic and critical analysis of the quality of care. There are three main forms of audit: structure, process and outcome.

1. *Structural audit* examines the organization of resources within a certain area. This may address the availability of human and/or equipment resources, e.g. a hospital's requirements for transcutaneous electrical nerve stimulation (TENS) machines, batteries and electrodes.

2. *Process audit* investigates the system of delivery of care, e.g. studying the methods of patient referral.

3. *Outcome audit* is the most clinically based audit. It examines the results of physiotherapy care, e.g. assessing whether the goals of treatment have been met within the stated time frames.

The audit process is cyclical. Firstly, a standard of care is defined. The actual practice is then audited in comparison with the agreed standard. Discrepancies provoke further discussion. Changes are then made to eliminate these discrepancies. After an appropriate length of time the cycle begins again.

EDUCATIONAL PROGRAMME

By using a structured system of problem oriented medical records and audit, the problem oriented medical system allows identification of areas where goals are not being met within an appropriate time frame. Audit may also reveal situations where the agreed standards are not met. In both instances staff education programmes will improve patient care.

CONCLUSION

Accurate assessment should reveal the exact nature of the patient's problems and delineate those that physiotherapy can improve. Only then can the best treatment be chosen for that patient. Subsequent reassessment is essential to ensure that treatment is specific, effective and efficient. This process ensures high-quality patient care.

REFERENCES

Ellis E 1985 Making a teaching stethoscope. Australian Journal of Physiotherapy 31: 244
Miller D L 1963 A study of techniques for the examination of sputum in a field survey of chronic bronchitis. American Review of Respiratory Disease 88: 473–483

Rubinstein I, Zamel N, DuBarry L, Hoffstein V 1990 Airflow limitation in morbidly obese, nonsmoking men. Annals of Internal Medicine 112: 828–832
Weed LL 1968 Medical records that guide and teach. New England Journal of Medicine 279: 593–600, 652–657

FURTHER READING

Bromley A I 1978 The patient care audit. Physiotherapy
64: 270–271

Forgacs P 1978 Lung sounds. Baillière Tindall, London

Heath J R 1978 Problem oriented medical systems.
Physiotherapy 64: 269–270

2

Thoracic imaging

Conor D. Collins   David M. Hansell

CHEST RADIOGRAPHY AND OTHER TECHNIQUES

Different types of chest radiograph

Chest radiographs have been used as the main radiological investigation of the chest ever since the discovery of X-rays by Röntgen in 1895 and they comprise 25–40% of all radiological investigations. Chest radiographs are indicated in almost any condition in which a pulmonary abnormality is suspected.

The majority of chest radiographs are obtained in the main radiology department. The radiograph is obtained with the patient standing erect. Patients who are immobile or too ill to come to the main department have a chest radiograph performed using a mobile machine (portable film); the resulting chest radiograph differs from a departmental film in terms of projection, positioning, exposure and film used, and is therefore not strictly comparable with a conventional posteroanterior (PA) film. Other types of chest radiograph are the lateral, lordotic, apical and decubitus views; these are generally taken in the main department.

Departmental films are referred to as 'posteroanterior' (or PA) chest radiographs and describe the direction in which the X-ray beam traverses the patient. The patient is positioned with his anterior chest wall against the film cassette and his back to the X-ray tube. The arms are abducted to rotate the scapulae away from the posterior chest and the radiograph is taken during full inspiration. The tube is centred at the spinous process of the fourth thoracic vertebra. For portable films which are taken in an anteroposterior (AP) projection, the patient's back is against the film cassette and the X-ray tube is positioned at a variable distance from the patient. As the heart is anteriorly placed within the chest it is further from the cassette, and is therefore magnified in an AP radiograph. The degree of magnification depends on the distance between the patient and the X-ray tube.

For a lateral radiograph the patient is turned 90° and the side of interest placed against the film cassette. The arms are extended forwards and the radiograph is again taken in full inspiration.

Lateral decubitus views are sometimes useful for the demonstration of small pleural effusions. For this projection the patient lies horizontally with the side in question placed downwards. The film cassette is positioned at the back of the patient and the X-ray beam is horizontal centred at midsternum. This provides a sensitive means of detecting small quantities of pleural fluid (50–100 ml) which cannot be identified on a frontal chest radiograph. However, ultrasonography is increasingly being used as a reliable means of confirming the presence of small pleural effusions.

Lordotic films are sometimes used to confirm middle lobe collapse and for demonstrating a questionable apical opacity otherwise obscured by the clavicle and ribs. For this AP projection the patient arches back so that the shoulders are touching the cassette with the centring point remaining the same. Linear tomography is another technique designed to reveal lesions otherwise hidden by the skeleton by blurring out everything over and under the lesion in question. This is achieved by having the X-ray tube and film cassette move at the same time but in opposite directions. These two techniques are less frequently used with the advent of computed tomography (CT).

Factors influencing the quality of a chest radiograph

The quality and thus diagnostic usefulness of a chest radiograph depends critically on the conditions under which it is obtained. Of particular importance are the radiographic exposure, the projection, the orientation of the patient relative to the film cassette, the X-ray tube to film distance, the depth of inspiration of the patient and the type of film-screen combination used.

The ideal chest radiograph provides an image of structures within the chest whilst exposing the patient to the lowest possible dose of radiation. Most radiology departments have a policy of obtaining either high kilovoltage (kVp) or low kilovoltage chest radiographs. Radiographs performed at high kilovoltage (e.g. 140 kVp) have much to recommend them. Even at total lung capacity with the patient erect, nearly a third of the lungs is partially obscured by the mediastinal structures, diaphragm and ribs. With the low kilovoltage technique (80 kVp or less) these areas are often poorly visualized. This problem is partially overcome by using films exposed at 140 kVp. The normal vessel markings and subtle differences in soft tissue densities are better demonstrated and a further advantage is the better penetration of the mediastinum which improves visualization of the trachea and main bronchi. The disadvantage of high kilovoltage radiographs is the relatively poor demonstration of calcified structures so that rib fractures and calcified pulmonary nodules or pleural plaques are less conspicuous.

During exposure the X-ray beam is modified according to the structures through which it passes. The photons that have passed through the patient carry the information which then must be converted into a visual form. Some of the photons emerging from the patient are aligned in a virtually parallel direction and other photons are scattered. These scattered photons degrade the final image but can be absorbed by using lead strips embedded in an aluminium sheet positioned in front of the cassette. This device is known as a grid. Photons that are travelling in parallel pass through the grid to form the image on the film.

The sensitivity of film to direct X-ray exposure is very low, and if used alone as the image receptor would result in a prohibitively large X-ray dose to the patient. Intensifying screens made of phosphorescent material are positioned on the inside of the cassettes and they convert the incident X-ray photons into visible light and it is this light which is recorded by the adjacent film. These phosphor screens are composed of either calcium tungstate or a rare earth containing compound. Rare earth phosphors emit more light in response to X-ray photons and, therefore, less radiation is necessary, compared with calcium tungstate screens, to produce the image. Similarly, improvements in the quality of X-ray film have also occurred over the years. Standard film emulsions tend to lack detail in the relatively under- or overexposed areas of the radiograph and newer emulsions have been developed so that detail is similar in all areas of the chest radiograph. The choice of film-screen combination has a crucial influence on the quality and 'look' of the radiograph produced. Further variations may result from film processing problems.

Over the years much effort has been expended on producing radiographs which are less affected by these factors so that differences present in serial radiographs on the same patient represent real differences and not technical variations. Newer devices designed to expose accurately the various parts of the chest using automatic exposure devices are now being installed. One of these, the advanced multiple beam equalization radiography (AMBER) system, produces chest radiographs which greatly improve the demonstration of mediastinal abnormalities and pulmonary nodules which would otherwise be obscured by the overlying heart or diaphragm (Fig. 2.1).

In the intensive care setting, portable chest radiographs are often taken in less than ideal conditions. Multiple tubes, lines and dressings in conjunction with an immobile, supine patient and the use of a mobile low-kilovoltage machine often result in suboptimal radiographs. One approach to this is the development of phosphor plate technology which is ultimately expected to replace conventional film-screen radiography. The phosphor plate is placed inside a conventional cassette and stores some of the energy of the incident X-ray photons as a latent image

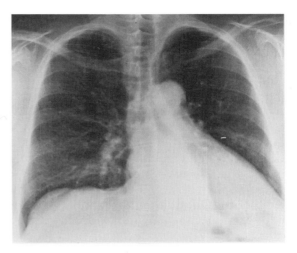

Fig. 2.1 Triangular opacity of left lower lobe collapse seen through the heart shadow on this AMBER chest radiograph.

(the image produced on a film or phosphor plate prior to development). The plate is scanned with a laser beam and the light emitted from the 'excited' latent image is detected by a photomultiplier. Thereafter this signal is processed in digital form. This digital image may be viewed either on a television monitor or on film (on which it has been laser printed). The great advantage of this system is that it can retrieve an image of diagnostic quality from a suboptimal exposure. Similar gross over- or underexposure would result in a non-diagnostic conventional radiograph. Manipulation of the digital image, particularly 'edge enhancement', aids the detection of linear structures such as the edge of a pneumothorax. However, conventional film radiography retains two important advantages. It has an extremely high spatial resolution (ability to resolve small objects) and the necessary equipment is reliable and relatively inexpensive.

Other techniques

Fluoroscopy

The patient is positioned, either standing or lying, in a screening unit which allows immediate radiographic visualization of the area in question on a television monitor. The patient can be turned in any direction and this technique can help to distinguish pulmonary from extra-pulmonary opacities. One of the main uses of fluoroscopy is to 'screen' the diaphragm to demonstrate paralysis or abnormal movement. It is also useful in needle placement during biopsy of lung masses.

Ultrasonography

High-frequency sound waves do not traverse air and the use of this technique is therefore limited in the chest. It is mainly used for cardiac work (echocardiography) and has become an essential technique in the investigation of patients with valvular and ventricular function problems. Outside the heart, ultrasonography is very useful in distinguishing between fluid above the diaphragm (pleural effusion; Fig. 2.2), fluid below the diaphragm (subphrenic collection), and pleural thickening. Chest radiography often cannot differentiate between pleural fluid and thickening with any certainty. Ultrasound can also be used to guide the placement of a drain into a pleural effusion.

Computed tomography

Computed tomography (CT) scanning depends on the same basic physical principle as conventional radiography, namely the absorption of X-rays by tissues of different densities. The basic components of a CT machine are a table on which the patient lies and a gantry through which the table slides. An X-ray tube and a series of detectors are housed within the gantry. The X-ray tube and detectors rotate around the patient. A computer is used to reconstruct the signals received by the detectors into an image. The images acquired are transverse (axial) cross-sections of the patient. In orienting the patient's right and left sides, it is the convention to view all CT images as if from the patient's feet.

Because of the cross-sectional nature of CT it can accurately localize lesions seen on only one

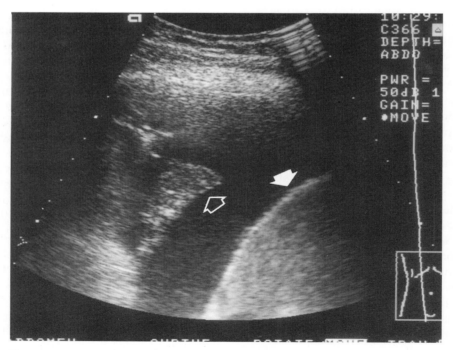

Fig. 2.2 Ultrasound of lower right hemithorax/upper abdomen demonstrating a right basal effusion with fluid interposed between collapsed right lower lobe (open arrow) and diaphragm (closed arrow).

view on plain chest radiographs. The superior contrast resolution of CT allows superb demonstration of mediastinal anatomy (e.g. lymph nodes and individual vessels) as well as calcification within a pulmonary nodule. Its ability to produce highly detailed thin sections of the lung parenchyma allows the complex morphology of many interstitial lung diseases to be defined more clearly. Its disadvantages are its relatively high cost and increased radiation exposure to the patient compared with chest radiography.

A relatively recent development has been the introduction of helical (spiral) CT scanning. Whereas conventional CT scanning involves alternating patient translation and exposure, helical CT involves simultaneous patient translation and X-ray exposure. The advantages are the elimination of respiratory misregistration artefacts, minimization of motion artefacts and production of overlapping images without additional radiation exposure. The technique is so named because the X-ray can be thought of as tracing a helix or spiral curve on the patient's surface.

Common indications for CT of the chest.

1. CT scanning is used to further evaluate hilar or mediastinal masses seen or suspected on a chest radiograph.

2. Within the lungs it can be used to further define the nature of a mass or cavitating lesion not clearly seen on the plain film.

3. In patients with normal chest radiographs but abnormal pulmonary function tests, thin section high-resolution CT sections of the lung may provide the first radiological evidence of parenchymal disease. This type of scanning is also very useful for assessing patients with suspected bronchiectasis.

4. CT is useful in patients with neoplasms, both in assessing their operability and their response to treatment.

Magnetic resonance imaging

The physical principles of magnetic resonance imaging (MRI) are more complex and very different from those governing CT scanning. The equipment consists of a sliding table on which the patient lies within the bore of a large magnet. A combination of the intense magnetic field and a series of radiofrequency waves produces an alteration in the alignment of protons (mostly in water) resulting in the emission of different signals which are detected and subsequently analysed for their intensity and position by a computer. The major advantages of MRI are that images may be obtained in any plane without the use of ionizing radiation. The disadvantages are its cost, limited availability and, in the chest, the images suffer from motion artefact due to breathing. As a result its application to chest imaging is as yet limited.

Interventional procedures

Percutaneous needle biopsy

Percutaneous needle biopsy of a pulmonary or mediastinal mass, to provide a histological specimen, is usually performed in patients in whom a bronchoscopic biopsy has failed or a thoracotomy is inappropriate. Different types of needle are used and the complication rate (pneumothorax and haemoptysis) bears some relation to the size of the needle. Contraindications to the procedure include any patient with poor respiratory reserve unable to withstand a pneumothorax, pulmonary arterial hypertension, and a previous contralateral pneumonectomy.

Pulmonary and bronchial arteriography: superior vena cavography

Pulmonary arteriography. This is usually undertaken in the investigation of suspected pulmonary embolism and pulmonary arteriovenous malformations. It requires puncture of either the femoral vein in the groin or the antecubital vein in the elbow and the guiding of a catheter through the right side of the heart under fluoroscopy. The tip of the catheter is positioned in the main pulmonary artery or selectively placed in a smaller pulmonary artery. Contrast is then injected. Arteriography remains the most specific method of identifying pulmonary emboli; these are shown as filling defects which cause non-filling of branches of the arterial tree. It is also the best and most appropriate technique for the demonstration of pulmonary arteriovenous malformations. These can be treated at the time of the arteriogram by the injection of occlusive materials (embolization).

Bronchial arteriography. Demonstration of the bronchial arteries requires catheterization of the femoral artery and passage of a catheter into the midthoracic aorta from where the bronchial arteries are selectively catheterized. The major indication for this procedure is recurrent or life-threatening haemoptysis in patients with a chronic inflammatory disease, usually bronchiectasis. Accurate placement of the catheter not only allows demonstration of the bleeding vessel but also allows embolization to be performed simultaneously.

Superior vena cavography. This is performed for the evaluation of superior vena caval (SVC) obstruction and the investigation of anatomical variants. More recently, patients with SVC compression due to tumour have been palliated by the insertion of an expandable metallic mesh wire stent at the site of the SVC narrowing, thus restoring flow and relieving symptoms.

THE NORMAL CHEST

Anatomy

On the normal posteroanterior radiograph (Fig. 2.3) the following structures can be identified:

- Outline of the mediastinum and heart
- The hila
- Pulmonary vessels and main bronchi
- Diaphragm
- Soft tissues and bones of the thoracic cage.

The heart and mediastinum

The mediastinum consists of the organs and soft tissues in the central part of the chest. These comprise the trachea, aortic arch and great vessels, superior vena cava and oesophagus. In children the thymus gland is a prominent component. On the two-dimensional chest radio-

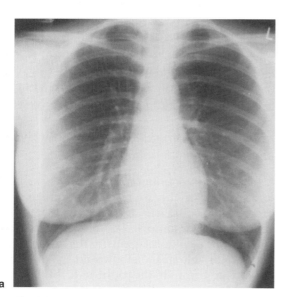
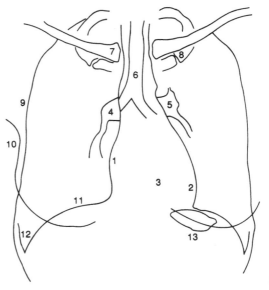

a   b

Fig. 2.3 a Normal PA chest radiograph. **b** Normal structures visible on a PA chest radiograph: 1, right atrium; 2, left ventricle; 3, right ventricle; 4, right pulmonary artery; 5, left pulmonary artery; 6, air within trachea; 7, clavicle; 8, first rib; 9, lateral border of hemithorax; 10, breast shadow; 11, right hemidiaphragm; 12, costophrenic angle; 13, gastric air bubble.

graph these structures are superimposed and cannot be clearly distinguished from each other. The mediastinum is conventionally divided into superior, anterior, middle and posterior compartments. Whilst the boundaries of the latter three are arbitrary, it is usual to divide them into equal thirds. The superior mediastinum is that portion lying above the aortic arch and below the root of the neck.

The mediastinal border on the right is formed superiorly by the right brachiocephalic vein and superior vena cava. The mediastinal shadow to the left of the trachea above the aortic arch comprises the left carotid and left subclavian arteries together with the left brachiocephalic and jugular veins. On a correctly exposed chest radiograph, air in the trachea can be seen throughout its length as it descends downwards deviating slightly to the right above the carina where it is displaced by the aortic arch.

The heart lies eccentrically in the chest, with one-third of the cardiac shadow to the right of the spine and two-thirds to the left. The density of the cardiac shadow on the left and right of the spine should be identical. The right cardiac border on a chest radiograph is formed by the right atrium. The left cardiac border is composed of the apex of the left ventricle and superiorly the left atrial appendage. The outline of the right ventricle, which is superimposed on the left ventricle, cannot be identified on a frontal radiograph. The maximum transverse diameter of the heart should be less than half the maximum transverse diameter of the thorax, as measured from the inside border of the ribs (the so-called 'cardiothoracic ratio').

The hila

Hilar shadows are a complex summation of the pulmonary arteries and veins with minor contributions from other components (the main bronchi and lymph nodes). In general, the hila are of equal density and are approximately the same size. Adjacent to the left hilum, the main pulmonary artery forms a localized bulge just above the left atrial appendage and just below the aortic arch. The area between the aortic arch and the main pulmonary artery is known as the 'aortopulmonary window'.

The superior pulmonary veins run vertically and converge on the upper and midhilum on both sides. It is not possible to distinguish arteries from veins in the outer two-thirds of the lungs. The inferior pulmonary veins run obliquely in a near horizontal plane below the lower lobe arteries to enter the left atrium beneath the carina (the division of the trachea into the right and left main stem bronchi). The hilar point is where the superior pulmonary vein on each side crosses the basal artery. This is more easily assessed on the right than on the left. Using this as an index point, the left hilum is normally 0.5–1.5 cm higher than the right one.

Abnormalities of the hilar shadows in the form of increased density or abnormal configuration are usually the result of lymph node or pulmonary artery enlargement. The detection of subtle hilar abnormalities is difficult and requires experience and knowledge of the many outlines that the hila may assume in normal individuals.

Fissures, vessels and segmental bronchi within the lungs

Each lung is divided into lobes surrounded by visceral pleura. There are two lobes on the left (the upper and lower, separated by the major (oblique) fissure) and three on the right (the upper, middle and lower lobes which are separated by the major (oblique) and minor (horizontal or transverse) fissures). In the majority of normal subjects some or all of the minor fissure is seen on a frontal radiograph. The major fissures are only identifiable on lateral projection. Each lobe of the lung contains a number of segments which have their own segmental bronchi. The walls of the segmental bronchi are invisible on the chest radiograph, except when seen end-on as ring shadows measuring up to 7 mm in diameter.

The pulmonary blood vessels are responsible for the branching and linear structures within the lungs. The diameter of the blood vessels beyond the hilum varies with the position of the patient and with haemodynamic factors. In the erect position there is a gradual increase in the diameter of the vessels, travelling from apex to base. This increase in size is seen in both the arteries and veins and is abolished if the patient lies supine.

The diaphragm

The interface between the lung and diaphragm should be sharp and, in general, the diaphragm is dome shaped with its highest point medial to the midclavicular line. The margin of the right hemidiaphragm at its highest point lies between the anterior ends of the fifth and seventh ribs. The right hemidiaphragm is higher than the left by up to 2 cm in the erect position. Laterally, the diaphragm dips downwards forming a sharp angle with the chest wall known as the 'costophrenic angle'. Filling in or blunting of these angles reflects pleural disease, either fluid or thickening.

Thoracic cage

On a high kilovoltage chest radiograph it should be possible to identify the edges of the vertebral bodies of the dorsal spine through the heart shadow. However, a high kilovoltage radiograph may 'burn out' the ribs, particularly the posterior portions. Because of this the chest radiograph may be an insensitive means of demonstrating rib abnormalities, particularly fractures.

Common anatomical variants

The trachea lies centrally, but in the elderly may deviate markedly to the right in its lower portion due to unfolding and dilatation of the aortic arch. A small ovoid soft tissue shadow just above the origin of the right main bronchus represents the azygos vein. This may be enlarged as a result of posture (supine position) or haemodynamic factors. It may be indistinguishable from an azygos lymph node.

Occasionally, extra fissures are seen in the lungs. The commonest of these is the azygos lobe fissure; this is seen as a fine white line running obliquely from the apex of the right lung to the azygos vein. Other accessory fissures are the superior and inferior accessory fissures, both of which are in the right lower lobe.

The surfaces of the two lungs abut each other anteriorly and posteriorly and give rise to two white lines projected over the vertebral column known as the 'anterior and posterior junction lines', respectively. Both of these may be seen overlying the trachea – the anterior line extending from the clavicles to the left main bronchus and the posterior line lying more medially and extending above the clavicles. The azygo-oesophageal recess line is a curved line projected over the vertebral column and extending from the azygos vein to the diaphragm. It represents the interface between the right lung and right oesophageal wall.

A small 'nipple' may occasionally be seen projecting laterally from the aortic knuckle due to the left superior intercostal vein. The term 'paraspinal line' refers to the line that parallels the left and right margin of the thoracic spine. The left is thicker than the right because of the adjacent aorta.

The lateral view

It is conventional to read the lateral film (Fig. 2.4) with the heart to the viewer's left and the dorsal spine to the right, irrespective of whether the film is labelled 'right' or 'left'. The chamber of the heart that touches the sternum is the right ventricle. Behind and above the heart lies lung, the density of which should be the same both behind the heart and behind the sternum. As the eye travels down the spine, the vertebral column should appear increasingly transradiant (Fig. 2.4a); the loss of this phenomenon suggests the presence of disease in the posterobasal segments of the lower lobes. In the middle of the lateral film lie the hilar structures with the main pulmonary artery anteriorly. The aortic arch should be easily identified, but only a variable proportion of the great vessels is visible depending on the degree of aortic unfolding. The brachiocephalic artery is most frequently identified arising anterior to the tracheal air column. The left and right brachiocephalic veins

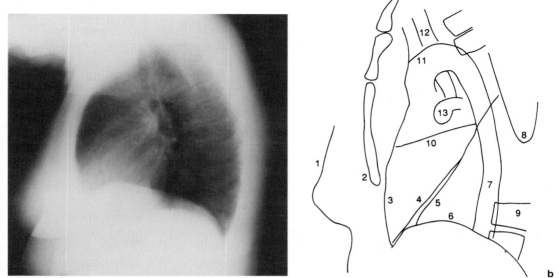

Fig. 2.4 **a** Normal lateral chest radiograph. **b** Normal structures visible on a lateral chest radiograph: 1, breast shadow; 2, sternum; 3, position of right ventricle; 4, right oblique fissure; 5, left oblique fissure; 6, hemidiaphragm; 7, descending aorta; 8, inferior angle of scapula; 9, dorsal vertebrae; 10, horizontal fissure; 11, aortic arch; 12, trachea; 13, pulmonary artery.

form an extrapleural bulge behind the upper sternum in about a third of individuals.

The course of the trachea is straight with a slight posterior angulation, but no visible indentation from adjacent vessels. The carina is not seen on the lateral view. The posterior wall of the trachea is always visible and is known as the 'posterior tracheal stripe'.

The oblique fissures are seen as fine diagonal lines running from the upper dorsal spine to the diaphragm anteriorly. The left is more vertically oriented and is visible just behind the right. The minor fissure extends forwards horizontally from the mid-right oblique fissure. Care must be taken not to confuse rib margins with fissure lines. As the fissures undulate, two distinct fissure lines may be generated by a single fissure. The fissures should be of no more than hairline width.

The scapulae are invariably seen in the lateral view and since they are incompletely visualized, lines formed by the edge of the scapula can easily be confused with intrathoracic structures. The arms are held outstretched in front of the patient on a lateral view and these give rise to soft tissue shadows projected over the anterior and superior mediastinum. A band-like opacity simulating pleural disease is often seen along the lower half of the anterior chest wall immediately behind the sternum. The left lung does not contact the most anterior portion of the left thoracic cavity at these levels because the heart occupies the space. This band-like opacity is known as the 'retrosternal line'.

Useful points in interpreting a chest radiograph

Documentary information. The name of the patient, and the time and date on which the radiograph was taken, particularly in relation to other films in a series, should all be noted. Often the film is annotated with the patient's date of birth. Of particular importance is the presence of the side markers ('right' or 'left'). The radiograph should also be marked 'AP' if the anteroposterior projection was used; departmental posteroanterior (PA) films are generally not marked as such.

Radiographic projection. A judgement as to whether a radiograph is AP or PA can be made from the following evidence:

1. The position of the label (this varies from department to department and is open to error).
2. The relationship of the scapulae to the lung margins (in the PA projection the scapulae are projected clear of the lungs and in AP projection they overlie the lungs).
3. The appearance of the vertebral bodies in the cervicodorsal region. The vertebral end plates are seen more clearly in the AP projection and the laminae are more clearly seen in the PA projection.

Supine versus prone position. It is important to know whether a chest radiograph was taken in the erect or supine position. In the supine position, blood flow is more evenly distributed throughout the lungs, making the upper zone vessels equal in size to those in the lower zones. This has implications in assessing the chest radiograph of a patient suspected of being in cardiac failure. In addition, fluid is distributed throughout the dependent part of the pleural space and any air–fluid levels that might be present on an erect film are impossible to detect. The position and contours of the heart, mediastinum and diaphragm are also different compared with an erect film. In the absence of any indication on the radiograph, one clue is the position of the gastric air bubble: if it is just under the left hemidiaphragm it is in the fundus and the patient is erect, whereas in the supine position air collects in the antrum of the stomach which lies centrally or slightly to the right of the vertebral column, well below the diaphragm.

Patient rotation. The patient may be rotated around one of three axes. Axial rotation is the commonest cause of unilateral transradiancy (one lung appearing darker than the other). It also distorts the mediastinal outline. The degree of rotation can be assessed by relating the medial ends of the clavicles to the spinous process of the vertebral body at the same level – they should be equidistant from the spinous processes.

Rotation about the horizontal coronal axis results in a more kyphotic or lordotic projection than normal. The main pulmonary artery and subclavian vessels may appear unduly prominent. Rotation around the horizontal sagittal axis usually leads to obvious tilt of the chest in relation to the edge of the radiograph which is assumed to be upright.

Physical attributes of the patient, such as a kyphoscoliosis or a depressed sternum (pectus excavatum), may also distort the appearance of the thoracic cage and its contents.

State of inspiration or expiration. The degree of inspiration is an important consideration for the correct interpretation of a chest radiograph. A poor inspiratory effort does not necessarily imply lack of patient cooperation and may as often be related to a pathological process. At full inspiration the midpoint of the right hemidiaphragm lies between the anterior end of ribs 5–7. A shallow inspiration affects the contour of the heart and mediastinum and may mimic the appearances of pulmonary congestion because the upper zone vessels will have the same diameter as the lower zone vessels.

Films taken deliberately with the patient in full expiration are invaluable in the investigation of air trapping. They are mandatory in any patient suspected of having inhaled a foreign body with consequent obstruction of a lobar bronchus. An expiratory film is also useful in accentuating a small pneumothorax.

Review areas. Several areas are difficult to assess on a frontal radiograph and should be scrutinized carefully. These review areas are:

- Apices
- Behind the heart
- Hilar regions
- Bones
- Lung periphery just inside the chest wall.

Detection and description of radiographic abnormalities should then be undertaken and a differential diagnosis listed based on the abnormalities detected. With experience the structured search gives way to the rapid identification of abnormalities and a search for confirmatory radiological signs and associated abnormalities.

COMMON RADIOLOGICAL SIGNS

Consolidation

'Consolidation' is the term used to describe lung in which the air-filled spaces are replaced by the products of disease, e.g. water, pus or blood. The two most important radiological signs of consolidation are (a) an air bronchogram, and (b) the silhouette sign. The causes of widespread consolidation may be divided into four categories (Table 2.1).

An air bronchogram is present when the airways contain air and appear as radiolucent (black) branching structures against a now white background of airless lung. The silhouette sign is present when the border of a structure is lost because the normally air-filled lung outlining the border is replaced by radio-opaque fluid or tissue. Recognition of this sign can help localize the affected area of abnormality within the chest. Thus, loss of a clear right heart border

Table 2.1 Causes of widespread pulmonary consolidation

Fluid transudation	Pulmonary oedema due to cardiac failure, renal failure, hepatic failure
Exudation	Infection, e.g. lobar pneumonia and bronchopneumonia, tuberculosis Adult respiratory distress syndrome (ARDS) Pulmonary haemorrhage due to contusion Pulmonary eosinophilia
Inhalation	Gastric contents Toxic fumes Oxygen toxicity
Infiltration	Lymphoma Alveolar cell carcinoma

is due to right middle lobe consolidation or collapse.

Localized areas of consolidation are usually due to infection. In some cases the borders of the consolidation are clearly demarcated. This usually corresponds to a fissure and the consoli-

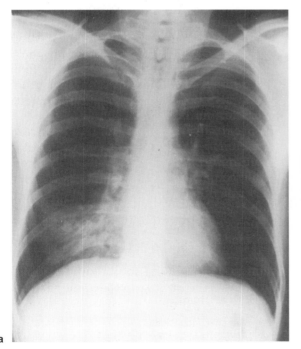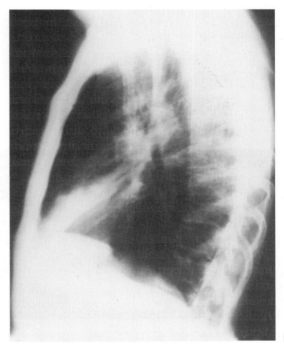

a   b

Fig. 2.5 Right middle lobe consolidation. **a** The right heart border is not seen clearly owing to adjacent consolidation. Note that the right hemidiaphragm is clearly visible as far as the vertebral column. **b** The lateral view confirms the presence of consolidation in the right middle lobe with the posterior aspect well demarcated by the oblique fissure.

dation is confined to one lobe (lobar pneumonia) (Fig. 2.5). If consolidation is slow to clear with treatment, it may be secondary to partial obstruction of a lobar bronchus, such as carcinoma of the bronchus. Consolidation may also be widespread and affect both lungs (Figs 2.6 and 2.7).

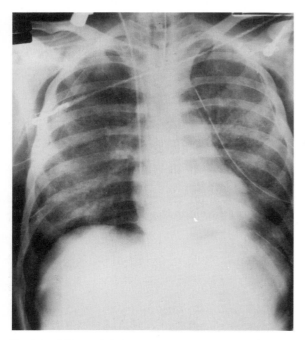

Fig. 2.6 Widespread airspace consolidation in a patient with adult respiratory distress syndrome (ARDS). There are multiple chest drains for bilateral pneumothoraces.

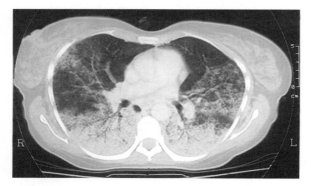

Fig. 2.7 Diffuse consolidation within apical segments of both lower lobes. Note prominent bilateral air bronchograms within consolidated lung. Infection due to *Pneumocystis carinii* and cytomegalovirus in an immunocompromised patient.

Collapse (atelectasis)

'Collapse' ('atelectasis') is the radiological term used when there is loss of aeration and, therefore, expansion in part or all of a lung. Collapse of a lobe or an entire lung is most frequently due to an endobronchial tumour, an inhaled foreign body, or a mucus plug.

Although collapse is most often thought of as occurring at a lobar level, focal areas of pulmonary collapse at a subsegmental level occur very commonly in postoperative patients. There are many signs of lobar collapse, but it is important to realize that not all these signs occur together. In addition, some non-specific signs may be present which indirectly point to the diagnosis and alert the observer to look for the more specific signs.

The most reliable and frequently present finding in lobar collapse is shift of the fissures, which invariably occurs to some extent. If air stays in the collapsed lobe, the contained blood vessels remain visible and appear crowded. If there is marked volume loss the density of the collapsed and airless lobe increases. The hila may show two types of change consisting either of gross displacement upwards or downwards or of rearrangement of individual hilar components (i.e. vessels and airways) leading to changes in shape and prominence. Elevation of the hemidiaphragm, reflecting volume loss, is most marked in collapse of a lower lobe. 'Peaking' of the mid-portion of the hemidiaphragm occurs in upper lobe collapse due to displacement of the oblique fissure. The signs associated with collapse are listed in Box 2.1.

Box 2.1   Signs associated with a collapsed lobe
• Increased density of the collapsed lobe • Shift of fissures • Silhouette sign • Hilar shift and distortion • Crowding of vessels and airways • Mediastinal shift • Crowding of the ribs • Elevation of hemidiaphragm

Collapse of individual lobes

Right upper lobe

On the posteroanterior (PA) radiograph there is elevation of the transverse fissure and of the right hilum. If the collapse is complete the non-aerated lobe is seen as an increased density along-side the superior mediastinum adjacent to the trachea (Fig. 2.8). On the lateral view the minor fissure moves upwards and the major fissure moves forwards. The retrosternal area becomes progressively more opaque and the anterior margin of the ascending aorta becomes effaced.

Right middle lobe

On the PA radiograph the lateral part of the minor fissure moves down and there is blurring of the normally sharp right heart border. This may be a subtle abnormality which is easily overlooked. On the lateral view the minor fissure moves downwards and the lower half of the

major fissure moves forwards, giving rise to a triangular shadow visible behind the lower sternum (Fig. 2.9).

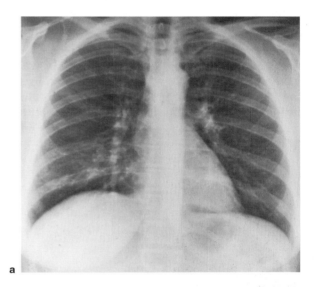

a

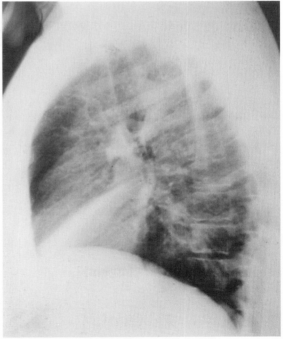

b

Fig. 2.8 Right upper lobe collapse. There is increased density medial to the elevated horizontal fissure. The cause was a large central tumour obstructing the right upper lobe bronchus.

Fig. 2.9 Right middle lobe collapse. **a** Loss of the right heart border is the only definite radiographic evidence of right middle lobe collapse. **b** The lateral view shows the typical triangular opacity overlying the cardiac shadow.

Right lower lobe

On the PA view there is an increase in density overlying the medial portion of the right hemidiaphragm and the right hilum is displaced inferiorly. The right heart border usually remains sharply defined since this is in contact with the aerated right middle lobe. On the lateral view the oblique fissure moves backwards, and with increasing collapse there is loss of definition of the right hemidiaphragm as well as increased density overlying the lower dorsal vertebrae (Fig. 2.10).

Left upper lobe

The main finding on the PA radiograph is of a veil-like increase in density, without a sharp margin, spreading outwards and upwards from the left hilum which is elevated. The aortic knuckle, left hilum and left heart border may have ill-defined outlines. As volume loss increases, the collapsed lobe moves closer to the midline and the lung apex may become lucent due to hyperinflation of the apical segment of the left lower lobe. A sharp border may also return to the aortic arch. On the lateral view the oblique fissure moves upwards and forwards, remaining relatively straight and roughly parallel to the anterior chest wall. With marked collapse there is herniation of the right lung across the midline giving an anterior band lucency to the retrosternal region and making the ascending aorta and arch sharp once again (Fig. 2.11). On the PA projection collapse (or consolidation) of the lingular segment of the left upper lobe should be suspected when the left cardiac border is ill-defined.

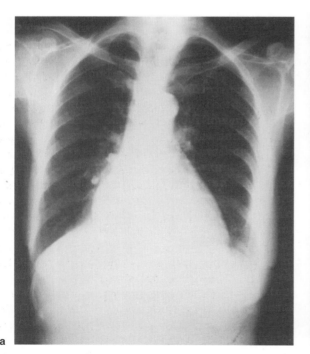
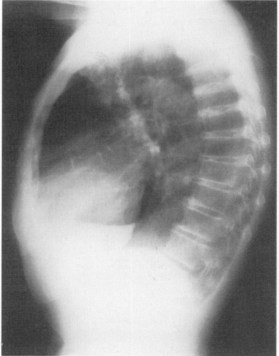

a

b

Fig. 2.10 Right lower lobe collapse. **a** The PA film shows loss of the outline of the medial portion of the right hemidiaphragm and there is increased density behind the right side of the heart. **b** On the lateral film the right hemidiaphragm is obscured posteriorly.

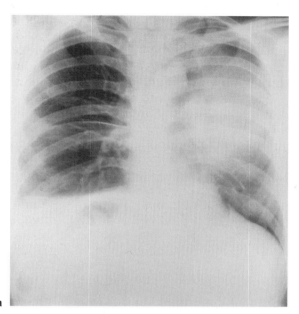 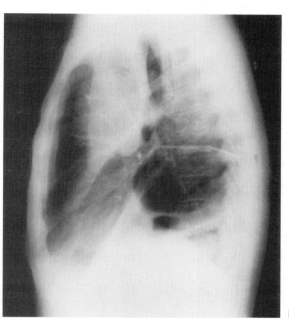

a   b

Fig. 2.11   Left upper lobe collapse. **a** There is a veil-like density in the left upper zone due to upper lobe collapse (the right hemidiaphragm is elevated due to previous trauma). **b** The lateral radiograph shows increased density anterior to the oblique fissure.

Left lower lobe

This is most commonly seen in patients following cardiac surgery and a thoracotomy due to the retention of secretions in the left lower lobe bronchus. On the PA view there is a triangular density behind the heart with loss of the medial portion of the left hemidiaphragm; if the PA radiograph is underexposed, it may be impossible to see this triangular opacity. On the lateral view there is displacement backwards of the oblique fissure and with increasing collapse there is increased density over the lower dorsal vertebrae. As non-aerated lung lies against the posterior hemidiaphragm this is now invisible (see Fig. 2.1).

Pneumothorax

When air is introduced into the pleural space, the resulting pneumothorax can be recognized radiographically. There are numerous causes of a pneumothorax, but the commonest include

penetrating injuries (e.g. stab wound, placement of a subclavian line) and breeches of the visceral pleura (e.g. spontaneous rupture of a subpleural bulla or mechanical ventilation with high pressures) (see Fig. 2.6). The cardinal radiographic sign is the visceral pleural edge: lateral to this edge no vascular shadows are visible and medial to this the collapsed lung is of higher density than the contralateral lung (Fig. 2.12). It is important to remember that in the supine position, the air of a small pneumothorax will collect anteriorly in the pleural space; thus on a portable supine chest radiograph, the pneumothorax will be visible as an area of relative translucency without a visceral pleural edge necessarily being identifiable.

If air enters the pleural space during inspiration but cannot leave on expiration (usually because of a check-valve effect of the torn flap of the visceral pleura), pressure increases rapidly and this results in a life-threatening tension pneumothorax. This can be recognized by a shift of the mediastinum to the opposite side and

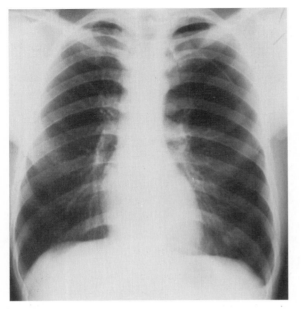

Fig. 2.12 Spontaneous pneumothorax: the visceral pleural edge is visible. There are no vascular shadows lateral to this edge and the partially collapsed left lung is of greater density than the right lung.

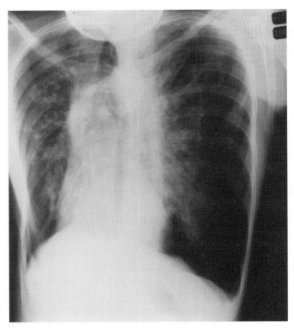

Fig. 2.13 Tension pneumothorax: this patient with cystic fibrosis has a left-sided tension pneumothorax. Note the shift of the mediastinum and straightening of the left dome of the diaphragm.

straightening of the ipsilateral diaphragm (Fig. 2.13).

The opaque hemithorax

If one-half of a chest is completely opaque (a white-out) it is due either to collapse of a lung or a large pleural effusion. If there is a shift of the mediastinum to the affected side it implies that volume loss in the lung (i.e. collapse) on that side must have occurred. Where there is no shift of the mediastinum, or it is shifted slightly to the side of the white-out, this is usually due to constricting pleural disease (including pleural tumour). A pleural effusion which is large enough to cause complete opacification of a hemithorax will displace the mediastinum away from the side of the white-out. Whilst penetrated posteroanterior and lateral films may help, it is sometimes surprisingly difficult to differentiate between the causes of an opaque hemithorax. Ultrasound and computed tomography allow the distinction

to be made with confidence, and the latter may give further information about the underlying disease.

Decreased density of hemithorax

The conditions outlined so far have all focused on increased density of the lungs on plain radiographs. However, there are a number of causes where one lung appears less dense than the other side. When a chest radiograph demonstrates greater radiolucency of one lung compared with the other, it is necessary first to determine whether this appearance is due to a pulmonary abnormality; the radiograph should be checked for patient rotation and for soft tissue asymmetry e.g. a mastectomy.

The pulmonary vessels are a helpful pointer to abnormalities causing a true decrease in density. In compensatory hyperinflation they are splayed apart. A search should also be made for a collapsed lobe. The vessels are considerably diminished or truncated in emphysema. Further radiological examination should include an expiration film if a pneumothorax is suspected. This will also demonstrate air trapping that occurs with bronchial obstruction. Computed tomography may also be useful in elucidating the cause of a hyperlucent lung. The lungs can be seen on computed tomography without the problem of overlying tissues, and any decrease in density is more readily apparent.

Elevation of the diaphragm

The right or left dome of the diaphragm may be elevated because it is paralysed, pushed up, or pulled up. However, there are a number of circumstances in which the diaphragm appears to be elevated without actually being so.

The radiographic evaluation of an apparently elevated diaphragm should begin with an assessment of the plain film, in particular evidence of prior surgery. Old radiographs are essential to determine whether the diaphragmatic elevation is long-standing. A decubitus film is particularly useful in ruling out a suspected subpulmonary effusion; in this instance the pleural effusion is confined to the space between the lung base and the superior surface of the diaphragm. The radiograph will show what appears to be an elevated hemidiaphragm. Ultrasound will assist in determining if fluid is present above and/or below the diaphragm. If the hemidiaphragm is paralysed, fluoroscopic examination is useful as it may demonstrate paradoxical movement on vigorous sniffing (instead of the diaphragm moving down it moves up). An important proviso is that a few normal individuals show this paradoxical movement of the diaphragm on sniffing. In congenital eventration part or all of the hemidiaphragm muscle is made up of a thin layer of fibrous tissue and it may be difficult to distinguish from paralysis even on fluoroscopy.

Pleural disease

Because the chest radiograph is a two-dimensional image, abnormalities of the pleura and chest wall are often difficult to assess. Gross pleural abnormalities are usually obvious on a chest radiograph, but even when there is extensive pleural pathology it may be difficult to distinguish between pleural fluid, pleural thickening (e.g. secondary to a previous inflammatory process) and a neoplasm of the pleura. In such cases a lateral decubitus film or ultrasound scan is useful in identifying the presence of fluid. Computed tomography can readily identify the encasing and constricting nature of a mesothelioma. Ultrasound is often better than computed tomography in distinguishing between pleural fluid and pleural thickening.

The pulmonary mass

Most pulmonary nodules or masses are discovered by plain chest radiography. It is important that previous films are obtained if at all possible. If the mass was present on the previous films and has not changed over a number of years, it can be assumed that the lesion is benign and no further action needs to be taken. However, if the nodule was not previously present or has increased in size, then further investigation is warranted.

Computed tomography (Fig. 2.14) will detect

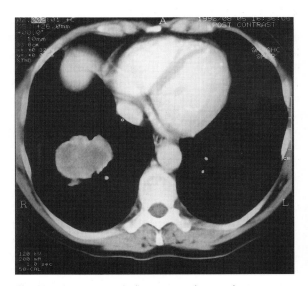

Fig. 2.14 Large necrotic (low attenuation area) tumour mass within right lower lobe.

or exclude the presence of other lesions within the lungs. The presence of calcification within the nodule, although often thought to be an indicator of benignity, will not exclude malignancy with complete certainty. In addition, computed tomography can be used to determine the presence of hilar or mediastinal lymph node enlargement as well as direct invasion of the adjacent mediastinum or chest wall. In patients in whom surgical resection of the pulmonary mass is not indicated, a cytological or histological specimen by percutaneous needle biopsy may be taken. This is usually reserved for small peripheral lesions that are not accessible by bronchoscopy. It can be performed under computed tomography guidance or fluoroscopy, but carries the complication of a pneumothorax (20%) or pulmonary haemorrhage (see other interventional techniques).

Pulmonary nodules

A large number of conditions are characterized by multiple pulmonary nodules (Fig. 2.15a). Combining the clinical information with an accurate description of the size and distribution of the nodules narrows down the list of differential diagnoses.

Metastatic deposits are by far the commonest cause of multiple pulmonary nodules of varying sizes in adult patients in the United Kingdom (Fig. 2.16), but this is not the case world-wide. In some parts of the United States of America, histoplasmosis is endemic and multiple lesions due to this condition may be more common than those due to malignancy. Making this important distinction may be difficult, and biopsy of one lesion may be the only reliable means of distinguishing a benign from a malignant cause for the multiple nodules.

Nodules are described as 'miliary' when they are less than 5 mm in diameter and are so numerous that they cannot be counted (Fig. 2.15b). The crucial diagnosis to consider, even if the patient is not particularly unwell, is miliary tuberculosis, since this life-threatening disease can be readily treated. If the patient is asymptomatic the differential diagnosis is more likely

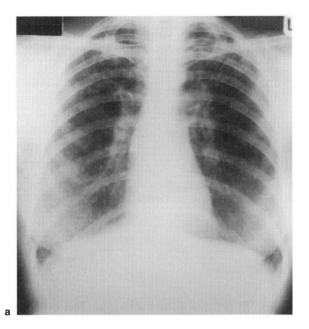

a

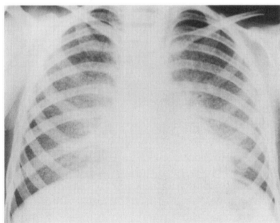

b

Fig. 2.15 **a** Multiple pulmonary nodules. The majority of these are greater than 5 mm in diameter. There is elevation of both hila secondary to fibrosis and volume loss in both upper lobes. The cause in this instance was sarcoidosis. **b** Multiple miliary nodules: these nodules are all less than 5 mm in diameter. The diagnosis was miliary tuberculosis.

to lie between sarcoidosis, metastatic disease or a coal worker's pneumoconiosis. As ever, previous radiographs showing the rate of growth of the nodules may give valuable clues to the likely nature of the disease.

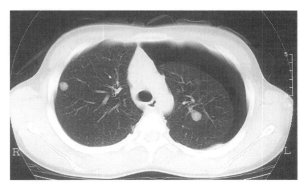

Fig. 2.16 Nodules within right and left upper lobes consistent with metastatic deposits. A left-sided pneumothorax is also present. (Primary tumour site – osteosarcoma of tibia.)

Cavitating pulmonary lesions

The radiological definition of cavitation is a lucency representing air within a mass or an area of consolidation. The cavity may or may not contain a fluid level, and is surrounded by a wall of variable thickness (Fig. 2.17).

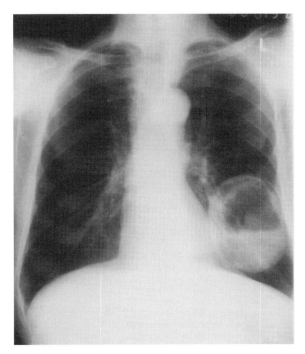

Fig. 2.17 Lung abscess: there is a thick-walled cavity containing a fluid level in the left lower lobe.

The two most likely diagnoses in an adult presenting with a cavitating pulmonary lesion on a chest radiograph are a cancer or a lung abscess. In children, infection is the commonest cause. Cavitation secondary to necrosis is well recognized in a variety of bacterial pneumonias, particularly those associated with tuberculosis, *Staphylococcus aureus*, anaerobes and *Klebsiella*. Diagnosis is usually by plain chest radiograph in the first instance, but computed tomography is also useful for localizing the abscess and sometimes to enable percutaneous aspiration to be undertaken. It also allows assessment of the relationship of the abscess to adjacent airways so that appropriate postural drainage can be planned.

In all age groups it is important to consider tuberculosis, especially if the cavitating lesions are in the lung apices. Linear or computed tomography may be necessary if the presence of cavitation is questionable; in addition computed tomography may show other features which help to narrow the differential diagnosis (e.g. pulmonary calcifications in tuberculosis, mediastinal lymph node enlargement in metastatic disease). In general, radiology alone cannot distinguish one cause of a cavitating mass from another.

SPECIFIC CONDITIONS

The postoperative and critically ill patient

In the context of intensive care medicine, the portable radiograph is one of the main means of monitoring critically ill patients. However, it is a far from perfect technique as the degree of inspiration is usually poor and may vary widely on serial radiographs. In addition, evaluation of cardiac size and the lung bases is, at best, difficult. This is often compounded by the rapidly changing haemodynamic state of the patient.

To some extent the advent of phosphor plate radiography has enabled more accurate assessments to be made because variations in exposure are not such a problem. Use of decubitus radiographs can be useful to evaluate the dependent side for fluid and the non-dependent side for small, but clinically important, pneumothoraces. For convenience it is useful to consider the various disease processes in the categories described below.

Support and monitoring apparatus

Careful radiographic monitoring of the position of various tubes and catheters used in the post-operative and critically ill patient is essential to decrease complications. Before evaluating the heart and lungs it is good practice to check each of these lines for proper positioning. The ideally placed central venous line ends in the superior vena cava (Fig. 2.18). Catheters terminating in the right atrium or ventricle may cause arrhythmias or perforation. Swan–Ganz catheters used to monitor pulmonary capillary wedge pressure are ideally sited in a main or lobar pulmonary artery. Drugs inadvertently injected directly into the wedged catheter may cause lobar pulmonary oedema or necrosis. Both catheters (central venous pressure line and Swan–Ganz) are inserted percutaneously and, therefore, share certain complications. The most frequent is a pneumothorax due to puncture of the lung at the time of subclavian vein insertion. If the catheter is inserted into the mediastinum or perforates a vein or artery, there may be dramatic widening of the superior mediastinum due to haematoma. If the catheter enters the pleural space, infused fluid rapidly fills the pleural space. Catheter perforation of the right atrium or ventricle may lead to cardiac tamponade which may be manifested as progressive enlargement of the heart shadow on serial radiographs.

The intra-aortic balloon pump is usually inserted via the femoral artery and is used in patients with intractable heart failure or in weaning the patient from cardiopulmonary bypass. On the frontal radiograph the tip of the catheter should be seen lying in the aortic arch.

A cardiac pacemaker wire is usually inserted via the external jugular, the cephalic or femoral vein and passed under fluoroscopic control into the apex of the right ventricle. Kinks or coils

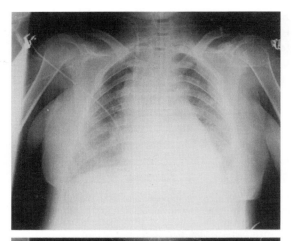

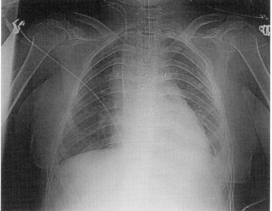

Fig. 2.18 Portable computed radiograph. This digital radiograph taken in an intensive care unit demonstrates the correct position of the tips of the two central venous lines and endotracheal tube. The upper image resembles a conventional radiograph and is used to examine the lungs; the lower image (the same radiograph) has been manipulated to make identification of lines easier.

of wire are undesirable and the wire should be examined carefully along its entire length.

The tip of a correctly positioned endotracheal tube (Fig. 2.18) lies in the midtrachea, approximately 5–7 cm above the carina. This distance is needed to ensure that it does not descend into the right main stem bronchus with flexion of the head and neck or ascend into the pharynx when the head and neck are extended. If the endotracheal tube is inadvertently passed into the right main stem bronchus (the more vertical of the two main bronchi), the left lung may collapse with a shift of the mediastinum to the left and hyperinflation of the right lung. If the endotracheal tube is positioned just below the vocal cords, the tube may retract into the pharynx, airway protection is lost and aspiration may occur. If the tube remains high in the trachea, inflation of the cuff may cause vocal cord damage. Delayed complications include focal tracheal necrosis leading ultimately to a localized stricture. It is worth noting that, even with correct positioning and cuff inflation, an endotracheal tube is not an absolute guarantee against aspiration of stomach contents into the airways.

Tracheostomy for long-term support has its own complications. A correctly placed tracheostomy tube should be parallel to the long axis of the trachea, approximately one-half to two-thirds the diameter of the trachea and end at least 5 cm from the carina. Marked subcutaneous or mediastinal emphysema may be due to tracheal injury or a large leak around the stoma. After prolonged intubation some tracheal scarring is inevitable. Symptomatic tracheal stenosis or collapse of a short length of the trachea is less common now owing to use of low-pressure occlusion cuffs on the endotracheal tubes. When positive end expiratory pressure (PEEP) is added, the patient's tidal volume and functional residual capacity increase. This is reflected in the radiograph as increased lung aeration. PEEP may open up areas of collapse and cause radiographic clearing. However, this may be spurious as any densities present will be less obvious owing to the increased lung volume. Similarly, when weaned off PEEP, the lung volume drops and the lungs may appear to be dramatically worse. Pulmonary barotrauma (air leakage due to elevated pressure) complicates approximately 10% of patients on positive pressure ventilation. If air continues to leak due to continued ventilation, a tension pneumothorax may develop. The chest radiograph is often the first indicator of this potentially fatal complication.

Collapse

Following laparotomy, at least half of all patients develop some postoperative pulmonary collapse. Volume loss is most often attributed to hypoventilation and retained secretions and it is most frequent in patients with chronic bronchitis, emphysema, obesity, prolonged anaesthesia or unusually heavy analgesia. The commonest radiographic manifestation is of linear densities which appear in the lower lung fields soon after surgery. Patchy, segmental or complete lobar consolidation is less common. When due to hypoventilation or large airway secretions, marked volume loss rather than dense consolidation is the usual appearance. Careful attention should be paid to unilateral elevation of the diaphragm and shifts of the minor fissure or hilar vessels. When collapse is due to multiple peripheral mucus plugs, the radiographic picture may be of pulmonary consolidation rather than volume loss. Areas of collapse tend to change rapidly and often clear with suction or physiotherapy. Postoperative collapse is not usually an infectious process, but if not treated promptly areas of collapse will usually become secondarily infected.

Aspiration pneumonia

Another frequent postoperative complication is the aspiration of gastric contents. A depressed state of consciousness and the presence of a nasogastric tube which disables the protective oesophagogastric sphincter are the most frequent predisposing factors. An endotracheal or tracheostomy tube does not always protect the patient from aspiration. The radiographic appearance of patchy, often bilateral, consolidation appears any time within the first 24 hours of aspiration and then progresses rapidly. In an uncomplicated case there is usually evidence of stability or regression by 72 hours, with complete clearing within 1–2 weeks. The infiltrates are usually patchy and diffuse and are most often seen at the lung bases, more commonly on the right. Complications include progression to adult respiratory distress syndrome (ARDS). Any worsening of the radiograph on the third day or thereafter should suggest the diagnosis of secondary infection.

Adult respiratory distress syndrome

Adult respiratory distress syndrome (ARDS) consists of progressive respiratory insufficiency following a major bodily insult and can be due to a large number of factors. Over the years it has been known as 'shock lung', 'stiff lung syndrome' and 'adult hyaline membrane disease'. At the pathophysiological level there is increased permeability of the pulmonary capillaries and the formation of platelet and fibrin microemboli. This results in alveolar oedema and haemorrhage which can affect the entire lung. After several days, hyaline membranes form within the distal air spaces. As a general rule, symptoms occur on the second day after insult or injury, but the radiograph remains normal during the initial hours of clinical distress. Interstitial oedema is the first radiographic abnormality, which may be of a faint, hazy ground-glass appearance (see Fig. 2.6), and this is followed rapidly by patchy air-space oedema. By 36–72 hours after insult, diffuse global air-space consolidation is evident. It is the timing of the radiographic changes relative to the insult and the onset of symptoms, rather than the radiological appearance alone, that suggest the diagnosis of ARDS. The radiographic pattern of established ARDS is identical to that of pulmonary oedema, i.e. bilateral extensive consolidation. The radiology of patients with ARDS rarely allows certain diagnosis of the underlying cause or supervening complications (e.g. aspiration or developing infections) to be made.

Pneumonia

Pulmonary infection may occur several days after surgery. Pneumonia may complicate collapse, but may result from aspiration or inhalation of infected secretions from the pharynx. The features of consolidation have already been covered, but the critically ill or postoperative patient frequently does not exhibit the expected features. Numerous factors, such as prior antibiotic therapy and coexistent heart or lung disease, conspire to modify the radiographic features. The radiographic appearance varies from a few ill-defined or discrete opacities to a pattern of coalescence and widespread patchy consolidation. Cavity or pneumatocele (a thin-walled air-filled space) formation is not infrequent.

Extrapulmonary air

The diagnosis of a pneumothorax is made by the identification of the thin line of the visceral pleura. Free air may also be found in the pulmonary interstitium, the mediastinum, the pericardial space and the subcutaneous tissues. In the intensive care setting, extrapulmonary air is most often due to barotrauma from mechanical ventilation or secondary to surgery or other iatrogenic procedures. Pulmonary interstitial emphysema is difficult to recognize radiographically and is invariably due to ventilator-induced barotrauma. Unlike air bronchograms, the interstitial air is seen as black lines and streaks radiating from the hila; they do not branch or taper towards the periphery. Interstitial emphysema usually culminates in a pneumomediastinum, and this is shown on a frontal radiograph as a radiolucent band against the mediastinum bordered by the reflected mediastinal pleura. Air may outline specific structures such as the aortic arch, the descending aorta or the thymus.

Cardiac failure

The radiographic diagnosis of early left ventricular failure is largely dependent on changes in the calibre of the pulmonary vessels in the erect patient. As the left atrial pressure rises, blood is shunted to the upper zones. This is the first and most important radiographic sign of elevated left ventricular pressure (Fig. 2.19); it is important to remember that, because of redistribution of blood flow in the supine position, a supine radiograph does not allow this criterion to be used.

Interstitial pulmonary oedema then follows; this is manifested by blurring of the vessel margins, a perihilar haze and a vague increased density over the lower zones. When fluid fills and distends the interlobular septa, Kerley B

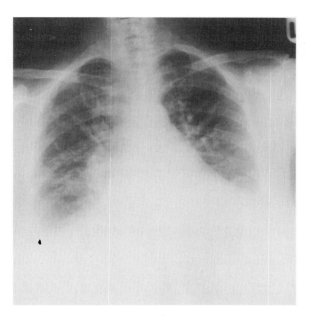

Fig. 2.19 Cardiac failure: the heart is enlarged with upper lobe blood diversion (prominent upper lobe vessels) and there are small basal pleural effusions.

lines (septal lines) may be visible. These are best visualized in the costophrenic angles as thin white lines arising from the lateral pleural surface. As the left ventricular pressure continues to rise, multiple small, ill-defined opacities occur in the lower half of the lungs. These represent alveoli filling with fluid. Alveolar oedema may also appear as poorly defined bilateral 'butterfly' perihilar opacification. Increasing cardiac size usually accompanies cardiac failure but, if it occurs following acute myocardial infarction or an acute arrhythmia, cardiac failure may be present without an increase in cardiac size. Bilateral pleural effusions often accompany cardiac failure.

Pulmonary embolism

The postoperative or critically ill patient has numerous risk factors for the development of deep venous thrombosis and thus pulmonary embolism. In this group, where respiratory distress is often multifactorial, the diagnosis of pulmonary embolism is extremely difficult.

Conventional radiographic findings are non-specific and include elevation of the diaphragm, collapse or segmental consolidation. A small pleural effusion may appear during the first 2 days following the embolus. It is important to recognize that a normal chest radiograph does not exclude a major pulmonary embolus; indeed a normal radiograph in a patient with acute respiratory distress is suggestive of the diagnosis. A radionuclide perfusion scan is of use because if it is normal a pulmonary embolus can be excluded; however, this is not a practical test for a patient in an intensive care unit and the decision to treat with anticoagulants is often made clinically.

The success of helical CT in the diagnosis of pulmonary embolism relates to its rapid scan time, volumetric data acquisition and high degree of vascular enhancement.

Kyphoscoliosis

Kyphoscoliosis makes assessment of the chest radiograph difficult and it is useful to reduce the distortion of thoracic contents due to the kyphoscoliosis by obtaining an oblique radiograph, positioning the patient in such a way that the spine appears at its straightest. Severe kyphoscoliosis may cause pulmonary arterial hypertension and cor pulmonale. Some congenital chest anomalies such as pulmonary agenesis (absence of a lung) and neurofibromatosis are associated with dorsal spine abnormalities. Because of the problems associated with getting a true posteroanterior and lateral view, computed tomography scanning is often the most satisfactory method of visualizing the lungs.

Bronchiectasis

This is a chronic condition characterized by local, irreversible dilatation of the bronchi, usually associated with inflammation. On a chest radiograph (Fig. 2.20a) the findings include: (a) the bronchial wall visible either as single thin lines or as parallel 'tram-lines'; (b) ring and curvilinear opacities which represent thickened airway walls

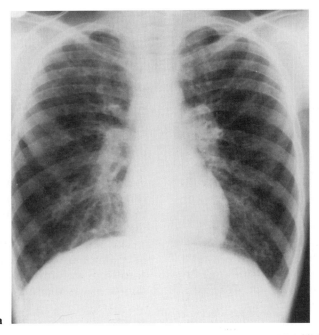

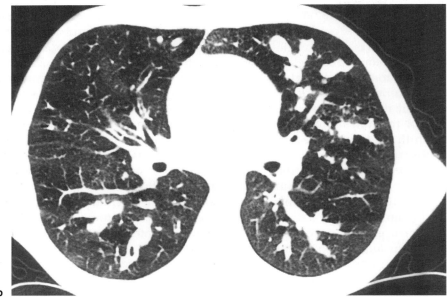

Fig. 2.20 **a** Cystic fibrosis: the lungs are over-inflated and there is widespread increased shadowing due to barely perceptible bronchial wall thickening and peribronchial consolidation. The proximal pulmonary arteries are enlarged due to a degree of pulmonary arterial hypertension. **b** Thin section computed tomography through the mid-zones showing widespread severe bronchiectasis with mucus plugging of many of the dilated airways.

seen end-on. These tend to range in size from 8 to 20 mm, have thin (hairline) walls, and may contain air–fluid levels; (c) dilated airways filled with secretions giving rise to broad band shadows some 5–10 mm wide and several centimetres long (seen end-on, these dilated fluid-filled airways produce rounded or oval nodular opacities); (d) overinflation throughout both lungs (particularly in cystic fibrosis); (e) volume loss where bronchiectasis is localized (this may give rise to crowding of bronchi or collapse due to mucus plugging that can be severe and result in complete collapse of a lobe); and (f) less specific signs include infective consolidation, scarring and pleural thickening.

The definitive diagnosis of bronchiectasis used to be made by bronchography (injection of contrast into the bronchial airway), but this is an invasive and unpleasant procedure and a viable alternative is high-resolution computed tomography (Fig. 2.20b). With this technique, thin slices are taken throughout both lungs and the findings are similar to those on the plain film (thickened bronchial walls, bronchial dilatation, ring opacities containing air–fluid levels). Comparing the diameter of the bronchial wall with the adjacent vessel is helpful, as both should be approximately the same size. Computed tomography may also be helpful in determining the optimum position for postural drainage. Upper lobe predominance is present in early cystic fibrosis, and after tubercle infection and allergic bronchopulmonary aspergillosis. The remainder affect predominantly the middle and lower lobes.

Chronic airflow limitation

This comprises three conditions which are present simultaneously in a given patient to a greater or lesser degree: chronic bronchitis, asthma and emphysema. The first is diagnosed by the patient's history and, strictly speaking, does not have any characteristic radiological features. In asthma the chest radiograph is normal in the majority of patients between attacks, but as many as 40% reveal evidence of hyperinflation during an acute severe episode.

In asthmatic children with recurrent infection, bronchial wall thickening occurs. Collapse of a lobe or an entire lung because of mucus plugging is another feature and may be recurrent affecting different lobes. Complications include a pneumomediastinum which arises secondarily to pulmonary interstitial emphysema and pneumothorax due to rupture of a subpleural bulla. Expiratory radiographs will aid detection of this as well as demonstrating any air trapping secondary to bronchial occlusion.

Emphysema is a condition characterized by an increase in air spaces beyond the terminal bronchiole owing to destruction of alveolar walls. Whilst it is strictly a pathological diagnosis, certain radiographic appearances are characteristic in more advanced cases. These include overinflation of the lungs, an alteration in the appearance of the pulmonary vessels, and the presence of bullae (Fig. 2.21). Overinflation results in flattening of the diaphragmatic dome and this results in an apparently small heart and a decreased cardiothoracic ratio. On the lateral chest radiograph the large retrosternal translucency caused by the hyperinflated lungs is particularly striking (Fig. 2.21b). The pulmonary vessels are abnormal: the smooth gradation in size of vessels from the hilum outwards is lost, with the hilar vessels being larger than normal and tapering abruptly, so-called 'pruning' of the vessels. However, the lungs are usually unevenly involved and this is mirrored by the uneven distribution of pulmonary vessels. When emphysema is predominantly basal in distribution, there is prominent upper lobe blood diversion which should not be mistaken for evidence of left-heart failure. Bullae are recognized by their translucency, their hairline walls and a distortion of adjacent pulmonary vessels. They vary greatly in size and are occasionally big enough to occupy an entire hemithorax. When large they are an important cause of respiratory distress. Complications of bullae formation are infection and haemorrhage, which are usually manifested as the presence of an air–fluid level. Pneumothorax is another complication and can on occasions be difficult to distinguish from a large bulla.

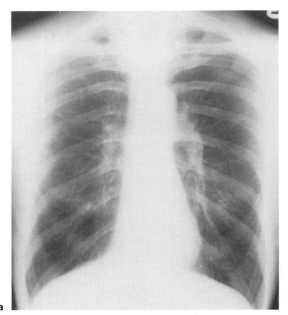
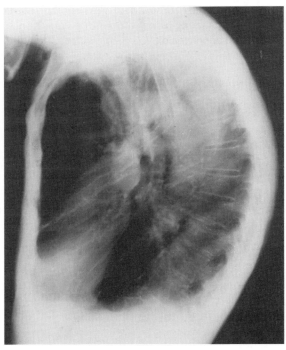

Fig. 2.21 Emphysema. **a** Both lungs are hyperinflated. There is dilatation of the proximal pulmonary arteries with pruning of the peripheral vasculature. **b** The retrosternal and retrocardiac areas are strikingly transradiant.

FURTHER READING

Armstrong P, Wilson A G, Dee P, Hansell D M 1995 Imaging of diseases of the chest. Year Book Medical Publishers, Chicago

Goodman L R, Putman C E 1991 Intensive care radiology: imaging of the critically ill, 3rd edn. W B Saunders, Philadelphia

Grainger R G, Allison D J 1996 Diagnostic radiology. An Anglo-American textbook of imaging, 3rd edn. Churchill Livingstone, Edinburgh

Keats T E 1988 Atlas of normal roentgen variants that may simulate disease, 4th edn. Year Book Medical Publishers, Chicago

Lipscombe D J, Flower C D R, Hadfield J W 1981 Ultrasound of the pleura: an assessment of its clinical value. Clinical Radiology 32: 289–290

Reed J C 1987 Chest radiology: plain film patterns and differential diagnosis, 2nd edn. Year Book Medical Publishers, Chicago

Simon G 1975 The anterior view chest radiograph – criteria for normality derived from a basic analysis of the shadows. Clinical Radiology 26: 429–437

Vix V A, Klatte E C 1970 The lateral chest radiograph in the diagnosis of hilar and mediastinal masses. Radiology 96: 307–316

Webb W R, Müller N L, Naidich D P 1996 High-resolution CT of the lung, 2nd edn. Lippincott-Raven, Philadelphia

3

Cardiopulmonary function testing

Michael D. L. Morgan   Sally J. Singh

INTRODUCTION

In health the human cardiorespiratory system has enormous reserve capacity to cope with the demands of exercise or illness. We are not normally aware of breathlessness or fatigue as a feature of resting activity. Furthermore, unless we harbour athletic ambitions we are unlikely to explore the boundaries of our physiological limitations, and assure ourselves that spare capacity would be present if it ever became necessary. The measurement of physiological capacity in health is, therefore, a matter of relevance only to the curious or the serious competitor who wishes to improve his performance. In patients with heart or lung disease the erosion of physiological reserve eventually imposes limitations upon the activities of daily life. Under these circumstances the measurement of cardiopulmonary function allows the accurate assessment of disability and of the effect of therapeutic intervention. This chapter examines the scientific basis of clinical measurement and its relevance to physiotherapy. In the current climate of clinical audit, physiotherapists must understand the need for objective demonstration of the effectiveness of their treatment.

The human body is an infinitely complex structure, the secrets of which are gradually being exposed by scientific investigation. Certain aspects of cardiopulmonary function can be assessed with some accuracy, but it must be remembered that such measurements are only a snapshot of a component of an organism which is constantly changing and may be influenced by the making of the measurement. It is therefore important to understand exactly what measurement is being made and under what circumstances it is valid before assessing its importance. Given this limitation, carefully made measurements are a valuable addition to clinical practice.

The cellular basis of respiration depends primarily on the production of energy and function from the aerobic metabolism of food. The requirements of an individual cell are simply the regular provision of oxygen and nutrients and the disposal of the acidic waste products of carbon dioxide and water. In a unicellular organism these requirements need only an environment for diffusion. By contrast, man requires a complex collection, distribution and disposal system to service the needs of the body. This system itself requires energy to function, and its capacity imposes a limit on the function of the whole organism. In man oxygen is extracted from the atmosphere by the lungs and delivered to the tissues via the blood. Cardiac function ensures the internal cellular delivery of oxygen and the removal of carbon dioxide back to the lungs for exhalation. The examination of the components of this system can be seen to be somewhat artificial in view of the interdependence of the activities. However, it is reasonable and conventional to consider the process in terms of three compartments. Firstly the lungs themselves, secondly the effectiveness of the integrated activity of gas exchange and acid–base balance, and finally the capacity of the circulatory system to deliver.

LUNG FUNCTION

The apparently simple function of the lung is to deliver oxygen to the gas-exchanging surface and exhaust carbon dioxide to the atmosphere. To achieve this, air is drawn by conductive flow into the alveoli and presented to the gas-exchanging surface where diffusion effects the process of exchange. The carriage of air through the airways depends on the patency of the tubes as well as on the consistency of the lung and the power of the respiratory muscles. These

aspects of pulmonary function are commonly measured in lung function laboratories.

General principles of measurement

Lung function measurements may be made for several reasons. They are useful in describing the lung for diagnostic purposes and subsequently in monitoring change. Accuracy and consistency are therefore very important, and conventions exist for the procedures of measurement and expression of results. In general, a measurement will only be accepted after multiple attempts have been scrutinized and expressed under standard conditions. These are usually body temperature and atmospheric pressure (BTPS). To guarantee accuracy, laboratory practice should include regular physical and biological calibration of the equipment. Standards for good laboratory conduct have been described (British Thoracic Society/Association of Respiratory Technologists and Physiologists 1994). In health there are several factors which influence the magnitude of lung function. These include height, sex and age, and to a lesser degree weight and ethnic origin (Anthonisen 1986, Cotes 1993). As a result, assessment of normality can only be made by comparison with reference values. The latter are obtained from the study of large numbers of normal people from the relevant population (European Community for Coal and Steel 1983). Once obtained, results can be expressed as percentage predicted or, more correctly, by comparison with the 95% confidence interval for that value.

Airway function

For the purposes of measurement the lung has only one portal of entry and exit, i.e. through the mouth, and airway function is assessed by quantification of gas flow or volume. The calibre of the airways reduces through their generations and the major resistance to gas flow is normally in the upper airway. The larger airways are supported by cartilage, while the smaller airways are held patent by the radial traction of the surrounding lung so that their calibre increases with the volume of the lung. The diameter of these airways is also controlled by neural tone which is predominantly parasympathetic. The disruption of airway function can occur through physical or rigid obstruction to a large airway by, for example, a tracheal tumour. It may also occur because of more widespread disease in asthma, when large numbers of smaller airways are affected by episodic alteration of their calibre by smooth muscle contraction, mucosal oedema and intraluminal secretions. In chronic bronchitis, obstruction occurs by mucosal thickening and mucous secretion, but in emphysema the mechanism is different. Though seldom occurring in isolation from other forms of airway obstruction, the result of parenchymal emphysema is to weaken the elastic structure which maintains radial traction on the airways and allows them to close too early in expiration. Tests of airway function measure airway calibre and are now well established in clinical practice. Most tests of airway patency examine expiratory function. There are three common methods:

- Spirometry (FEV_1 and FVC)
- Flow–volume curves
- Peak expiratory flow (PEF).

Production of the spirogram from a maximal forced expiration following a full inspiration is reliable and provides the forced expiratory volume in 1 second (FEV_1) and the forced vital capacity (FVC) (Fig. 3.1). The measurement is usually made using a spirometer which measures volume, or derived from a flow signal obtained from a pneumotachograph or turbine. Most commonly, the FEV_1 and FVC are measured during the same manoeuvre, but a greater vital capacity may be obtained in patients with airway disease if it is performed slowly. Reduction in FEV_1 with relative preservation of FVC or vital capacity (VC) is known as an 'obstructive' pattern, which indicates and grades airway obstruction: $FEV_1/FVC < 75\%$ is graded as mild, $< 60\%$ as moderate, and $< 40\%$ as severe impairment (American Thoracic Society 1986). Simultaneous reduction in both FEV_1 and FVC with an increase in the FEV_1/FVC ratio is called a 'restrictive' defect and is usually associated with a reduction in lung volume. Abnormal values are defined as those recognized to be outside the normal range of two standard deviations for sex, height and age. This usually requires a reduction of about 15% from predicted values. Thus simple spirometry can detect and quantify airway obstruction, but gives no indication of the cause.

Measurement of the flow–volume curve is now commonplace and can provide information about the nature of airway obstruction. In this

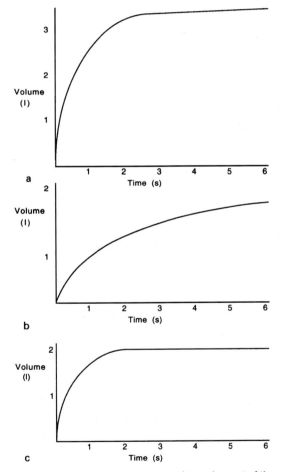

Fig. 3.1 **a** In the normal spirogram the major part of the vital capacity (FVC) is expelled in 1 s (FEV_1). **b** In patients with airway obstruction the FEV_1 is reduced to a greater degree than the FVC. This pattern is known as 'obstructive'. **c** When the lungs are small and empty quickly the pattern is known as 'restrictive'.

test, the gas flow from a full maximum expiration is plotted against the expired volume as the lung empties (Fig. 3.2). The flow of gas from the lung reaches a peak expiratory flow (PEF) after about 100 milliseconds and then declines linearly as the lung empties. If the measurement is continued into the subsequent full inspiration, a flow–volume 'loop' is produced and inspiratory flow rates can be measured. The shape of the expiratory and inspiratory portions are different, since in expiration the active expulsion is assisted by the elastic recoil of the lung while inspiratory flow rates are a reflection of airway calibre and inspiratory muscle strength only. Something of the nature of the airway obstruction can be learnt from consideration of the actual and relative values of PEF, peak inspiratory flow (PIF) and the values of expiratory flow at 50% and 75% vital capacity (MEF_{50} and MEF_{75}). Simple inspection of the loop is often sufficient to distinguish between rigid upper

airway obstruction, intraluminal obstruction in chronic bronchitis and asthma, and the 'pressure-dependent' collapse seen in pure emphysema with relative preservation of inspiratory flow rates.

The PEF is one component of the flow–volume manoeuvre which has been used with increasing popularity. This has been encouraged by the availability of simple devices for its measurement. Provided that the patient does not have weak respiratory muscles and has made a maximum effort, the PEF will reflect airway calibre. The absolute values obtained are not particularly helpful unless they are extremely low, but the easily repeated measurements can be used to obtain valuable insight into the mechanisms of variable airway obstruction in asthma. There is a normal diurnal variation in airway calibre of about 50 l/min which is exaggerated in patients with poorly controlled asthma (Fig. 3.3) (Benson 1983). Wider variation will be seen

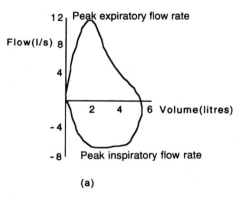

(a)

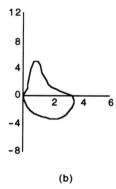

(b)

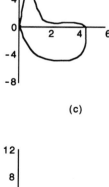

(c)

Fig. 3.2 **a** The normal flow–volume loop has a characteristic shape. **b** Airway obstruction from asthma or chronic bronchitis appears as a concave expiratory limb and reduced inspiratory flows. **c** In emphysema the expiratory flows are suddenly attenuated, but the inspiratory flows are relatively well preserved. **d** A rigid obstruction to a major airway can produce an oval loop. **e** Inspiratory flows are reduced in diaphragm weakness or extrathoracic tracheal obstruction.

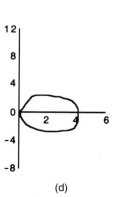

(d)

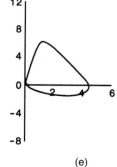

(e)

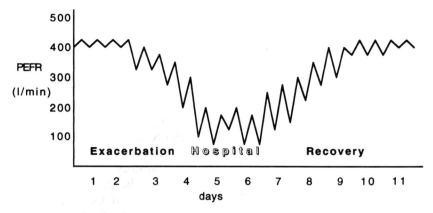

Fig. 3.3 A reconstruction of a peak flow chart from an asthmatic patient. As an attack develops, the normal diurnal variation increases and the mean values drop until treatment reverses the pattern in recovery. The decline and recovery may take several days.

approaching or recovering from an attack and following exposure to trigger factors. The real value of the PEF lies in its repeatability and its portability. The issue of meters to patients with asthma allows domiciliary and occupational investigation of asthma. It also provides a tool for patients to use to monitor their asthma objectively as part of a self-management plan. In past years, the PEF chart has been used during hospital admissions to record the progress and predict the discharge of patients with airway disease. Although this is valuable in asthma where the airway obstruction is variable, it can show no change at all in patients with chronic airflow limitation in spite of a clinical improvement. In this case the twice-weekly measurement of FEV_1 and FVC is more likely to mirror progress than will the slavish recording of the PEF chart (Gibson 1995).

The physical properties of the lung

The two lungs contain millions of alveoli within a fibroelastic matrix. They do not have a very rigid structure and are held in contact with the rib cage by surface-tension forces at the apposition of the two pleural surfaces. The resting volume of the lung (the functional residual capacity (FRC)) is thus determined by the outward spring of the rib cage and the inward elastic recoil of the lung matrix. Expansion and contraction of the lung therefore involves the controlled stretching or relaxation of the lung by the respiratory muscles away from FRC. The position of FRC can be influenced if the lung is stiffer than usual (as in interstitial disease), or if it is more compliant (as when damaged by emphysema). The measurement of the lung's volume can therefore give some insight into these conditions.

The actual volume of the lung must be measured indirectly in life since the lungs obviously cannot be removed for the measurement. There are several techniques which measure slightly different aspects of volume. The most familiar method is helium dilution, which involves rebreathing through a closed circuit a mixture of gases containing a known concentration of helium which is not absorbed into the circulation. The measurement of the final concentration of helium is used to calculate the gas dilution, or the 'accessible' volume, of the lung. An alternative method uses the Boyle's law principle – gas in the chest is compressed and the change in pressure is used to calculate the volume of gas within the chest. This method requires a large airtight box or plethysmograph. In both methods the actual volume that is estimated is the

FRC, and total lung capacity (TLC) and residual volume (RV) are obtained from an additional spirometric trace. A further method involves the calculation of the total volume of the lung from the dimensions of a chest radiograph. This volume includes the total volume of gas, tissue and blood. Since the techniques do measure different aspects of volume, consistency in sequential measurements is important. In normal lungs the results are very similar, but where there is airway obstruction the values may be disparate. Such disparity can be used to advantage, e.g. in calculating the degree of trapped gas as the difference between the plethysmographic and helium dilution lung volumes.

The chest wall and the respiratory muscles

To maintain their shape the lungs depend on the support of the rib cage and the patency of the airways and alveoli. The expansion of the rib cage by the respiratory muscles is responsible for the tidal flow of gas into and out of the lungs. Over the past few years there has been increasing awareness of the importance of dysfunction of the respiratory muscles and the bony rib cage in contributing to respiratory failure. Such conditions include myopathies and polio as well as skeletal malformations such as scoliosis which decrease rib cage compliance and reduce the effectiveness of the musculature. The respiratory muscles include the diaphragm as the major muscle of inspiration and the intercostal muscles and scalenes. The latter together with the sternomastoids are known as the 'accessory muscles', but actually have a stabilizing role in tidal breathing. The combination of the respiratory muscles and the bony rib cage is called the 'chest wall' and conceptually is considered as the organ which inflates the lungs. Weakness of the respiratory muscles will eventually lead to ventilatory failure which may first become apparent during the night as an exaggeration of the normal nocturnal hypoventilation (Shneerson 1988) (Fig. 3.4).

The function of the respiratory muscles is difficult to study directly since the muscles have complex origins and insertions. Furthermore, their product, which is the pressure generated within the thoracic cavity, depends on the co-ordinated action of many muscles the individual functions of which may be difficult to distinguish in life. It is possible to make some assessment of both the strength and endurance of the muscles and also to separate the diaphragm from the other muscles. The simple strength that the inspiratory and expiratory muscles can generate as pressure is easy to measure. The maximum inspiratory pressure (PiMax) and expiratory pressure (PeMax) are easy to measure with a manometer or electronic gauge. The normal values of approximately $-100\ cmH_2O$ and $+120\ cmH_2O$ (Black & Hyatt 1971) are well in excess of that needed to inflate the lungs (5–$10\ cmH_2O$) and, therefore, provide a sensitive measure of developing muscle weakness. These measurements do have a learning requirement and are not suitable for monitoring of patients with rapidly developing muscle weakness such as in Guillain–Barré syndrome. Under these circumstances the sequential measurement of the vital capacity is much more reliable, since a failure to maintain it will predict ventilatory failure.

The strength of the diaphragm can be separated from the other muscles by measuring the pressure gradient across it. This is achieved by using balloons attached to pressure transducers to estimate the pressure in the oesophagus and the stomach. The gradient across the diaphragm during a maximum inspiration or sniff is an indirect measure of the strength of the diaphragm. Normal values for sniff pressures have now been published (Uldry & Fitting 1995). If required, a value free of volition can be obtained by electrical stimulation of the phrenic nerve in the neck, or even by magnetic stimulation of the cerebral cortex. Fortunately, measurements of separate diaphragm strength are seldom required in clinical practice. A simple guide to diaphragm function can be obtained by observation of the change in vital capacity with posture. When supine, the vital capacity normally falls by 8–10%, but when diaphragm weakness is present it may fall by more than 30%.

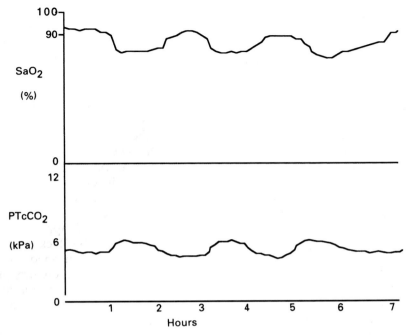

Fig. 3.4 A sleep study from a patient with kyphoscoliosis demonstrates periodic falls in SaO₂ associated with rapid eye movement (REM) sleep. The lower panel shows the simultaneous rises in transcutaneous carbon dioxide (PTcCO₂) associated with the episodes of hypoventilation.

The measurement of the supine vital capacity is, therefore, a good screening test of diaphragm function (Green & Laroche 1990). More recently the measurement of sniff pressures at the mouth or nose has become recognized as a reflection of pure diaphragmatic activity.

The respiratory muscles are duty bound to contract regularly through life to sustain it. Consequently, the prediction of fatigue or the measurement of endurance capacity would have more relevance to clinical practice. The identification of fatigue is not very reliable and there is no simple test that can be applied at the bedside. There are, however, several ways of estimating respiratory muscle endurance capacity. The simplest is the maximum voluntary ventilation (MVV), while other methods include breathing through resistances. One of the more interesting examples of the latter is incremental threshold loading, where increasing resistances are added until they can no longer be sustained. This makes a test for the respiratory muscles which is similar to the exercise tests used for the systemic musculature (Martyn et al 1987).

Gas exchange and oxygen delivery

The requirements of the average cell for oxygen are quite modest, and a mitochondrion may need a PO_2 of as little as 1 kPa (7.5 mmHg) to function effectively. At sea level the atmospheric PO_2 is 20 kPa (150 mmHg) (FiO₂ = 0.21) and in the process of delivering oxygen to the cell there is a loss along this gradient. This is illustrated in Figure 3.5. The first step is the dilution of inspired air with expired air within the alveolus. Each tidal breath (V_T) contains a portion of gas which will remain within the airways and not come into contact with the alveoli. This is known as the 'dead space ventilation' (V_D) and must be achieved before any effective alveolar ventilation ($\dot{V}_A$) can take place:

$$V_T = V_D + \dot{V}_A$$

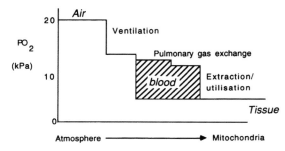

Fig. 3.5 A gradient of PO_2 from the air to the tissues is determined by losses in the initial ventilation of the lungs, circulation in the blood and transfer across the interstitial fluid. Fortunately, the mitochondrial oxygen requirements are very small.

Alveolar gas therefore contains a mixture of fresh gas and some expired CO_2, and the alveolar PO_2 is reduced to about 16 kPa (120 mmHg) before gas exchange begins.

At the alveolar level, gas exchange involves the transfer across the alveolar–capillary membrane of oxygen molecules to the blood and the reverse transfer of carbon dioxide. This is achieved by simple diffusion, which is amplified in the case of oxygen by the affinity of haemoglobin. It normally takes mixed venous blood about 300 milliseconds (ms) to traverse a capillary, and complete equilibrium usually occurs in about 100 ms. This aspect of oxygen transfer from the lung to the blood can be tested using carbon monoxide. Carbon monoxide has a very strong affinity for haemoglobin, follows the same path into the blood and can be measured easily. This principle forms the basis of the carbon monoxide transfer test which measures the amount of carbon monoxide which can be transferred to the blood in the course of a single breath (TLCO). This gives a rough indication of the gas-transferring ability of the lung as a whole and is reduced in conditions like fibrosing alveolitis, emphysema and pneumonectomy where the quality or quantity of the gas-exchanging surface is reduced. If the total TLCO is corrected for lung volume then the subsequent value is known as the 'coefficient of gas transfer' (KCO) and describes the gas-exchanging quality of the lung that is available for ventilation. For example, a very large

normal man and small child should have different TLCOs but their KCO values should be identical.

The carbon monoxide transfer test can give some information about the ability of the lung to transfer gas, but there is not a direct relationship between the TLCO and arterial oxygenation. The lung contains millions of alveolar capillary units, and adequate oxygenation depends on the coordinated, satisfactory function of the whole unit. The pulmonary causes of arterial hypoxaemia have four major origins:

- Hypoventilation
- Interference with pulmonary diffusion
- Ventilation/perfusion imbalance
- True shunt.

Hypoventilation is fairly easy to recognize because the fall in arterial PO_2 is associated with a rise in arterial PCO_2. This occurs in ventilatory failure associated with airway obstruction, chest wall disease and drug intoxication. Interference with pulmonary diffusion is quite rare because the process is very efficient. However, the system may be stretched at altitude or in the presence of disease such as fibrosing alveolitis. Even in this disease the hypoxia is related to increased pulmonary capillary transit time rather than to diffusion failure. The most common contribution to hypoxaemia in many diseases is ventilation/perfusion ($\dot{V}/\dot{Q}$) imbalance. Since effective lung function depends on the coordination of equivalent ventilation and perfusion to all units, it is not surprising that failure of the local matching mechanisms can cause trouble. The most extreme example would be a pulmonary embolus where ventilation continues in an area with no circulation. In other conditions such as asthma, the patchy distribution of airway obstruction will have similar but less dramatic effects. Some blood passes through the lung without coming into contact with the gas-exchanging surface. Normally this is a very small quantity (< 5%), but effective shunts can be considerable in pneumonia and other conditions where the alveoli are blocked by inflammatory exudate although the circulation continues through the ineffective portion of the lung. This results in extreme hypoxia which cannot easily be corrected by additional oxygen.

Oxygen carriage and arterial blood gases

Oxygen and carbon dioxide are carried in the blood in different ways. Oxygen is immediately bound to haemoglobin and released in the tissues under conditions of low oxygen tension or acidosis. Very little oxygen is carried in solution in the blood under conditions of normal pressure, although this can be increased in a hyperbaric chamber. By contrast, carbon dioxide is carried in the blood entirely in solution, mostly as bicarbonate. The difference between the two forms of carriage of the metabolic gases is fundamental to the interpretation of the measurement of arterial blood gases. The individual cell requires oxygen to survive, but the carriage of oxygen in the blood will have no effect on the body other than the delivery. By contrast, the chemistry involved in the carriage of carbon dioxide controls the short-term acid–base state of the body. When considering blood gas measurements, it is best to examine these functions separately.

The normal atmospheric PO_2 is approximately 20 kPa (150 mmHg) falling to 16 kPa (120 mmHg) within the alveolus. The arterial PO_2 (PaO_2) is usually about 14 kPa (105 mmHg) in a healthy subject. Although we are used to these values they are only true at sea level and really only have relevance because the partial pressure is easy to measure. What matters to the individual cell is the quantity of oxygen that it receives, not the partial pressure. Oxygen delivery to the tissues depends on other factors which include the amount of haemoglobin, the degree of saturation of haemoglobin with oxygen and the rate at which oxygenated blood is delivered to the tissues. Assuming that the haemoglobin and the cardiac output are normal, then the measurement of oxygen saturation of haemoglobin is more relevant to oxygen delivery than is the PaO_2. The PaO_2 is related to oxygen saturation in a complex manner determined by the properties of haemoglobin and known as the 'oxygen

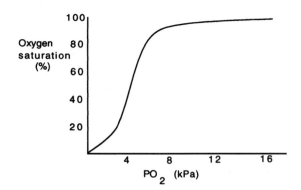

Fig. 3.6 The oxygen dissociation curve relates oxygen saturation to ambient PO_2. In lung disease it is important to recognize that oxygen delivery is assured if PaO_2 is in excess of 8 kPa.

dissociation curve' (Fig. 3.6). This relationship demonstrates that, under most conditions, once PaO_2 reaches 8 kPa (60 mmHg), haemoglobin is fully saturated and cannot carry more oxygen. Thus an arterial PO_2 above that value is only an insurance measure. The availability of pulse oximeters has made the non-invasive measurement of oxygen saturation (SaO_2) commonplace. Pulse oximeters work by transcutaneous examination of the colour spectrum of haemoglobin which changes with its degree of saturation. These instruments are reasonably accurate over the top range of saturation, but become unreliable below about 50% (Tremper & Barker 1989). The measurement of SaO_2 is an extremely valuable tool for monitoring patients' safety. There are, however, some important aspects of interpretation of its use which may be potentially hazardous. Oximetry provides information about oxygen saturation and this will relate to ventilation only if the inspired oxygen level is normal. Monitoring oxygen saturation will not detect underventilation and a rising $PaCO_2$. In patients who are breathing additional oxygen, a false sense of security can be given by a normal SaO_2 even though the $PaCO_2$ is rising. Furthermore, accurate recording of SaO_2 requires a good peripheral circulation which may often be compromised in patients who are hypovolaemic.

The assessment of acid–base status requires

the measurement of arterial blood gas tensions. The average blood gas analyser measures PO_2, PCO_2 and pH. It subsequently calculates from the Henderson–Hasselbalch equation the values of bicarbonate, standard bicarbonate and base excess. The appreciation of the acid–base state requires examination of $PaCO_2$ and pH. Abnormalities are usually described in terms of their generation (Fig. 3.7). For example, a respiratory acidosis resulting from underventilation will display a low pH and an elevated $PaCO_2$. If this has been present for any length of time the serum bicarbonate will have become elevated and acid is excreted by the kidneys to compensate. In cases of nocturnal hypoventilation the daytime PaO_2 may be normal, but the elevation of the base excess gives a clue to the ventilatory history. If an alkalosis (high pH) is associated with a low $PaCO_2$, then this could be due to voluntary hyperventilation and is termed a 'respiratory alkalosis'. The build-up of acid products in diabetes or renal failure will result in a low pH and bicarbonate together with a low $PaCO_2$ in an attempt to compensate for a metabolic acidosis. Finally, the loss of acid from the stomach in prolonged vomiting can produce a metabolic alkalosis which is characterized by

high pH, high bicarbonate and normal $PaCO_2$. These sketches of blood gas disturbance are superficial interpretations, but they provide a useful framework for clinical management under most circumstances.

Respiratory failure

Respiratory failure is defined as inadequate oxygen delivery. As we have seen, this can be due to a variety of circumstances and may or may not be accompanied by a disturbance of the CO_2 level. The critical PaO_2 level is about 8 kPa (60 mmHg), since a lower pressure than this will prejudice oxygen saturation and delivery. Therefore, respiratory failure is defined by convention as $PaO_2 < 7.3$ kPa (54.8 mmHg). If the $PaCO_2$ is elevated above 6.5 kPa (48.8 mmHg), this is termed 'ventilatory failure' and is associated with chronic airflow limitation or other forms of hypoventilation. The understanding of respiratory failure has changed in recent years with the recognition that it is seldom due to a single malfunction of the respiratory system (Fig. 3.8). For example, the rise in $PaCO_2$ and hyperinflation associated with worsening airway obstruction may adversely affect the respiratory

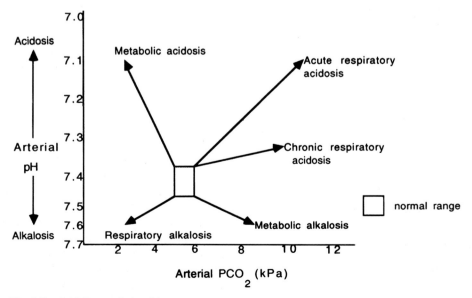

Fig. 3.7 Acid–base relationships.

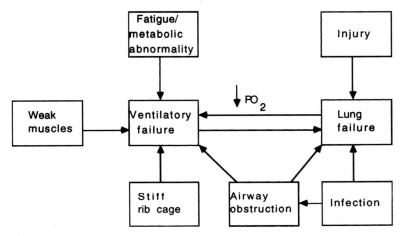

Fig. 3.8 Respiratory failure results from damage to the lung or inability to ventilate it. However, most situations have contributions from several mechanisms which result in a fall in PaO_2.

muscles and introduce a chest wall contribution to failure. Conversely, the loss of lung volume associated with muscle weakness may lead to atelectasis and decreased pulmonary compliance, which will in turn put a greater load on the lung. Understanding of the complexities of chronic respiratory failure has helped to improve the outlook for some groups of patients, e.g. patients with ventilatory failure due to chest wall disease or obstructive sleep apnoea. In these conditions there are abnormalities of breathing during sleep, which may result in nocturnal hypoventilation or transient apnoea, that produce periods of oxygen desaturation which may spill over to the daytime. Recognition of this by oximetry and other more detailed somnography may result in effective treatment by nocturnal nasal intermittent positive pressure ventilation or continuous positive airway pressure (CPAP) (see Ch. 6). By extension these techniques may also have a role in the acute management of selected patients with COPD who have diminished respiratory drive (Wedzicha 1996).

Posture and thoracic surgery

A knowledge of the effect of posture and thoracic surgery on pulmonary function is obviously very important to the physiotherapist. The circum-stances of treatment make this knowledge of practical benefit. Lung function measurements are usually made sitting or standing, but the major postural effect occurs due to gravity in the supine position. There is a small fall in vital capacity (VC) (8%) and a reduction in functional residual capacity (FRC) while lying down which results from repositioning of the diaphragm and pooling of blood in the chest. This change can be used to advantage to identify patients with covert diaphragm weakness where the VC may drop by more than 30%. Gravity also produces a change in the distribution of ventilation and perfusion within the lungs. In the supine posture ventilation and perfusion is preferentially directed to the dependent zones (Kaneko et al 1966). This is important in adults if the lung disease is unilateral since oxygenation will be better if the good lung is dependent.

Physiotherapists are often involved in the assessment of patients for cardiothoracic surgery and their subsequent management. Some thoracic surgery such as bullectomy or decortication improves lung function, but most procedures impair the lung. The mechanisms of impairment include the anaesthetic, the thoracotomy and pulmonary resection. Following anaesthesia there is an immediate loss of FRC and subsequently VC which reaches a trough of about 40% at 24 hours and may take up to 2 weeks to recover (Jenkins et al 1988). This immediate loss of volume is associated with a widened gradient across the lung (A–aDO$_2$) and potential hypoxia which is worsened by obesity, age and smoking. Thoracotomy itself, without pulmonary surgery, will reduce the VC by approximately 10%, which recovers over a period of 3 months. There are no strong arguments for the benefit of median sternotomy over thoracotomy as far as recovery of long-term lung function is concerned. In the short term the physiotherapist should be cautious during treatment when gas exchange will be impaired if the patient is lying on the thoracotomy side.

The surgical removal of lung tissue does not necessarily have the predictable effects on function that might be imagined. Following pneumonectomy the functional state of the patient is remarkably stable, and in the long term the VC and total lung capacity (TLC) become slightly larger than expected for one lung. The TLCO eventually settles to 80% predicted and the KCO may be high since the whole pulmonary blood flow now travels through one lung. The changes after lobectomy are surprisingly different. The long-term effects may be small but in the postoperative phase the disruption may be unexpectedly large. The contusion of lung adjacent to the lobectomy sets up $\dot{V}/\dot{Q}$ disturbances which may in the short term be as significant as removal of the whole lung.

The physiological assessment of patients for thoracic surgery is not really very straightforward (Zibrak et al 1990, Olsen 1992). There is no single test which allows a distinction to be made between success and failure. It is important to consider the nature of the operation and the preoperative function as well as general health, weight and smoking habit. If there is any doubt about the suitability of a candidate from his spirometry and history (particularly cough, sputum and breathlessness) then some assessment of exercise capacity is advisable.

Lung volume reduction surgery

There has been a recent resurgence of interest

in this technique which can potentially make a dramatic improvement to the function of patients with more diffuse pulmonary emphysema. The technique is a development of bullectomy which removes approximately 30% of the substance of the lung which results in deflation of the chest wall. Surprisingly this operation can produce improvements in FEV$_1$ and elastic recoil pressure while reducing hyperinflation. Although the techniques have not yet been adequately assessed, they appear promising in selected patients with more heterogeneous emphysema who have marked symptomatic hyperinflation (Cooper et al 1995, American Thoracic Society 1996).

The effect of growth and ageing on lung function

The respiratory system reaches its peak in the third decade of life. Development of the lung continues from birth until the end of adolescence and starts to deteriorate after the age of 25 years. Fortunately, in the absence of disease there is sufficient reserve capacity to see out old age without discomfort!

The actual measurement of pulmonary function in childhood is problematic because of the obvious lack of cooperation. It is possible to measure lung volume and partial flow–volume curves in infancy by using an adapted plethysmograph. This is possible in the sedated child by producing a pneumatic 'hug' as an alternative to active expiration. In older children it is difficult to obtain cooperation for measurements until they are about 8 years old. After this age lung function can be measured easily, but there are difficulties in interpretation and production of reference values. The inconsistency of the timing of puberty and rapid growth spurts make comparisons difficult, but normal ranges have been produced for these age groups (Polgar & Promadhat 1971).

The most obvious differences between children and adults lie in the development of airway function. The airways develop faster than the alveoli which may not reach maturity until about the seventh year. As the lung matrix develops, the airway walls remain strong and relatively patent. As a result expiratory flow rates, although lower than in adulthood, are relatively high. For example, the FEV_1/FVC ratio may be greater than 90% and the expiratory flow–volume curve may have a flat or convex appearance. In addition to airway patency there are also developments in the behaviour of the chest wall with growth. In childhood the musculoskeletal structures are immature and flexible. Rib cage distortion is often seen in childhood during illness, but disappears with growth and muscularization. The combination of airway patency and plasticity of the chest wall allows an interesting experiment. In childhood the residual volume (RV) is not determined by airway closure but by the strength of the expiratory muscles. Thus if children or young adults are hugged at the end of a forced expiration more air can be expelled. After the age of 25 years, RV is determined by premature airway closure and the lungs cannot be emptied further.

Life after 25 years is all downhill for the respiratory system. As with general ageing, the tissues become less elastic and the lung elastic recoil diminishes. TLC tends to remain static but RV rises as the FEV_1 and FVC fall with age. Arterial PO_2 and $A-aDO_2$ worsen but do not reach critically low values. Exercise capacity, as judged by oxygen consumption, shows a decline with age but it can be retarded by regular activity. As general levels of activity reduce with age, these effects are not usually important, but the changes may be accelerated by smoking or disease.

Interpretation of lung function tests

The value of lung function tests lies in the description of pathophysiology which may give a guide to diagnosis. Once a baseline has been established, changes in function can be used to assess progress with natural history or treatment. Although there may be some investigations which are specific to various diseases it is seldom possible to rely on a single investigation for the purpose. The usual description of disease requires the combination of spirometry, lung volume and gas transfer measurement. The addition of bronchodilator response, a flow–

volume loop and blood gases would provide further information, while additional specific tests are requested as indicated. The additional tests may include an exercise study or respiratory muscle function test to examine the relevant aspect. Interpretation of the tests involves the comparison of the values to the reference population and a description of the pattern of abnormality if present. A helpful report will also give some guidance on the accuracy of the clinical diagnosis and suggest confirmatory investigations if the diagnosis is unclear. Some examples of clinical cases and the patterns of abnormal lung function are given in Table 3.1.

The measurement of disability and exercise testing

Static lung function tests can describe the physical properties of the lungs, but do not always reflect the performance of the cardiopulmonary system in action. The relationship between disability and, for example, spirometry is only a general one and individual predictions about exercise performance cannot be made. To assess disability it must generally be measured by some form of exercise test or inferred from questioning the patient. Exercise tests are valuable in making an objective assessment of disability and in observing the physiological response to exercise in order to assist diagnosis. Tests of exercise performance can either be performed in a complex manner in the laboratory or simply by observation of walking achievement down a hospital corridor. The former generally examine the detailed physiological response while walking tests can give a useful and reproducible assessment of disability. A further value of exercise testing is to use the stimulus to provoke bronchoconstriction where exercise-induced asthma is suspected. In this use the exercise should be performed in an environment as close as possible to that which produces the symptoms.

Questionnaires

One of the difficulties in assessing lung disease through interview is the problem of silent

Table 3.1 Conclusions from pulmonary function tests are best derived from the examination of several measurements. **a** A 66-year-old man with chronic airflow limitation. There is an increase in lung volumes, or hyperinflation of TLC and RV. The spirometry is obstructive but there is good bronchodilator reversibility, especially in the vital capacity. TLCO is slightly reduced but not as low as would be found in severe emphysema. The picture is one of smoking-related airflow obstruction, with the potential for some improvement. **b** A 49-year-old man with cryptogenic fibrosing alveolitis. There is a 'restrictive' defect with loss of lung volumes. Spirometry is not restrictive because of coexisting smoking-related airway obstruction. After treatment with prednisolone (10 March 1992) all values improved. **c** A 40-year-old woman with severe muscle weakness. There is a 'restrictive' picture, but the KCO is elevated because gas exchange is relatively normal. Respiratory muscle strength is reduced.

a

	Predicted	Observed	Post-bronchodilator
FEV_1 (l)	2.86	1.15	1.30
FVC (l)	4.11	2.80	3.55
FEV_1/FVC (%)	70	41	37
TLC (l)	6.98	7.47	
RV (l)	2.54	4.24	
TLCO ($mmol \cdot min^{-1} \cdot kPa^{-1}$)	8.80	6.72	
KCO ($mmol \cdot min^{-1} \cdot kPa^{-1} \cdot l^{-1}$)	1.33	1.06	
VA (l)		6.33	

b

	Predicted	23 April 1991	10 March 1992
FEV_1 (l)	3.75	1.70	2.45
FVC (l)	4.94	2.40	3.30
FEV_1/FVC (%)	75	71	74
TLC (l)	7.59	4.34	5.55
RV (l)	2.41	1.67	2.10
TLCO ($mmol \cdot min^{-1} \cdot kPa^{-1}$)	10.97	5.82	7.36
KCO ($mmol \cdot min^{-1} \cdot kPa^{-1} \cdot l^{-1}$)	1.57	1.38	1.77
VA (l)		4.06	4.20

c

	Predicted	Observed
FEV_1 (l)	2.27	0.8
FVC (l)	2.83	1.10
FEV_1/FVC (%)	77	73
TLC (l)	4.25	1.89
RV (l)	1.22	0.85
TLCO ($mmol \cdot min^{-1} \cdot kPa^{-1}$)	7.49	3.84
KCO ($mmol \cdot min^{-1} \cdot kPa^{-1} \cdot l^{-1}$)	1.79	2.44
VA (l)	4.15	1.58
PeMax (cmH_2O)	59–127	50
PiMax (cmH_2O)	29–117	40

deterioration. As disease affects the lung its impact on daily life may go unnoticed until there has been considerable loss of physiological capacity. Most people simply do not ordinarily stress the lungs to the extent of disclosure. Furthermore, patients with exercise limitation adopt a restricted lifestyle which may hide their disability. Sometimes simple questions can identify the disruption of normal activity. The more useful questions include inquiry about exercise tolerance in terms of walking distance on the flat before stopping for a rest, and ability to cope with hills and stairs. A more subtle approach is to ask whether patients can keep up with their spouse or continue a conversation while walking.

Human performance and quality of life are heavily influenced by mood and other psychological influences. An overall picture of disability can be judged by application of a detailed questionnaire designed to cover either general features of disability or those which relate to specific examples. There are disease-specific questionnaires available for chronic lung disease. The Chronic Respiratory Disease Questionnaire (CRDQ) and St George's Questionnaire have been validated for patients with COPD and asthma, respectively (Guyatt et al 1987, Jones 1991). These questionnaires are quite good at distinguishing change after an intervention but not so good at comparisons between patients or absolute assessment. This is particularly true of the CRDQ which uses individualized questions to obtain sensitivity. The Breathing Problems Questionnaire is another self-administered, disease-specific instrument which can provide a good comparative description of disability (Hyland et al 1994).

Laboratory estimation of exercise capacity

Observation of the physiological response to exercise in the laboratory is the gold standard measurement of disability. This is usually performed during a progressive maximal test which is completed when the subject is unable to continue. Sometimes, more detailed information about endurance or the pathophysiology can be obtained from a steady-state performance at a fixed workload. The vehicle for exercise is usually a treadmill or a cycle ergometer. The latter provides a stable platform and more accurate assessment of workload, while the walking action on the treadmill will be more familiar to most patients. The choice of platform is often determined by local circumstances but some care must be taken in the comparison. In health a greater $\dot{V}O_2$ is achieved on the treadmill, but this is not necessarily the case in severe COPD where the cycle may be a greater exercise stimulus. Under these circumstances the context should be taken into account and retest comparisons made on the same platform (Mathur et al 1995).

While the exercise is progressing the basic physiological response is observed by measuring ventilation, heart rate and oxygen uptake and carbon dioxide production. Other measurements such as oxygen saturation or cardiac output can be made if necessary. The test is conducted in such a fashion as to obtain a symptom-limited duration of about 10 minutes with the increments of workload increased every minute by about 50 watts (W) for healthy subjects (10 W or less for patients with COPD). During this period the heart rate will rise linearly with workload. Ventilation also rises linearly until about 60% of maximum workload when it increases disproportionately. Oxygen uptake ($\dot{V}O_2$) will also rise linearly until the same point above which the rate of uptake slows and eventually reaches a plateau at the maximum oxygen uptake ($\dot{V}O_2$max) (Fig. 3.9). The $\dot{V}O_2$max is determined in health by the cardiovascular delivery of oxygen to the muscles and is a crude estimate of capacity and cardiopulmonary fitness. The point of inflection of pulmonary ventilation on the $\dot{V}_E$ versus $\dot{V}O_2$ slope, is known as the anaerobic threshold. It is usually measured by the gas exchange method ($\dot{V}O_2$ v $\dot{V}CO_2$ plot). The concept of anaerobic threshold is in dispute but is thought to identify the spare potential capacity that could be improved by physical training. It can also help to distinguish cardiac from lung disease. In unfit people the $\dot{V}O_2$max can be improved with training, but this soon reaches a ceiling and further fitness is achieved by im-

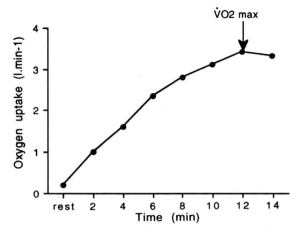

Fig. 3.9 The relationship between work and oxygen uptake during progressive exercise.

provement of anaerobic threshold or endurance capacity (Astrand & Rodahl 1986).

In patients with lung disease the limits to maximal exercise may be different. For example, maximal performance may be limited by low muscle mass, ventilation, respiratory muscle impairment and gas exchange. For this reason patients with COPD do not demonstrate a true $\dot{V}O_2$max because performance is terminated prematurely by the ventilatory limit imposed by airway obstruction. Fatigue from limb muscle weakness may also be a significant factor in these patients.

The value of exercise testing in lung disease lies in the measurement of the degree of functional impairment by assessment of the maximal workload and $\dot{V}O_2$max in comparison with reference values. If a patient fails to achieve his predicted performance the mode of failure can help to identify the mechanism. For example, in patients with lung disease the early rise of $\dot{V}_E$ may be characteristically in excess of expected but reach a premature limit imposed by the physical constraints of damaged lungs. Concurrently the heart rate response may be attenuated, in contrast to patients with cardiac disease where the test may have to be terminated because of early attainment of maximum predicted heart rate or chest pain. It is always important to determine why the subject stops at the end of a test. This is best achieved by the visual presentation of a scale of breathlessness or fatigue at regular intervals. In health, maximum performance is limited by oxygen uptake or motivation, while in lung disease the limit may be ventilatory and in cardiac disease it may be due to inadequate cardiac output. Usually these mechanisms can be distinguished, although it must be remembered that patients with cardiac or pulmonary disease become inactive and unfit.

The value of exercise testing:

- Differential diagnosis of dyspnoea
- Objective assessment of disability
- Assessment of therapeutic intervention
- Identification of exercise-induced asthma.

Field exercise tests

Laboratory tests of performance are the most accurate but are not always available and require expensive equipment. As an alternative, several field tests have been developed which can measure performance, and the results of such tests relate quite well to laboratory estimates. Such tests are popular with physiotherapists, athletic coaches and the military since they can be applied easily to large numbers of subjects and do not need dedicated equipment or training. There are two main categories of field test – those which are unpaced and those where the speed of activity is imposed.

One of the first unpaced tests was the 12-minute running test which was developed to assess the fitness of military personnel. This concept was adapted to the needs of the respiratory patient by downgrading the activity to a walk along a hospital corridor. Later, a reduction of the time to 6 minutes appeared to have no disadvantages. The 12- and 6-minute walks have become familiar forms of assessment for respiratory patients (McGavin et al 1976, Butland et al 1982). The test procedure is extremely simple, with a course marked out along the corridor and the patient given the simple instruction to cover as much ground as possible in the time permitted. These tests have proven value but

also have some limitations. There is quite a large learning effect and the reproducibility only becomes acceptable after two or more attempts (Mungall & Hainsworth 1979, Knox et al 1988). In addition, no two patients will attack the test in the same way and the relative stresses may not allow direct comparison. Lastly, the lack of pace constraint makes the test performance vulnerable to mood and encouragement. Nevertheless, these simple tests require no equipment and, within their limitations, provide valuable information about general exercise capacity and major therapeutic changes.

The second type of field exercise test imposes a pace on the patient which reduces the effect of motivation and encouragement. An endurance walking test instructs the patient to walk at a constant fast pace for an unlimited distance and measures the time and distance travelled. Another form of constrained exercise is the step test where the subject steps up and down a couple of steps in time to a metronome signal. Inability to continue, signals the end of the test and could be due to fatigue or breathlessness. This test has the capacity for incremental progression by increasing the pacing rate, but is a rather unnatural form of exercise.

An attempt to combine the comprehensive nature of incremental laboratory tests and the flexibility of the 6-minute walk has been made in the shuttle walk test. This is an adaptation of the 20 m shuttle running test where a subject runs between two cones 20 m apart with the pace determined by a series of audio signals (Léger & Lambert 1982). At intervals the pace increases until the subject can continue no longer. For patients with lung disease the shuttle distance is reduced to 10 m and the pace increments altered to provide a comfortable start and reasonable range (Fig. 3.10) (Singh et al 1992). Under these circumstances the test provides a similar physiological stimulus and can be combined with measurements of heart rate and breathlessness to obtain almost as much information as provided by the laboratory standard. These functional walking tests are very useful in the context of pulmonary rehabilitation where mass laboratory testing is impractical; they pro-

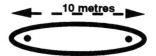

Level	Shuttles /level	Speed (mph)
1	3	1.12
2	4	1.50
3	5	1.88
4	6	2.26
5	7	2.64
6	8	3.02
7	9	3.40
8	10	3.78
9	11	4.16
10	12	4.54
11	13	4.92
12	14	5.30

a

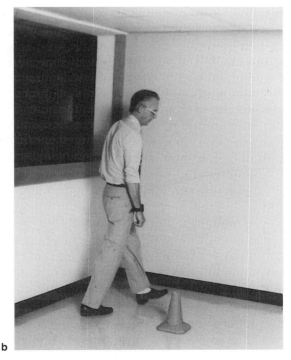

b

Fig. 3.10 **a** The shuttle walk test involves the perambulation of an oval 10 m course. The walking speeds are increased every minute and thereby increase the number of shuttles per level. **b** The subject turns around the cone in the shuttle walk in time with an audio signal. This subject is wearing a heart rate telemeter on his wrist.

vide a baseline measure of disability and have been shown to be sensitive to change (Lacasse et al 1996).

CARDIAC FUNCTION

In many respects the heart is a more simple organ than the lung and much of its function is accessible to measurement. It is, however, a less forgiving organ and minor abnormalities of coronary artery or cardiac muscle function may have dramatic effects. The major components of the heart include the myocardial muscle pump, the electrical conduction pathways, the internal valvular system and the coronary vasculature which supplies the muscle. Apart from congenital defects in the structure of the heart, disease can affect any of these components. Like the lung, the heart has a relatively limited symptomatic response to injury, and disease will present as chest pain, breathlessness, disturbance of heart rhythm or overt peripheral oedema. Cardiac failure occurs when the heart is unable to supply the expected demand of cardiac output. This may occur naturally at extremes of vigorous exercise when the cardiovascular delivery of oxygen cannot be maintained. When cardiac function cannot be maintained on moderate exercise or at rest then cardiac failure is present.

Although the two sides of the heart must be in overall balance, the pattern of failure will depend on the site of pathology. Left ventricular failure occurs when that ventricle cannot empty effectively and the resulting pulmonary venous hypertension may lead to pulmonary oedema. By contrast, the relative failure of the right ventricle leads to engorgement of the systemic venous system, resulting in peripheral oedema, ascites and elevated neck veins. The combination of left and right ventricular disorder is known as 'biventricular' or 'congestive' cardiac failure. Investigation of cardiac function includes examination of its structural, electrical and haemodynamic aspects. As for the lung, these features can be examined at rest or during exercise in order to uncover cardiac reserve.

MANCHESTER ROYAL INFIRMARY
SCHOOL OF PHYSIOTHERAPY

Cardiac imaging

In recent years there have been advances in the technology available for the functional study of the heart. Apart from conventional radiology the heart is accessible to imaging by ultrasound, and by radionuclide and magnetic resonance techniques which complement each other. The simple chest radiograph can still provide valuable functional information about the presence of failure and is probably the most useful clinical tool for monitoring its progress (Fig. 3.11). Enlargement of the heart on a radiograph either represents increased muscle bulk or, more commonly, dilatation resulting from increased fibre length in failure. Pulmonary venous pooling will fill the upper lobe vessels as the first sign of trouble, followed by definition of the interlobular lymphatics which become visible as Kerley B lines. If the pulmonary venous pressure rises above about 25 mmHg there is a risk of interstitial oedema. This is first visible as loss of definition of the hilum, but subsequently may produce widespread shadowing. If congestive failure is present the picture may be complicated by pleural effusions. The radiograph can therefore provide a useful picture of dysfunction.

Ultrasound examination of the heart has become an invaluable asset to cardiac investigation and has superseded many invasive techniques. Standard echocardiography provides a sound image of the structure of the heart, while Doppler echo is able to identify flow patterns and pressure gradients within the chambers. The conventional echocardiogram is performed in M mode ('Motion' mode) and two-dimensional imaging. The original M mode technique uses a narrow single beam of sound to image a portion of the heart. It remains valuable in the examination of mitral and aortic valve function where the rapid movements of the leaflets can be scanned. Indirect estimates of function can be obtained by measurement of valve closure rates and patterns. In a significant proportion of patients, particularly those with coexistent lung disease, it is impossible to obtain a satisfactory picture. Two-dimensional or cross-sectional echocardiography uses a fan array of

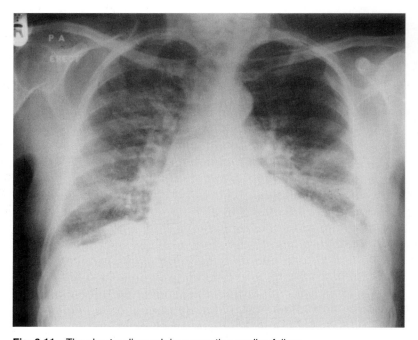

Fig. 3.11   The chest radiograph in congestive cardiac failure.

transducers to obtain a cross-sectional image of the heart. This provides much clearer pictures of the relationships between the heart's structures. It can also use the dimensional changes through the cardiac cycle to calculate the ejection fraction and estimate the cardiac output. Such measurements are not extremely accurate because they are based on stable geometric assumptions, but they can be useful. It may be difficult to guarantee images in some patients, but the recent development of transoesophageal probes has improved the scope of cross-sectional imaging. Doppler echocardiography has added a new dimension to functional imaging. The Doppler principle uses the flow of blood through the heart to calculate its velocity. It is able to detect turbulent flow and use its presence to estimate the pressure gradient across the valves. Sometimes it is also possible to measure pulmonary artery pressure. As confidence is growing with this technique the requirement for direct invasive measurement of cardiac function is less common.

Imaging of the heart and its circulation by using nuclear isotopes is also a well-developed technique. Two main techniques are in regular use. Injection of thallium-201 into the bloodstream leads to rapid distribution of the isotope through the tissues in proportion to the local blood flow. The coronary circulation is no different and the isotope is distributed within the heart. If the isotope is injected during exercise, areas of underperfusion relating to coronary artery disease are highlighted. This technique is more sensitive than exercise cardiography, but cannot be specific about the site of arterial disease. Another use of nuclear isotopes in the assessment of cardiac function involves the labelling of the red blood cell with technetium-99m. The radioactivity contained within the circulation allows examination of passage through the heart and calculation of the ejection fractions of both ventricles. The images are obtained with a conventional gamma camera, but the timing of the capture is determined by gating to the electrocardiogram (ECG). This technique is called a 'MUGA scan' (multigated acquisition scan) and is one of the most accurate, non-

invasive methods of measuring ejection fraction. An alternative radionuclide method of obtaining ejection fraction depends on a more complex capture of first pass isotope, but this is not widely used.

Magnetic resonance imaging (MRI) is a developing field which holds promise for the functional exploration of the heart. The images of the heart and great blood vessels are often striking in their clarity. The magnetic properties of oxygen in blood promise the possibility of detailed, non-invasive measurement of function. At present the technique is still held back from its potential by the necessity for long scan times and ECG gating, but advances in this field are rapid.

The electrical function of the heart

The electrocardiogram (ECG) is the most established of the modern cardiological investigations. In fact, it has become so familiar that it could be considered as an extension of the clinical examination. The ECG can provide information about the function of the intracardiac conducting tissue and reflects the presence of cardiac disease through its electrical properties. Some conditions produce characteristic patterns of ECG abnormality. Examples include myocardial infarction and ischaemia, pericarditis and pulmonary embolism. In diseases which affect the conducting tissue the arrhythmias that they produce can be identified. The presence of heart failure cannot be determined from the ECG alone. However, inferences can be made from the presence of large complexes due to ventricular hypertrophy or very small complexes in pericardial effusion.

The standard ECG is not always helpful in patients with palpitations, particularly if it does not capture the arrhythmia. In these circumstances the provision of 24- or 48-hour recording may be helpful. If the problem is likely to occur with even less frequency, the ECG can be recorded at home during an event and 'phoned in'.

The exercise ECG has developed an importance of its own in the assessment of ischaemic heart disease. In this investigation the ECG is recorded during a progressive exercise test. This is usually a treadmill test, but cycle and step tests have been used. In the UK the most popular treadmill protocol is the Bruce (p. 394) variety where both the speed and the gradient of the treadmill are increased every 3 minutes. Other protocols such as the Balke or Naughton (Jones 1988) are just as acceptable for producing the stimulus. There is a difference here in the protocols compared with those used for the study of metabolic gas exchange in lung disease. Cardiac protocols are deliberately provocative whereas maximal performance is best coaxed from the subject with a more gentle increment towards the end of the test. The indications for exercise electrocardiography include the investigation of angina and post-myocardial infarction assessment as well as the postoperative examination of bypass surgery. The most common abnormalities associated with ischaemic heart disease on exercise are ST segment changes. False positive changes are quite common, but the exercise ECG has become quite a sensitive guide to the presence of ischaemic heart disease and a good predictor of prognosis after myocardial infarction.

Haemodynamic function

Access to the chambers and blood vessels of the heart is available through cardiac catheterization. This technique was originally developed as a research tool to examine the physiology of the circulation by measuring intracardiac pressures. The passage of catheters into the heart is now commonplace in cardiological investigation and on intensive care units. Its value no longer lies solely in the measurement of function but it can also provide a vehicle for therapeutic intervention in the form of balloon valvuloplasty or angioplasty.

The assessment of function during cardiac catheterization employs the measurement of pressure, the injection of contrast media or the sampling of blood. These objectives are achieved by insertion of the catheter into the left or right heart via a femoral or brachial blood vessel.

A right heart catheter is passed into the right ventricle from a peripheral vein and can be guided further into the pulmonary artery. The left ventricle is accessible from the femoral artery by crossing the aortic valve. Both coronary arteries are also entered by this route. The pressure in the left atrium may be difficult to obtain directly unless there is a perforation in the atrial septum. An approximation to the left atrial pressure can be obtained by wedging the right heart catheter in a small pulmonary artery. A special flow-directed catheter, the Swan–Ganz catheter, with a balloon attached to the tip has been developed to facilitate the passage into the pulmonary circulation.

Knowledge of the pressures within the heart is useful to assess the need for surgery in patients with valvular disease. The demonstration of a significant gradient across the mitral or aortic valve will confirm the clinical or ultrasound impression. The pulmonary artery wedge pressure (PAWP) is a guide to the left atrial pressure and can predict the likelihood of pulmonary oedema or guide complex fluid replacement in intensive care units or operating theatres.

Injection of radiological contrast can either outline the coronary blood vessels (angiogram) or the cavity of the ventricle. The former is the standard assessment in ischaemic heart disease, while the latter is the most informative method for describing the motion of the heart and for calculating the ejection fraction. In general, angiography is more descriptive of the structure rather than the function of the heart.

The estimation of cardiac output can be made non-invasively by a variety of, sometimes inventive, methods. However, to be of value the estimate should be accurate and is obtained by catheterization. The classical method is called the 'Fick principle' where the result is computed from the total oxygen uptake and the arteriovenous oxygen difference. Although this method is accurate it is unacceptably invasive. The most popular method now uses a modified pulmonary artery catheter to measure output by thermodilution. In this case a known bolus of cold saline is injected into the superior vena cava and the temperature drop is recorded in the pulmonary artery. The cardiac output is calculated by using a bedside computer. Knowledge of the cardiac output and its changes can be a very powerful clinical tool. It is especially useful in the management of very sick patients where the manipulation of cardiac output by combination of inotrope drugs and vasodilators can ensure optimal oxygen delivery for the tissues. Another example of its value is the exploration of cardiac reserve of output during exercise or electrical pacing or pharmacological stimulation.

REFERENCES

American Thoracic Society 1986 Evaluation of impairment/disability secondary to respiratory disorders. American Review of Respiratory Disease 133: 1205–1209

American Thoracic Society 1996 Lung volume reduction surgery. American Journal of Respiratory and Critical Care Medicine 154: 1151–1152

Anthonisen N R 1986 Tests of mechanical function. In: Fishman A P (ed) Handbook of respiratory physiology, the respiratory system III. American Physiological Society, Bethesda

Astrand P-O, Rodahl K 1986 Textbook of work physiology, 3rd edn. McGraw-Hill, New York, pp 753–784

Benson M K 1983 Diseases of the airways. In: Weatherall D J, Ledingham J G G, Warrel D A (eds) Oxford textbook of medicine. Oxford University Press, Oxford, vol 2, pp 15.60–15.70

Black L F, Hyatt R E 1971 Maximal static respiratory pressures in generalised neuromuscular disease. American Review of Respiratory Disease 103: 641–650

British Thoracic Society/Association of Respiratory Technologists and Physiologists 1994 Guidelines for the measurement of respiratory function. Respiratory Medicine 88: 165–194

Butland R J A, Pang J, Gross E R et al 1982 Two-, six-, and 12-minute walking tests in respiratory disease. British Medical Journal 284: 1607–1608

Cooper J D, Trulock E P, Triantafillou A N et al 1995 Bilateral pneumectomy (volume reduction) for chronic obstructive pulmonary diseases. Journal of Thoracic and Cardiovascular Surgery 109: 106–119

Cotes J E 1993 Lung function: assessment and application in medicine, 5th edn. Blackwell Scientific, Oxford

European Community for Coal and Steel 1983 Standardized lung function testing. Bulletin Européen de Physiopathologie Respiratoire 19(suppl 5): 1–95

Gibson G J 1995 Respiratory function tests. In: Brewis R A L, Corrin B, Geddes D M, Gibson G J (eds) Respiratory medicine, 2nd edn. W B Saunders, London, pp 229–243

Green M, Laroche C M 1990 Respiratory muscle weakness. In: Brewis R A L, Corrin B, Geddes D M, Gibson G J (eds) Respiratory medicine. W B Saunders, London, pp 1373–1387

Guyatt G H, Berman L B, Townsend M et al 1987 A measure of the quality of life for clinical trials in chronic lung disease. Thorax 42: 773–778

Hyland M E, Bott J, Singh S J, Kenyon C A P 1994 Domains, constructs and the development of the breathing problems questionnaire. Quality of Life Research 3: 245–256

Jenkins S C, Soutar S A, Moxham J 1988 The effects of posture on lung volumes in normal subjects and in patients pre- and post-coronary artery surgery.

Physiotherapy 74: 492–496

Jones N L 1988 Clinical exercise testing, 3rd edn. W B Saunders, Philadelphia

Jones P W 1991 Quality of life measurement for patients with disease of the airway. Thorax 46: 676–682

Kaneko K M, Milic-Emili J, Dolovich M B et al 1966 Regional distribution of ventilation and perfusion as a function of body position. Journal of Applied Physiology 21: 767–777

Knox A J, Morrison J F J, Muers M F 1988 Reproducibility of walking test results in chronic obstructive airways disease. Thorax 43: 388–392

Lacasse Y, Wong E, Guyatt G H et al 1996 Meta-analysis of respiratory rehabilitation in chronic obstructive pulmonary disease. Lancet 348: 1115–1119

Léger L A, Lambert J 1982 A multi-stage 20-m shuttle run test to predict VO_2 max. European Journal of Applied Physiology 49: 1–12

McGavin C R, Gupta S P, McHardy G J R 1976 Twelve-minute walking test for assessing disability in chronic bronchitis. British Medical Journal 1: 822–823

Martyn J B, Moreno R H, Pare P D, Pardy R L 1987 Measurement of inspiratory muscle performance with incremental threshold loading. American Review of Respiratory Disease 135: 919–923

Mathur R S, Revill S M, Vara D D et al 1995 Comparison of peak oxygen consumption during cycle and treadmill exercise in severe chronic airflow obstruction. Thorax 50: 829–833

Mungall I P F, Hainsworth R 1979 Assessment of respiratory function in patients with chronic obstructive airways disease. Thorax 34: 254–258

Olsen G N 1992 Pre-operative physiology and lung resection. Chest 101: 300–301

Polgar G, Promadhat V 1971 Pulmonary function testing in children: techniques and standards. W B Saunders, Philadelphia

Shneerson J 1988 Disorders of ventilation. Blackwell Scientific, Oxford, pp 78–85

Singh S J, Morgan M D L, Scott S et al 1992 The development of the shuttle walking test of disability in patients with chronic airways obstruction. Thorax 47: 1019–1024

Tremper K K, Barker S J 1989 Pulse oximetry. Anesthesiology 70: 98–108

Uldry C, Fitting J W 1995 Maximal values of sniff nasal inspiratory pressure in healthy subjects. Thorax 50: 371–375

Wedzicha J A 1996 Domiciliary ventilation in chronic obstructive pulmonary disease: where are we? Thorax 51: 455–457

Zibrak D J, O'Donnell C R, Marton K 1990 Indications for pulmonary function testing. Annals of Internal Medicine 112: 763–771

FURTHER READING

American College of Sports Medicine 1991 Guidelines for exercise testing and prescription, 4th edn. Lea & Febiger, Philadelphia

British Thoracic Society / Association of Respiratory Technologists and Physiologists 1994 Guidelines for the measurement of respiratory function. Respiratory Medicine 88: 165–194

Cotes J E 1993 Lung function: assessment and application in medicine, 5th edn. Blackwell Scientific, Oxford

Gibson G J 1996 Clinical tests of respiratory function, 2nd edn. Chapman & Hall, London

Jones N L 1988 Clinical exercise testing, 3rd edn. W B Saunders, Philadelphia

Hampton J R 1992 ECG made easy, 4th edn. Churchill Livingstone, Edinburgh

Muller W F, Scacci R, Gast L R 1987 Laboratory evaluation of pulmonary function. J B Lippincott, Philadelphia

Nunn J F 1987 Applied respiratory physiology, 3rd edn. Butterworths, London

West J B 1990 Respiratory physiology, 4th edn. Williams & Wilkins, Baltimore

West J B 1992 Pulmonary pathophysiology, 4th edn. Williams & Wilkins, Baltimore

4

Monitoring and interpreting medical investigations

John S. Turner

MONITORING

Introduction

There has been an explosion of computer and video technology in recent years, and patient monitoring has benefited from this in no small way. The ability to detect and rapidly react to changes in physiology is now possible, and it is this that has become the essence of modern intensive care.

The ideal monitoring system is not yet a reality (although several major manufacturers would deny this), but it is coming closer all the time. This system would need to be accurate, precise, and reliable. It would be sensitive to small changes in the parameters it monitors, yet able to distinguish and eliminate artefacts. It would preferably be non-invasive for the sake of safety. It would function on a real-time rather than an intermittent basis. It would have a memory for previous data and would be able to show trends. Its memory module would be moveable to allow it to capture data in the ward, in transport, and in another environment such as an operating theatre. It would also almost certainly be extremely expensive!

Conventional observations

Back to reality. Nursing observations have for many years included the taking of the patient's temperature, pulse, respiratory rate, and blood pressure. These are performed manually and carefully charted at intervals varying from quarter-hourly to 6-hourly to daily, being performed more frequently in high-care areas. These practices are quite adequate for general ward situations where patients are not critically ill, and are even useful in intensive care units (ICUs), both for making physical contact with the patient and for checking the invasively monitored observations.

The major limitation of intermittently performed observations is that they may only establish the presence of an abnormality some time after it has developed. Thus the ability to react immediately to the development of an abnormality is lost. More frequently performed observations are obviously superior in this regard, but real-time continuous monitoring is the ultimate goal of monitoring.

Non-invasive monitoring

Non-invasive monitoring of a variety of parameters is now routinely practised in many areas, especially ICUs and operating theatres. Commonly monitored parameters include temperature, heart rate, blood pressure and oxygen saturation. Respiratory rate may be measured by some monitoring systems, and in certain circumstances end-tidal CO_2 and transcutaneous PO_2 and PCO_2 monitoring may be performed. These may all be displayed on a single monitor screen. Technical problems and artefacts can occur with the display of any of these parameters, so the patient's clinical status must be checked before acting on a monitor display abnormality.

Temperature

Temperature is continuously monitored by means of an oesophageal or rectal probe. This determines core temperature, which is usually at least 1°C higher than axillary temperature and may be more in shock. Problems are rarely encountered with this method. The oesophageal temperature may be lower if the gases for respiratory support are unwarmed and the rectal probe may occasionally fall out without being noticed, leading to an erroneously low temperature being

displayed. A rectum full of faeces may also lead to a lower temperature being recorded.

Heart rate

Heart rate is measured from the electrocardiogram (ECG) trace. Artefacts are common. Interference (usually from patient movement or a warming blanket) may confuse the monitor into showing the presence of a tachycardia or arrhythmia, while small complexes may be interpreted as asystole. Physiotherapy may also cause movement artefacts. On the ECG trace, large T waves (and occasionally P waves or a pacemaker spike) may be interpreted as QRS complexes, leading to the displayed heart rate being double the actual rate. Detached or dried-out electrodes will lead to asystole being displayed. Sinus tachycardia, sinus bradycardia, and atrial fibrillation are described below.

Respiratory rate

Respiratory rate may be measured by making use of the changing impedance across the chest wall as it moves with respiration. In systems which offer this parameter, the sensors are built into the ECG leads. The heart rate and other movements of the chest can cause overreading of respiratory rate, while electrodes placed too far apart may not give a reading at all.

Appropriate physiotherapy treatment (e.g. for lobar lung collapse) may reduce a rapid respiratory rate, but it must be emphasized that an already tachypnoeic patient should not be allowed to become exhausted during treatment as he may rapidly decompensate. This may even necessitate emergency intubation. Close contact with the medical and nursing staff should therefore be maintained in such cases.

Blood pressure

Blood pressure is monitored with a pressure cuff around the upper arm. An oscillometric method is used to measure blood pressure, with automatic cuff inflation and deflation. The accuracy of such systems is generally good, but the cuff needs to be applied correctly and be of the appropriate size for the arm. The system also needs to be calibrated correctly against a mercury column. Non-invasive blood pressure monitoring is performed intermittently, but the interval between readings may be as short as 1 minute.

Physiotherapy treatment may cause a patient to become hypertensive, especially if the treatment causes pain or anxiety. The hypotensive patient may occasionally become more unstable, and here the risks and benefits of treatment need to be carefully balanced.

Oxygen saturation

Oxygen saturation (Clark et al 1992) is continuously measured by a pulse oximeter with a probe on a finger or ear lobe. There are two methods: the functional method which measures the difference between oxyhaemoglobin and deoxyhaemoglobin, and the fractional method which measures all types of haemoglobin over a wide spectrum of light absorption. The former method may record erroneously high saturations if there is a high concentration of carboxyhaemoglobin (the combination of carbon monoxide and haemoglobin) in the blood, while the latter method will be inaccurate if a light-emitting diode (LED) or ultraviolet light (including sunlight) is close to the probe. Saturations are generally accurate between 100% and 80%, but may be inaccurate at lower levels. The saturation trace must be observed to correspond with the heart rate; if this is not so the reading may be erroneous. Low saturations with either method may be due to poor peripheral perfusion, painted or nicotine-stained fingernails, pierced ears, intravenous contrast medium, or injected dyes.

Hypoxaemia has been shown to occur both during and after chest physiotherapy (Tyler 1982); awareness and careful monitoring are therefore important. A patient on a ventilator and on high inspired oxygen concentrations or positive end-expiratory pressure may become dangerously hypoxaemic during tracheal suctioning. Strategies to limit this risk include preoxygenation and use of a sealed suction port (as used for fibreoptic bronchoscopy).

End-tidal CO_2

End-tidal CO_2 (ETCO$_2$) may be measured on an intubated patient. The method works by the principle of absorption of infrared light. A probe from the monitor is inserted into the ventilator circuit close to the end of the endotracheal tube. ETCO$_2$ correlates well with PCO_2 in normal lungs, but less well in diseased lungs (Clark et al 1992). It is used widely in anaesthesia and for the ventilation of head-injured patients, but its use in other contexts is less well defined.

In paediatric (especially neonatal) patients, transcutaneous PO_2 and PCO_2 measurements are practised in many centres. The transcutaneous electrode is fixed to the skin which it heats and makes permeable to gas transport. Local hyperaemia arterializes the capillary blood. Good correlation between transcutaneous and arterial measurements has been shown. However, transcutaneous measurements have been shown to be sensitive but not specific indicators of blood gas status as they may be influenced not only by the partial pressure of the gas but also by a reduction in cardiac output or local blood flow. They have not gained acceptance in adult critical care practice.

Invasive monitoring

This requires the use of an invasive catheter, which is inserted into an artery, a central vein, the pulmonary artery or, in some neurosurgical centres, the extradural space (for intracranial pressure (ICP) monitoring). The catheter is connected to a transducer which is in turn connected to a pressure monitor (Fig. 4.1). The monitor displays pressure wave-forms and values on a real-time basis (Fig. 4.2). We have become accustomed to seeing these displays (often in a variety of bright colours), and usually blindly accept that each component of the system is working correctly and accurately; this is unhappily not always the case and we may be lulled into a false and dangerous sense of security. Inaccuracies may (and commonly do) occur from any one (or a combination) of the following:

- The catheter may be incorrectly positioned.

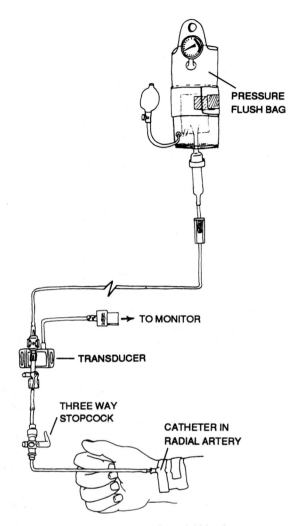

Fig. 4.1 Invasive monitoring of arterial blood pressure.

- The catheter may be partially blocked or kinked.
- The connecting tubing may be partially blocked or kinked, or it may allow too much resonance in the system leading to exaggerated pressure wave forms (under-damping).
- The transducer may be faulty or incompatible with the other equipment.
- The monitor may be incorrectly calibrated.
- The pressure bag (which pressurizes the system for flushing and to prevent backflow) may not be properly inflated.

All these aspects of invasive pressure monitoring need to be checked regularly, especially if the readings do not correlate with the clinical appearance of the patient. In many cases, potentially harmful treatment has been instituted on the basis of totally incorrect information.

Common invasively monitored parameters include arterial blood pressure and central venous pressure (CVP). *Arterial cannulation* allows continuous monitoring of blood pressure as well as easy access for blood gas analysis. The radial artery on the non-dominant side is the most common site of insertion; other sites include brachial, dorsalis pedis, and femoral arteries. The femoral artery is especially useful in states of shock, when peripheral pulses may be impalpable. The catheter is usually inserted percutaneously, but may be introduced by surgical cut-down. Complications of arterial cannulation are uncommon and include infection and, rarely, thrombosis. Disconnection of the catheter from the line can easily occur with movement of the patient; vigorous bleeding will follow and exsanguination is a real risk. These lines should always therefore remain visible and care should be taken when moving the patient. Should disconnection occur, reconnection should be quickly performed; should displacement occur, firm pressure should be applied to the bleeding site.

CVP measurement involves placement of a catheter into a central vein (generally the superior vena cava), usually via the subclavian or internal jugular vein. The basilic, external jugular, and femoral veins may also be used for access; the advantage of these sites is that there is no risk of pneumothorax and that bleeding is easier to control. Disadvantages of these routes include difficulty with accurate placement and a higher incidence of thrombosis. The CVP represents the state of filling of the vasculature and heart, more specifically the right side of the heart. If correctly interpreted, it can yield valuable diagnostic information and guide fluid therapy. The complications associated with all central venous catheters are not insubstantial: they include vascular erosion, air embolism, bleeding, thrombosis, and infection. Again, dis-

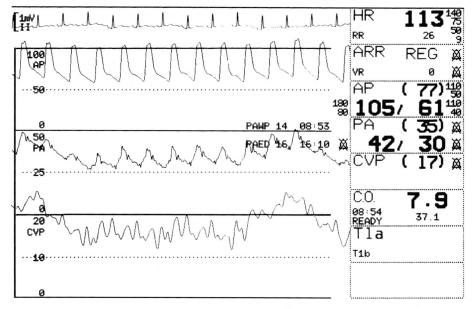

Fig. 4.2 Display of pressure wave forms and ECG trace on monitor screen: HR, heart rate; ARR, arrhythmia monitoring; REG, regular; AP, arterial pressure; PA, pulmonary artery pressure; CVP, central venous pressure; CO, cardiac output.

connection can occur with movement. Bleeding will occur if the end of the catheter is below the level of the heart, while air may be sucked into the system and air embolism may result if the end of the catheter is above that level. Air embolism is a very serious event and can result in immediate collapse and death.

With a *pulmonary artery catheter*, pulmonary capillary wedge pressure (PCWP) may be monitored and cardiac output (CO) may be measured by means of the thermodilution technique. Systemic vascular resistance (SVR), pulmonary vascular resistance (PVR), oxygen delivery, and oxygen consumption may also be calculated.

The pulmonary artery catheter is inserted via a central vein through the right side of the heart into the pulmonary artery. At its tip it has a balloon which is inflated when the catheter is in the heart and this allows the catheter to be carried through the heart chambers by the flow of blood (Fig. 4.3). When the inflated balloon occludes the pulmonary artery, the catheter no longer measures pulmonary artery pressure but PCWP. By a series of extrapolations, left atrial

pressure and, therefore, left ventricular preload can be gauged (Fig. 4.4). This gives valuable information over and above CVP measurement when the left and right sides of the heart are not functioning equally. The left heart alone may fail in anterior myocardial infarction and the right heart alone may fail in pulmonary embolism, cor pulmonale, pericardial constriction, and right ventricular infarction. In all these settings, measurement of CVP alone may give totally misleading information about left ventricular filling. The interpretation of the PCWP is not always straightforward and has many pitfalls for the unwary (Raper & Sibbald 1986).

Measurement of cardiac output is an integral part of pulmonary artery catheterization. The resultant calculations of SVR, oxygen delivery, and oxygen consumption give an enormous amount of information about the state of the heart and circulation. Manipulation of these variables by vasoactive drugs is useful in a variety of disease states, including sepsis, pulmonary oedema, adult respiratory distress syndrome, and cardiogenic shock.

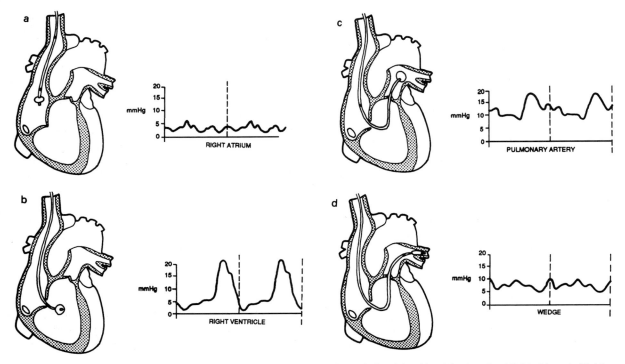

Fig. 4.3 Pressure traces as the pulmonary artery catheter passes through the right side of the heart. **a** Right atrium. **b** Right ventricle. **c** Pulmonary artery. **d** Pulmonary capillary wedge pressure.

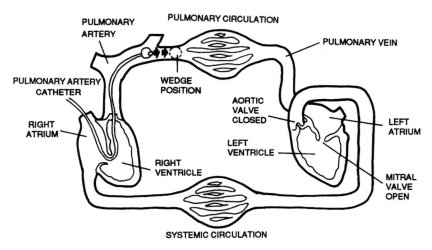

Fig. 4.4 In diastole, with the mitral valve open, pulmonary capillary wedge pressure corresponds to left atrial pressure.

Left atrial pressure may be measured directly by means of a catheter inserted into the left atrium at the time of cardiac surgery. The catheter is brought out through the chest wall and monitoring takes place in the conventional way. All the above mentioned complications may occur; in addition, displacement may occasionally result in pericardial tamponade.

Intracranial pressure monitoring may be performed in patients with head injuries, brain surgery, intracranial and subarachnoid haemorrhage, and cerebral oedema from other causes. However, the frequency of use of this technique depends on the enthusiasm of individual units. Such monitoring may give an indication of a rise in ICP before it becomes clinically evident, thus allowing therapeutic manoeuvres (hyperventilation, mannitol, surgery) to be initiated before cerebral damage occurs. The importance of ICP measurement is that it provides an estimate of cerebral perfusion pressure (cerebral perfusion pressure = mean arterial pressure – ICP) which

in turn relates to cerebral blood flow (CBF). Raised ICP causes reduced CBF which leads to tissue hypoxia and acidosis, raised PCO_2, cerebral vasodilatation, and oedema, all of which cause a further rise in ICP.

ICP may be measured by means of an extradural or subarachnoid bolt, an intraventricular catheter (inserted through the skull into the lateral ventricle), or an epidural catheter. The former methods are the most widely used (Fig. 4.5). The intraventricular catheter has the additional advantage of being able to drain cerebrospinal fluid, thereby relieving raised ICP. All these methods are invasive and the potential complications are not insignificant, the most serious being infection.

ECG monitoring

It is beyond the scope of this chapter to cover arrhythmia recognition and management, but the more common arrhythmias are discussed and

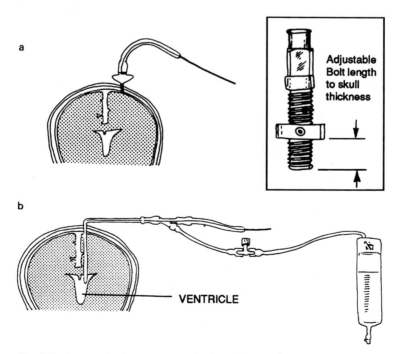

Fig. 4.5 Intracerebral pressure monitoring. **a** Extradural or subarachnoid bolt. **b** Intraventricular catheter with cerebrospinal fluid drainage bag.

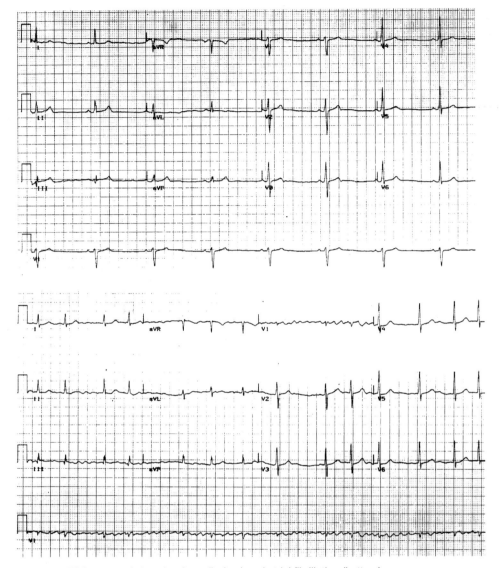

Fig. 4.6 ECG traces of sinus bradycardia (top) and atrial fibrillation (bottom).

examples of ECG traces given (Fig. 4.6). Physiotherapy procedures may both cause arrhythmias (Hammon et al 1992) and may worsen those already present. Great awareness and care is needed, especially in those patients at risk of developing arrhythmias.

1. *Sinus bradycardia* is a sinus rhythm below 60 beats/min. The common causes are drugs (e.g. beta blockers) and hypoxaemia; bradycardia may be a warning sign that the latter is occurring and, as such, should be taken very seriously. Vagal stimuli from tracheal suctioning may also be implicated. Care with suctioning and generous preoxygenation may be necessary; occasionally it is reassuring to have atropine drawn up and ready to inject.

2. *Sinus tachycardia* is a sinus rhythm above

100 beats/min. Pain and anxiety are common causes, but occasionally it may be precipitated by haemodynamic instability or respiratory distress. Procedures should be carefully explained to the patient, and adequate analgesia should be given before physiotherapy begins.

3. *Atrial fibrillation* is a common arrhythmia in critically ill patients. It is a totally irregular rhythm that may reach a ventricular rate of up to 200 beats/min and cause haemodynamic instability. It may be paroxysmal. The cause is usually multifactorial, but common precipitating factors include hypokalaemia, hypoxaemia, dehydration or overhydration, ischaemic heart disease, and cardiac surgery.

Patients at risk of developing arrhythmias often have ischaemic heart disease or a history of arrhythmias. However, critically ill patients may suddenly develop a rhythm disturbance, the cause of which is usually multifactorial. A patient may have recently had an arrhythmia (often of short duration) so it is vital to check the charts and to communicate with the doctors and nurses looking after the patient.

The present state of development is that most good monitoring systems today have memory capacity and can display past values on a minute-to-minute basis. Trends can be graphically displayed and analysed. A printer link may allow ECG or pressure traces to be printed and retained. Already in use in some centres are systems that utilize a specialized software package which enables the rapid recording, storage, display and reporting of a wide range of clinical data. Data are either downloaded directly from the patient monitors or entered manually. Hard copies of relevant data are produced using a printer. This system totally replaces nursing charts and is an extremely attractive option in terms of labour saving, accuracy, convenience and immediacy.

INTERPRETING MEDICAL INVESTIGATIONS

A number of blood and microbiological tests are regularly performed on patients in hospital, leading to an enormous amount of data which need to be responsibly interpreted (even when it is sometimes irresponsibly requested!). It is clearly vital to know the normal values for these tests, which abnormalities are important and which are not, and how to respond to any abnormalities which need treatment. The more commonly performed haematological, biochemical, and microbiological tests are discussed with these issues in mind. Normal values depend on the test technique, the units in which the result is given, and the local reference values.

Haematology

Full blood count

This is usually performed in an automated blood analyser which produces a printout of results. Included in most analysers are the following (the abbreviations given are commonly used).

Haemoglobin (Hb). Haemoglobin is the red oxygen-carrying pigment in red blood cells (RBCs). Its primary function is the transport of oxygen. Hb is easy to measure (it can be measured in the ward with a Spencer haemoglobinometer) and is an indirect measure of the number of RBCs in the circulation and, therefore, of the total red cell mass. In states of dehydration or overhydration Hb may be falsely raised or lowered.

A reduced red cell mass is referred to as 'anaemia', while an increased red cell mass is known as 'polycythaemia' or 'erythrocytosis'. There are many causes of anaemia, but those most commonly seen are acute or chronic blood loss, iron deficiency, and chronic illness or inflammation. Polycythaemia may be primary (from a disorder of the bone marrow) or secondary (owing to chronic hypoxaemic lung disease or cyanotic heart disease, renal carcinoma, cerebellar haemangioblastoma, or uterine fibroids).

Mean corpuscular volume (MCV). This is a measure of the size of the RBCs. A low MCV (small RBCs) is referred to as 'microcytosis': the most common cause is iron deficiency. A high MCV is referred to as 'macrocytosis', and is most often caused by vitamin B_{12} or folate deficiency. The MCV is useful in narrowing down the differential diagnosis of anaemia and other blood disorders.

Mean corpuscular haemoglobin (MCH). This is calculated by dividing the Hb by the total red cell count. It reflects the amount of Hb in the RBCs.

White cell count (WCC). The white blood cells, or leukocytes, perform a variety of functions in the body. Their major role is to defend the body against infection, and their interaction in achieving this goal is remarkable. The neutrophils (the predominant type of leukocyte) perform the immediate response to infection by phagocytosing offending organisms. Lymphocytes are involved in the production of antibodies, and play a pivotal role in both cell-mediated and humoral immunity. The monocyte–macrophage cell line is also involved in immunity, primarily by processing antigens and presenting them to immunocompetent lymphocytes. They also have an important phagocytosing and scavenging function, and incidentally play a role in the regulation of haematopoiesis.

The functions of eosinophils and basophils are poorly understood, but eosinophils seem to be important in the defence against parasitic infections and in allergic disorders.

Platelet count (Plt). Platelets circulate in the bloodstream as tiny discs less than half the size of RBCs and are an essential component in blood clotting. They are part of the first-line reaction to a breach in the vascular endothelium. A reduction in the platelet count is known as 'thrombocytopenia' while an increase is called 'thrombocytosis'. There are many causes for thrombocytopenia, but the common ones seen in critically ill patients include sepsis, disseminated intravascular coagulopathy (see below), drug-related causes, and consumption by dialysis machines or other extracorporeal circuits.

Differential count

This looks primarily at the white cells in the blood, but at the same time the morphology of the red blood cells and the platelets may be commented upon. A drop of blood is smeared smoothly across a glass slide; this is then stained and examined under a microscope. The different cells are counted in a high power field and the numbers are given as a percentage. Absolute numbers of cells will thus depend upon the total white cell count. The differential count may be useful in diagnosis of specific infections or infiltrations, allergic or parasitic disorders, and assessing immune status.

Clotting profile

This is generally performed in a patient who is either bleeding or is at high risk of developing a bleeding problem. Indices measured include prothrombin time, partial thromboplastin time (PTT), platelets, fibrinogen, and fibrin degradation products (FDPs). There is a wide variety of bleeding disorders with an even wider variety of causes; patients may be at risk for spontaneous haemorrhage or haemorrhage caused by minor trauma (and this may include physiotherapy procedures).

Prothrombin time and partial thromboplastin time measure the integrity of different limbs of the clotting cascade. The prothrombin time is now usually given as the ratio of measured time over control time, with international standardization of the reagents used: it is thus referred to as the 'international normalized ratio' (INR).

In acutely ill patients, there are two commonly found disorders of coagulation. Firstly, a dilutional coagulopathy may occur from massive blood transfusions without the addition of clotting factors. The INR and PTT are prolonged, and platelets and fibrinogen are reduced. Secondly, disseminated intravascular coagulopathy (DIC) may be caused by a wide variety of precipitating events, including sepsis, trauma, and incompatible blood transfusions (Bick 1988). Clotting factors are consumed by inappropriate intravascular coagulation, and there is thus a deficiency of them which leads to bleeding. Again INR and PTT are prolonged, platelets and fibrinogen are low (they may be extremely low), and FDPs are present in large amounts, representing the fibrinolysis (clot breakdown) that is taking place intravascularly.

Patients with a DIC or thrombocytopenia

(especially when the platelet count is less than 20) may be at risk of pulmonary haemorrhage. Great care should be taken during suctioning and physiotherapy, and the potential benefits should be weighed against this risk.

Biochemistry

Arterial blood gases

These not only give an indication of oxygenation and carbon dioxide clearance, but also of acid–base status. Most automated blood gas machines measure only pH, PO_2 and PCO_2, and extrapolate from these values the bicarbonate and oxygen saturation. These extrapolations are accurate under most circumstances, but oxygen saturation may be fallacious in the presence of carboxyhaemoglobin. Hypoxaemia (PaO_2 of less than 8 kPa or 60 mmHg at sea level) and hypercarbia ($PaCO_2$ of more than 6 kPa or 45 mmHg) are easy to recognize and their causes are not discussed here. The metabolic and respiratory causes of acidosis and alkalosis are a little more complex and may cause confusion.

In simple terms, in acidosis the pH is always low (normal pH is 7.36–7.44) and in alkalosis the pH is always high (remember that pH is an inverse and logarithmic expression of hydrogen ion concentration). Metabolic causes of acidosis and alkalosis involve a primary change of the bicarbonate concentration, and respiratory causes involve a change of $PaCO_2$. The different disorders are discussed further below, a systematic approach to blood gases follows, and some rather simplistic examples are given in Table 4.1.

Metabolic acidosis. This is probably the most serious acid–base disorder. It may be caused by either an excess of acid (lactate, ketoacids, metabolites, or poisons) or a loss of bicarbonate by the small intestine or the kidneys. Lactate accumulates in states of inadequate oxygen delivery to the tissues; this is usually seen in shock of any cause. Ketoacids accumulate in diabetic ketoacidosis which is always associated with a raised blood glucose. Both lactate and ketoacids may be measured in the laboratory. In renal failure, tubular dysfunction reduces bicarbonate generation; in addition, there are unmeasured acidic anions in the blood, and glomerular dysfunction leads to a reduction in the amount of sodium available for exchange with hydrogen ions. Poisons or drugs in overdose may be acidic, e.g. ethylene glycol and aspirin.

Compensation for the acidosis occurs by hyperventilation with a resultant fall in $PaCO_2$. This accounts for the deep sighing respiration (Kussmaul breathing) often seen in metabolic acidosis.

Treatment of metabolic acidosis is controversial. For many years bicarbonate was the mainstay of treatment, but evidence is now accumulating that its effects are mainly cosmetic and may be harmful (Cooper et al 1990). These include shifting the oxygen dissociation curve thereby inhibiting the release of oxygen, causing hypernatraemia and hyperosmolarity, and provoking an intracellular acidosis (Ritter et al 1990). It would seem that treatment of the cause of the acidosis should be the primary objective.

Respiratory acidosis. The primary problem is a raised $PaCO_2$. This is the result of alveolar

Table 4.1 Examples of acid–base disturbances and the compensatory mechanisms

Disorder	pH	$PaCO_2$	Bicarbonate	Compensation
Metabolic acidosis	7.2	5	18	CO_2
Compensation	7.4	3	18	
Respiratory acidosis	7.2	8	26	Bicarbonate
Compensation	7.4	8	36	
Metabolic alkalosis	7.5	5	34	CO_2
Compensation	7.4	7	34	
Respiratory alkalosis	7.5	3	26	Bicarbonate
Compensation	7.4	3	20	

hypoventilation, the cause of which may be inadequate minute volume (as in a weak or tired patient) or increased dead space (as in severe chronic obstructive airways disease). Often these occur in combination. Compensation occurs by an increase in plasma bicarbonate; this is done mainly by the kidneys, which increase bicarbonate reabsorption in the tubules.

The plasma bicarbonate level may be useful in differentiating acute from chronic respiratory acidosis. In the acute state bicarbonate is normal, while in the chronic state it is raised owing to the aforementioned compensatory mechanisms. This distinction may have important clinical consequences, for example in differentiating severe asthma from chronic lung disease.

Metabolic alkalosis. This may be caused by an excess of bicarbonate (always iatrogenic) or a loss of acid (either from the stomach or the kidneys). Acid may be lost from the stomach in cases of upper gastrointestinal tract obstruction or ileus; litres of fluid may be lost daily. The most common cause of acid loss by the kidneys is hypokalaemia. Here there is an inadequate amount of potassium ions available for exchange with sodium ions; hydrogen ions are sacrificed in their place.

Respiratory alkalosis. Here the primary problem is a low $PaCO_2$, which is always a result of hyperventilation. This may occur in a spontaneously breathing person who is anxious, in pain, or has a respiratory disorder (causes include asthma, pneumonia, pulmonary embolus, and adult respiratory distress syndrome). Rarely, neurological disorders (affecting the respiratory centre) will cause hyperventilation. It may also be seen in a mechanically ventilated patient who is being given too large a minute volume or who is tachypnoeic for any of the reasons mentioned above.

A systematic approach to blood gases follows. First look at the PaO_2. Determine whether it is normal or whether the patient is hypoxaemic. The PaO_2 is essentially independent of the other variables. Next look at the pH. Establish acidosis, alkalosis, or normal. If abnormal, check if the problem relates to the $PaCO_2$ or the bicarbonate. It is sometimes said to be confusing as to which

of these is the problem and which is the compensatory effect. It really is very easy. The one that correlates with the pH (i.e. acidosis, low bicarbonate) has to be the cause; the other is therefore the compensation (see examples in Table 4.1).

Electrolytes

Sodium and potassium are often measured as part of an automated biochemistry run, although many ICUs will have a separate electrolyte analyser that works on the principle of ion-selective electrodes. These analysers may be more accurate for potassium measurements than for sodium. Their advantage is obviously their immediacy.

Hyponatraemia has a variety of causes, but is more commonly caused by relative excess of water than deficiency of sodium. This is often iatrogenic, following excessive administration of hypotonic fluids. Another common cause is the syndrome of inappropriate antidiuretic hormone (ADH) secretion, in which ADH is secreted despite hypotonicity of the serum. The result is water retention and, thereby, hyponatraemia. The causes of this syndrome are numerous and include malignancies, pulmonary disorders, and disturbances of central nervous system function. The treatment of hyponatraemia has been well described (Swales 1991).

Hypernatraemia is most often caused by water depletion. A true sodium excess is uncommon and is always iatrogenic. Both hyponatraemia and hypernatraemia may cause neurological signs ranging from confusion to coma.

Hypokalaemia, on the other hand, is potentially far more dangerous. It may predispose to cardiac arrhythmias, especially if combined with hypoxaemia. Hyperkalaemia may predispose to ventricular tachycardia and fibrillation. Physiotherapy treatment may have to be postponed until these abnormalities have been corrected.

Glucose

This needs to be regularly monitored in diabetics and in all critically ill patients. Blood glucose can easily be measured in the ward by means of reagent strips. A very high blood glucose level is almost always caused by diabetes mellitus or an intravenous infusion of high glucose content, while a slightly raised value may be caused by stress. The causes of a low blood glucose include starvation, liver failure (failure to produce glucose), insulin therapy, or an insulin-secreting tumour.

Renal function tests

These include urea and creatinine. Urea is formed mainly from protein breakdown and creatinine mainly from muscle breakdown; there are obligatory amounts of both of these that need to be handled by the kidneys daily. If formation increases or excretion decreases, serum levels will rise. Renal failure causes both urea and creatinine to rise, though often at different rates. In hypovolaemic or low cardiac output states, urea rises more than creatinine, whilst in rhabdomyolysis (breakdown of skeletal muscle) creatinine rises faster than urea.

Liver function tests

Very few so-called 'liver function tests' actually measure liver function. Instead they simply represent the result of liver damage: raised enzymes reflect damage to cells and raised bilirubin may reflect a variety of abnormalities, not all of which actually occur in the liver.

Enzymes such as lactate dehydrogenase (LDH) and aspartate aminotransferase (AST) are not specific to liver tissue, and even when they are produced by damaged liver cells give little clue to the underlying pathology. Gamma glutamyl transferase (GGT) and alanine aminotransferase (ALT) are found in few other tissues, but again do not reflect causation. Alkaline phosphatase (ALP) is also not specific to liver cells, but that fraction which comes from the liver is concentrated in bile ducts and, as such, gives a clue to biliary disease or obstruction.

Bilirubin is a pigment that is produced from the breakdown of haem (from the haemoglobin in red blood cells). The liver takes up circulating bilirubin, conjugates it and excretes it in bile via the biliary tract. The clinical manifestation of a raised plasma bilirubin level is jaundice. In most hepatic disorders, both the conjugated and unconjugated fractions of bilirubin are raised. However, a predominantly unconjugated hyperbilirubinaemia (raised levels of unconjugated bilirubin in the blood) is often due to massive breakdown of red blood cells as in haemolysis or haematoma. Conjugated hyperbilirubinaemia is commonly seen in hepatitis or biliary tract obstruction; in the latter the classical clinical triad of dark urine, pale stools, and pruritus is seen.

In critical illness, two distinct syndromes of liver dysfunction have been described (Hawker 1991). These are ischaemic hepatitis, occurring early and characterized by a massive rise in AST and ALT with only a slight rise in bilirubin, and ICU jaundice, which develops later, is part of the syndrome of multiple organ failure, and is characterized by a progressive rise in bilirubin with only a slight enzyme rise.

Tests that reflect the synthetic capacity of the liver are more useful in determining actual liver function. Protein synthesis is one of the major functions of the liver; these proteins include clotting factors, albumin, and globulins. Thus, measuring the INR (see above) and serum albumin can give a good idea of the synthetic function of the liver, provided there are no other reasons for these tests to be abnormal.

Cardiac enzymes

Enzymes are released by all damaged muscle cells. Cardiac enzyme estimations are therefore performed to confirm myocardial damage, usually caused by a myocardial infarct but occasionally caused by chest trauma. There is a characteristic pattern of enzyme rise, with creatine kinase (CK) rising first, followed by AST and then LDH. For more specificity, isoenzymes (specific fractions of the enzymes) of CK and LDH may be measured. CK is also present in skeletal muscle, so the myocardial fraction (MB fraction) is measured to exclude skeletal muscle damage (from surgery, trauma, or intramuscular injections) as a source. LDH is present in many other tissues, including skeletal muscle, red blood cells, liver, and lung. The LD1 and LD2 fractions are specific for cardiac muscle or red blood cells (the distinction is easily made clinically).

Electrical cardioversion has been said to cause CK (and specifically the MB fraction) to rise. This may be important in determining whether a patient has had a myocardial infarct. The evidence is that measurable myocardial damage rarely follows cardioversion, and that when CK MB is raised, the elevation is small (Ehsani et al 1976).

Microbiology

Introduction

Infection control is becoming more and more important as more nasty and often antibiotic-resistant organisms are seen in hospitals, especially in ICUs. The importance of hand-washing between going from one patient to another cannot be overemphasized. This is the simplest and still the most effective method of preventing cross-infection. Organisms such as methicillin-resistant *Staphylococcus aureus* (MRSA) and more recently vancomycin-resistant enterococcus (VRE) are becoming major problems in hospitals and have even caused closure of specialized units. In ICUs, Gram-negative organisms such as pseudomonas and acinetobacter have become particular problems, becoming impossible to eradicate.

Blood cultures

These are usually taken when the patient is pyrexial, in an attempt to isolate microorganisms which may be present in the bloodstream. The blood is drawn (usually from a forearm vein) in strictly aseptic conditions, placed in a special culture medium, incubated at 37°C, and then cultured in the laboratory. A positive result is almost always of serious consequence, although contaminants may occur, usually from poor aseptic technique. A positive blood culture does not identify the site of sepsis, although the type of organism cultured may give a clue. The source of the sepsis needs to be found and dealt with in its own right.

Sputum/tracheal aspirate

Sputum is produced when a non-intubated patient coughs up pulmonary secretions, while a tracheal aspirate is a suctioned specimen from an endotracheal tube or tracheostomy. There is always a risk that a sputum specimen may contain mainly saliva, and that it may be contaminated by oral organisms. Tracheal aspirates, on the other hand, represent the microflora of the lower airways, and are much less likely to be contaminated, although after prolonged mechanical ventilation the tracheobronchial tree is often colonized by oral organisms. Physiotherapists are often requested to obtain these specimens, upon which future treatment may be based, and great care should be taken to get adequate and representative samples.

Newer methods of obtaining uncontaminated specimens which accurately reflect the microbiology of a specific lung segment include protected specimen brushing with quantitative colony counts and bronchoalveolar lavage (Chastre et al 1995).

A sputum or tracheal aspirate specimen is stained with Gram's stain, examined under a microscope, and cultured. Antibiotic sensitivities are performed on a positive culture. One must be aware that the presence of organisms on tracheal aspirate may not be indicative of pulmonary infection, but may simply represent colonization. To make the diagnosis of pulmonary infection (and, therefore, to start antibiotics) one needs to have most of the following criteria: purulent secretions, white blood cells on Gram's stain of tracheal aspirate, organisms on culture of tracheal aspirate, fever, raised white blood cell count, infiltrates on the chest radiograph, and a reduction in PaO_2.

Community-acquired pneumonia has been well studied in many countries and the organisms accounting for most cases have been established. *Streptococcus pneumoniae* is the commonest organism by far, followed by *Myco-plasma pneumoniae* (in epidemics) and influenza virus. The logical antibiotic management of community-acquired pneumonia has been described (American Thoracic Society 1993).

Diagnosis of pneumonia in a patient already on a ventilator is often much more difficult, although some of the newer diagnostic methods mentioned above are useful (Meduri 1995). Clinical judgement may still be necessary to differentiate colonization from infection.

Swabs and specimens from other sites

These may be taken from superficial wounds or from deep sites. Positive superficial cultures may represent skin colonization, so it is important to look for local (redness, pus) and systemic (pyrexia, raised white blood cell count) evidence of sepsis before starting antibiotic therapy. Local therapy with frequent cleaning and dressings is usually all that is required for superficial sepsis. Specimens obtained from needle aspiration or during operative procedures (i.e. from the abdominal cavity or chest) are not likely to represent colonization, and such infections cannot be treated topically – surgical drainage and antibiotic therapy are needed.

Urine

Urine specimens may be contaminated with perineal flora, so they are either taken by a midstream urine collection with strict attention to aseptic technique or from a urinary catheter. The urine is spun down in a centrifuge, and then stained, examined, and cultured in the same way as sputum. Although patients with long-term indwelling urinary catheters may develop bacterial bladder colonization with no clinical consequence, in other patients urinary tract infections may be a considerable source of morbidity.

REFERENCES

American Thoracic Society 1993 Guidelines for the initial management of adults with community-acquired pneumonia: diagnosis, assessment of severity, and initial antimicrobial therapy. American Review of Respiratory Disease 148: 1418–1426

Bick R L 1988 Disseminated intravascular coagulation and related syndromes: a clinical review. Seminars in Thrombosis and Haemostasis 14: 299–338

Chastre J, Fagon J Y, Bornet-Lesco M et al 1995 Evaluation of bronchoscopic techniques for the diagnosis of nosocomial pneumonia. American Journal of Respiratory and Critical Care Medicine 152: 231–240

Clark J S, Votteri B, Ariagno R L et al 1992 State of the art. Noninvasive assessment of blood gases. American Review of Respiratory Disease 145: 220–232

Cooper D J, Walley K R, Wiggs B R, Russell J A 1990 Bicarbonate does not improve haemodynamics in critically ill patients who have lactic acidosis. Annals of Internal Medicine 112: 492–498

Ehsani A, Ewy G A, Sobel B E 1976 Effects of electrical countershock on serum creatine phosphokinase (CPK) isoenzyme activity. American Journal of Cardiology 37: 12–18

Hammon W E, Connors A F, McCaffree 1992 Cardiac arrhythmias during postural drainage and chest percussion of critically ill patients. Chest 102: 1836–1841

Hawker F 1991 Liver dysfunction in critical illness. Anaesthesia and Intensive Care 19: 165–181

Meduri G U 1995 Diagnosis and differential diagnosis of ventilator-associated pneumonia. Clinics in Chest Medicine 16: 61–94

Raper R, Sibbald W J 1986 Misled by the wedge? The Swan–Ganz catheter and left ventricular preload. Chest 89: 427–434

Ritter J M, Doktor H S, Benjamin N 1990 Paradoxical effect of bicarbonate on cytoplasmic pH. Lancet 335: 1243–1246

Swales J D 1991 Management of hyponatraemia. British Journal of Anaesthesia 67: 146–153

Tyler M L 1982 Complications of positioning and chest physiotherapy. Respiratory Care 27: 458–466

FURTHER READING

Hampton J R 1986 The ECG in practice. Churchill Livingstone, Edinburgh

Lee G R et al 1993 Wintrobe's clinical haematology, 9th edn. Lea & Febiger, Philadelphia

Mandell G L 1995 Mandell, Douglas and Bennett's Principles and practice of infectious diseases. Churchill Livingstone, New York

Sherlock S, Dooley J 1993 Diseases of the liver and biliary system, 9th edn. Blackwell Scientific, Oxford

Zilva J F, Pannall P R, Mayne P D 1988 Clinical chemistry in diagnosis and treatment, 5th edn. Edward Arnold, London

5

Mechanical support

John S. Turner

INTRODUCTION

Medical technology has advanced in quantum leaps over the last 40–50 years and efficient mechanical support of lungs, heart and kidneys is now available. The gastrointestinal tract may be supported by means of total parenteral nutrition and the haemopoietic system by cell transfusion and colony-stimulating factors (such as granulocyte–macrophage colony-stimulating factor). There is as yet no effective form of hepatic support, although liver transplantation is being performed in the acute setting as is heart and lung transplantation. The indications for these dramatic and heroic measures are, however, limited.

This chapter covers respiratory, cardiac, and renal support, with most of the emphasis being placed on respiratory support including newer forms of ventilation and weaning.

RESPIRATORY SUPPORT

Respiratory failure is usually defined as the inability to maintain a PaO_2 of more than 8 kPa (60 mmHg) or a $PaCO_2$ of less than 6 kPa (45 mmHg). The causes are numerous and some of the more common ones are listed below in the section on indications for mechanical ventilation. Respiratory support aims to correct these biochemical abnormalities. This can be performed in a number of ways.

Oxygen therapy

Oxygen is delivered by means of face mask or nasal cannulae. Oxygen therapy will correct the majority of less severe cases of hypoxia, but obviously cannot correct hypercarbia.

Continuous positive airway pressure

In the technique of continuous positive airway pressure (CPAP), oxygen is delivered by a system that maintains a positive pressure in the circuitry and airways throughout inspiration and expiration. CPAP is useful in cases where lung volumes are reduced, in particular the functional residual capacity (Fig. 5.1). Examples of this include subsegmental lung collapse, pneumonia, and adult respiratory distress syndrome. Again hypercarbia cannot be corrected and may be worsened as dead-space ventilation may be increased. CPAP usually improves ventilation–perfusion ($\dot{V}/\dot{Q}$) mismatch and, by improving lung compliance, it may reduce the work of breathing.

There are two basic methods of providing CPAP: continuous-flow or demand-flow. Continuous-flow systems have gas flowing through the circuit throughout the respiratory cycle. A high gas flow (50–100 l/min) is necessary to maintain this flow during the initial phase of inspiration. There is no demand valve to open, but the system is noisy and uses large volumes

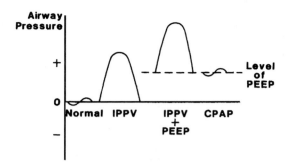

Fig. 5.2 Pressure–time curves of various modes of ventilation.

of oxygen and air. On the other hand, demand-flow systems (including the CPAP mode on ventilators) allow gas to flow only when inspiration is initiated and a demand valve is thereby opened. This is a quieter system and uses less gas, but a certain amount of work is required of the patient in order to open the demand valve. Some systems are worse than others in this regard (Bersten et al 1989), although a modification of the demand-flow system known as 'flow-by' seems to present the patient with little additional work. This system is becoming more widely available. When CPAP is combined with positive pressure ventilation, it is generally known as 'positive end-expiratory pressure' (PEEP) (Fig. 5.2).

Conventional mechanical ventilation

Mechanical ventilation has evolved from negative pressure ventilators used in the polio epidemic of the 1950s. Positive pressure ventilators that followed are now controlled by sophisticated microprocessor technology. The physiology, principles and practice of mechanical ventilation have been reviewed in detail (Hubmayr et al 1990, Schuster 1990).

The basic principles of how a ventilator works remain unchanged. Very simply, *inspiration* may be generated by application of either a constant pressure or a constant flow of gas to the lungs, and *expiration* may be allowed when either a set pressure has been reached, a set volume has been delivered, or a set time has passed. Modern

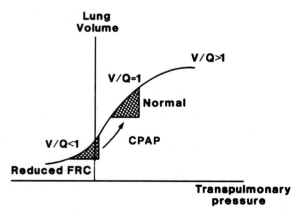

Fig. 5.1 Continuous positive airway pressure (CPAP) increases a reduced functional residual capacity (FRC).

ventilators have a variety of ventilation modes which allow for comfortable patient–ventilator interaction. Ventilation modes commonly employed and available on most modern ventilators include the following:

1. *Controlled mandatory ventilation (CMV)* – here the patient has no control over ventilation. Breaths are delivered at a rate and volume that are determined by adjusting the ventilator controls, regardless of the patient's attempts to breathe. If the patient is not unconscious or paralysed, CMV may be extremely uncomfortable.

2. *Intermittent mandatory ventilation (IMV)* – here respiratory rate and tidal volume are set as above, but the patient may breathe spontaneously between the mandatory breaths, which still are delivered at the preset regular intervals.

3. *Synchronized intermittent mandatory ventilation (SIMV)* – the mandatory breaths are delivered in synchrony with the patient's breathing. Again the patient may breathe on his own, but the mandatory breaths will be delivered at a time in the ventilatory cycle that is convenient for the patient (a breath will therefore not be delivered while the patient is breathing out). Patient comfort is improved.

4. *Inspiratory pressure support (IPS)* – this is a relatively new ventilatory technique, introduced in 1981. Its use and application have not yet been fully evaluated, and remain controversial (Kacmarek 1989). It is a pressure-limited form of ventilation, with each breath being triggered by the patient. Once a breath is triggered, a flow of gas enters the circuit, with the pressure rapidly reaching the preset level. This pressure is maintained until the flow decreases to a ventilator-specific level, at which time expiration is allowed. The patient has full control over the respiratory rate. IPS can deliver the same level of ventilation (as assessed by gas exchange) as SIMV, often with lower peak airway pressures, as long as the patient has an adequate respiratory drive. Alone or in combination with SIMV, it can make ventilation more comfortable for the patient. Theoretically, by allowing some degree of muscle training without permitting fatigue, IPS would be helpful in weaning patients from

mechanical ventilation. To date, clinical trials addressing this issue have shown conflicting results.

5. *Inverse ratio ventilation* – this is ventilation where the inspiratory phase is longer than the expiratory phase. It may be volume or pressure regulated, the latter (pressure-controlled inverse ratio ventilation or PCIRV) being the most widely used. The technique has been well described (Tharratt et al 1988) but there are no clinical trials comparing it with other forms of ventilation. It is now widely used but requires expertise and careful monitoring of haemodynamic and respiratory parameters.

Non-invasive ventilation

Non-invasive ventilation (ventilation without an endotracheal tube or tracheostomy) can be delivered by negative or positive pressure techniques. Negative pressure ventilation is epitomized in the large and frightening 'iron lung', used in the 1950s for the ventilation of patients with poliomyelitis. Newer and much more compact and comfortable negative pressure ventilators are now available (Shneerson 1991), and domiciliary ventilation with them is feasible. A review by Branthwaite (1991) covers the practical aspects of this form of ventilation. Non-invasive ventilation is considered further in Chapter 6.

Indications for mechanical ventilation

The indications for ventilation vary for different disorders and are rarely absolute. In practical (and somewhat simplistic) terms they include the following:

Adult respiratory distress syndrome. A patient who has a PaO_2 of less than 8 kPa (60 mmHg) on oxygen and CPAP.

Pneumonia. A patient who is unable to clear secretions or who has a PaO_2 of less than 8 kPa (60 mmHg) on oxygen and CPAP.

Asthma. A patient who is becoming exhausted or confused, usually with a rising $PaCO_2$.

Chronic obstructive airways disease. Similar to asthma, but a higher $PaCO_2$ may be normal for the patient. Non-invasive ventilation may be an option in these patients (Elliott et al 1990) in selected circumstances and with the necessary expertise.

Respiratory muscle weakness. A patient who is unable to clear secretions, who has lost bulbar function, or who cannot produce a vital capacity of more than 15 ml/kg.

Blunt chest trauma. A patient who, despite adequate analgesia, cannot produce a vital capacity of more than 15 ml/kg, or is unable to clear secretions, or who has a PaO_2 of less than 8 kPa (60 mmHg) on oxygen and CPAP.

Pulmonary oedema. This is largely a clinical decision, as pulmonary oedema tends to improve very quickly with appropriate medical treatment. Patients who are moribund or not responding to treatment will need ventilation, as will patients who have had a large myocardial infarct.

Other system involvement. Patients may be ventilated simply to support the respiratory system when they have a life-threatening disorder of another system, e.g. multiple trauma or septic shock.

Elective postoperative ventilation. Some patients may be electively ventilated postoperatively, either because of the magnitude of the surgery or because they have impaired pulmonary function.

Aims and complications of respiratory support

The first and most important aim of respiratory support is to oxygenate the patient. This is initially done by increasing the inspired oxygen concentration. Oxygen concentrations of above 50% are toxic to the lungs if used for any length of time, with toxicity increasing exponentially as the concentration rises further. Positive end-expiratory pressure (PEEP) may be added to improve oxygenation. Once levels of PEEP above 10 cmH_2O are used, a pulmonary artery catheter may be needed to measure oxygen delivery. PEEP may depress cardiac output more than it improves oxygenation, and oxygen delivery may therefore be compromised. Increasing the inspiratory time to allow for higher mean airway

pressures but lower peak inspiratory pressure (PIP) may improve oxygenation. Sedation and occasionally muscle relaxants may be necessary to ventilate a critically ill patient.

Barotrauma, which is related to PIP, needs to be avoided. There is no pressure which is absolutely safe, but barotrauma occurs with significant frequency once the PIP exceeds 50 cmH_2O, and increases exponentially as pressures rise above this level. Manoeuvres to lower PIP include reducing the tidal volume, reducing PEEP, and allowing a longer inspiratory time (even to inverse ratio ventilation).

The importance of carbon dioxide removal has decreased recently. Patients with severe respiratory failure have been ventilated in a way that allows the $PaCO_2$ to rise to up to 8 kPa (60 mmHg) or more (Hickling et al 1990). This concept of 'permissive hypercapnia' has been used in a variety of situations and generally allows a smaller tidal volume and minute volume to be used, reducing the incidence of barotrauma and oxygen toxicity.

Patient comfort and acceptability can be achieved by carefully matching patient and ventilator. Tidal volume, rate, and inspiratory time can be manipulated to make the patient comfortable. This is an art, and demands patience and understanding. Occasionally, sedation is needed, but this should be a last resort.

Respiratory support is not without complications, some of which are minor and some of which may be lethal. The more commonly occurring complications include barotrauma, haemodynamic disturbances, nosocomial infections, alteration in gastrointestinal motility, and a positive fluid balance (Pingleton 1988).

Weaning from respiratory support

Criteria for weaning from mechanical ventilation were first described in the 1970s. They are adequate in most cases, but their relatively high failure rate has led investigators to look at other predictors of a successful wean. These include work of breathing (Fiastro et al 1988), and more recently the 'CROP index' and rapid shallow breathing index (Yang & Tobin 1991).

The latter is simple to perform and is by far the most practically useful of the above. It is calculated by allowing the patient to breathe room air through a spirometer for 1 minute while the respiratory rate is counted. The minute volume (measured on the spirometer) is divided by the respiratory rate to give an average tidal volume. The index is calculated by dividing the respiratory rate by the tidal volume (in litres). Weaning is unlikely with an index above 100, and likely with an index below 100.

Conventional weaning criteria involve clinical, mechanical, and biochemical parameters:

Clinical

- The clinical condition of the patient is improving.
- The patient is cooperative and alert and able to clear secretions.
- There is no abdominal distension, cardiovascular instability, or likelihood of prolonged immobility.
- The respiratory rate is less than 30 breaths/min.

Mechanical

- Vital capacity is more than 15 ml/kg.
- Maximal inspiratory mouth pressure is more than 20 cmH_2O.
- Minute volume is less than 10 l/min.

Biochemical

- Normal pH and $PaCO_2$.
- PaO_2 more than 8 kPa (60 mmHg) on no more than 40% oxygen and 5 cm PEEP.

Once the above criteria are satisfied, weaning may be started. Before and during the weaning period, meticulous attention needs to be paid to nutrition, electrolyte status, control of infection and bronchospasm, and mobilization of the patient. The last factor is probably the most important, and the physiotherapist will be very involved in sitting and then standing and walking the patient. Even patients with many lines, tubes, and catheters can be mobilized with

a little ingenuity. Weaning can be performed in two different ways. Either the proportion of breathing performed by the ventilator can be gradually reduced, letting the patient perform a greater and greater amount of breathing until he is independent of the ventilator (IMV was the first ventilatory mode to allow this), or the patient can be allowed to breathe spontaneously for progressively longer periods with full ventilation between them (the so-called 'T-piece method'). Both methods have their proponents, although there is probably little to choose between them. The latter method is commonly used in difficult weans.

Common problems which may cause difficulties with weaning (Branthwaite 1988) include the following:

- Impaired ventilatory drive
- Upper and lower airway incompetence, obstruction, or secretions
- Lung parenchymal fluid or infection
- Pleural effusion or pneumothorax
- Chest wall abnormality, instability, or respiratory muscle weakness
- Electrolyte or nutritional problems
- Cardiovascular insufficiency.

Unconventional respiratory support

Less conventional modes of respiratory support include extracorporeal membrane oxygenation (ECMO), extracorporeal carbon dioxide removal (ECCO$_2$R), intravenacaval oxygenation (IVOX) and high-frequency jet ventilation (HFJV). These modes are only available in major centres, are costly and extremely labour intensive, and have not yet been shown in controlled studies to hold any advantage over conventional ventilation (Evans & Keogh 1991). They have their enthusiasts, however, and in their hands the results are impressive.

Extracorporeal membrane oxygenation

This is a well-established and useful technique in neonatal respiratory distress syndrome, but has not shown advantages over conventional ventilation in controlled trials in adults. However, it may still be a useful technique for short periods, especially as a bridge to transplantation, an indication for which it has been used successfully. The technique involves a high-flow extracorporeal circuit from the inferior vena cava to the aorta using cannulae in the femoral vein and artery. A membrane oxygenator is used in the circuit to provide oxygenation and carbon dioxide removal. The extracorporeal blood flow is up to 80% of the cardiac output, and vital organs may be poorly perfused with non-pulsatile blood flow.

Extracorporeal carbon dioxide removal

An uncontrolled trial has shown startling results with the $ECCO_2R$ technique (Gattinoni et al 1986), with a survival rate of 47% in 55 patients with adult respiratory distress syndrome in whom the mortality was predicted to be more than 90%. A low flow venovenous circuit is used with a membrane oxygenator and the patient is ventilated at a slow rate with very small tidal volumes. Complications are less common than with ECMO. A controlled trial comparing $ECCO_2R$ with conventional ventilation has shown the newer mode to be no better (Morris et al 1994). Enthusiasts are still getting excellent results however.

Complications of extracorporeal gas exchange (ECMO and $ECCO_2R$) include haemorrhage, thrombosis and thromboembolism, sepsis, and multiple organ failure, although the latter complication may merely reflect the organ failure associated with the respiratory failure for which the technique is used.

Intravenacaval oxygenation

Intravenacaval oxygenation (IVOX) has been recently developed (Conrad et al 1993) and clinical trials have shown it to be a useful adjunctive therapy. A catheter with multiple fine tubes within it is placed in the inferior vena cava. Oxygen is passed through these at subatmospheric pressure and gas exchange takes place by passive diffusion.

High-frequency jet ventilation

In high-frequency jet ventilation (HFJV), small pulses of gas at a rate of 60–600 per minute are delivered from a jet nozzle at the proximal end of the endotracheal tube, with humidified warmed air being entrained from a bias gas source. Lung volume is maintained with a higher mean airway pressure, thereby improving oxygenation. There are several theories as to how gas exchange can occur with such an unphysiological method of ventilation. Diffusion of gas and regional convective currents seem to play a major role. Although a controlled clinical trial has shown no advantage over conventional ventilation (Carlon et al 1983), the technique has been shown to be safe, and newer computer-controlled prototypes are showing promise.

Nitric oxide administration

Administration of this gas via the ventilator was recently shown to reduce pulmonary artery pressures and improve arterial oxygenation in patients with severe respiratory failure (Rossaint et al 1993). It appears that ventilation–perfusion matching is improved without systemic vasodilatation. Data about outcome are not yet available but a number of clinical trials are currently being performed.

CARDIAC SUPPORT

Even before heart transplantation was pioneered in 1967, the need for an artificial heart had been identified. This could be used for short-term support of the heart while waiting for it to recover from an acute insult (such as myocardial infarction or cardiac surgery) or for a donor heart to become available for transplantation, or for long-term cardiac support. There are modalities available which provide partial to complete support, but they are expensive and may have significant side-effects.

Intra-aortic balloon pump

The intra-aortic balloon pump (IABP) comprises a sausage-shaped balloon (15 mm $\times$ 280 mm

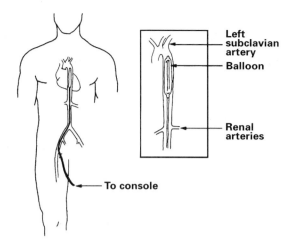

Fig. 5.3 Placement of the intra-aortic balloon pump.

and inflated by 40 ml of gas) mounted on a dual-lumen catheter. The balloon is introduced via the femoral artery, either percutaneously or by surgical dissection and direct vision, to the thoracic aorta (Fig. 5.3). Correct positioning of the catheter is confirmed by fluoroscopy or chest radiography. The catheter is attached to a console with a helium gas source for balloon inflation. The IABP is triggered by the electrocardiogram (ECG) to deflate during ventricular systole and to inflate during diastole. By so doing it improves cardiac performance (the left ventricle ejects into an 'empty' aorta) and improves myocardial perfusion (which occurs during diastole and is enhanced by the blood not running off into the aorta).

Indications for the use of the IABP include cardiogenic shock (after myocardial infarction), unstable angina, weaning from cardiopulmonary bypass, and stabilization of patients with acute mitral regurgitation or ventricular septal defect following myocardial infarction. In these cases it is used as a bridge to definitive surgery, although the mortality for these defects remains in the region of 50%. The IABP cannot generate a cardiac output independent of the heart, and a minimum cardiac output of about 1.5 l/min is needed for it to be effective.

The IABP is clearly a major invasive device, and complications may be serious. They include aortic dissection, arterial perforation, limb ischaemia, thrombocytopenia, and dislodgement of atherosclerotic emboli. Air embolism may occur if the balloon bursts. Major bleeding may occur following removal of the IABP.

Ventricular assist device

A ventricular assist device (VAD) is simply a pump that functions in parallel with the heart. Blood is withdrawn from the venous side of the circulation and returned to the arterial side, usually with a catheter in the left atrium and the left ventricle (left ventricular assist device or LVAD). Occasionally, both sides of the heart need support and this is achieved with a biventricular assist device (BIVAD). The VAD can provide most of the cardiac output, but the flow it delivers is not pulsatile, which may adversely affect vital organs such as the kidneys. Indications for its use include failure to wean from cardiopulmonary bypass (Adamson et al 1989) and bridging to heart transplantation (Hill 1989). It is not without significant complications, with haemorrhage, thromboembolism, and septicaemia being the most common.

RENAL SUPPORT

Before the advent of dialysis and transplantation, chronic renal failure (CRF) was invariably fatal and acute renal failure (ARF) usually fatal. Today, although ARF still carries a high mortality rate, especially when part of the complex of multiple organ failure, CRF can be effectively managed in dialysis and renal transplantation programmes.

The aims of renal support are very simple. They include control of fluid, electrolytes, and acid–base status, and elimination of uraemic toxins and drugs. These aims can be carried out in a number of ways which are detailed below.

General principles of dialysis

All forms of dialysis involve diffusion of solute across a semipermeable membrane and down a concentration gradient. In peritoneal dialysis the membrane is the peritoneum and the blood flow is provided by the capillaries supplying it. In all forms of haemodialysis, the membrane is composed of cellophane or cuprophane and blood flow is provided by an extracorporeal circuit.

Conventional haemodialysis

Haemodialysis (HD) was first described in 1960 and is now the most commonly used dialysis therapy for both ARF and CRF. Blood is pumped through an extracorporeal system which in-cludes a filter with a semipermeable membrane, and dialysate (usually water mixed with pre-determined concentrations of electrolytes and buffer) flows in a countercurrent direction through the filter, on the other side of the mem-brane. A gradient is thus created for electrolytes and metabolic waste products to diffuse across the membrane, and fluid is driven across by hydrostatic pressure.

Vascular access is obtained by intravenous catheters or by the surgical creation of arterio-venous fistulae or shunts. HD is generally performed for 4–6 hours at a time, either daily or on alternate days. Although HD allows rapid correction of fluid and electrolyte abnormalities, it may not be well tolerated in critically ill, haemodynamically unstable patients. Hypoten-sion may develop and cause further ischaemic insult to the kidney. Hypoxaemia almost in-variably occurs; it is caused by neutrophil aggre-gation in the lungs and complement activation in the filter membrane.

Continuous forms of renal support

Conventional haemodialysis is not well tolerated in critically ill patients as it may produce rapid changes in intravascular volume, blood pressure, PaO_2, and pH. Slower but continuous forms of haemodialysis were developed to address this problem. Outcome data are impressive when compared with historical controls (Bellomo & Boyce 1993). The terminology is confusing; terms such as CAVH, CAVHD, CVVH, and CVVHD (see below) perplex the uninitiated. The treat-ment choices differ in several ways (Schetz et al

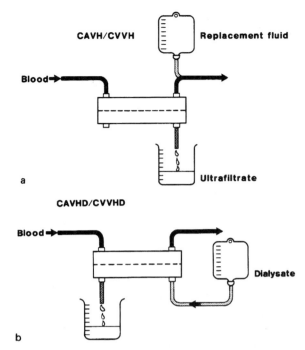

Fig. 5.4 Continuous renal support: the concepts of filtration and dialysis. **a** Haemofiltration alone. **b** Haemofiltration with dialysis.

1989). Access to the circulation may be by both arterial and venous cannulae (arteriovenous) or by venous cannulae (venovenous). The blood flow through the circuit may be pumped by an external pump or by the patient's own arterial pressure as in arteriovenous systems. Pure haemofiltration may be performed, or may be combined with dialysis (Fig. 5.4). Whatever the method, the extracorporeal circuit needs to be anticoagulated to prevent the blood from clotting.

Continuous haemofiltration

In continuous haemofiltration (Paradiso 1989), blood flow in the extracorporeal circuit may be driven by a pump with vascular access provided by venous catheters (continuous venovenous haemofiltration or CVVH) or may be driven by the patient's own arterial pressure with an arterial and a venous catheter (continuous arteriovenous haemofiltration or CAVH). The hydrostatic pressure created in either system drives filtrate through the semipermeable membrane. This filtrate is essentially plasma water, but as it moves across the membrane it drags solutes with it by the process of convection. Large amounts of filtrate may be removed (up to 1 l/hour), and this fluid (the ultrafiltrate) is replaced with a fluid that has an electrolyte composition similar to plasma.

Continuous haemofiltration with dialysis

The terminology for continuous haemofiltration with dialysis (Miller et al 1990) is similar to the above, with the variants being continuous venovenous haemofiltration with dialysis (CVVHD) and continuous arteriovenous haemofiltration with dialysis (CAVHD). Here dialysis fluid is pumped through the filter in a countercurrent direction to the blood flow (similar to HD outlined above). Greater solute clearance can be achieved, and as the hydrostatic pressure does not need to be as high as in CVVH, less ultrafiltrate is formed and less replacement fluid is needed. As CAVHD does not involve actively pumping blood into the extracorporeal circuit, it can be used in haemodynamically very unstable patients and is probably the technique of choice in that situation.

Peritoneal dialysis

The peritoneum is an excellent semipermeable membrane and is used as such in peritoneal dialysis (PD). A catheter is inserted percutaneously into the peritoneal cavity and dialysate (usually 1–2 l) is allowed to run in, remain in the peritoneal cavity for a period of time, and then run out. Dialysate comes in premixed bags and its composition allows for the removal of electrolytes and uraemic waste products. Solute clearance is determined by dialysate flow rate, peritoneal permeability, peritoneal vascularity, and blood flow. Dialysate with a high glucose concentration allows large amounts of fluid to be removed by osmosis.

The most common complication of PD is abdominal discomfort caused by raised intra-abdominal pressure and splinting of the diaphragm; this may result in basal subsegmental lung collapse and hypoxaemia. Peritonitis is a more serious problem, and usually relates to contamination of the dialysate at the time of bag changes. Prompt recognition and the instillation of intraperitoneal antibiotics are the mainstays of treatment. Other complications include bowel perforation (usually at the time of catheter insertion) and hyperglycaemia.

The main advantage of PD is that correction of fluid and metabolic abnormalities is gradual and there is minimal haemodynamic disturbance (although ventilation may be compromised by the intra-abdominal fluid). However, clearance of uraemic toxins is generally less efficient than with HD, and this may be a problem in critically ill hypermetabolic patients. In addition, PD cannot be used in patients with acute intra-abdominal pathology or recent abdominal surgery.

Indications for renal support

Acute renal failure

The indications for renal support in acute renal failure are generally based on clinical parameters rather than on biochemistry alone. They include the speed of deterioration of renal function, the general clinical scenario, and the likely rapidity of recovery. Absolute indications for urgent renal support are fluid overload, hyperkalaemia, or acidosis unresponsive to conventional treatment. The urea and creatinine values are useful as a guide to starting renal support, but absolute values are controversial. As a rough rule, dialysis is often started when urea is greater than 40 mmol/l, creatinine is greater than 500 μmol/l, or when potassium is greater than 6 mmol/l.

Chronic renal failure

The decision to initiate renal support in a patient with chronic renal failure is usually made by the renal unit in a major hospital. It is almost always coupled with entering the patient onto a waiting list for renal transplantation, using renal support as a bridge until a live related or cadaver transplant can be performed. Patients are fully assessed for their suitability to enter such a programme by a team that generally includes physicians, nurses, a social worker, and a psychiatrist.

Potential hazards for physiotherapists

Mechanical problems

These include kinking of support lines, disconnection of different parts of the circuit and, worst of all, displacement of catheters from artery or vein. The former will cause the system to stop functioning or to function less well, but the latter can cause spectacular haemorrhage which may be fatal if not noticed immediately. Disconnection may also cause air embolism. Great care should therefore be taken when moving patients on dialysis.

Haemodynamic

Patients on renal support may be relatively depleted of intravascular fluid and changes in posture may produce hypotension and, occasionally, cardiac arrhythmias.

Infection

Renal failure produces a state of relative immunosuppression with patients being more susceptible to infection. Meticulous care therefore needs to be taken with sterile techniques such as suctioning and even manual hyperinflation.

Respiratory

Patients on dialysis are prone to hypoxaemia (for the reasons mentioned above) and may desaturate rapidly during suctioning or turning.

REFERENCES

Adamson R M, Dembitsky W P, Reichman R T et al 1989 Mechanical support: assist or nemesis? Journal of Thoracic and Cardiovascular Surgery 98: 915–921

Bellomo R, Boyce N 1993 Acute continuous hemodiafiltration: a prospective study of 110 patients and a review of the literature. American Journal of Kidney Disease 21: 508–518

Bersten A D, Rutten A J, Vedig A E, Skowronski G A 1989 Additional work of breathing imposed by endotracheal tubes, breathing circuits, and intensive care ventilators. Critical Care Medicine 17: 671–677

Branthwaite M A 1988 Problems in practice. Getting a patient off the ventilator. British Journal of Diseases of the Chest 82: 16–22

Branthwaite M A 1991 Non-invasive and domiciliary ventilation: positive pressure techniques. Thorax 46: 208–212

Carlon G C, Howland W S, Ray C et al 1983 High frequency jet ventilation. A prospective randomised evaluation. Chest 84: 551–559

Conrad S A, Eggerstede J M, Morris V F, Romero M D 1993 Prolonged intracorporeal support of gas exchange with an intravenacaval oxygenator. Chest 103: 158–161

Elliott M W, Steven M H, Phillips G D, Branthwaite M A 1990 Non-invasive mechanical ventilation for acute respiratory failure. British Medical Journal 300: 358–360

Evans T W, Keogh B F 1991 Extracorporeal membrane oxygenation: a breath of fresh air or yesterday's treatment. Thorax 46: 692–694

Fiastro J F, Habib M P, Shon B Y, Campbell S C 1988 Comparison of standard weaning parameters and the mechanical work of breathing in mechanically ventilated patients. Chest 94: 232–238

Gattinoni L, Pesenti A, Mascheroni D et al 1986 Low frequency positive pressure ventilation with extracorporeal CO_2 removal in severe acute respiratory failure. Journal of the American Medical Association 256: 881–886

Hickling K G, Henderson S J, Jackson R 1990 Low mortality associated with low volume pressure limited ventilation with permissive hypercapnia in severe adult respiratory distress syndrome. Intensive Care Medicine 16: 372–377

Hill J D 1989 Bridging to cardiac transplantation. Annals of Thoracic Surgery 47: 167–171

Hubmayr R D, Abel M D, Rehder K 1990 Physiologic approach to mechanical ventilation. Critical Care Medicine 18: 103–113

Kacmarek R M 1989 Inspiratory pressure support: does it make a clinical difference? Intensive Care Medicine 15: 337–339

Miller R, Kingswood C, Bullen C, Cohen S 1990 Renal replacement therapy in the ICU: the role of continuous arteriovenous haemodialysis. British Journal of Hospital Medicine 43: 354–362

Morris A H, Wallace C J, Menlove R L et al 1994 Randomized clinical trial of pressure-controlled inverse ratio ventilation and extra-corporeal CO_2 removal for adult respiratory distress syndrome. American Journal of Respiratory and Critical Care Medicine 149: 295–305

Paradiso C 1989 Hemofiltration: an alternative to dialysis. Heart & Lung 18: 282–290

Pingleton S K 1988 State of the art. Complications of acute respiratory failure. American Review of Respiratory Disease 137: 1463–1493

Rossaint R, Falke K J, Lopez F et al 1993 Inhaled nitric oxide for the adult respiratory distress syndrome. New England Journal of Medicine 328: 399–405

Schetz M, Lauwers P M, Ferdinande P 1989 Extracorporeal treatment of acute renal failure in the intensive care unit: a critical view. Intensive Care Medicine 15: 349–357

Schuster D P 1990 A physiologic approach to initiating, maintaining, and withdrawing ventilatory support during acute respiratory failure. The American Journal of Medicine 88: 268–278

Shneerson J M 1991 Non-invasive and domiciliary

ventilation: negative pressure techniques. Thorax 46: 131–135

Tharratt R S, Allen R P, Albertson T E 1988 Pressure controlled inverse ratio ventilation in severe adult respiratory failure. Chest 94: 755–762

Yang K L, Tobin M J 1991 A prospective study of indexes predicting the outcome of trials of weaning from mechanical ventilation. New England Journal of Medicine 324: 1445–1450

6

Non-invasive ventilation

Amanda J. Piper   Elizabeth R. Ellis

INTRODUCTION

The application of non-invasive ventilatory support to improve ventilation is not a new idea. The tank ventilator or 'iron lung', which provides negative pressure to the chest wall, was first developed in the 19th century (Woollam 1976). Further developments and modifications occurred, but it was not until the poliomyelitis outbreaks of the 1940s and 1950s that such devices became widely used. Continuous positive airway pressure through a face mask for patients with pulmonary oedema and other forms of acute respiratory failure was extensively described in the 1930s (Poulton & Oxon 1936, Barach et al 1938). However, with the development of positive pressure ventilators and the introduction of the endotracheal tube in the 1960s, use of non-invasive forms of ventilatory support for acute respiratory failure declined. Negative pressure devices continued to be used in patients with severe respiratory muscle impairment following poliomyelitis, and in other patient groups presenting with chronic respiratory failure where long-term ventilatory support in the home was required (Weirs et al 1977, Garay et al 1981). Since the mid-1980s, interest in non-invasive ventilatory support has again flourished, specifically the use of positive airway pressure devices and face mask interfaces. Although this interest had its genesis in the area of sleep disordered breathing and chronic respiratory failure, clinicians have rapidly recognized the value of this therapy in acute medical and surgical conditions where respiratory failure develops, in weaning from conventional ventilatory support and as an adjunct to established respiratory care programmes. In this chapter we will outline the mechanisms by which abnormal sleep-breathing contributes to the development of awake respiratory failure and the role nocturnal ventilatory support plays in reversing this. We will also look at the potential application of this technique in a broadening range of clinical conditions.

BREATHING, SLEEP AND RESPIRATORY FAILURE

It has been recognized for many years that significant changes in breathing and ventilation can occur during sleep (Gastaut et al 1966). However, it has only been in the past 15 years or so that the contribution abnormal breathing during sleep can play in the development of awake hypercapnia has been more fully appreciated. Our understanding of what happens to breathing during sleep has been greatly enhanced by three major developments in technology. The first is the routine use of accurate oximeters (Trask & Cree 1962, Saunders et al 1976) which have allowed the continuous monitoring of arterial oxygenation over prolonged periods of time. Secondly, the development of a comfortable and acceptable nasal mask interface (Sullivan et al 1981) has provided a simple but effective means by which abnormalities of nocturnal breathing can be reversed. The last is the relatively recent development of portable ventilatory support systems for home use. These developments made it possible to continuously monitor changes in breathing associated with sleep state, and to provide patients with a treatment intervention which was both effective and acceptable on a long-term basis.

Changes in breathing during sleep

Sleep is associated with a number of normal physiological events which have little effect on individuals with normal respiratory drive and mechanics. However, in patients with a range of respiratory abnormalities, sleep can lead to worsening respiratory function and gas exchange.

The awake state itself is associated with an additional stimulus to breathe, over and above that determined by the metabolic control system. This is known as the wakefulness drive to breathe and is lost with the onset of sleep. General postural muscle tone is also reduced at sleep onset, resulting in increases in upper airway resistance and reductions in ventilatory drive. At the same time, ventilatory responses to both hypoxia and hypercapnia are reduced so that there is an attenuated response to changes in gas exchange compared to wakefulness. As a result, a small fall in ventilation occurs with sleep in the range of 10–15% (Douglas et al 1982).

Although reduced, ventilation during non-rapid eye movement (NREM) sleep is steady, particularly during periods of slow wave sleep. However, even in normal subjects there is substantial variation in breathing during rapid eye movement (REM) sleep, most pronounced during periods of phasic eye movements. During these episodes, alveolar ventilation may fall by as much as 40% (Douglas et al 1982, Gould et al 1988). REM sleep is also associated with alterations in respiratory control, caused by descending inhibition of alpha and gamma motor neurons. This produces hypotonia of postural muscles, including the intercostal and accessory respiratory muscles, and a reduction in the rib cage contribution to ventilation. As a result, ventilation during REM sleep becomes heavily reliant on diaphragmatic activity.

In patients with severely compromised lung function or significant inspiratory muscle weakness, recruitment of other inspiratory and accessory muscles, including the abdominals, may occur to augment breathing. By this compensatory mechanism, individuals are usually able to maintain adequate ventilation during wakefulness and NREM sleep for prolonged periods. In those with significant lung disease, recruitment of the intercostal muscles occurs not only to augment ventilation but to maintain end-expiratory lung volume, thereby preventing small airway closure. With the transition into REM sleep, this postural muscle activity will be lost, resulting in a reduction in minute ventilation, worsening ventilation–perfusion relationships and a deterioration in gas exchange. Falls in saturation will be more severe in those patients with awake saturation values already near the steep portion of the oxyhaemoglobin dissociation curve. The degree of abnormal breathing which then occurs will depend upon the patient's arousal response. Arousal causes a change in state from sleep to transient wakefulness, permitting the re-emergence of accessory muscle activity and restoration of ventilation, albeit briefly. In this way, arousal acts as a defensive mechanism, limiting the degree of gas exchange abnormality which is permitted to occur. However, this response also leads to sleep fragmentation, which in itself can alter respiratory drive and arousal thresholds, so that eventually more extreme blood gas derangement must occur before the arousal response is activated.

The role of sleep in the development of awake hypercapnic respiratory failure

It is now well recognized that decompensated breathing first becomes apparent in REM sleep (Bye et al 1990). However, as REM sleep takes up only a relatively small proportion of total sleep time, patients with REM hypoventilation, even if severe, may remain clinically stable for months or even years before significant daytime hypercapnia becomes apparent. Initially, ventilation and sleep between periods of REM hypoventilation are usually normal, often through the recruitment of accessory respiratory muscles. In addition, the arousal mechanism operates to defend ventilation by limiting the amount of time spent in REM sleep, and therefore the degree of abnormal gas exchange which occurs. Characteristically, awake blood gases remain normal during this initial stage.

Progression of abnormal breathing into NREM sleep heralds the second stage in the evolution of sleep-induced respiratory failure (Piper & Sullivan 1994a). Mechanisms responsible for this progression include not only a deterioration of the underlying disease itself, but the appearance of other factors which may load breathing such as ageing, weight gain, upper airway dysfunction or the development of an intercurrent illness such as a chest infection. Sleep fragmentation from abnormal breathing events has the capacity to further alter respiratory control and depress arousal. These factors allow more severe sleep disordered breathing to occur, with less arousal between events. This begins a vicious cycle whereby resetting the sensitivity of the ventilatory control system occurs so that higher levels of carbon dioxide and lower levels of oxygen are tolerated without stimulating a change in respiration, not only asleep but during wakefulness as well. During this stage, daytime CO_2 retention becomes apparent (Fig. 6.1).

The final stage in the development of sleep-induced hypercapnia is characterized by unstable respiratory failure both awake and asleep. During this stage, changes in blood gases during sleep are extreme, and sleep architecture may be profoundly disturbed. By this stage, the clinical condition of the patient may deteriorate considerably, which can be mistaken for a progression of the underlying disease process. However, by supporting breathing during sleep, significant improvements in awake blood gases, reduction in hospital admissions, improved exercise tolerance and improved quality of life can be achieved.

INDICATIONS FOR NON-INVASIVE VENTILATION
Chronic respiratory failure

From the above analysis it is clear that sleep disordered breathing causing unstable respiratory failure and severe daytime symptoms is an obvious indication for non-invasive ventilatory support. There are a number of disorders where nocturnal respiratory failure occurs, producing awake hypercapnia (Table 6.1). The following features are indicators that sleep hypoventilation may be occurring and where nocturnal ventilatory support should be considered:

- Daytime hypercapnia $PaCO_2 > 6$ kPa (45 mmHg)

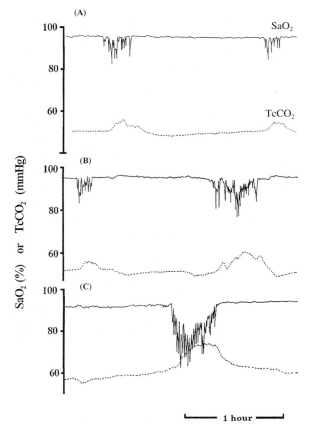

Fig. 6.1 Serial recordings of oxygen saturation (SaO$_2$) and transcutaneous carbon dioxide (TcCO$_2$) from a patient with Duchenne muscular dystrophy showing the progressive nocturnal respiratory failure. Panel (A) illustrates mild sleep disordered breathing, with modest falls in SaO$_2$. Eight months later (B), more substantial oxygen desaturation was apparent during REM sleep, with rises in carbon dioxide. By panel (C), severe REM desaturation was occurring, with failure of SaO$_2$ to return to baseline values between periods of abnormal breathing. This was accompanied by large rises in CO$_2$. Over the same period, awake CO$_2$ had risen from 40 to 45 mmHg (5.3 to 6.0 kPa), with no change in inspiratory muscle pressures.

- Severe nocturnal hypoxaemia
- Excessive daytime sleepiness
- Severe early morning headaches.

However, for many patients the onset of nocturnal respiratory failure occurs over an extended period of time, in some cases even years. With such an insidious onset, the signs and symptoms of chronic hypoventilation may be overlooked,

Table 6.1 Conditions where nocturnal hypercapnic respiratory failure is likely to occur

Neuromuscular	Myopathies
	Duchenne muscular dystrophy
	Acid maltase deficiency
	Neuropathies
	Poliomyelitis
	Motor neurone disease
	Bilateral phrenic nerve palsy
Chest wall	Kyphoscoliosis
	Thoracoplasty
Impaired ventilatory control	Obesity hypoventilation syndrome
	Brain stem injury
	Primary alveolar hypoventilation
Airway obstruction	Severe obstructive sleep apnoea
Lung disease	Chronic obstructive pulmonary disease
	Cystic fibrosis
	Bronchiectasis

or incorrectly attributed to the ongoing progression of the primary disease process.

More difficult questions arise in patients with milder conditions, and there are specific issues that affect individuals with particular diseases or syndromes. In all cases the feasibility of non-invasive ventilation depends on whether the presentation is acute or chronic. The capacity of an individual to maintain adequate ventilation during sleep depends on a balance between the respiratory load placed on the respiratory muscles and the ability of the respiratory muscles to sustain that load. Chronic adaptations (as described earlier) which occur in response to the failure to maintain adequate ventilation can complicate this balance.

The kinds of loads that are placed on the respiratory muscles include those that occur during sleep, such as upper airway resistance, which may be considerable, and the relative inefficiency of the rib cage when the intercostal muscles are inhibited during REM. These changes may occur on a background of high work of breathing from increased airways resistance, from decreased respiratory compliance from chest wall deformities or lung disease, or from the relative inefficiency of muscle contraction from hyperinflation.

On the other hand, the respiratory muscles may be unable to sustain the work of breathing because of inherent problems of their own. Respiratory muscle performance can be adversely affected by hypoxaemia, hypercapnia, malnutrition, biomechanical alterations, trauma or disease.

Factors affecting muscle performance and respiratory load can present differently in each patient. Therefore, it is important to analyse each case as it helps to predict how effective different types of intervention are likely to be. For example, a patient may have a normal work of breathing but very weak muscles as occurs in neuromuscular disease. The condition of these patients is often complicated by lung and chest wall stiffness as a chronic adaptation to low lung volumes. Alternatively, a patient may have normal muscles but a very high work of breathing. This high work of breathing may be generalized throughout the respiratory system, as in restrictive lung disease, or it may be localized, as in upper airway obstruction. In other instances, the patient may have 'weak' muscles with an increase in the work of breathing, such as in obstructive lung disease with significant hyperinflation, hypoxaemia and malnutrition.

Assessment of chronic hypoventilation

Although a number of investigators have tried to use daytime pulmonary function tests as a predictor of the degree of abnormal breathing occurring during sleep, no strong correlation has been found (Bye et al 1990). However, we do know that a low vital capacity, a significant fall in vital capacity from erect to supine or a maximum inspiratory pressure of less than 30 cmH_2O are all indicators that sleep disordered breathing and hypoventilation may be present (Bye et al 1990). Each of these tests can be easily carried out at the bedside as part of the overall assessment of a patient presenting in respiratory failure. Strong use of the accessory respiratory muscles at rest, including the sternomastoid and the abdominal muscles should raise the possibility that respiratory function during sleep may worsen.

In general, if there is awake hypercapnia then there will be substantial sleep-linked worsening of respiratory failure (Piper & Sullivan 1994a), although the converse does not necessarily hold true. Many subjects with awake CO_2 within the normal range will have significant sleep-linked respiratory failure.

The limitations of daytime indices as predictors of nocturnal hypoventilation mean that detailed sleep studies are required in order to accurately assess the severity and nature of the disorder. Sleep studies should include measurement of the standard sleep parameters such as electroencephalogram (EEG), electrooculogram (EOG) and submental electromyogram (EMG). The extent and quality of sleep is essential information for gauging the likely impact that the disordered breathing may have on cognitive and other functions. In addition, comprehensive cardiac and respiratory monitoring should be carried out, including electrocardiogram (ECG), oximetry, airflow, diaphragm EMG, rib cage and abdominal movement, and transcutaneous CO_2.

Types of ventilators

There are currently two types of ventilator systems available for mask ventilation: volume preset and pressure preset devices. Each type of device has its own advantages and limitations. A successful outcome using mask ventilation will depend upon the clinician's understanding of the underlying pathological processes which have contributed to the patient's respiratory deterioration, and choosing a machine and mode of ventilatory support which best meets the respiratory needs of the patient. Criteria for choosing a ventilator are discussed later.

Kyphoscoliosis

The final stages of severe kyphoscoliosis have been characterized by progressive respiratory failure associated with severe nocturnal hypoventilation (Ellis et al 1988). The REM hypoventilation is probably caused by a combination of a very high work of breathing for a diaphragm that is at a significant mechanical disadvantage.

Table 6.2 Comparison of volume and pressure preset home ventilators (Adapted, with permission, from Respir Care 1994; 39(5): 504)

	Volume preset	Pressure preset
Tidal volume	Constant	Variable
Pressure	Variable	Constant
Leak compensation	No (need to increase TV)	Yes (if mild to moderate)
Constant EEP	No	Yes
Internal battery	Usually	No
Portability	+	++
Comfort	+	++
Alarms	Usually	No

In some patients sleep disordered breathing is also complicated by upper airway obstruction. Nose mask ventilation is particularly suitable for these patients as other methods of assisted ventilation are very difficult. Tracheostomy can be difficult because of the loss of the extrathoracic trachea and the fitting of a cuirass is made exceptionally difficult by the chest wall deformity. Non-invasive ventilation can be readily achieved with a nose mask in this group despite the stiffness of the chest wall and the additional requirement of positive expiratory pressures (Ellis et al 1988).

Cystic fibrosis

The beneficial effects of nocturnal non-invasive ventilation for patients with end-stage cystic fibrosis (CF) are only beginning to be recognized. Non-invasive ventilation has been shown to be of value during periods of acute deterioration, where marked pulmonary deterioration occurs despite maximum conventional therapy (Piper et al 1992). Use of nasal ventilatory support in this setting can correct hypoxaemia without inducing additional CO_2 retention.

This technique may be used to stabilize the patient in the short-term while donor organs become available (Hodson et al 1991), or on a longer-term basis, allowing the patient to return home (Piper et al 1992). Although in initial reports volume preset machines were used, bilevel pressure devices also have a role, but are probably more effective at an earlier stage of lung deterioration.

Some patients report improved sputum clear-ance after initiation of nasal ventilatory support, possibly related to better tolerance of longer chest physiotherapy sessions (Piper et al 1992). Improved lung expansion and chest wall excursion while on the machine may also play a role.

Duchenne muscular dystrophy

Ventilatory support is often reluctantly prescribed for patients with progressive neuromuscular disease, owing to a perceived lack of quality of life for these patients. However, quality of life is often underestimated in such patients. The use of long-term non-invasive ventilation has been shown to stabilize pulmonary function and prolong life expectancy in patients with Duchenne muscular dystrophy (DMD) and awake hypercapnia (Vianello et al 1994). In contrast, Raphael and co-workers (1994) trialled non-invasive ventilation as a preventive measure in DMD patients free of daytime respiratory failure. They found no benefit from early intervention with this technique, with the treated group showing a similar rate of deterioration in blood gases and pulmonary function as a control group. Further, there was a higher death rate in the treated group, although the reasons for this were not entirely clear.

Chronic obstructive pulmonary disease

Nocturnal nasal ventilation has been used effectively in selected patients with stable chronic obstructive pulmonary disease (COPD). However, this form of therapy is not tolerated as well as in other diagnostic groups (Strumpf et al 1991), and longer-term outcomes are not as favourable as in patients with neuromuscular and chest wall disorders (Simonds & Elliott 1995). Those patients most likely to benefit from nocturnal ventilatory support appear to be those with significant daytime hypercapnia, who have symptomatic sleep problems and in whom nocturnal hypercapnia can be successfully reduced by overnight ventilation. Recently, Meecham Jones et al (1995) reported a randomized crossover study of nasal pressure support ventilation plus oxygen therapy compared with domiciliary oxygen therapy alone in 18 hypercapnic patients with COPD. Improvements in daytime arterial blood gas tensions, overnight $TcCO_2$, total sleep time and sleep efficiency were seen during non-invasive ventilation and oxygen therapy compared with oxygen therapy alone, suggesting that control of hypoventilation with non-invasive ventilation can be achieved. These authors found that those who showed the greatest reduction in nocturnal hypercapnia with ventilation were likely to gain the greatest benefit from the treatment.

Acute respiratory failure

In order to reduce the problems associated with endotracheal intubation and ventilation, an increasing number of centres are now using non-invasive ventilation as a treatment alternative for patients with acute respiratory failure. It avoids the complications of endotracheal intubation, is more comfortable for the patient, allowing speech and swallowing and avoids the need for sedation and immobilization. Treatment does not have to be instituted in the intensive care or emergency department environment, and is increasingly commenced on general medical or surgical wards (Bott et al 1993, Servera et al 1995, Piper & Willson 1996).

Appropriate patient selection is essential for a successful treatment outcome. Non-invasive ventilation should be seen as a therapy to prevent the need for intubation rather than an alternative to it. Therefore, when undertaking this therapy it is important to be able to identify those patients who are unlikely to respond well, in order that a delay in mandatory intubation does

---

Box 6.1 Characteristics of patients with acute respiratory failure unlikely to do well on non-invasive ventilation (Vitacca et al 1993, Soo Hoo et al 1994, Brochard et al 1995, Kramer et al 1995)

- Agitation, encephalopathic, uncooperative
- Severe illness, including extreme acidosis (pH <7.2)
- Presence of excessive secretions or pneumonia
- Multiple organ failure
- Haemodynamic instability
- Inability to maintain a lip seal
- Inability to protect the airway
- Overt respiratory failure requiring immediate intubation

---

not occur (Box 6.1). The ideal patient should be cooperative enough to tolerate a mask and to follow simple instructions. A successful outcome depends to a large degree on the ability to rapidly correct acidosis, decrease CO_2 and reduce respiratory rate (Soo Hoo et al 1994). This in turn will be influenced by the ability of the patient and the therapist to minimize mouth leaks and to coordinate breathing with the ventilator. If hypercapnia and acidosis fail to improve within the first few hours of treatment, longer term success is unlikely (Soo Hoo et al 1994, Ambrosino et al 1995).

In patients who are hypoxaemic but retain carbon dioxide, the use of non-invasive ventilation permits higher levels of inspired oxygen to be introduced without unduly worsening hypercapnia. Under these circumstances, the use of non-invasive ventilation supports patients until their acute deterioration can be reversed (Conway et al 1993).

The majority of studies reported to date have involved patients with chronic obstructive pulmonary disease (COPD) during an acute exacerbation. It appears that the type of ventilator (volume preset or bilevel pressure support) or the type of interface chosen (nose or full face mask) is not pivotal in determining the success of treatment. However, results will be influenced by the patient's tolerance and adaptation to the machine, and some patients may find the bilevel pressure support devices easier to adapt to (Vitacca et al 1993). Very dyspnoeic patients tend to be mouth breathers, and where it is not possible for the patient to maintain lip closure, a full face mask needs to be used to ensure machine–patient synchronization and that an effective tidal volume is delivered.

Use of non-invasive ventilatory support in COPD patients during acute respiratory failure has shown very encouraging outcomes. In a large study by Brochard and colleagues (1995), only 26% of the non-invasive ventilation group required intubation compared to 74% of the standard treatment group. Further, hospital stay was significantly longer, and the mortality and complication rate higher in the group receiving standard treatment. However, an important caveat exists when interpreting these data. Only 31% of all patients with COPD admitted during the study period were considered suitable for enrolment, emphasizing that success with this form of therapy relies heavily on appropriate patient selection. Several recent studies have also provided data which suggest that the early administration of non-invasive ventilatory support during episodes of acute respiratory failure may improve the long-term outcome in patients with COPD. Improved 12-month survival and a reduction in the number of further ICU or hospital admissions has been reported in patients treated with mask ventilation compared to those undergoing either conventional therapy (Confalonieri et al 1996) or intubation and ventilation (Vitacca et al 1996).

Although patients with acute respiratory failure from causes other than COPD may also be successfully ventilated with non-invasive ventilation (Pennock et al 1994), more recent prospective randomized studies have not been so positive (Kramer et al 1995). Where acute respiratory deterioration is on the basis of pneumonia or congestive heart failure, outcomes using mask ventilation have not been as favourable (Ambrosino et al 1995, Wysocki et al 1995, Meduri et al 1996). Although the reasons for this are unclear, it may relate to problems with clearing secretions, poor lung compliance requiring high pressure or the inhomogeneity of gas exchange in some disorders. Those patients presenting with acute respiratory failure and hypercapnia respond better to non-invasive ventilatory support than those with hypoxaemia alone (Wysocki et al 1995).

We are increasingly seeing patients who develop postoperative respiratory failure following major surgery. Many of these patients are overweight, and probably have pre-existing sleep disordered breathing. The affects of anaesthesia and analgesia may worsen an already compromised upper airway, producing apnoea and its sequelae such as hypoxaemia and blood pressure fluctuations. In addition, diaphragm inhibition after upper abdominal surgery can exacerbate REM hypoventilation. These patients generally respond well and rapidly to bilevel pressure support, primarily used during sleep.

Another group who respond very rapidly and positively to non-invasive ventilation are those patients with obesity hypoventilation. This syndrome is characterized by obesity, a long history of snoring, excessive daytime sleepiness and severe derangement of awake blood gases. These patients frequently present grossly decompensated with right heart failure, lower limb oedema and hypercapnia. Use of non-invasive ventilatory support in these patients results in improved awake blood gases and clinical condition within days of commencing therapy, without the need for intubation and its associated complications. In most patients, transfer to more simple devices such as CPAP can be achieved for long-term domiciliary use (Piper & Sullivan 1994b).

Although some investigators have described nasal ventilation in the acute phase as a time-consuming procedure (Chevrolet et al 1991), more recent experience suggests that this is not necessarily the case (Bott et al 1993, Kramer et al 1995). It has also been shown that the use of this technique can be transferred to the general ward environment without a reduction in efficacy (Pennock et al 1994). However, training of staff regarding the management of patients undergoing this therapy is essential. This includes the need for continuous monitoring, not only to check the efficacy of the technique, but to ensure the safety of the patient. Sudden death may occur if an accidental disconnection from the ventilator occurs (Kramer et al 1995).

Non-invasive ventilation is usually continued until blood gases have stabilized for several hours, then trial periods off the mask are commenced. The patient's response to spontaneous ventilation is monitored, and mask ventilatory support reinstituted if breathing deteriorates. In some cases, almost continuous use of the mask during the first day or two may be necessary. There is then a gradual withdrawal of awake ventilatory support to nocturnal use only. Prior to hospital discharge, investigation into the need for domiciliary therapy and the type of therapy required will be needed.

Weaning

Although most patients are able to be weaned from mechanical ventilation without incident, a small number will require a prolonged weaning period. In many cases, a history of underlying lung, chest wall or neuromuscular disease will be found. Although a number of weaning strategies have been developed to facilitate the resumption of spontaneous breathing, some patients will not tolerate removal of ventilatory support without developing unacceptably high levels of carbon dioxide retention. Non-invasive ventilatory support can be a useful tool in the weaning of such patients from conventional mechanical ventilation (Udwadia et al 1992). Nasal mask ventilation has also been used in the immediate post-extubation period in patients thought likely to have weaning difficulties (Restrick et al 1993), or who develop acute respiratory failure shortly after extubation (Wysocki et al 1995).

In patients already tracheostomized and on partial ventilatory support, nasal mask ventilation can be substituted for tracheal support (Restrick et al 1993). This is usually commenced on a continuous basis, with the patient removing the mask for short periods for eating, speaking and coughing. Periods of spontaneous breathing are then interspersed with periods on the nasal mask, the balance being determined by patient tolerance and clinical response. Once nasal ventilatory support has been shown to be acceptable and to effectively support ventilation, the tracheostomy tube is removed. Non-invasive ventilation is then continued nocturnally and

for any rest/sleep period during the day as required. Although some patients may be weaned entirely from the mask, most patients have an underlying process which features sleep disordered breathing, and so discharge home on nocturnal ventilatory support is necessary.

PRACTICAL ISSUES IN THE APPLICATION OF NON-INVASIVE VENTILATION

Criteria for choosing a ventilator

A number of factors need to be considered when choosing a machine and mode of ventilatory support. These include the clinical condition of the patient on presentation, the diagnosis, the patient's respiratory drive, the compliance of the lungs and chest wall, the degree of synchronization that can be achieved between the patient and the device, and the familiarity of the staff with the equipment. Sleep study data are useful in patients requiring long-term ventilation in identifying any degree of upper airway dysfunction which may be present as well as determining the patient's respiratory drive during sleep. Understanding the features and limitations of the various machines available and the modes of ventilatory support in which they can operate will assist in selecting the appropriate system to meet the patient's needs. In some centres, the choice of device will also be influenced by cost. However, the final decision should come down to how effective the device is in supporting ventilation and maintaining gas exchange in the individual.

Type of ventilator

Ventilator systems available for non-invasive positive pressure support fall into two categories. Volume preset machines such as the PLV 100 (Lifecare, Lafayette, Colorado, USA), the PV 501 (Breas, Sweden) or the Bromptonpac (PneuPAC Ltd., Luton, Beds, UK) operate as time cycled flow generators, and deliver a fixed tidal volume irrespective of the airway pressure generated, as long as leaks from the system are minimized.

Pressure preset systems include bilevel positive pressure devices, the most widely recognized being the BiPAP machine (Respironics, Murrysville, Pennsylvania, USA). Other pressure preset devices include the NIPPY (Thomas Respiratory Systems, England), the DP90 (Taema, France) and the VPAP II (ResMed, Australia). With these devices, tidal volume will vary according to the inspiratory pressure set, the inspiratory–expiratory pressure difference, and the chest wall/lung compliance of the patient.

In studies comparing the efficacy of these two systems, little difference has been found either in acute (Vitacca et al 1993) or chronic respiratory failure (Meecham Jones & Wedzicha 1993). However, there may be differences in patient acceptance, particularly during acute respiratory failure (Vitacca et al 1993), with many patients finding the bilevel pressure support devices easier to tolerate. Poor tolerance to volume preset devices may be related to increased airway resistance causing elevated inspiratory pressure in the mask that will be uncomfortable or cause leaks that limit the effectiveness of ventilation (Soo Hoo et al 1994). On the other hand, in patients with low chest wall compliance higher airway pressures may be needed to maintain optimal ventilation, particularly during REM sleep. In these patients, volume preset ventilators can prove more reliable and effective in delivering a stable tidal volume despite changing chest wall mechanics. A change to a volume preset device should always be considered if hypoventilation persists on bilevel ventilatory support.

Bilevel devices are said to compensate better for mild to moderate leaks from the mask and mouth than volume preset devices. Clinical experience has shown that mouth leaks are common during mask ventilation, particularly during sleep, and that these leaks may adversely affect the quality of ventilation even with bilevel positive pressure devices (Meecham Jones et al 1994; Piper & Willson 1996).

Settings

Machines may be used in assist/control (volume preset) or spontaneous modes (bilevel devices), where the machine cycles into inspiration in response to the patient's spontaneous inspiratory effort. However, the volume preset and a number of the bilevel devices such as the BiPAP, can also be set to deliver a preset respiratory rate should the patient fail to trigger the device. Titration of inspiratory pressures for patients on a bilevel device or tidal volume for a patient using volume preset is made on the basis of patient tolerance and the effect such a pressure has on ventilation and gas exchange. However, when setting pressures or volumes it should be borne in mind that excessively high inspiratory pressures will promote leakage of air from the mouth, reducing the effectiveness of ventilatory support. Excessive hyperventilation can also occur, which may induce upper airway obstruction, and the appearance of central apnoea. More recent evidence suggests that the timed mode of ventilation using bilevel devices is less predictable and less stable than nasal ventilation with volume preset devices and may produce periodic breathing during both wakefulness and sleep, related to glottic closure (Parreira et al 1996).

The use of end-expiratory pressures (EPAP) may be advantageous in a number of clinical conditions, including controlling upper airway closure, recruiting collapsed alveoli or to overcome intrinsic end-expiratory pressure. Bilevel positive pressure devices are more reliable in maintaining end-expiratory pressure than volume preset machines. However, setting of the EPAP reduces the differential pressure between inspiration and expiration, which may affect the degree to which minute ventilation is augmented. Elliott & Simonds (1995) found that the addition of $5 \, cmH_2O$ of EPAP in patients with neuromuscular disease reduced the severity of gas exchange abnormalities during sleep, but had no effect in patients with COPD. Further, they found the use of EPAP had deleterious effects on sleep quality in some patients. Similarly, the use of expiratory pressure in patients with COPD during acute exacerbations did not confer any additional benefit and was found to be poorly tolerated (Meecham Jones et al 1994).

In some cases the bilevel device may fail to adequately reduce CO_2 despite increasing minute ventilation and decreasing respiratory effort. This has been explained by CO_2 rebreathing in patients with exhaled flow rates that exceed the leak rate of the exhalation port at the set expiratory pressure (Ferguson & Gilmartin 1995). This is most likely to occur in patients with high respiratory rates where the duration of expiration is short. Although this can be eliminated by using EPAP pressures of 8 cm or more (Ferguson & Gilmartin 1995), the majority of patients are unlikely to need or tolerate these pressures. Further, IPAP pressure would need to be increased to maintain the IPAP–EPAP pressure difference, which may not produce greater ventilatory support because of increased mouth leaks (Fernandez et al 1993). There are now a number of different types of expiratory valves available such as the Plateau exhalation device or the non-rebreathing valve (Respironics, USA) which are effective in minimizing CO_2 rebreathing (Ferguson & Gilmartin 1995).

These considerations regarding ventilator settings highlight the need for monitoring of the patient during initial trials of non-invasive ventilation in order to determine response to therapy. In this way a change in the mode or type of ventilator can be made if ventilation is not being adequately supported. Although some centres have based machine settings on ventilation achieved during wakefulness (Strumpf et al 1991), such settings may not be adequate during sleep. This may relate to changes in the behaviour of the glottis, mouth leaks, alteration in respiratory drive or compliance of the respiratory system associated with changes in sleep state. It is recommended that ventilator parameters are based on patient tolerance and gas exchange while awake, and then nocturnal monitoring is used to ensure that such settings are also appropriate to maintain adequate sleep ventilation (see Initiating therapy, p. 112).

Humidification and oxygen therapy

In some patients, the high flows of cold dry air across the nasal passages can cause distress-ing nasal symptoms which may affect compliance with therapy, or increase nasal resistance (Richards et al 1996) which will affect the amount of ventilation delivered. Patients may report sneezing, nasal stuffiness or rhinorrhoea, and erroneously believe they are developing a head cold. The use of an in-line humidifier such as an HC-100 (Fisher-Paykel, New Zealand), which can both warm and moisten the air, will largely improve these symptoms. However, as nasal symptoms frequently point to the presence of significant mouth leaks, this should be attended to, as leaks may reduce the effectiveness of ventilation. In patients with bronchial hypersecretion, such as CF or bronchiectasis, the addition of in-line humidification whilst using nasal ventilatory support may be useful in ensuring secretions are well hydrated. Patients with acute respiratory failure may become dehydrated, and can also benefit from additional humidification of the airways.

In patients who require ventilatory support on a continuous basis, nebulized bronchodilators and normal saline can be given during mask ventilatory support, either via a mouthpiece whilst the nasal mask is in place, or added in-line to the system close to the nasal mask. Bilevel ventilatory support devices have been used to deliver aerosolized β_2-agonists in the emergency department for patients with bronchospasm, and have been shown to be associated with a greater increase in the peak expiratory flow rates compared to aerosols delivered by small volume nebulizers alone (Pollack et al 1995).

Generally, supplemental oxygen is not required in those patients with chronic respiratory failure from neuromuscular or chest wall disorders. However, in patients with parenchymal disease or those with acute respiratory failure, additional oxygen is likely to be needed, and can be added either into the ventilator tubing or into a port on the mask itself. The flow rate needed will be determined by the oxygen saturation achieved.

Interfaces

Either nasal or full face masks may be used

to deliver ventilatory support (Figs 6.2 and 6.3). It is recommended that a nasal mask be tried initially, transferring to a full face mask if mouth leaks cannot be controlled adequately with a

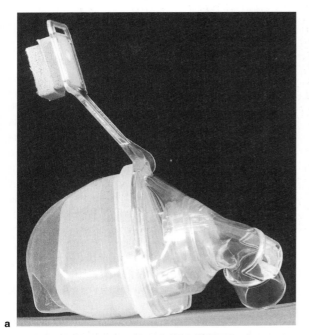

a

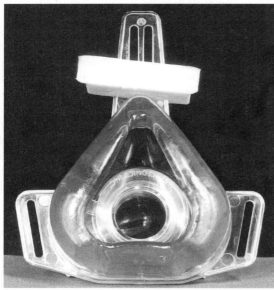

b

Fig. 6.2 Examples of commercially available nasal mask systems: **a** the Series 2 Bubble Mask (ResMed, Australia); **b** the Gel Mask (Respironics, USA).

chin strap (Figs 6.4 & 6.5). A review of the available literature suggests that successful outcomes in acute respiratory failure can be achieved with both types of interface (Bott et al 1993, Soo Hoo et al 1994), although the full face mask has been preferred by some groups in the acute setting to better control mouth leaks (Brochard et al 1990, Fernandez et al 1993). Nasal masks tend to be more comfortable, have a lower dead space and allow easier access for secretion removal and speech. Individually moulded masks can be constructed for those patients difficult to fit with standard commercial masks, or those using mask ventilation on a long-term basis. However, a high degree of skill and experience is needed to ensure comfort and fit, and frequent refitting may be necessary.

Initiating therapy

At present there is no consensus as to when non-invasive ventilatory support should be commenced in patients with documented nocturnal hypoventilation. The decision is not a difficult one if a patient presents with awake hypercapnia or has overt symptoms of sleep disordered breathing. However, the identification of isolated REM desaturation may be a more difficult one. Intervening too early may result in the patient rejecting therapy.

Patients may need time to adapt to the idea of assisted ventilation as it may signal to them the beginning of the 'end'. The difficulty is that in some patients who are deteriorating rapidly this may be the case. With most, however, it should signal a new beginning. There are many reasons for rejecting the idea of the ventilator. Some patients do not believe in altering the natural course of events. Some may find it beyond their resources and capabilities to acquire and manage the technology. Some find the thought of sleeping with a machine totally foreign or too disruptive to their circumstances. Some believe that they will become ventilator dependent or that it will weaken their muscles.

Each of these beliefs needs to be explored and discussed without judgement. They can be resolved in a number of ways. Patients need to

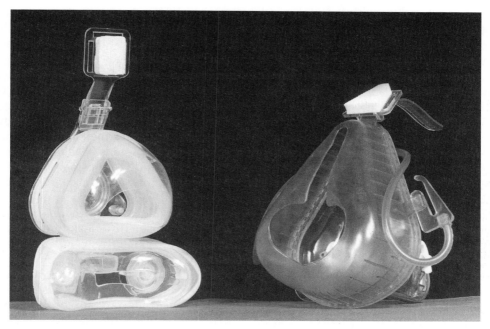

Fig. 6.3   Two types of full face mask suitable for non-invasive ventilatory support. The nose-mouth mask (ResMed, Australia) on the left, and the Spectrum Face Mask (Respironics, USA) on the right.

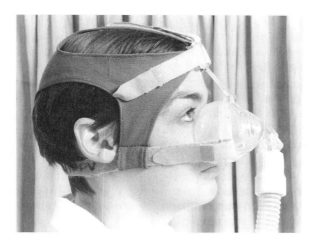

Fig. 6.4   Nasal mask and headgear system (ResMed, Australia).

be allowed to make their own choice and when the symptoms of respiratory failure or sleep deprivation become severe enough they may then seek relief. Alternatively patients can be counselled, often with the help of other patients,

that the benefits outweigh any real or perceived detriments. Patients have to be willing for trials to be successful and it is helpful if a member of the family or someone in the household can manage the equipment. For most patients, compliance is usually dependent on relief of symptoms. Paulus & Willig (1993) surveyed 34 patients with neuromuscular disorders ventilated nasally. Over half the patients considered nocturnal ventilation to be constraining, but felt that these constraints were more than acceptable if the benefits outweighed any inconveniences.

Kramer et al (1995) reported that approximately 18% of patients are intolerant of non-invasive therapy during acute respiratory failure, although compliance appears to be slightly better with bilevel pressure support devices than volume preset (Vitacca et al 1993). Failure rates in patients with chronic respiratory failure have been reported between 19 and 36% (Gay et al 1991, Strumpf et al 1991). However, acceptance of therapy may differ depending on the underlying pathology, the patient's response to therapy and relief of symptoms. Initial experience with mask ventilation may also influence outcome. A number of groups commence ventilation on an inpatient basis to provide the patient with maximum support whilst minimizing problems (Meecham Jones et al 1995, Piper & Willson 1996). This permits intensive coaching of patients to enable them to synchronize with the ventilator, and to adjust the ventilator settings so there is better matching with the patient's own breathing pattern. It also provides the opportunity to determine any problems that are arising which could affect patient response to therapy, and adversely affect their acceptance of treatment.

After acclimatizing the patient to the mask and flow from the ventilator, the ventilator is then adjusted to match the patient's own respiratory pattern and timing. Further adjustments are then made to ensure blood gases are maintained or improved. Where inspiratory time or flow can be set, this will be based on the patient's own respiratory pattern, taking into account the effect short inspiratory times can have on gas exchange. In patients where the compliance of the alveoli is heterogeneous, much of the delivered tidal volume will be directed towards those alveoli with short filling times, producing an overdistension of already inflated units, and not contributing to improved gas exchange. Prolonging the inspiratory time allows the recruitment of alveoli with slower filling times, so that increased ventilation can contribute to improved gas exchange.

Adverse effects

There are many complications or adverse effects which can arise during attempts to establish patients on non-invasive ventilation. Mouth leaks during the inspiratory phase of the ventilator cycle are probably the most common problem and probably occur in all patients at some time but remain a significant problem in approximately 60% of patients. This leak can reduce effective ventilation and may only be obvious during certain sleep stages. Leaks may be seen in the presence of upper airway obstruction,

if asynchrony between the patient and the ventilator develops or if the lips and palate fail to provide a seal. If the leak is significant it can usually be remedied by the use of a chin strap which should cradle the chin and hold the lower jaw up. The chin strap is designed to have elastic sections on the sides so that patients can still move their jaw comfortably and call out and breathe should their nose become blocked, or the ventilator fails. Other solutions for this problem include, repositioning of the neck, taping the lips, mouth guards and full face masks. Full face masks are usually preferred once the patient's confidence has been established. The presence of leaks will not only reduce the degree of effective ventilation reaching the lungs, but may also cause sleep fragmentation.

Upper airway obstruction can occur particularly if the cycling pressure is allowed to drop below the closing pressure of the upper airway. It is very difficult to establish effective ventilation when this occurs, although it can, in some very mild cases, be reduced by positioning the patient's head so that the neck is slightly more extended. Sometimes a chin strap alone is effective in lifting the jaw and thereby opening the upper airway. An increase in end-expiratory pressure usually ensures adequate ventilation. For some patients, the added expiratory pressures are only required in the first few days of assisted ventilation until there is some restoration of upper airway tone.

Mask leaks commonly occur on either side of the bridge of the nose and can cause significant irritation to the eyes. If the leak is small it can be compensated for by the machine and this is preferable to pulling the mask too tightly onto the face. Patients usually learn to eliminate the leaks by repositioning the mask or by adjusting the strap alignment. Elastic straps of the head harnesses usually need regular replacement to ensure effective mask pressures. Other solutions include custom-built masks and a change in sleeping posture.

Mask pressure can cause pressure sores or pressure marks on the bridge of the nose or across the top lip in particular. These are best prevented by careful selection of mask for size and skin sensitivity. The areas respond well to standard pressure care including gentle massage, being left clean, dry and open and getting a regular amount of sunshine. The bridge of the nose often becomes thick and tough with time, although some people have recurring problems. For these patients the bridge of the nose can be protected with special pressure-absorbing materials that are commonly used with prostheses. The mask can be adapted to reduce pressure by inserting a spacer on the top bar of the mask. Alternatively the patient may need to use a mouthpiece or nasal plugs (e.g. Puritan Bennett, Lenexa, KS, USA) which fit securely into the nares without pressure on the nasal bridge, permitting pressure areas to heal. Head harness or strap pressure can cause abrasions over the back of the neck or over the ears. This can be simply relieved by redesigning the head harness to realign the straps or to include cotton wadding or a pad over the tender parts.

Abdominal distension can be caused by air in the stomach particularly when high cycling pressures are required for effective ventilation. This problem is more likely to be seen in volume cycled ventilators. It appears that air can track through the stomach to the bowel and cause considerable discomfort. Every effort should be made to lower the cycling pressure without compromising effective ventilation. Some patients find relief from lying on their left side at night, some from having an empty stomach and some resort to medications including charcoal tablets and acidophilus tablets.

Monitoring

When commencing mask ventilation in the acute situation, careful monitoring is mandatory in order to gauge the effectiveness of ventilatory support. Oximetry and transcutaneous carbon dioxide should be used to monitor trends in gas exchange continuously (Fig. 6.5). Direct measurements of arterial blood gases should be taken

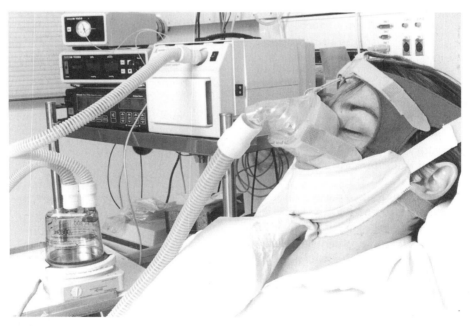

Fig. 6.5 Nasal mask set up. Oximeter and transcutaneous carbon dioxide monitors in the background are used to measure the physiological response to nasal ventilatory support. An active humidifier has been placed in the circuit between the bilevel ventilator and the patient (bottom left-hand corner).

prior to commencing ventilation, then again at 1 hour, 6 hours, 24 hours and as needed depending on the patient's clinical condition. In addition, heart rate, respiratory rate and the fraction of inspired oxygen should be recorded hourly for the first few hours until the patient is stable. Blood pressure measurements may also be necessary, particularly if there is any question of the patient's haemodynamic stability.

These monitored trials are the only way of differentially diagnosing problems and resolving them promptly. In patients with chronic respiratory failure, acclimatization to the mask and machine can be carried out during the day, with monitoring of oxygen saturation and preferably CO_2, either end-tidal or transcutaneous. Frequently the patient will fall asleep during these initial trials, and problems such as mouth leaks or the development of upper airway obstruction may be identified at this time. Once the patient is able to sleep for a number of hours on the machine, a sleep study, if possible, is performed to gauge the degree to which the patient and machine are synchronized, the stability in gas exchange, any technical problems which may occur and the effect of therapy on sleep. During these studies, a number of respiratory variables will be monitored in addition to the signals needed for sleep staging. Various centres will measure mask pressure, chest wall motion, diaphragmatic and other respiratory muscle electromyograms, or inspiratory/expiratory tidal volumes to provide information about the efficacy of ventilatory support.

Ideally, the initial trials should have full polysomnography, respiratory monitoring and an expert therapist in attendance. After this the degree of monitoring can be reduced and the patients encouraged to manage the equipment themselves and solve any problems that may arise. Patients should be independent and confident in managing the equipment and their own care throughout the night prior to discharge from hospital. Alternatively, if individuals remain dependent on some assistance the home carers should be brought in for at least part of the night to develop skills in setting up and trouble shooting.

Home management

Most ventilator users adapt well to ongoing ventilatory support in the home, and would choose ventilation again if required to do so (Goldstein et al 1995). However, it is important to provide full information to patients and families at the time of considering ongoing ventilation to ensure that an informed choice is made, especially in patients with progressive disorders. Family and community support is extremely valuable for a patient on nocturnal ventilatory support. Family acceptance of the therapy is important for ongoing compliance and for adequate maintenance of the equipment. Many patients report that they feel very isolated because there are so few people within the community with the same problem. This can manifest itself in at least two ways. Firstly, they feel that no one in their peer group really understands what they are experiencing and secondly they feel that health care providers in their local community do not understand their condition or their needs.

While patients are able to travel and stay with family and friends, they are often reluctant to do so because of the extra demands in terms of noise and setting up the ventilator. This can be particularly difficult for young people who wish to stay with friends and yet dread the consequences of being different. The noise of the equipment can be dampened with a soundproof casing which should be designed to still allow adequate air into the inlet port and prevent overheating.

Care and maintenance of equipment

While patients are not ventilator dependent, many express considerable anxiety about the risk of being without the ventilator even for one night. They are anxious about the symptoms of sleep deprivation and hypercapnia. Those who are geographically isolated or live alone are particularly vulnerable to equipment failure. Back-up systems and emergency plans are valuable and need to be worked out with each individual. Patients should be encouraged to enter into a regular maintenance agreement with the companies or hospitals supplying the equipment. All relevant instructions for cleaning and maintenance should be provided in writing and in their preferred language.

PHYSIOTHERAPY INTERVENTION DURING NON-INVASIVE VENTILATION

Physiotherapists have been involved in the application of non-invasive ventilation since the polio epidemics of the 1950s. Through until the mid-1970s physiotherapists routinely administered respiratory medications by intermittent positive pressure breathing (IPPB) through a mask or mouthpiece. This mode of treatment was also used by physiotherapists to improve ventilation or reduce dyspnoea associated with a high work of breathing. A considerable amount of research has been done and reviewed by physiotherapists which contributed to rationalizing the use of this technique (Bennett et al 1976, Berend et al 1978).

By the late 1970s and through the 1980s IPPB was being used predominantly to increase ventilation in patients with severe pain or with poor ventilatory control. It was also an excellent tool to provide hyperoxygenation and hyperinflation prior to and after nasopharyngeal or oropharyngeal suctioning. It has also been effective for sputum removal and for improving ventilation in specific groups (Starke et al 1979) particularly those who do not have sufficient conscious control of ventilation to increase their tidal volume independently. CPAP and bilevel positive pressure devices have replaced IPPB in many centres, being used on both medical and surgical wards as part of an overall strategy to increase ventilation, clear secretions and improve gas exchange.

By the mid- to late 1980s the potential advantages of non-invasive ventilation in the management of chronic respiratory failure began to be realized (Grunstein et al 1991). Since that time physiotherapists have been closely involved in the application of this technique and investigation into its role in a wide range of clinical situations (Ellis et al 1987, 1988, Piper et al 1992,

Bott et al 1993, Conway et al 1993, Keilty et al 1994, Piper & Sullivan 1994b, Piper & Willson 1996).

Physiotherapists may become involved with the application of this technique at a number of different levels (Box 6.2). Their skills and knowledge base regarding respiratory disease and its management place them in a good position to be key members in any non-invasive ventilation service. Physiotherapists are experienced in assessing breathing patterns, and coaching patients to alter breathing in order to improve ventilation. When implementing non-invasive ventilatory support, training of the patient to accept the mask and flow from the device is essential for eventual acceptance. There is also the need for close bedside monitoring of the patient, with ongoing ventilator adjustments to optimize ventilatory support and maximize patient comfort. Such adjustments require

---

Box 6.2 Role of the physiotherapist

Assessment of the patient
- Identification of symptoms of sleep disordered breathing
- Bedside pulmonary function testing including respiratory muscle strength
- Exercise tolerance (e.g. 6-minute walking test, shuttle walking test)
- Level of dyspnoea during daily activities

Initiating therapy
- Choice of device and setting
- Acclimatizing patient to mask and machine
- Education of patient and family regarding therapy
- Monitoring response to therapy

Planning a concurrent rehabilitation programme
- Need for oxygen and the level required during activities
- Upper limb and whole body training
- Lifestyle modification
- Use of ventilatory support as part of secretion clearance

Discharge planning
- Training patient and/or care givers in the care and operation of the equipment
- Home exercise programme
- Ongoing appointments and emergency plans

Follow-up
- Pulmonary function testing
- Exercise tolerance
- Trouble shooting problems: technical problems versus changes in clinical condition

a solid understanding of respiratory physiology as well as good clinical skills in assessing the response of the patient to therapy.

The use of non-invasive ventilation should be seen as an adjunct to other physiotherapeutic techniques as part of an overall rehabilitation programme. Use of this modality has been reported to improve secretion clearance and increase tolerance to other physiotherapy procedures (Piper et al 1992). It permits patients to adopt positions for postural drainage that they would otherwise not be able to adopt due to breathlessness. In patients with severe muscle weakness and poor cough, mask ventilation may be used to assist deep breathing and mobilization of secretions. Anecdotally, patients report being able to tolerate longer physiotherapy sessions when using ventilatory support, which is important in patients who tire easily but who have retained or copious secretions. The tidal volume or inspiratory pressure of the device may be increased during physiotherapy sessions to aid chest wall expansion and assist the mobilization of secretions. The use of mask ventilation in this situation should be seen as an integral part of the patient's respiratory care regimen, and used in conjunction with other physiotherapeutic techniques.

By the time patients with chronic respiratory failure present for nocturnal ventilatory support they are usually severely debilitated. Their presentation is usually characterized by severe shortness of breath on exertion, excessive daytime sleepiness, fatigue, prolonged illness and regular hospitalization. Because of all of these factors it is very likely that significant peripheral deconditioning has occurred which limits their tolerance to daily activities and exercise performance. After a period of nocturnal ventilatory support, patients are able to perform a great deal more work without fatigue and are capable of a reconditioning programme which should improve their quality of life further.

The beneficial effects of positive pressure during exercise in patients with severe lung disease have been reported (Keilty et al 1994). Benefits include reduced breathlessness, increased exercise time and improved oxygen saturation. However, the benefits of routine application of this technique during exercise training remain unclear and await further investigation.

SUMMARY

Non-invasive ventilation is a technique which can improve gas exchange and reduce the work of breathing and is becoming increasingly used to manage both chronic and acute respiratory failure. Physiotherapists will continue to have a significant role in the effective management of these patients.

REFERENCES

Ambrosino N, Foglio K, Rubini F, Clini E, Nava S, Vitacca M 1995 Noninvasive mechanical ventilation in acute respiratory failure due to chronic obstructive pulmonary disease: correlates for success. Thorax 50: 755–757

Barach A L, Martin J, Eckman M 1938 Positive-pressure respiration and its application to the treatment of acute pulmonary edema. Annals of Internal Medicine 12: 754–795

Bennett L, Heath J, Mitchell R 1976 An inpatient observation and comparison of the Bennett's IPPB and aerosol methods of administering salbutamol. Australian Journal of Physiotherapy 23: 111–113

Berend N, Webster J, Marlin E E 1978 Salbutamol by pressure-packed aerosol and by intermittent positive pressure ventilation in chronic obstructive bronchitis. British Journal of Diseases of the Chest 72: 122–124

Bott J, Carroll M P, Conway J H, Keilty S E J, Ward E M, Brown A M, Paul E A et al 1993 Randomised controlled trial of nasal ventilation in acute ventilatory failure due to chronic obstructive airways disease. Lancet 341: 1555–1557

Brochard L, Isabey D, Piquet J 1990 Reversal of acute exacerbations of chronic obstructive lung disease by inspiratory assistance with a face mask. New England Journal of Medicine 323: 1523–1530

Brochard L, Mancebo J, Wysocki M, Lofaso F, Conti G, Rauss A, Simonneau G et al 1995 Noninvasive ventilation for acute exacerbations of chronic obstructive pulmonary disease. New England Journal of Medicine 333: 817–822

Bye P T P, Ellis E R, Issa F G, Donnelly P D, Sullivan C E 1990 The role of sleep in the development of respiratory failure in patients with neuromuscular disease. Thorax 45: 241–247

Chevrolet J C, Jolliet P, Abajo B, Toussi A, Louis M 1991 Nasal positive pressure ventilation in patients with acute respiratory failure. Difficult and time-consuming procedure for nurses. Chest 100: 775–782

Confalonieri M, Parigi P, Scartabellati A, Aiolfi S, Scorsetti S, Nava S, Gandola L 1996 Noninvasive mechanical ventilation improves the immediate and long-term outcome of COPD patients with acute respiratory failure. European Respiratory Journal 9: 422–430

Conway J H, Hitchcock R A, Godfrey R C, Carroll M P 1993 Nasal intermittent positive pressure ventilation in acute exacerbations of chronic obstructive pulmonary disease – a preliminary study. Respiratory Medicine 87: 387–394

Douglas N J, White D P, Pickett C K, Weil J V, Zwillich C W 1982 Respiration during sleep in normal man. Thorax 37: 840–844

Elliott M W, Mulvey D A, Moxham J, Green M, Branthwaite M A 1991 Domiciliary nocturnal nasal intermittent positive pressure ventilation in COPD: mechanisms underlying changes in blood gas tensions. European Respiratory Journal 4: 1044–1052

Elliott M W, Simonds A K 1995 Nocturnal assisted ventilation using positive airway pressure: the effect of expiratory positive airway pressure. European Respiratory Journal 8: 436–440

Ellis E R, Bye P T P, Bruderer J W, Sullivan C E 1987 Treatment of respiratory failure in patients with neuromuscular disease. American Review of Respiratory Disease 135: 148–152

Ellis E R, Grunstein R R, Chan C S, Bye P T P, Sullivan C E 1988. Treatment of nocturnal respiratory failure in kyphoscoliosis. Chest 94: 811–815

Fernandez R, Blanch L, Valles J, Baigorri F, Artigas A 1993 Pressure support ventilation via face mask in acute respiratory failure in hypercapnic COPD patients. Intensive Care Medicine 19: 456–461

Ferguson G T, Gilmartin M 1995 CO_2 rebreathing during BIPAP ventilatory assistance. American Journal of Respiratory and Critical Care Medicine 151: 1126–1135

Garay S M, Turino G M, Goldring R M 1981 Sustained reversal of chronic hypercapnia in patients with alveolar hypoventilation syndromes: long-term maintenance with noninvasive mechanical ventilation. American Journal of Medicine 70: 269–274

Gastaut H, Tassinari C A, Duron B 1966 Polygraphic study of the episodic diurnal and nocturnal manifestations of the Pickwick syndrome. Brain Research 1: 167–186

Gay P C, Patel A M, Viggiano R W, Hubmayr R D 1991 Nocturnal nasal ventilation for treatment of patients with hypercapnic respiratory failure. Mayo Clinical Proceedings 66: 695–703

Goldstein R S, Psek J A, Gort E H 1995 Home mechanical ventilation. Demographics and user perspectives. Chest 108: 1581–1586

Gould G A, Gugger M, Molloy J, Tsara V, Shapiro C M, Douglas N J 1988 Breathing pattern and eye movement density during REM sleep in humans. American Review of Respiratory Disease 138: 874–877

Grunstein R R, Ellis E R, Hillman D, McEvoy R D, Robertson C F, Saunders N A 1991 Treatment of sleep disordered breathing. The Medical Journal of Australia 154: 355–359

Hodson M E, Madden B P, Steven M H, Tsang V T, Yacoub M H 1991 Non-invasive mechanical ventilation for cystic fibrosis patients – a potential bridge to transplantation. European Respiratory Journal 4: 524–527

Keilty S E J, Ponte J, Fleming T A, Moxham J 1994 Effect of inspiratory pressure support on exercise tolerance and breathlessness in patients with severe stable chronic obstructive pulmonary disease. Thorax 49: 990–994

Kramer N, Meyer T J, Mehang J, Cece R D, Hill N S 1995 Randomized, prospective trial of noninvasive positive pressure ventilation in acute respiratory failure. American Journal of Respiratory and Critical Care Medicine 151: 1799–1806

Meduri G U, Turner R E, Abou-Shala N, Wunderink R, Tolley E 1996 Non-invasive positive-pressure ventilation via face mask: first-line intervention in patients with acute hypercapnic and hypoxemic respiratory failure. Chest 109: 179–193

Meecham Jones D J, Wedzicha J A 1993 Comparison of pressure and volume preset nasal ventilator systems in stable chronic respiratory failure. European Respiratory Journal 6: 1060–1064

Meecham Jones D J, Paul E A, Grahame-Clarke C, Wedzicha J A 1994 Nasal ventilation in acute exacerbations of chronic obstructive pulmonary disease: effect of ventilation mode on arterial blood gas tensions. Thorax 49: 1222–1224

Meecham Jones D J, Paul E A, Jones P W, Wedzicha J A 1995 Nasal pressure support ventilation plus oxygen compared with oxygen therapy alone in hypercapnic COPD. American Journal of Respiratory and Critical Care Medicine 152: 538–544

Parreira V F, Jounieaux V, Aubert G, Dury M, Delguste P E, Rodenstein D O 1996 Nasal two-level positive-pressure ventilation in normal subjects. Effects on the glottis and ventilation. American Journal of Respiratory and Critical Care Medicine 153: 1616–1623

Paulus J, Willig T N 1993 Nasal ventilation in neuromuscular disorders: respiratory management and patient's experience. European Respiratory Review 3: 245–249

Pennock B E, Crawshaw L, Kaplan P D 1994 Noninvasive nasal mask ventilation for acute respiratory failure. Institution of a new therapeutic technology for routine use. Chest 105: 441–444

Piper A J, Sullivan C E 1994a Sleep breathing in neuromuscular disease. In: Saunders N, Sullivan C E (eds) Sleep and breathing, 2nd edn. Marcel Dekker, New York, pp 761–821

Piper A J, Sullivan C E 1994b Effects of short-term NIPPV in the treatment of patients with severe obstructive sleep apnea and hypercapnia. Chest 105: 434–440

Piper A J, Willson G 1996 Nocturnal nasal ventilatory support in the management of daytime hypercapnic respiratory failure. Australian Journal of Physiotherapy 42(1): 17–29

Piper A J, Parker S, Torzillo P J, Sullivan C E, Bye P T P 1992 Nocturnal nasal IPPV stabilizes patients with cystic fibrosis and hypercapnic respiratory failure. Chest 102: 846–850

Pollack C V, Fleisch K B, Dowsey K 1995 Treatment of acute bronchospasm with beta-adrenergic agonist aerosols delivered by a nasal bilevel positive airway pressure circuit. Annals of Emergency Medicine 26: 552–557

Poulton E P, Oxon D M 1936 Left-sided heart failure with pulmonary edema – its treatment with the 'pulmonary plus pressure machine'. Lancet 231: 981–983

Raphael J C, Chevret S, Chastang C, Bouvet F 1994 Randomised trial of preventive nasal ventilation in Duchenne muscular dystrophy. Lancet 343: 1600–1603

Restrick L J, Scott A D, Ward E M, Feneck R O, Cornwell W E, Wedzicha J A 1993 Nasal intermittent positive-pressure ventilation in weaning intubated patients with chronic respiratory failure from assisted intermittent, positive-pressure ventilation. Respiratory Medicine 87: 199–204

Richards G N, Cistulli P A, Ungar G, Berthon-Jones M, Sullivan C E 1996 Mouth leak with nasal continuous positive airway pressure increases nasal airway resistance. American Journal of Respiratory and Critical Care Medicine 154: 182–186

Saunders N A, Powles A C P, Rebuck A S 1976 Ear oximetry: accuracy and practicability in assessment of arterial oxygenation. American Review of Respiratory Disease 113: 745–749

Servera E, Perez M, Marin J, Vergara P, Castano R 1995 Noninvasive nasal mask ventilation beyond the ICU for an exacerbation of chronic respiratory insufficiency. Chest 108: 1572–1576

Simonds A K, Elliott M W 1995 Outcome of domiciliary nasal intermittent positive pressure ventilation in restrictive and obstructive disorders. Thorax 50: 604–609

Soo Hoo G W, Santiago S, Williams A J 1994 Nasal mechanical ventilation for hypercapnic respiratory failure in chronic obstructive pulmonary disease: Determinants of success and failure. Critical Care Medicine 22: 1253–1261

Starke I D, Webber B A, Branthwaite M A 1979 IPPB and hypercapnia in respiratory failure. Anaesthesia 34: 283–287

Strumpf D A, Millman R P, Carlisle C C, Grattan L M, Ryan S M, Erickson A D, Hill N S 1991 Nocturnal positive-pressure ventilation via nasal mask in patients with severe chronic obstructive pulmonary disease. American Review of Respiratory Disease 144: 1234–1239

Sullivan C E, Berthon-Jones M, Issa F G, Eves L 1981 Reversal of obstructive sleep apnea by continuous positive airway pressure applied through the nose. Lancet 1: 862–865

Trask C H, Cree E M 1962 Oximeter studies on patients with chronic obstructive emphysema, awake and during sleep. New England Journal of Medicine 266: 639–642

Udwadia Z F, Santis G K, Steven M H, Simonds A K 1992 Nasal ventilation to facilitate weaning in patients with chronic respiratory insufficiency. Thorax 47: 715–718

Vianello A, Bevilacqua M, Salvador V, Cardaioli C, Vincenti E 1994 Long-term nasal intermittent positive pressure ventilation in advanced Duchenne's muscular dystrophy. Chest 105: 445–448

Vitacca M, Rubini F, Foglio K, Scalvini S, Nava S, Ambrosino N 1993 Noninvasive modalities of positive pressure ventilation improve the outcome of acute exacerbations in COLD patients. Intensive Care Medicine 19: 450–455

Vitacca M, Clini E, Rubini F, Nava S, Foglio K, Ambrosino N 1996 Non-invasive mechanical ventilation in severe chronic obstructive lung disease and acute respiratory failure: short- and long-term prognosis. Intensive Care Medicine 22: 94–100

Weirs P W J, LeCoultre R, Dallinga O T, Van Dijl W, Meinesz A F, Sluiter H J 1977 Cuirass respirator treatment of chronic respiratory failure in scoliotic patients. Thorax 32: 221–228

Woollam C H M 1976 The development of apparatus for intermittent negative pressure respiration (1) 1832–1918. Anaesthesia 31: 537–547

Wysocki M, Tric L, Wolff M A, Millet H, Herman B 1995 Noninvasive pressure support ventilation in patients with acute respiratory failure. A randomized comparison with conventional therapy. Chest 107: 761–768

FURTHER READING

Meduri G U 1996 Noninvasive positive pressure ventilation in patients with acute respiratory failure. Clinics in Chest Medicine 17: 513–553

Simonds A K 1996 Non-invasive respiratory support. Chapman & Hall, London

7

The effects of positioning and mobilization on oxygen transport

Elizabeth Dean

INTRODUCTION

The purpose of this chapter is to provide a framework for clinical decision making with respect to positioning and mobilizing patients with cardiopulmonary dysfunction. 'Cardiopulmonary dysfunction' refers to impairment of one or more steps in the oxygen transport pathway. First, the oxygen transport pathway and the factors that contribute to impairment of oxygen transport are described. Second, three clinically significant effects of positioning and mobilization are distinguished:

1. To improve oxygen transport in acute cardiopulmonary dysfunction
2. To improve oxygen transport in the post-acute and chronic stages of cardiopulmonary dysfunction
3. To prevent the negative effects of restricted mobility, particularly those that adversely affect oxygen transport.

In addition, the physiological and scientific rationale for use of positioning and mobilization for each of the above effects is described. Conceptualizing cardiopulmonary dysfunction as impairment of the steps in the oxygen transport pathway and exploiting positioning and mobilization as primary interventions in remediating this impairment will maximize physiotherapy efficacy.

The following terms (Ross & Dean 1989) have been adopted in this chapter:

1. *Body positioning* refers to the application of

positioning to optimize oxygen transport, primarily by manipulating the effect of gravity on cardiopulmonary and cardiovascular function.

2. *Mobilization and exercise* refer to the application of progressive exercise to elicit cardiopulmonary and cardiovascular responses to enhance oxygen transport. In the context of cardiopulmonary physiotherapy, 'mobilization' refers to low-intensity exercise for typically acutely ill patients or those with severely compromised functional work capacity.

3. *Optimizing oxygen transport* is the goal of positioning and mobilization. The 'adaptation' or 'training-sensitive' zone defines the upper and lower limits of the various indices of oxygen transport needed to elicit the optimal adaptation of the steps in the oxygen transport pathway. This zone is based on an analysis of the factors that contribute to cardiopulmonary dysfunction, and thus is specific for each patient.

CONCEPTUAL FRAMEWORK FOR CLINICAL DECISION MAKING

The oxygen transport pathway

Optimal cardiopulmonary function and gas exchange reflect the optimal matching of oxygen demand and supply (Dantzker 1983, Weber et al 1983). The efficiency with which oxygen is transported from the atmosphere along the steps of the oxygen transport pathway to the tissues determines the efficiency of oxygen transport overall (Fig. 7.1). The steps in the oxygen transport pathway include ventilation of the alveoli, diffusion of oxygen across the alveolar capillary membrane, perfusion of the lungs, biochemical reaction of oxygen with the blood, affinity of oxygen with haemoglobin, cardiac output, integrity of the peripheral circulation, and oxygen extraction at the tissue level (Johnson 1973). At rest, the demand for oxygen reflects basal metabolic requirements. Metabolic demand normally changes in response to gravitational (positional), exercise, and psychological stressors. When one or more steps in the oxygen transport pathway is impaired secondary to cardiopulmonary dysfunction, oxygen demand

at rest and in response to stressors can be increased significantly. Impairment of one step in the pathway may be compensated by other steps, thereby maintaining normal gas exchange and arterial oxygenation. However, with more severe impairment involving several steps, arterial oxygenation may be reduced, the work of the heart and lungs increased, tissue oxygenation impaired and, in the most extreme situation, multisystem organ failure may ensue.

While the oxygen transport pathway ensures that an adequate supply of oxygen meets the demands of the working tissues, the carbon dioxide pathway ensures that carbon dioxide, a primary by-product of metabolism, is eliminated. This pathway is basically the reverse of the oxygen transport pathway in that carbon dioxide is transported from the tissues via the circulation to the lungs for elimination. Carbon dioxide is a highly diffusible gas and is readily eliminated from the body. However, carbon dioxide retention is a hallmark of diseases in which the ventilatory muscle pump is operating inefficiently or the normal elastic recoil of the lung parenchyma is lost.

Factors contributing to cardiopulmonary dysfunction

Cardiopulmonary dysfunction, in which oxygen transport is threatened or impaired, results from four principal factors, namely, the underlying disease pathophysiology, bed rest/recumbency and restricted mobility, extrinsic factors imposed by the patient's medical care, and intrinsic factors relating to the patient (Box 7.1) (Dean 1993a, Dean & Ross 1992a). An analysis of those factors that contribute to cardiopulmonary dysfunction provides the basis for positioning and mobilization to enhance oxygen transport for a given patient. The treatment is then directed at the specific underlying contributing factors. In some cases, e.g. low haemoglobin, the underlying impairment of oxygen transport cannot be affected by physical intervention. However, because such factors influence treatment outcome, they need to be considered when planning, modifying and progressing treatment.

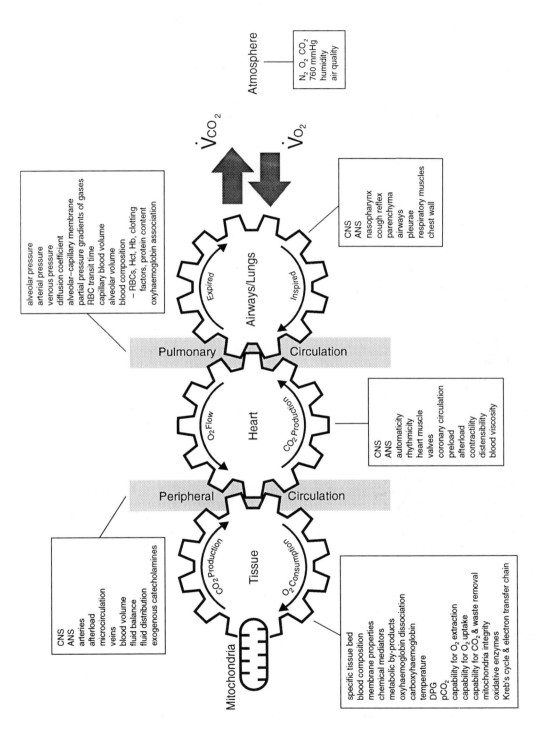

Fig. 7.1 A scheme of the components of ventilatory–cardiovascular–metabolic coupling underlying oxygen transport. Modified from Wasserman et al (1987). CNS, central nervous system; ANS, autonomic nervous system; DPG, diphosphoglycerate; RBC, red blood cell; Hct, haematocrit; Hb, haemoglobin.

Box 7.1 Factors contributing to cardiopulmonary dysfunction, i.e. factors that compromise or threaten oxygen transport (adapted from Dean 1993a, Dean & Ross 1992a and Ross & Dean 1992)

- **Cardiopulmonary pathophysiology**
  Acute
  Chronic – primary
        – secondary
  Acute and chronic

- **Bed rest/recumbency and restricted mobility**

- **Extrinsic factors**
  Reduced arousal
  Surgical procedures
  Incisions
  Dressings and bindings
  Casts/splinting devices/traction
  Invasive lines/catheters
  Monitoring equipment
  Medications
  Intubation
  Mechanical ventilation
  Suctioning
  Pain
  Anxiety
  Hospital admission

- **Intrinsic factors**
  Age
  Gender
  Ethnicity
  Congenital abnormalities
  Smoking history
  Occupation
  Air quality
  Obesity
  Nutritional deficits
  Deformity
  Fluid and electrolyte balance
  Conditioning level
  Impaired immunity
  Anaemia/polycythaemia
  Thyroid abnormalities
  Multisystem complications
  Previous medical and surgical history

Multisystem organ dysfunction and failure may lead to or result from cardiopulmonary dysfunction; thus they are associated with significant mortality and morbidity. In these conditions, multiple factors impair multiple steps in the oxygen transport pathway; hence, identifying which steps are affected and amenable to physiotherapy interventions is tantamount to optimal treatment outcome (Dean & Frownfelter 1996).

THERAPEUTIC EFFECTS OF POSITIONING AND MOBILIZATION

To improve oxygen transport in acute cardiopulmonary dysfunction

Positioning and mobilization have profound acute effects on cardiopulmonary and cardiovascular function, and hence on oxygen transport (Table 7.1). These effects translate into improved gas exchange overall: reduction in the fraction of inspired oxygen, pharmacological and ventilatory support (Svanberg 1957, Burns & Jones 1975, Dean 1985). Such effects need to be exploited in the management of acute cardiopulmonary dysfunction with the use of positioning and mobilization as *primary* treatment interventions to enhance oxygen transport and as between-treatment interventions (Dean & Ross 1992b, Ross & Dean 1992).

Positioning

Physiological and scientific rationale. The distributions of ventilation ($\dot{V}_A$), perfusion ($\dot{Q}$), and ventilation and perfusion matching in the lungs are primarily influenced by gravity, hence, body position (Clauss et al 1968, West 1962, 1977). The intrapleural pressure becomes less negative down the upright lung. Thus, the apices have a greater initial volume and reduced compliance than do the bases. Because the bases are more compliant in this position, they exhibit greater volume changes during ventilation. In addition to these gravity-dependent interregional differences in lung volume, ventilation is influenced by intraregional differences which are dependent on regional mechanical differences in the compliance of the lung parenchyma and the resistance to airflow in the airways. Perfusion increases down the upright lung such that the $\dot{V}_A/\dot{Q}$ ratio in the apices is disproportionately high compared with that in the bases. Ventilation and perfusion matching is optimal in the mid-lung region. Manipulating body position, however, alters both interregional and intraregional determinants of ventilation and perfusion and their matching. When considering specific positions to enhance arterial oxygenation for a given

Table 7.1 Acute effects of upright positioning and mobilization an oxygen transport (adapted from Dean & Ross (1992a) and Imle & Klemic (1989))

Systemic response	Stimulus	
	Positioning (supine to upright)	Mobilization
Cardiopulmonary	↑ Total lung capacity ↑ Tidal volume ↑ Vital capacity ↑ Functioning residual capacity ↑ Residual volume ↑ Expiratory reserve volume ↑ Forced expiratory volumes ↑ Forced expiratory flows ↑ Lung compliance ↓ Airway resistance ↓ Airway closure ↑ PaO_2 ↑ AP diameter of chest ↓ Lateral diameter of rib cage and abdomen Altered pulmonary blood flow distribution ↓ Work of breathing ↑ Diaphragmatic excursion ↑ Mobilization of secretions	↑ Alveolar ventilation ↑ Tidal volume ↑ Breathing frequency ↑ $A–aO_2$ gradient ↓ Pulmonary arteriovenous shunt ↑ $\dot{V}_A/\dot{Q}$ matching ↑ Distension and recruitment of lung units with low ventilation and low perfusion ↑ Mobilization of secretions ↑ Pulmonary lymphatic drainage ↑ Surfactant production and distribution
Cardiovascular	↑ Total blood volume ↓ Central blood volume ↓ Central venous pressure ↓ Pulmonary vascular congestion ↑ Lymphatic drainage ↓ Work of the heart	↑ Cardiac output ↑ Stroke volume and heart rate ↑ Oxygen binding in blood ↑ Oxygen dissociation and extraction at the tissue level

AP, anteroposterior; ↑, increases; ↓, decreases.

patient, one needs to consider the underlying pathophysiology impairing cardiopulmonary function, the effects of bed rest/ recumbency and restricted mobility, aspects of the patient's care and unique aspects of the patient.

Although the negative effects of the supine position have been well documented for several decades (Dripps & Waters 1941, Dean & Ross 1992b), supine or recumbent positions are frequently assumed by patients in hospital. These positions are non-physiologic and are associated with significant reductions in lung volumes and flow rates, and increased work of breathing (Craig et al 1971, Hsu & Hickey 1976). The decrease in functional residual capacity (FRC) contributes to closure of the dependent airways and reduced arterial oxygenation (Ray et al 1974). This effect is accentuated in older persons (Leblanc et al 1970), patients with cardiopulmonary disease (Fowler 1949), patients with abdominal pathology, smokers and obese individuals.

The haemodynamic consequences of the supine position are also remarkable. The gravity-dependent increase in central blood volume may precipitate vascular congestion, reduced compliance and pulmonary oedema (Sjostrand 1951, Blomqvist & Stone 1983). The commensurate increase in stroke volume increases the work of the heart (Levine & Lown 1952). Within 6 hours, a compensatory diuresis can lead to a loss of circulating blood volume and orthostatic intolerance, i.e. haemodynamic intolerance to the upright position. Bed rest deconditioning has been attributed to this reduction in blood volume and the impairment of the volume-regulating mechanisms rather than physical deconditioning per se (Hahn-Winslow 1985). Thus, the upright position is essential to maximize lung volumes and flow rates, and this position is the only means of optimizing fluid shifts such that the circulating blood volume and the volume-regulating mechanisms are maintained. The upright position coupled with movement is necessary to promote normal fluid regulation and balance (Lamb et al 1964).

Side-to-side positioning is frequently used in the clinical setting. If applied in response to assessment rather than routinely (Chuley et al 1982), the benefits derived from such positioning can be enhanced. Adult patients with unilateral lung disease may derive greater benefit when the affected lung is uppermost (Remolina et al 1981). Arterial oxygen tension is increased secondary to improved ventilation of the unaffected lung when this lung is dependent. Patients with uniformly distributed bilateral lung disease may derive greater benefit when the right lung is lowermost (Zack et al 1974). In this case, arterial oxygen tension is increased secondary to improved ventilation of the right lung, which may reflect the increased size of the right lung compared with the left and that, in this position, the heart and adjacent lung tissue are subjected to less compression. Although various studies have shown beneficial effects of side lying, positioning should be based on multiple considerations including the distribution of disease if optimal results are to be obtained.

The prone position has considerable physiological justification in patients with cardiopulmonary compromise (Douglas et al 1977). The beneficial effects of the prone position on arterial oxygenation may reflect improved lung compliance, tidal ventilation, diaphragmatic excursion and FRC, and reduced airway closure (Dean 1985). A variant of the prone position, prone abdomen free, has shown additional benefits over prone abdomen restricted. In the prone abdomen free position, the patient is positioned such that the movement of the abdomen is unencumbered by the bed. This can be achieved either by raising the patient's body in relation to the bed so that the abdomen falls free, or by using a bed with a hole cut out at the level of the abdomen. Despite compelling evidence to support the prone position, this position may be poorly tolerated in some patients, or may be contraindicated in haemodynamically unstable patients. In these situations, intermediate positions approximating prone

may produce many of the beneficial effects and minimize any potential hazard.

Positioning for drainage of pulmonary secretions may be indicated in some patients (Kirilloff et al 1985). Historically, these positions have been based on the anatomical arrangement of the bronchopulmonary segments to facilitate drainage of a particular segment. The bronchiole to the segment of interest is positioned perpendicular to facilitate drainage with the use of gravity. The efficacy of postural drainage compared with deep breathing and coughing induced with mobilization/exercise and repositioning of the patient, has not been established. However, the fact that mobilization impacts on more steps in the oxygen transport pathway including the airways, to effect secretion clearance, supports the exploitation of mobilization coupled with deep breathing manoeuvres and coughing as a *primary* treatment intervention.

Assessment and treatment planning. Body positioning, i.e. the specific positions selected, the duration of time spent in each position, and the frequency the position is assumed, is based on a consideration of the factors that contribute to cardiopulmonary dysfunction and treatment response. Understanding of the physiology of cardiopulmonary and cardiovascular function and the effects of disease, highlight certain positions that are theoretically ideal. However, these positions need to be modified or may be contraindicated for a given patient, based on other considerations (Box 7.1). For example, if extreme positional changes are contraindicated, small degrees of positional rotation performed frequently can have significant benefit on gas exchange and arterial oxygenation. A three-quarters prone position may produce favourable results when the full prone position is contraindicated or is not feasible. This modification may simulate the prone abdomen free position which has been shown to augment the effect of the traditional prone abdomen restricted position (Douglas et al 1977). Furthermore, a three-quarters prone position may be particularly beneficial in patients with obese or swollen abdomens who may not tolerate other variations of the prone position. With

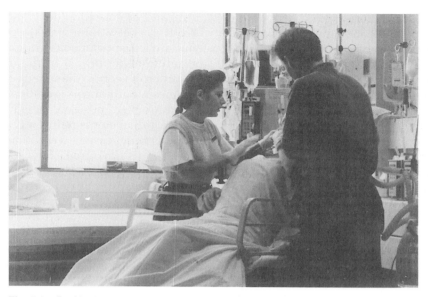

Fig. 7.2 Positioning a critically ill patient may require several people and continual monitoring of the patient's response. Even though a position (particularly an upright position) may only be tolerated for a short period of time, the physiological benefits are considerable.

attention to the patient's condition, invasive lines and leads, and appropriate monitoring, a patient can be aggressively positioned (Fig. 7.2).

The time which a patient spends in a position and the frequency with which that position is assumed over a period of time are based on the indications for the position and treatment outcome. Objective measures of the various steps that are compromised in the oxygen transport pathway as well as indices of oxygen transport overall, are used in making these decisions. Subjective evaluation based on clinical judgement also has a place. A specific position can be justified, provided there is objective and subjective evidence of improvement. Signs and symptoms of deterioration need to be monitored so that deleterious positions can be avoided and deterioration secondary to excessive time in any one position can be detected. Prolonged duration in any single position will inevitably lead to compromise of the function of dependent lung zones.

The ratio of treatment to between-treatment time is low. Typically, between-treatment time consists of some combination of positioning and mobilization. Positioning and mobilizing patients between treatments may be incorporated as an extension of treatment. Patients require monitoring and observation during these periods, as well as treatments. Between-treatment time may incorporate the use of maximally restful positions that do not compromise oxygen transport. Lastly, patients are positioned and mobilized between treatments to prevent the negative effects of restricted mobility and recumbency.

Special consideration (e.g. with respect to specific positioning and the use of supports) needs to be given to positioning patients who are comatose or paralysed in that their joints and muscles are relatively unprotected and prone to trauma.

Progression. Progression of positioning involves decision making to incorporate new positions or modify previous positions, to modify the duration spent in each position and the frequency with which each position is assumed over a period of time. These decisions are also based on the factors that contribute to cardiopulmonary dysfunction and objective and subjective indices of change in the patient's cardiopulmonary status. With improvement in cardiopulmonary status, the patient spends more time in erect positions and is mobilized more frequently and independently.

Physiologic 'stir-up' is an objective of positioning (Dean 1996a). The purpose is to effect the normal gravitational stress on cardiopulmonary and cardiovascular function that is experienced in health. This is best simulated if patients are positioned from one extreme position to another, e.g. supine to prone or upright, rather than from half to full side lying which is associated with a lesser 'stir-up' effect. Haemodynamically unstable patients, however, require greater monitoring during extreme position changes, and may not tolerate some position changes well.

Mobilization

Physiological and scientific rationale. The acute response to mobilization/exercise reflects a commensurate increase in oxygen transport to provide oxygen to the working muscles. The increase is dependent on the intensity of the mobilization/exercise stimulus. The demand for oxygen and oxygen consumption ($\dot{V}O_2$) increases as exercise continues, with commensurate increases in minute ventilation ($\dot{V}_E$), i.e. the amount of air inhaled per minute, cardiac output, and oxygen extraction at the tissue level. Relatively low intensities of mobilization can have a direct and profound effect on oxygen transport in patients with acute cardiopulmonary dysfunction (Lewis 1980, Dull & Dull 1983, Dean & Ross 1992a) and need to be instituted early after the initial pathological insult (Orlava 1959, Wenger 1982). The resulting exercise hyperpnoea, i.e. the increase in $\dot{V}_E$, is effected by an increase in tidal volume and breathing frequency. In addition, ventilation and perfusion matching is augmented by the distension and recruitment of lung zones with low ventilation and low perfusion. Spontaneous exercise-induced deep breaths are associated with improved flow rates, and mobilization of pulmonary secretions (Wolff et al 1977). In clinical populations, these effects elicit spontaneous coughing. When mobilization is performed in the upright position, the anteroposterior diameter of the chest wall assumes a normal configuration compared with the recumbent position in which the anteroposterior diameter is reduced and the transverse diameter is increased. In addition, diaphragmatic excursion is favoured, flow rates augmented and coughing is mechanically facilitated. The work of breathing may be reduced with caudal displacement of the diaphragm and the work of the heart is minimized by the displacement of fluid away from the central circulation to the legs.

With respect to cardiovascular effects, acute mobilization/exercise increases cardiac output (CO) by increasing stroke volume and heart rate. This is associated with increased blood pressure and increased coronary and peripheral muscle perfusion.

Passive movement of the limbs may augment deep breaths and heart function. There is little scientific evidence, however, to support any additional benefit from various facilitation techniques (Bethune 1975). Thus, time allocated to the use of passive manoeuvres may compete with time for positioning and mobilization, i.e. interventions with demonstrated clinical efficacy. Although passive movements have a relatively small effect on cardiopulmonary function, they have several important benefits for neuromuscular and musculoskeletal function which support their use provided they do not replace active movement.

Assessment and treatment planning. For practical and ethical considerations, the mobilization plan for the patient with acute cardiopulmonary dysfunction cannot be based on a standardized exercise test, as is the case for patients with chronic conditions. However, response to a mobilization/exercise stimulus can be assessed during a patient's routine activities, such as turning or moving in bed, activities of daily living or responding to routine nursing and medical procedures (Dean 1996b). Comparable to prescribing exercise for the patient with chronic cardiopulmonary dysfunction, the parameters are specifically defined so that the stimulus is optimally therapeutic. The optimal stimulus is that which stresses the oxygen transport capacity of the patient and effects the greatest adaptation without deterioration or excessive distress.

To promote adaptation of the steps in the oxygen transport pathway to the stimulation of acute mobilization, the stimulus is administered in a comparable manner to that in an exercise programme prescribed for chronic cardiopulmonary dysfunction. The components include a pre-exercise period, a warm-up period, a steady-state period, a cool-down period and a recovery period (Blair et al 1988). These components optimize the response to exercise by preparing the cardiopulmonary and cardiovascular systems for steady-state exercise, and by permitting these systems to re-establish resting conditions following exercise. The cool-down period, in conjunction with the recovery period, ensures that exercise does not stop abruptly and allows for biochemical degradation and removal of the by-products of metabolism. Mobilization consists of discrete warm-up, steady-state and cool-down periods; the components need to be identified, even in the patient with a very low functional capacity, i.e. a critically ill patient who may be only able to sit up over the edge of the bed. In such cases, preparing to sit up constitutes a warm-up period for the patient; the stimulus of sitting unsupported for several minutes while being aroused and encouraged to talk, constitutes a steady-state period. Returning to bed constitutes the cool-down period. In the recovery period, the patient continues to be observed to ensure that mobilization is tolerated well and that the indices of oxygen transport return to resting levels. This information is then used as the basis for mobilization in the next treatment.

Valid and reliable monitoring practices provide the basis for the parameters of mobilization, assessing the need for progression, and defining the adaptation or training-sensitive zone. Monitoring is also essential given that subjecting patients to mobilization/exercise stimulation is inherently risky, particularly for patients with cardiopulmonary dysfunction. Indices of overall oxygen transport in addition to indices of the function of the individual steps in the oxygen transport pathway provide a detailed profile of the patient's cardiopulmonary status. In critical care settings, the physiotherapist has access to a wide range of measures to assess gas exchange. Minimally, in the general ward setting, measures of breathing frequency, arterial blood gases, arterial saturation, heart rate, blood pressure and clinical observation provide the basis for ongoing assessment, mobilization/exercise, and progression. With appropriate attention to the patient's condition, invasive lines and leads, and appropriate monitoring, a patient can be aggressively mobilized and ambulated (Fig. 7.3).

A fundamental requirement in defining the parameters for mobilization is that the patient's oxygen transport system is capable of increasing the oxygen supply to meet an increasing metabolic demand. If not, mobilization is absolutely contraindicated and the treatment of choice to optimize oxygen transport is body positioning. However, in the case of a patient being severely haemodynamically unstable, even the stress of positioning may be excessive. Thus, although critically ill patients may be treated aggressively, every patient has to be considered individually, otherwise the patient may deteriorate or be seriously endangered.

Progression. Progression and modification of the mobilization stimulus occur more frequently in the management of the patient with acute cardiopulmonary dysfunction compared with the progression of the exercise stimulus for the patient with chronic illness. The status of acutely ill patients can vary considerably within minutes or hours. Whether the mobilization stimulus is increased or decreased in intensity depends on the patient's status and altered responses to mobilization. The mobilization stimulus is adjusted such that it remains optimal despite the patient's changing metabolic needs. Capitalizing on narrow windows of opportunity for therapeutic intervention must be exploited 24 hours a day with respect to the type of mobilization stimulus, its intensity, duration

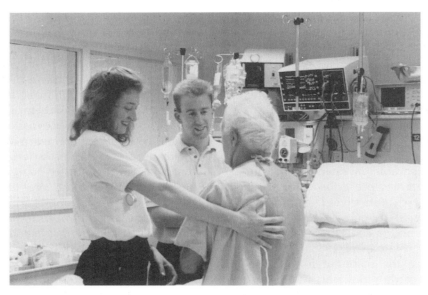

Fig. 7.3 Example of mobilizing a patient to a self-supported upright sitting position. Mobilizing a critically ill patient needs to be a priority wherever possible. Short frequent sessions to the erect position (sitting or standing if possible) with continual monitoring of the patient's response should be the goal. As the patient progresses, sessions increase in intensity and duration, and reduce in frequency.

and frequency, particularly in the critically ill patient.

The 'immovable' patient. Given the well-documented negative effects of restricted mobility, the 'immovable' patient deserves special consideration. Although bed rest is ordered for patients frequently without reservation, the risks need to be weighed against the benefits. Restricted mobility coupled with recumbency constitutes a death knell for many severely compromised patients. Thus, an order for bed rest needs to be evaluated and challenged to ensure that this order is physiologically justified.

Kinetic beds and chairs. Advances in furniture technology to facilitate positioning and mobilizing patients have lagged behind advances in clinical medicine, particularly in the critical care area. Conventional hospital beds are designed to be stationary, and their widths and heights are often non-adjustable, making them difficult for the patient to get in and out of bed. Kinetic beds and chairs have become increasingly available over the past decade; however, they are not widely used clinically. These devices

were originally designed to facilitate positioning and moving heavy and comatose patients. Some beds are designed to rotate on their long axis from side to side over several minutes. Other beds simulate a side to side movement with inflation and deflation of the two sides of an air-filled mattress. Although these beds have potential cardiopulmonary benefit (Glavis et al 1985, Kyle et al 1992), they do not replace active positioning and movement. Mechanically adjustable bedside chairs constitute an important advance. These chairs adjust to a flat horizontal surface that can be adjusted to bed height and positioned beneath the patient lying on the bed. The device with the patient on top is then wheeled parallel to the bed where it can be adjusted back into a chair, and thus the patient assumes a seated position. The degree of recline can be adjusted to meet the patient's needs and for comfort. This chair also facilitates returning the patient to bed. The disadvantages of kinetic beds and chairs include the expense and the potential for overreliance on them. Without these devices, a heavy patient may require several people and several minutes to position in a chair which may be only tolerated for a few minutes. However, the cardiopulmonary benefits of the stimulation of preparing to be moved, the reflex attempts of the patient to assist and adjust to changing position, as well as actually sitting upright in a chair, are not reproduced by bed positioning alone or by a kinetic bed. Research is needed to determine the indications and potential benefits of kinetic beds and chairs so that they can be judiciously used in the clinical setting as an integral therapeutic intervention.

To improve oxygen transport in post-acute and chronic cardiopulmonary dysfunction

In post-acute and chronic cardiopulmonary dysfunction, a primary consequence of impaired oxygen transport is reduced functional work capacity (Wasserman & Whipp 1975, Belman & Wasserman 1981). Work capacity can be improved with long-term exercise which improves the efficiency of the steps in the oxygen transport pathway, and promotes compensation within the pathway as well as by other mechanisms. To optimize the patient's response, exercise can be carried out in judicious body positions in which oxygen transport is favoured.

Exercise is the treatment of choice for patients whose impaired oxygen transport has resulted from chronic cardiopulmonary dysfunction. Body positioning, however, may have some role in severe patients in optimizing oxygen transport at rest. Barach & Beck (1954), for example, reported that emphysematous patients were less breathless, had reduced accessory muscle activity and had a significant reduction in ventilation when positioned in a 16° head-down position. Some patients exhibited greater symptomatic improvement than in the upright position with supplemental oxygen. Classic relaxation positions, e.g. leaning forward with the forearms supported, can also be supported physiologically. Coupling such physiologically justifiable positions with mobilization/exercise will augment the benefits of exercise.

Physiological and scientific rationale. Although the physiological responses to long-term exercise in patients with chronic cardiopulmonary disease may differ from those in healthy persons, patients can significantly improve their functional work capacity (Table 7.2). In healthy persons, an improvement in aerobic capacity reflects improved efficiency of the steps in the oxygen transport pathway to adapt to increased oxygen demands imposed by exercise stress. This adaptation is effected by both central (cardiopulmonary) and peripheral (at the tissue level) changes (Wasserman & Whipp 1975, Dean & Ross 1992a). Such aerobic conditioning is characterized by a training-induced bradycardia secondary to an increased stroke volume and increased oxygen extraction capacity of the working muscle. These adaptation or training responses result in an increased maximal oxygen uptake and maximal voluntary ventilation, and reduced submaximal $\dot{V}_E$, cardiac output, heart rate, blood pressure and perceived exertion. Patients with chronic lung disease, however, are often unable to exercise at the intensity required to elicit an aerobic training response. Their functional work capacity is improved by

Table 7.2 Chronic effects of mobilization/exercise on oxygen transport

Systemic response	
Cardiopulmonary	↑ Capacity for gas exchange ↑ Cardiopulmonary efficiency ↓ Submaximal minute ventilation ↓ Work of breathing
Cardiovascular	Exercise-induced bradycardia ↑ Maximum $\dot{V}O_2$ ↓ Submaximal heart rate, blood pressure, myocardial oxygen demand, stroke volume, cardiac output ↓ Work of the heart ↓ Perceived exertion ↑ Plasma volume Cardiac hypertrophy ↑ Vascularity of the myocardium
Tissue level	↑ Vascularity of working muscle ↑ Myoglobin content and oxidative enzymes in muscle ↑ Oxygen extraction capacity

↑, increases; ↓, decreases.

other mechanisms, e.g. desensitization to breathlessness, improved motivation, improved biomechanical efficiency, increased ventilatory muscle strength and endurance or some combination (Belman & Wasserman 1981, Loke et al 1984). Patients with chronic heart disease such as patients with infarcted left ventricles may be able to train aerobically; however, training adaptation primarily results from peripheral rather than central factors (Bydgman & Wahren 1974, Hossack 1987, Ward et al 1987).

Planning an exercise programme. The exercise programme is based on the principle that oxygen delivery and uptake is enhanced in response to an exercise stimulus which is precisely defined for an individual in terms of the type of exercise, its intensity, duration, frequency and the course of the training programme. These parameters are based on an exercise test in conjunction with assessment findings. Exercise tests are performed on a cycle ergometer, treadmill or with a walk test. The general procedures and protocols are standardized to maximize the validity and reliability of the results (Blair et al 1988, Dean et al 1989). The principles of and guidelines for exercise testing and training patients with chronic lung and heart disease have been well documented (Dean 1993b). The training-sensitive zone is defined by objective and subjective measures of oxygen transport determined from the exercise test. The components of each exercise training session include baseline, warm-up, steady-state portion, cool-down and recovery period (Blair et al 1988, Dean 1993b). The cardiopulmonary and cardiovascular systems are gradually primed for sustaining a given level of exercise stress, whilst in addition the musculoskeletal system adapts correspondingly. Following the steady-state portion of the training session, the cool-down period permits a return to the resting physiological state. Cool-down and recovery periods are essential for the biochemical degradation and elimination of the metabolic by-products of exercise.

Progression. Progression of the exercise programme is based on a repeated exercise test. This is indicated when the exercise prescription no longer elicits the desired physiological responses – specifically, when the steady-state work rate consistently elicits responses at the low end or below the lower limit of the training-sensitive zone for the given indices of oxygen transport. This reflects that maximal adaptation of the steps in the oxygen transport pathway to the given exercise stimulus has occurred. The degree of conditioning achieved is precisely matched to the demands of the exercise stimulus imposed.

To prevent the negative effects of restricted mobility

Although physiologically distinct, the effects of immobility are frequently confounded by the effects of recumbency in the hospitalized patient. Restricted mobility and the concomitant reduction in exercise stress affect virtually every organ system in the body with profound effects on the cardiovascular and neuromuscular systems. Recumbency and the elimination of the vertical gravitational stress exerts its effects primarily on the cardiovascular and cardiopulmonary systems (Dock 1944, Harrison 1944, Blomqvist & Stone 1983). The most serious consequences of restricted mobility and recumbency are those resulting from the effects on the cardiopulmonary and cardiovascular systems, and hence on oxygen transport. Although other consequences of restricted mobility, e.g. increased risk of infection, skin breakdown, and deformity, may not constitute the same immediate threat to oxygen transport and tissue oxygenation, they can have significant implications with respect to morbidity and mortality (Rubin 1988). Thus, restricted mobility and recumbency need to be minimized, and mobility and the upright position maximized to avert the negative consequences of restricted mobility, the risk of morbidity associated with these effects, and the direct and indirect cardiopulmonary and cardiovascular effects. These negative consequences are preventable with frequent repositioning and mobilizing of the patient (Table 7.3). The prevention of these effects is a primary goal of positioning and mobilizing patients between treatments.

Table 7.3 Effects of positioning and mobilization that prevent the negative effects of restricted mobility and recumbency*

Systemic response	
Cardiopulmonary	↑ Alveolar ventilation
	↓ Airway closure
	Alters the distributions of ventilation, perfusion and ventilation and perfusion matching
	Alters pulmonary blood volume
	Alters distending forces on uppermost lung fields
	↓ Secretion pooling
	Secretion mobilization and redistribution
	Alters chest wall configuration and pulmonary mechanics
	Varies work of breathing
Cardiovascular	Alters cardiac compression (positioning), wall tensions, filling pressures
	Alters preload, afterload, and myocardial contraction
	Alters lymphatic drainage
	Varies work of the heart
	Promotes fluid shifts
	Stimulates pressure- and volume-regulating mechanisms of the circulation
	Stimulates vasomotor activity
	Maintains normal fluid balance and distribution
Tissue level	Alters hydrostatic pressure and tissue perfusion
	Maintains oxygen extraction capacity (mobilization)

*Some of the preventive effects of body positioning and mobilization are comparable; however, the magnitude of these effects in response to mobilization tends to be greater than with body positioning.

SUMMARY AND CONCLUSION

Cardiopulmonary dysfunction refers to impairment of one or more steps in the oxygen transport pathway which can impair oxygen transport overall. Factors that can impair the transport of oxygen from the atmosphere to the tissues include cardiopulmonary pathology, bed rest, recumbency, and restricted mobility, extrinsic factors related to the patient's medical care, intrinsic factors related to the patient or some combination of these factors. Positioning and mobilization are two interventions that have potent and direct effects on several of the steps in the oxygen transport pathway. These interventions have a *primary* role in improving oxygen transport in acute and chronic cardiopulmonary dysfunction, and in averting the negative effects of restricted mobility and recumbency particularly those related to cardiopulmonary and cardiovascular function.

The principal goal of physiotherapy in the management of cardiopulmonary dysfunction is to optimize oxygen transport. A systematic approach to achieving this goal consists of:

1. Distinguishing the specific steps in the oxygen transport pathway which are impaired or threatened.

2. Establishing which factors contribute to this impairment.

3. Distinguishing which factors are (a) amenable to positioning and mobilization and (b) not directly amenable to positioning and mobilization, as these factors will modify treatment.

4. Specifying the parameters for positioning and mobilization so that they directly address the factors responsible for the cardiopulmonary dysfunction wherever possible, i.e. to elicit the acute effects of these interventions to enhance oxygen transport, or to elicit the long-term effects on oxygen transport, i.e. training responses and improved functional work capacity.

5. Avoiding the multisystem consequences of restricted mobility and recumbency, particularly those that impair or threaten oxygen transport.

6. Recognizing when positioning or mobilizing a patient needs to be modified to avoid a deleterious outcome.

Conceptualizing cardiopulmonary dysfunction as deficits in the steps in the oxygen transport pathway, and identifying the factors responsible for each impaired step provides a systematic approach to clinical decision making in cardiopulmonary physiotherapy. Positioning and mobilization can then be specifically directed at the mechanisms underlying cardiopulmo- nary dysfunction wherever possible. Such an approach will maximize the efficacy of position- ing and mobilizing patients with cardiopulmo- nary dysfunction and enhance the outcome of medical management overall.

REFERENCES

Barach A L, Beck G J 1954 Ventilatory effect of head-down position in pulmonary emphysema. American Journal of Medicine 16: 55–60

Belman M J, Wasserman K 1981 Exercise training and testing in patients with chronic obstructive pulmonary disease. Basics of Respiratory Disease 10: 1–6

Bethune D D 1975 Neurophysiological facilitation of respiration in the unconscious patient. Physiotherapy Canada 27: 241–245

Blair S N, Painter P, Pate R R et al 1988 Resource manual for guidelines for exercise testing and prescription. Lea & Febiger, Philadelphia

Blomqvist C G, Stone H L 1983 Cardiovascular adjustments to gravitational stress. In: Shepherd J T, Abboud F M (eds) Handbook of physiology. Section 2: circulation. American Physiological Society, Bethesda, vol 2, pp 1025–1063

Burns J R, Jones F L 1975 Early ambulation of patients requiring ventilatory assistance. Chest 68: 608

Bydgman S, Wahren J 1974 Influence of body position on the anginal threshold during leg exercise. European Journal of Clinical Investigation 4: 201–206

Chuley M, Brown J, Summer W 1982 Effect of postoperative immobilization after coronary artery bypass surgery. Critical Care Medicine 10: 176–178

Clauss R H, Scalabrini B Y, Ray R F, Reed G E 1968 Effects of changing body position upon improved ventilation– perfusion relationships. Circulation 37(suppl 2): 214–217

Craig D B, Wahba W M, Don H F 1971 'Closing volume' and its relationship to gas exchange in seated and supine positions. Journal of Applied Physiology 31: 717–721

Dantzker D R 1983 The influence of cardiovascular function on gas exchange. Clinics in Chest Medicine 4: 149–159

Dean E 1985 Effect of body position on pulmonary function. Physical Therapy 65: 613–618

Dean E 1993a Bedrest and deconditioning. Neurology Report 17: 6–9

Dean E 1993b Advances in rehabilitation for older persons with cardiopulmonary dysfunction. In: Katz P R, Kane R L, Mezey M D (eds) Advances in long-term care. Springer-Verlag, New York, ch 1, pp 1–71

Dean E 1996a Body positioning. In: Frownfelter D, Dean E (eds) Principles and practice of cardiopulmonary physical therapy, 3rd edn. Mosby, St Louis

Dean E 1996b Mobilization and exercise. In: Frownfelter D, Dean E (eds) Principles and practice of cardiopulmonary physical therapy, 3rd edn. Mosby, St Louis

Dean E, Frownfelter D 1996 Clinical case study guide to accompany principles and practice of cardiopulmonary physical therapy, 3rd edn. Mosby, St Louis

Dean E, Ross J 1992a Mobilization and exercise conditioning. In: Zadai C (ed) Pulmonary management in physical therapy. Churchill Livingstone, New York

Dean E, Ross J 1992b Discordance between cardiopulmonary physiology and physical therapy: toward a rational basis for practice. Chest 101: 1694–1698

Dean E, Ross J, Bartz J, Purves S 1989 Improving the validity of exercise testing: the effect of practice on performance. Archives of Physical Medicine and Rehabilitation 70: 599–604

Dock W 1944 The evil sequelae of complete bed rest. Journal of the American Medical Association 125: 1083–1085

Douglas W W, Rehder K, Froukje B M 1977 Improved oxygenation in patients with acute respiratory failure: the prone position. American Review of Respiratory Disease 115: 559–566

Dripps R D, Waters R M 1941 Nursing care of surgical patients. I. The 'stir-up'. American Journal of Nursing 41: 530–534

Dull J L, Dull W L 1983 Are maximal inspiratory breathing exercises or incentive spirometry better than early mobilization after cardiopulmonary bypass? Physical Therapy 63: 655–659

Fowler W S 1949 Lung function studies. III. Uneven pulmonary ventilation in normal subjects and patients with pulmonary disease. Journal of Applied Physiology 2: 283–299

Glavis C, Sparacino P, Holzemer W, Skov P 1985 Effect of a rotating bed on mechanically ventilated critically ill patients. Presented at the Third Kinetic Therapy Seminar, San Antonio

Hahn-Winslow E 1985 Cardiovascular consequences of bed rest. Heart & Lung 14: 236–246

Harrison T R 1944 The abuse of rest as a therapeutic measure for patients with cardiovascular disease. Journal of the American Medical Association 125: 1075–1078

Hossack K F 1987 Cardiovascular responses to dynamic exercise. In: Hanson P (ed) Exercise and the heart. W B Saunders, Philadelphia, pp 147–156

Hsu H O, Hickey R F 1976 Effect of posture on functional residual capacity postoperatively. Anesthesiology 44: 520–521

Imle P C, Klemic N 1989 Changes with immobility and methods of mobilization. In: Mackenzie C F (ed) Chest physiotherapy in the intensive care unit, 2nd edn. Williams & Wilkins, Bethesda, pp 188–214

Johnson R L 1973 The lung as an organ of oxygen transport. Basics of Respiratory Disease 2: 1–6

Kirilloff L H, Owens H R, Rogers R M, Mazzocco M C 1985 Does chest physical therapy work? Chest 88: 436–444

Kyle K, Jackiw A, Schroeder S et al 1992 Cardiopulmonary effects of kinetic bed therapy in mechanically ventilated patients. Presented at the American Thoracic Society Meeting, San Antonio

Lamb L E, Johnson R L, Stevens P M 1964 Cardiovascular deconditioning during chair rest. Aerospace Medicine 23: 646–649

Leblanc P, Ruff F, Milic-Emili J 1970 Effects of age and body position on airway closure in man. Journal of Applied Physiology 28: 448–451

Levine S A, Lown B 1952 'Armchair' treatment of acute coronary thrombosis. Journal of the American Medical Association 148: 1365–1369

Lewis F R 1980 Management of atelectasis and pneumonia. Surgical Clinics of North America 60: 1391–1401

Loke J, Mahler D A, Man S F P 1984 Exercise improvement in chronic obstructive pulmonary disease. Clinics in Chest Medicine 5: 121–143

Orlava O E 1959 Therapeutic physical culture in the complex treatment of pneumonia. Physical Therapy Review 39: 153–160

Ray J F, Yost L, Moallem S et al 1974 Immobility, hypoxemia, and pulmonary arteriovenous shunting. Archives of Surgery 109: 537–541

Remolina C, Khan A V, Santiago T V, Edelman N H 1981 Positional hypoxemia in unilateral lung disease. New England Journal of Medicine 304: 523–525

Ross J, Dean E 1989 Integrating physiological principles into the comprehensive management of cardiopulmonary dysfunction. Physical Therapy 69: 255–259

Ross J, Dean E 1992 Body positioning. In: Zadai C (ed) Pulmonary management in physical therapy. Churchill Livingstone, New York

Rubin M 1988 The physiology of bed rest. American Journal of Nursing 88: 50–56

Sjostrand T 1951 Determination of changes in the intrathoracic blood volume in man. Acta Physiologica Scandinavica 22: 116–128

Svanberg L 1957 Influence of position on the lung volumes, ventilation and circulation in normals. Scandinavian Journal of Laboratory Investigation 25(suppl): 7–175

Ward A, Malloy P, Rippe J 1987 Exercise prescription guidelines for normal and cardiac populations. Cardiology Clinics 5: 197–210

Wasserman K, Whipp B J 1975 Exercise physiology in health and disease. American Review of Respiratory Disease 112: 219–249

Wasserman K, Hansen J E, Sue D Y, Whipp B J 1987 Principles of exercise testing and interpretation. Lea & Febiger, Philadelphia

Weber K T, Janicki J S, Shroff S G, Likoff M J 1983 The cardiopulmonary unit: the body's gas transport system. Clinics in Chest Medicine 4: 101–110

Wenger N K 1982 Early ambulation: the physiologic basis revisited. Advances in Cardiology 31: 138–141

West J B 1962 Regional differences in gas exchange in the lung of erect man. Journal of Applied Physiology 17: 893–898

West J B 1977 Ventilation and perfusion relationships. American Review of Respiratory Disease 116: 919–943

Wolff R K, Dolovich M B, Obminski G, Newhouse M T 1977 Effects of exercise and eucapnic hyperventilation on bronchial clearance in man. Journal of Applied Physiology 43: 46–50

Zack M B, Pontoppidan H, Kazemi H 1974 The effect of lateral positions on gas exchange in pulmonary disease. American Review of Respiratory Disease 110: 49–55

FURTHER READING

American College of Sports Medicine 1991 Guidelines for exercise testing and prescription, 4th edn. Lea & Febiger, Philadelphia

Bates D V 1989 Normal pulmonary function. Respiratory function in disease, 3rd edn. W B Saunders, Toronto

Convertino V A 1987 Aerobic fitness, endurance training, and orthostatic intolerance. Exercise and Sports Sciences Review 15: 223–259

Dantzker D R 1991 Cardiopulmonary critical care, 2nd edn. W B Saunders, Philadelphia

McArdle W D, Katch F I, Katch V L 1996 Exercise physiology. Energy, nutrition, and human performance, 4th edn. Lea & Febiger, Philadelphia

Pollack M L, Wilmore J H 1990 Exercise in health and disease, 2nd edn. W B Saunders, Philadelphia

Reinhart K, Eyrich K (eds) 1989 Clinical aspects of oxygen transport and tissue oxygenation. Springer-Verlag, London

West J B 1990 Ventilation, blood flow and gas exchange, 5th edn. Blackwell Scientific, Oxford

West J B 1995 Respiratory physiology: the essentials, 5th edn. Williams & Wilkins, Baltimore

8

Physiotherapy techniques

Barbara A. Webber   Jennifer A. Pryor

Delva D. Bethune
(Neurophysiological facilitation of respiration*)

Helen M. Potter
(Musculoskeletal dysfunction)

Debbie McKenzie
(Transcutaneous electrical nerve stimulation, Acupuncture)

BREATHING CONTROL

Breathing techniques can be divided into normal breathing, known as 'breathing control', where minimal effort is expended, and breathing exercises where either inspiration is emphasized as in thoracic expansion exercises or expiration is emphasized as in the huff of the forced expiration technique.

Breathing control is normal tidal breathing using the lower chest with relaxation of the upper chest and shoulders. This used to be known as 'diaphragmatic breathing', but this term is a misnomer as during normal tidal breathing there is activity not only in the diaphragm but also in the internal and external intercostal muscles, the abdominal and scalene muscles (Green & Moxham 1985).

To be taught breathing control, the patient should be in a comfortable well-supported position either sitting (Fig. 8.1) or in high side lying (Fig. 8.2). The patient is encouraged to relax his upper chest, shoulders and arms while using the lower chest. One hand, which may be either the patient's or the physiotherapist's, or one hand of each, can be positioned lightly on the upper abdomen. As the patient breathes in, the hand should be felt to rise up and out; as the patient breathes out, the hand sinks down and in. Inspiration is the active phase, expiration should be relaxed and passive and

---

*Reprinted with permission from Bethune 1991 in Pryor J A (ed) Respiratory care. Churchill Livingstone, Edinburgh.

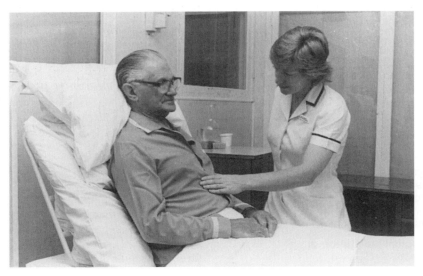

Fig. 8.1 Breathing control in sitting.

both inspiration and expiration should be barely audible. Inspiration through the nose allows the air to be warmed, humidified and filtered before it reaches the upper airways. If the nose is blocked, breathing through the mouth will reduce the resistance to the flow of air and will reduce the work of breathing. If the patient is very breathless breathing through the mouth will reduce the anatomical dead space.

Some patients reflexly use pursed-lip breathing. Breathing through pursed lips has the effect of generating a small positive pressure during expiration which may reduce to some extent the collapse of unstable airways, for example in emphysema (see Ch. 14, p. 382). This technique increases the work of breathing, particularly if it has become a forced noisy manoeuvre, and many patients no longer need to use pursed-lip breathing when they have relearned breathing control (normal breathing), which minimizes the work of breathing.

There are positions which optimize the length tension status of the diaphragm (Sharp et al 1980, O'Neill & McCarthy 1983, Dean 1985). By sitting or standing leaning forward, the abdominal contents raise the anterior part of the diaphragm, possibly facilitating its contraction during inspiration. A similar effect can be seen in the side lying and high side lying positions where the curvature of the dependent part of the diaphragm is increased. This effect combined with relaxation of the head, neck and shoulders promotes the pattern of breathing control.

Any breathless patient, for example patients with emphysema, asthma, pulmonary fibrosis or lung cancer, will benefit from using breathing control in positions which encourage relaxation of the upper chest and shoulders and allow movement of the lower chest and abdomen. One of the most useful positions is high side lying (Fig. 8.2). For maximal relaxation of the head, neck and upper chest, the neck should be slightly flexed and the top pillow should be above the shoulder, supporting only the head and neck. Other useful positions are:

- Relaxed sitting (Fig. 8.3)
- Forward lean standing (Fig. 8.4)
- Relaxed standing (Fig. 8.5)
- Forward lean sitting (Fig. 8.6)
- Breathless children may prefer a kneeling position (Fig. 8.7).

These positions discourage the tendency of breathless patients to push down or grip with their hands, which causes elevation of the

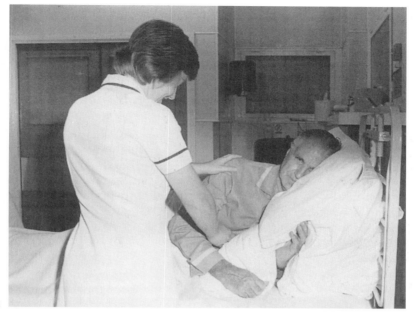

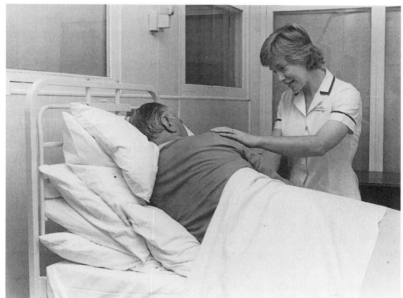

Fig. 8.2 Breathing control in high side lying.

shoulders and overuse of the accessory muscles of breathing. Figure 8.3b shows a position that is often preferred by patients who are overweight.

Breathing control is also used to improve exercise tolerance in breathless patients when walking up slopes, hills and stairs (Fig. 8.8). Breathless patients tend to hold their breath on exertion and rush, for example up a flight of stairs, arriving at the top extremely breathless and unable to speak. The simple technique of

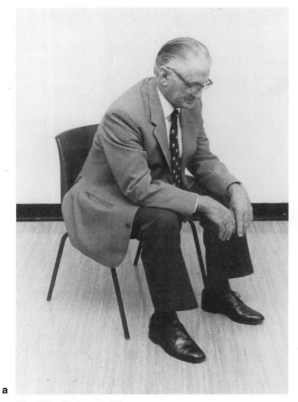

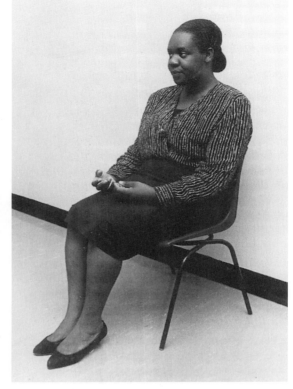

a

b

Fig. 8.3 Relaxed sitting.

relaxing the arms and shoulders, reducing the walking speed a little and using the pattern of breathing *in* on climbing one step and breathing *out* on climbing the next step can lead to a marked reduction in breathlessness and the ability to converse on arrival at the top of the flight of stairs (Webber 1991). When this technique has been mastered, some patients, on days when they are less breathless, may find breathing *in* for *one* step and *out* for *two* steps more comfortable.

The severely breathless patient may find the combination of breathing control with walking also helpful when walking on level ground. A respiratory walking frame (Fig. 8.9) with or without portable oxygen can be used to assist ambulation in the severely breathless patient.

Breathing control is an integral part of the active cycle of breathing techniques and is also used to control a bout or paroxysm of coughing.

AIRWAY CLEARANCE TECHNIQUES

The active cycle of breathing techniques

The active cycle of breathing techniques (ACBT) is used to mobilize and clear excess bronchial secretions. It has been shown to be effective in the clearance of bronchial secretions (Pryor et al 1979, Wilson et al 1995) and to improve lung function (Webber et al 1986). It neither causes or increases hypoxaemia (Pryor et al 1990), nor increases airflow obstruction (Thompson & Thompson 1968, Pryor & Webber 1979, Pryor et al 1994).

In the management of children with cystic fibrosis in the Ukraine, the physiotherapy techniques used had been very uncomfortable. The introduction of the ACBT during a 6-month period led to subjective improvements and significant improvements in oxygen saturation (Phillips et al 1996).

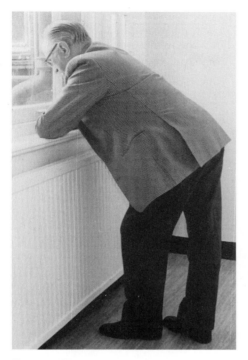

Fig. 8.4   Forward lean standing.

The ACBT is a flexible method of treatment which can be adapted for use in any patient, young or old, medical or surgical, where there is a problem of excess bronchial secretions. It can be used with or without an assistant.

It is a cycle of breathing control, thoracic expansion exercises and the forced expiration technique (FET). The original studies on 'the forced expiration technique' (Pryor et al 1979, Webber et al 1986, Hofmeyr et al 1986) used this cycle of techniques, but people began to use a regimen of huffing alone or other variations on the FET (Falk et al 1984, Reisman et al 1988) and the literature became confusing. In order to emphasize the use of thoracic expansion exercises and the periods of breathing control, in addition to the FET, the whole regimen was renamed the active cycle of breathing techniques (ACBT) (Webber 1990). The regimen did not change in practice and the early studies on the FET were randomized controlled trials of the ACBT.

Thoracic expansion exercises

Thoracic expansion exercises are deep breathing exercises emphasizing inspiration. Inspiration is active and may be combined with a 3-second hold before the passive relaxed expiration. The postoperative manoeuvre of a 3-second hold at full inspiration has been said to decrease collapse of lung tissue (Ward et al 1966). This 'hold' may also be of value in some patients with medical chest conditions, but it is probably inappropriate in the very breathless patient.

In the normal lung the resistance to airflow via the collateral ventilatory system is high, but with increasing lung volume and in the presence of lung pathology the resistance decreases, allowing air to flow via the collateral channels – the pores of Kohn, channels of Lambert and channels of Martin (Menkes & Traystman 1977) (Fig. 8.10). Air behind secretions may assist in mobilizing them.

The effectiveness of thoracic expansion exercises in re-expanding lung tissue and in mobilizing and clearing excess bronchial secretions can also be explained by the phenomenon of interdependence (Mead et al 1970). This is the effect of the expanding forces exerted between adjacent alveoli. At high lung volumes the expanding forces between alveoli are greater than at tidal volume and assist in re-expansion of lung tissue.

Three or four expansion exercises are usually appropriate before pausing for a few seconds for a period of breathing control. Any more deep breaths could produce the effects of hyperventilation or could tire the patient.

Thoracic expansion exercises can be encouraged with proprioceptive stimulation by placing a hand, either the patient's or the physiotherapist's, over the part of the chest wall where movement of the chest is to be encouraged. There is no evidence to support an increase in ventilation to the lung underlying the hand (Martin et al 1976), but there is an increase in chest wall movement and an increase in lung volume.

Sometimes an additional increase in lung volume can be achieved by using a 'sniff' manoeuvre at the end of a deep inspiration. This manoeuvre may not be appropriate in patients

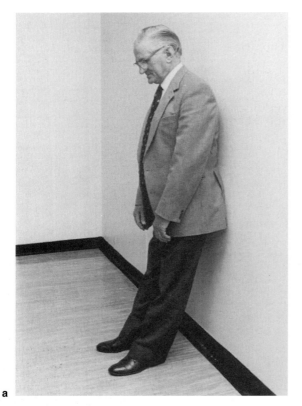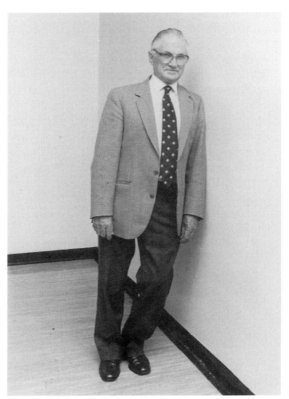

a   b

Fig. 8.5 Relaxed standing.

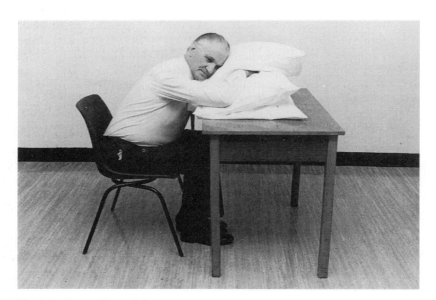

Fig. 8.6 Forward lean sitting.

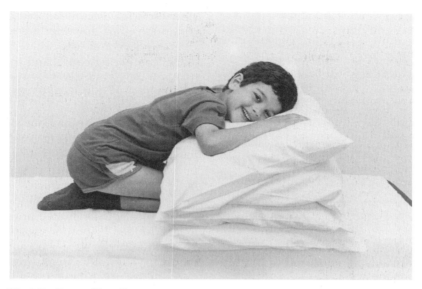

Fig. 8.7 Forward kneeling.

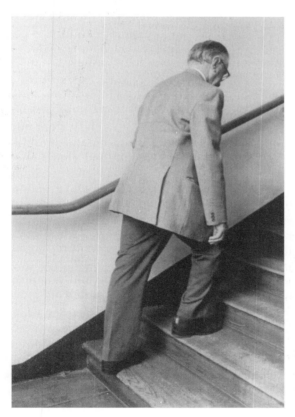

Fig. 8.8 Breathing control while stair climbing.

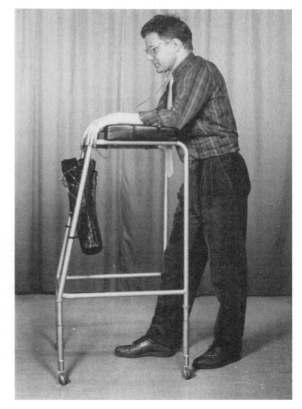

Fig. 8.9 Respiratory walking frame in use.

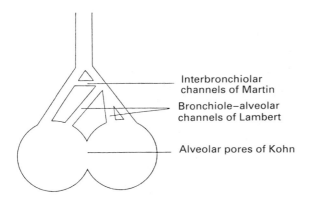

Fig. 8.10 Collateral ventilation pathways.

who are hyperinflated, but for surgical patients who need further motivation to increase their lung volume it can be a useful technique.

Thoracic expansion exercises may be combined with chest shaking, vibrations, and/or chest clapping. These techniques may further assist in the clearance of secretions (pp. 147–151).

The forced expiration technique (FET)

The forced expiration technique is a combination of one or two forced expirations (huffs) and periods of breathing control. Huffing to low lung volumes will move the more peripherally situated secretions and when secretions have reached the larger more proximal upper airways a huff or cough from a high lung volume can be used to clear them.

With any forced expiratory manoeuvre there is dynamic compression and collapse of the airways downstream (towards the mouth) of the equal pressure point (West 1992). This is an important part of the clearance mechanism of either a huff or a cough.

As lung volume decreases during a forced expiratory manoeuvre the equal pressure points move more peripherally, and below functional residual capacity they move towards the alveoli. At lung volumes above functional residual capacity the equal pressure points are located in lobar or segmental bronchi (Macklem 1974). A series of coughs without intervening inspirations was advocated by Mead et al (1967) to

clear bronchial secretions, but clinically a single continuous huff down to the same lung volume is as effective and less exhausting. Hasani et al (1994) comparing cough and the FET concluded that both were equally effective in clearing lung secretions, but that the FET required less effort from the patients.

The mean transpulmonary pressure during voluntary coughing is greater than during a forced expiration. This results in greater compression and narrowing of the airways which limits airflow and reduces the efficiency of bronchial clearance (Langlands 1967). In 1989, Freitag et al demonstrated an oscillatory movement, 'hidden' vibrations, of the airway walls in addition to the squeezing action produced by the forced expiratory manoeuvre.

The viscosity of mucus is shear dependent (Lopez-Vidriero & Reid 1978) and the shear forces generated during a huff should reduce mucus viscosity. This together with the high flow of a forced expiratory manoeuvre would also be expected to aid mucus clearance and the expectoration of sputum.

When mobilizing and clearing peripheral secretions it is an unnecessary expenditure of energy to start the huff from a high lung volume. A huff from mid-lung volume is more efficient and probably more effective. To huff from mid-lung volume a medium-sized breath should be taken in, and with the mouth and glottis open, the air is squeezed out using the chest wall and abdominal muscles. It should be long enough to loosen secretions from the more peripherally situated airways and should not just be a clearing noise in the back of the throat. However, if the huff is continued for too long it may lead to unnecessary paroxysmal coughing. Too short a huff may be ineffective (Partridge et al 1989), but when the secretions have reached the upper airways, a shorter huff or a cough from a high lung volume is used to clear them.

The huff is a forced but not violent manoeuvre. To be maximally effective the length of the huff and force of contraction of the expiratory muscles should be altered to maximize airflow from the periphery and to minimize airway collapse.

A peak flow mouthpiece, or similar piece

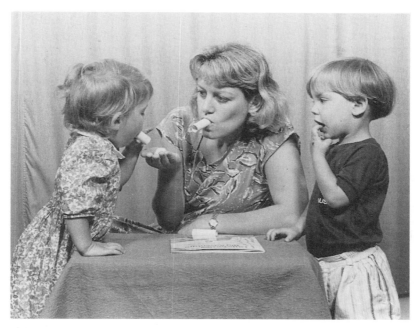

Fig. 8.11 Huffing games.

of tubing, may improve the effectiveness of the huff as it helps to keep the glottis open. Some people find that huffing through a tube at a tissue or cotton-wool ball is helpful in perfecting the technique.

The huff can be introduced to children as blowing games (Thompson 1978) and from about the age of 2 years they are usually able to copy others huffing (Fig. 8.11).

An essential part of the forced expiration technique is the pause for breathing control after one or two huffs which prevents any increase in airflow obstruction. The length of the pause will vary from patient to patient. In a patient with bronchospasm or unstable airways, or in one who is debilitated and fatigues easily, longer pauses (perhaps 10–20 seconds) may be appropriate. In patients with no bronchospasm the periods of breathing control may be considerably shorter (perhaps two or three breaths or 5–10 seconds).

In the tetraplegic patient, clearance of secretions from the upper airways is difficult because maximum lung volume cannot be achieved and the equal pressure points will therefore never

reach the largest airways (Morgan et al 1986). Secretions can be cleared from the smaller airways, but accumulate in the larger upper airways.

Application of the active cycle of breathing techniques

The cycle of breathing control, thoracic expansion exercises and the forced expiration technique is adapted for each patient (Fig. 8.12). Sometimes one set of thoracic expansion exercises will be followed by the forced expiration technique (Fig. 8.12a and b), but if secretions loosen slowly it may be more appropriate to use two sets of thoracic expansion exercises (Fig. 8.12c). The surgical patient will probably benefit from the 3-second hold with the thoracic expansion exercises (Fig. 8.13), but there is probably no indication for the use of chest clapping, and wound support may be more suitable than chest compression during huffing and coughing (Fig. 8.14).

In many patients the active cycle of breathing techniques will effectively clear secretions in the

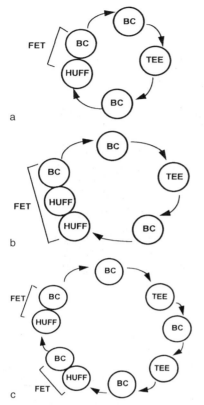

Fig. 8.12 Examples to demonstrate the flexibility of the active cycle of breathing techniques: BC, breathing control; TEE, thoracic expansion exercises; FET, forced expiration technique.

sitting position, but in others gravity-assisted positions will be required.

For patients with a moderate amount of bronchial secretions, for example with bronchiectasis or cystic fibrosis, a minimum of 10 minutes in any productive position is usually necessary. For patients with minimal secretions, for example some asthmatics, some chronic bronchitics or following surgery, less time is required. The 'end-point' of a treatment session can be recognized, either by the physiotherapist or the patient treating himself, when an effective huff to low lung volume in two consecutive cycles has been dry sounding and non-productive. The sicker patient may not reach this end-point before tiring and should stop when fatigue is recognized.

It is important to introduce the concept of self-treatment at an early stage. Patients in hospital should be encouraged to take some responsibility for their treatment (Fig. 8.15). Surgical patients should continue their breathing exercises in between the treatment sessions with the physiotherapist. Medical patients can perhaps start by doing their own evening treatment. If the patient takes responsibility for his treatment before discharge home, both the patient and physiotherapist will have the confidence that treatment will be continued effectively. It is, however,

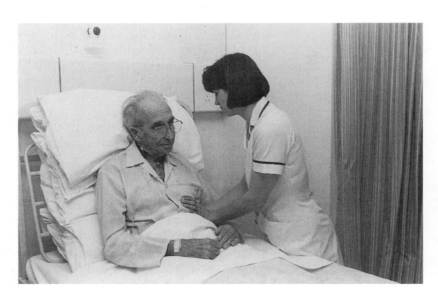

Fig. 8.13 Thoracic expansion exercises.

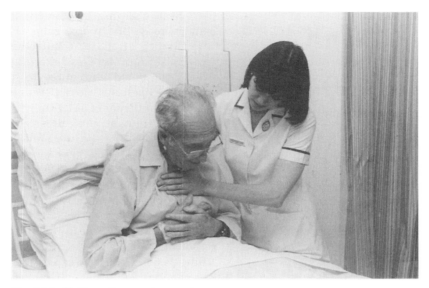

Fig. 8.14   Huffing with wound support.

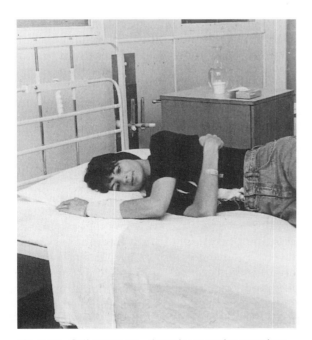

Fig. 8.15   Self-treatment – thoracic expansion exercises.

important to negotiate rather than prescribe a physiotherapy home programme to increase compliance with treatment (Carr et al 1996).

Revision of techniques at appropriate intervals

is necessary to assess the effectiveness of the treatment regimen, and to correct and update techniques as necessary. Currie et al (1986) recognized the importance of reassessment in maintaining patient compliance.

Chest clapping

Chest clapping is performed using a cupped hand with a rhythmical flexion and extension action of the wrist. The technique is often done with two hands (Fig. 8.16) but, depending on the area of the chest, it may be more appropriate to use one hand. For the infant chest clapping is performed using two or three fingers of one hand. Single-handed chest clapping is probably the technique of choice for self-chest clapping.

Chest clapping should never be uncomfortable and should be done over a layer of clothing to avoid sensory stimulation of the skin. It should not be necessary to use extra layers of clothing or towelling as the force of the chest clapping should be adapted to suit the individual.

Mechanical percussion has been shown to increase intrathoracic pressure (Flower et al 1979) and chest clapping may have a similar effect but this change in intrathoracic pressure has not

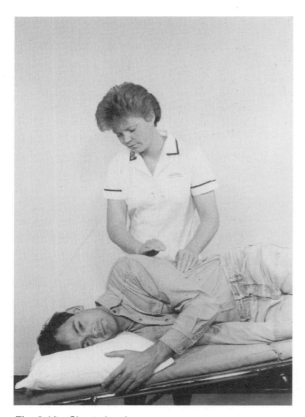

Fig. 8.16 Chest clapping.

been correlated with an increase in the clearance of bronchial secretions. Andersen (personal communication, 1987) hypothesized that the air-filled alveoli would buffer increases in intrathoracic pressure and markedly reduce the mechanical effect of chest clapping.

Some studies (Campbell et al 1975, Wollmer et al 1985) have demonstrated an increase in airflow obstruction when chest clapping is included in the regimen, but other studies (Pryor & Webber 1979, Gallon 1991) have shown no increase in airflow obstruction with chest clapping.

In infants and small children not yet old enough to do voluntary breathing techniques, and in patients with neuromuscular weakness or paralysis, and the intellectually impaired, chest clapping is a useful technique to stimulate coughing probably by the mobilization of secretions.

Chest clapping has been shown to cause an increase in hypoxaemia (Falk et al 1984, McDonnell et al 1986), but when short periods of chest clapping (less than 30 seconds) have been combined with three to four thoracic expansion exercises no fall was seen in oxygen saturation (Pryor et al 1990).

In a group of clinically stable patients with cystic fibrosis no advantage was shown when self-chest clapping was used in addition to thoracic expansion exercises (Webber et al 1985), but this cannot be extrapolated to either all medical chest conditions or to acute chest problems. Single-handed chest clapping (Fig. 8.17) is advocated in self-treatment as it is difficult to coordinate two-handed clapping at the same time as using thoracic expansion exercises.

If a patient feels that self-chest clapping is beneficial, but the physiotherapist thinks that it is tiring and may be causing hypoxaemia, the patient could be monitored using an oximeter. If oxygen desaturation of clinical significance occurs during the self-chest clapping the patient should be encouraged to omit the clapping, but to continue with the thoracic expansion exercises. Patients studied by Carr et al (1995) felt that self-chest clapping was useful when they were clinically stable, but more particularly when they were unwell. The benefits of chest clapping remain uncertain, but if chest clapping is considered to be clinically beneficial for an individual it should be continued, provided there are no adverse effects.

There is probably no indication for chest clapping in postoperative patients and in patients following chest injury. Severe osteoporosis and frank haemoptysis are contraindications, although chest clapping is unlikely to increase bleeding when bronchial secretions are lightly streaked with blood.

Vigorous and rapid chest clapping may lead to breath holding and may induce bronchospasm in a patient with hyperreactive airways. There is no evidence that alteration in the rate of chest clapping increases or decreases the mobilization of bronchial secretions. A rhythmical comfortable rate for both patient and physiotherapist is probably the most appropriate.

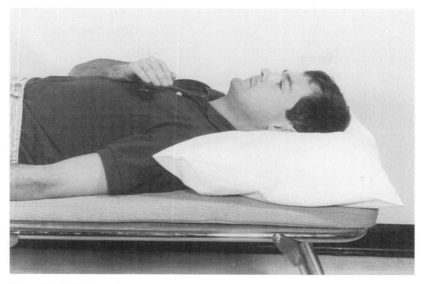

Fig. 8.17 Self-chest clapping.

Chest shaking, vibrations and compression

The hands are placed on the chest wall and, during expiration, a vibratory action in the direction of the normal movement of the ribs is transmitted through the chest using body weight. This action augments the expiratory flow and may help to mobilize secretions. It is unknown whether airway closure will be increased if the vibratory action is continued into the expiratory reserve volume, but the techniques are frequently combined with thoracic expansion exercises which would counteract any resulting airway closure.

The vibratory action may be either a coarse movement (chest shaking) or a fine movement (chest vibrations). Little work has been done on the effects of either coarse or fine vibrations and physiotherapists have tended to adopt the techniques that they find the most helpful clinically.

In infants, vibrations are performed using two fingers in contact with the chest wall. Chest vibrations and shaking should never be uncomfortable and should be adapted to suit the individual patient. Some patients doing their own chest physiotherapy find self-chest vibra-

tions helpful. One hand is placed on top of the other on the appropriate part of the chest wall and vibrations or shaking are carried out during expiration. With the hands in a similar position chest compression throughout expiration is often helpful (Fig. 8.18) to augment the forced expiratory manoeuvre of the huff. When in side lying self-compression can be given over the side of the chest with the upper arm and elbow and the hand of the other arm (Fig. 8.19).

The physiotherapist or other carer may give compression during huffing or coughing. Some patients find this helpful, but others prefer to be unsupported. Postoperative patients usually find that supporting the wound facilitates both huffing and coughing. With fractured ribs and other chest injuries shaking of the chest wall would be inappropriate, but compressive support may assist the clearance of secretions.

In the paralysed patient the technique of rib springing may be used where compression of the chest wall is continued throughout expiration and overpressure is applied at the end of the breath out. By releasing the hands quickly inspiration is encouraged. This technique is inappropriate in the non-paralysed patient and may be harmful as compression against a reflexly

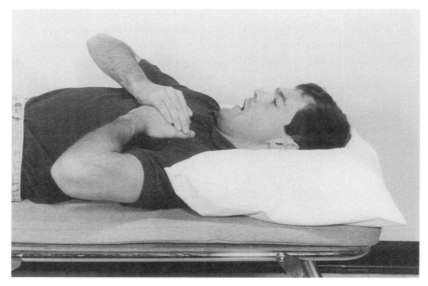

Fig. 8.18 Self-chest compression.

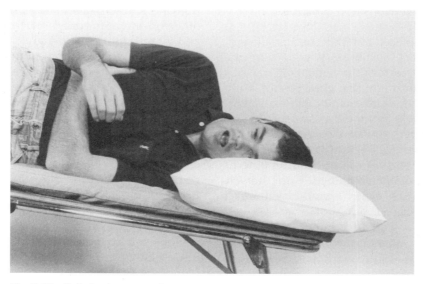

Fig. 8.19 Self-chest compression.

splinted chest wall may produce rib fractures. Assisted coughing for the paralysed patient is described in Chapter 17.

In the drowsy, semicomatose patient (for example, the chronic bronchitic in respiratory failure with sputum retention), chest compres-sion similar to, but less vigorous than, rib springing may stimulate a deeper inspiration.

Chest shaking or chest vibrations can also be used during the expiratory phase of a manual hyperinflation treatment (Ch. 11, p. 285) to assist the clearance of secretions.

Care must be taken when using the techniques of chest shaking, vibrations and compression if there are signs of osteoporosis or metastatic deposits affecting the ribs or vertebral column.

Gravity-assisted positions

Gravity can be used to assist the clearance of bronchial secretions (Sutton et al 1983, Hofmeyr et al 1986). Nelson (1934) described the use of positioning for draining secretions, based on the anatomy of the bronchial tree. The recognized positions (Thoracic Society 1950) (Fig. 8.20) are shown in Figures 8.21 to 8.31 and described in Table 8.1.

Some patients cannot tolerate the recognized positions and for others they may be contra-indicated. Modified positions such as high side lying (Fig. 8.32) or side lying (Fig. 8.15) may be more appropriate. At school, college, work or when on holiday modified positions may be easier, more convenient and likely to encourage patient compliance (Figs 8.15 and 8.33).

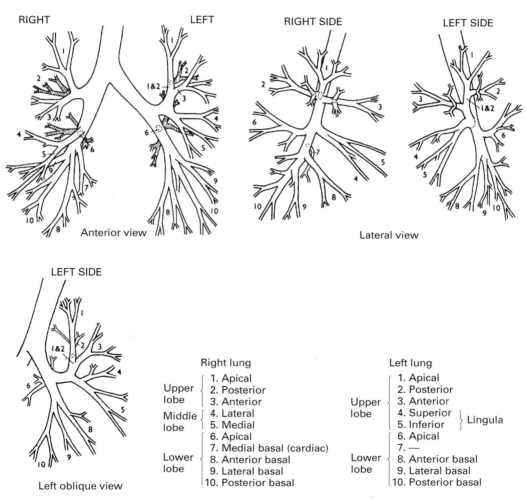

	Right lung			Left lung
Upper lobe	1. Apical 2. Posterior 3. Anterior		Upper lobe	1. Apical 2. Posterior 3. Anterior 4. Superior ⎫ Lingula 5. Inferior ⎭
Middle lobe	4. Lateral 5. Medial			
Lower lobe	6. Apical 7. Medial basal (cardiac) 8. Anterior basal 9. Lateral basal 10. Posterior basal		Lower lobe	6. Apical 7. — 8. Anterior basal 9. Lateral basal 10. Posterior basal

Fig. 8.20 Diagram illustrating the bronchopulmonary nomenclature approved by the Thoracic Society (1950) (reproduced by permission of the Editor of *Thorax*).

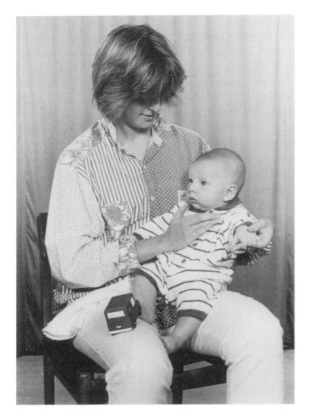

Fig. 8.21 Apical segments upper lobes.

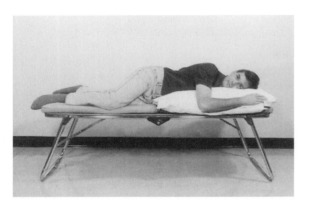

Fig. 8.22 Posterior segment right upper lobe.

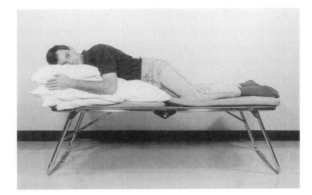

Fig. 8.23 Posterior segment left upper lobe.

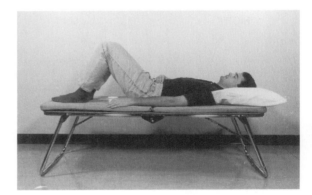

Fig. 8.24 Anterior segments upper lobes.

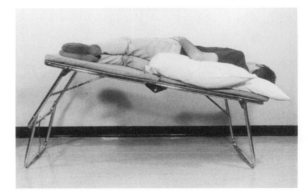

Fig. 8.25 Lingula.

Individual assessment will indicate whether gravity-assisted drainage positions are of clinical benefit. In some patients with very tenacious secretions gravity is unlikely to help and a com-

fortable position in which effective breathing techniques can be carried out is likely to be the most beneficial.

It is inappropriate to use the downward chest

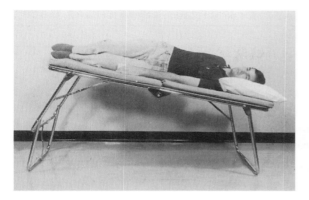

Fig. 8.26 Right middle lobe.

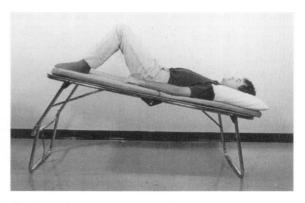

Fig. 8.29 Anterior basal segments.

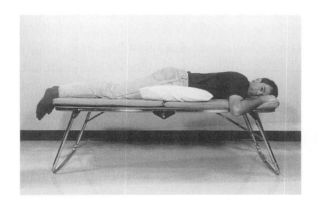

Fig. 8.27 Apical segments lower lobes.

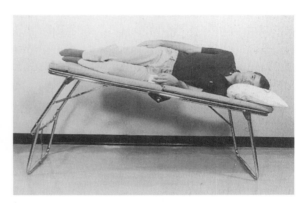

Fig. 8.30 Lateral basal segment right lower lobe.

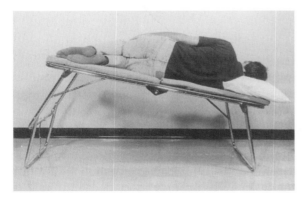

Fig. 8.28 Right medial basal and left lateral basal segments lower lobes.

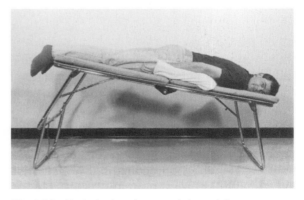

Fig. 8.31 Posterior basal segments lower lobes.

Table 8.1 Gravity-assisted drainage positions (numbers refer to Fig. 8.20 and patient position is shown in Figs 8.21 to 8.31)

	Lobe		Position	
Upper lobe	1	Apical bronchus	1	Sitting upright
	2	Posterior bronchus		
		(a) Right	2a	Lying on the left side horizontally turned 45° on to the face, resting against a pillow, with another supporting the head
		(b) Left	2b	Lying on the right side turned 45° on to the face, with three pillows arranged to lift the shoulders 30 cm (12 in) from the horizontal
	3	Anterior bronchus	3	Lying supine with the knees flexed
Lingula	4	Superior bronchus	4 & 5	Lying supine with the body a quarter turned to the right maintained by a pillow under the left side from shoulder to hip. The chest is tilted downwards to an angle of 15°
	5	Inferior bronchus		
Middle lobe	4	Lateral bronchus	4 & 5	Lying supine with the body a quarter turned to the left maintained by a pillow under the right side from shoulder to hip. The chest is tilted downwards to an angle of 15°
	5	Medial bronchus		
Lower lobe	6	Apical bronchus	6	Lying prone with a pillow under the abdomen
	7	Medial basal (cardiac) bronchus	7	Lying on the right side with the chest tilted downwards to an angle of 20°
	8	Anterior basal bronchus	8	Lying supine with the knees flexed and the chest tilted downwards to an angle of 20°
	9	Lateral basal bronchus	9	Lying on the opposite side with the chest tilted downwards to an angle of 20°
	10	Posterior basal bronchus	10	Lying prone with a pillow under the hips and the chest tilted downwards to an angle of 20°

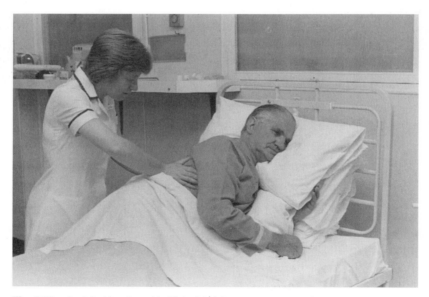

Fig. 8.32 Assisted treatment in high side lying.

tilted positions immediately following meals and in the following conditions: cardiac failure, severe hypertension, cerebral oedema, aortic and cerebral aneurysms, severe haemoptysis, abdominal distension, gastro-oesophageal reflux (infants may be an exception, p. 336), and after recent surgery or trauma to the head or neck.

Ventilation/perfusion. When positioning a

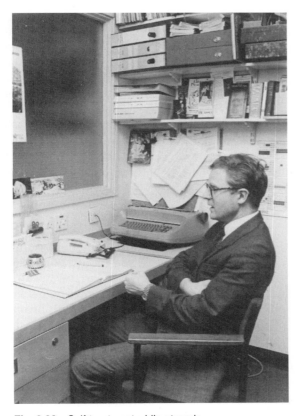

Fig. 8.33 Self-treatment while at work.

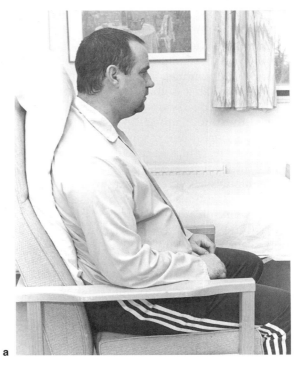

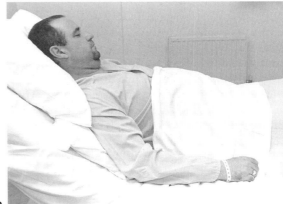

Fig. 8.34 Positioning: **a** sitting upright; **b** slumped sitting.

patient for drainage of secretions, it is also important to remember the effect of gravity on ventilation and perfusion (see Ch. 7). In the adult, both ventilation and perfusion are preferentially distributed to the dependent parts of the lung (West 1992) whereas in children this differs (p. 332). In adults with unilateral lung disease gas exchange may be improved by using the side lying position with the unaffected lung dependent (Zack et al 1974). Postoperatively the easiest method of increasing functional residual capacity (FRC) and preventing lung collapse is appropriate positioning and early ambulation (Jenkins et al 1988). Most patients can sit out of bed the day after surgery (Fig. 8.34a). If they cannot sit in a chair, they should be encouraged to either sit upright in bed or adopt a side lying position, but they should not be in a slumped sitting position (Fig. 8.34b).

Autogenic drainage

Autogenic drainage (AD) aims to maximize airflow within the airways to improve the clearance of mucus and ventilation (David 1991). Chevaillier developed this concept in Belgium in the late 1960s, but little was published until 1979 (Dab & Alexander 1979). Autogenic drainage is breathing at different lung volumes and an active expiration is used to mobilize the mucus.

Chevaillier described three phrases: 'unstick', 'collect' and 'evacuate' (Schöni 1989). Breathing at low lung volumes is said to mobilize peripheral mucus. This is the first or 'unstick' phase. It is followed by a period of tidal breathing which is said to 'collect' mucus in the middle airways. Then, by breathing at higher lung volumes, the 'evacuate' phase, expectoration of secretions from the central airways is promoted. A huff from high lung volume is now encouraged to clear the secretions from the trachea (Chevaillier 1995). Coughing is discouraged.

AD has been altered in Germany (David 1991) and is not split into the three phases as the patients were found to be uncomfortable breathing at low lung volumes. This technique is known as modified autogenic drainage (M AD) (Kieselmann 1995). The patient breathes around tidal volume while breath holding for 2–3 seconds at the end of each inspiration. Coughing is used to clear mucus from the larynx (Kieselmann 1995).

The flow–volume curve is frequently used to support an increase in airflow with the unforced expiratory manoeuvre of autogenic drainage (Schöni 1989). However, it must be remembered that it is only possible to go outside the flow–volume curve if pressure-dependent collapse exists.

Autogenic drainage is usually practised in the sitting position. It takes 10–20 hours to teach the main principles and sessions of 30–45 minutes twice a day are necessary (David 1991). Children under the age of about 8 years would find it difficult to concentrate for any length of time on the different levels of breathing involved.

In a long-term study of patients with cystic fibrosis AD was compared with 'conventional' percussion and postural drainage. AD was found to be at least as effective as the conventional treatment and the patients had a marked preference for AD (Davidson et al 1992).

Positive expiratory pressure

The positive expiratory pressure (PEP) mask was described by Falk et al (1984) who found an increase in sputum yield and an improvement in transcutaneous oxygen tension when compared with postural drainage, percussion and breathing exercises. It was suggested that the increase in sputum yield was produced by the effect of PEP on peripheral airways and collateral channels.

The PEP apparatus consists of a face mask and a one-way valve to which expiratory resistances can be attached. A manometer is inserted into the system between the valve and resistance to monitor the pressure which should be between 10 and 20 cmH$_2$O during mid-expiration (Falk & Andersen 1991).

The patient sits leaning forward with his elbows supported on a table and holding the mask firmly over the nose and mouth (Fig. 8.35). A mouthpiece and nose clip can be used in place of the mask if this is preferred. The patient breathes at tidal volume with a slightly active expiration for about six to ten breaths and the lung volume should be kept up by avoiding complete expiration. This is followed by the forced expiration technique to clear the secretions that have been mobilized. The duration and frequency of treatment are adapted to each individual, but treatment is usually performed for 15 minutes twice a day in patients with

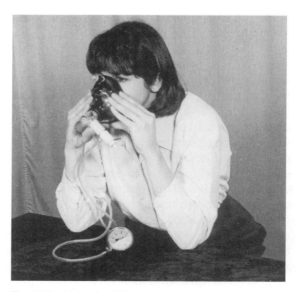

Fig. 8.35 Using the PEP mask.

stable chest disease with excess bronchial secretions (Falk & Andersen 1991). In postoperative patients short periods of PEP used every hour as a prophylactic treatment have been described by Ricksten et al (1986).

The study by Falk et al (1984) in patients with cystic fibrosis compared an assisted 'conventional' postural drainage treatment with an unassisted PEP mask regimen and found that the PEP mask regimen was more effective and the one preferred by the patients. In order to reduce the variables studied, Hofmeyr et al (1986) compared the unassisted treatment of PEP combined with the forced expiration technique, with thoracic expansion exercises combined with the forced expiration technique (the active cycle of breathing techniques). This study could not show any advantage in using the PEP mask, more sputum being produced when the active cycle of breathing techniques was used.

Falk & Andersen (1991) suggest that with the PEP treatment the increase in lung volume may allow air to get behind secretions blocking small airways and assist in mobilizing them. This effect may also be achieved by the thoracic expansion exercises.

van der Schans et al (1991) studied mucus clearance with PEP using a radio-aerosol technique in patients with cystic fibrosis. They showed that PEP temporarily increased lung volume, but did not lead to an improvement in mucus transport.

High-pressure PEP is a modified form of PEP mask treatment described for the treatment of patients with cystic fibrosis by Oberwaldner et al (1986). By using high pressures of PEP (50–120 cmH$_2$O), secretions may be mobilized more easily in patients with unstable airways. While sitting upright the patient holds the mask firmly against the face. Six to ten rhythmical breaths at tidal volume are followed by an inspiration to total lung capacity and then a forced expiratory manoeuvre against the resistance to low lung volume which usually results in the expectoration of sputum (Oberwaldner et al 1991).

An individual optimum expiratory resistance is carefully determined by spirometry. It is the resistance that allows the patient to expire to a volume greater than his usual forced vital capacity. The technique is only recommended for use where full lung function equipment is available for regular reassessment of the appropriate expiratory resistance for each individual. Meticulous care must be taken as an incorrect resistance can lead to a deterioration in lung function.

Flutter

The Flutter is a small, simple portable device (Fig. 8.36) used to assist the clearance of bronchial secretions. It is pipe-shaped with a single opening at the mouthpiece and a series of small outlet holes at the top of the bowl. The bowl contains a high-density stainless steel ball-bearing enclosed in a small cone. During expiration the movement of the ball along the surface of the cone creates a positive expiratory pressure (PEP) and an oscillatory vibration of the air within the airways. The device is held horizontally and tilted slightly downwards until a maximal oscillatory effect can be felt. The Flutter combines the techniques of oral high-frequency oscillation (OHFO) and PEP. It can be used in the sitting position or in the position of supine lying.

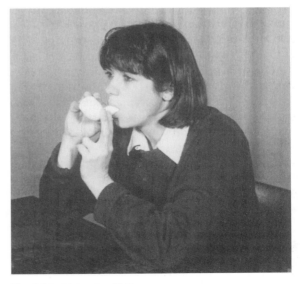

Fig. 8.36 Using the Flutter.

The Flutter is placed in the mouth and inspiration is either through the nose or through the mouth by breathing around the Flutter (it is not possible to breathe in through the Flutter). A slow deep breath in with a breath hold of 3–5 seconds is followed by a breath out, through the Flutter, at a faster rate than normal. After four to eight of these breaths many patients use huffing either through the Flutter or without the Flutter. This may precipitate expectoration and should be followed by a pause for breathing control.

Originally the recommended technique for the Flutter was a gentle exhalation through the device. Treatment was continued for a period of 10 minutes. Secretions were expectorated by spontaneous coughing. It was this regimen that was shown by Pryor et al (1994) to be less effective than the ACBT. The inclusion of huffing, as described in the regimen above, is likely to increase the effectiveness of airway clearance.

Konstan et al (1994) compared three regimens: the Flutter, voluntary coughing and a regimen of postural drainage which included up to 10 positions. Each session lasted 15 minutes. The Flutter regimen was the most effective as measured by the weight of sputum expectorated, but PEP (Falk et al 1984) had been shown to be more effective than a similar postural drainage regimen. In a subsequent study the ACBT was shown to be more effective than PEP (Hofmeyr et al 1986).

When autogenic drainage was compared with the Flutter it was concluded that both regimens were equally effective, but the Flutter was easier to teach (Lindemann 1992). A clinical trial was undertaken using the Flutter in patients following thoracotomy, but no advantage could be found in its inclusion (Chatham et al 1993).

The use of the Flutter in airway clearance may improve compliance in some patients, especially children. Care must be taken to wash and dry the parts of the device after use to minimize the risk of infection.

Mechanical percussion, vibration, oscillation and compression

Mechanical percussors have been shown to increase intrathoracic pressure (Flower et al 1979), but Pryor et al (1981) could not demonstrate any increase in sputum clearance or improvement in lung function with mechanical percussion.

Goodwin (1994) has undertaken a review of mechanical percussion, vibration, high-frequency oscillation and chest wall compression in airway clearance. He concluded that mechanical vibration may increase mucociliary clearance and that high-frequency chest wall compression (Arens et al 1994, Hansen et al 1994) was more promising than oral high-frequency oscillation (George et al 1985, Pryor at al 1989, van Hengstum et al 1990). Further work needs to be undertaken on the frequency of the vibration and it may be patient dependent.

In some parts of the world, for example North America, high-frequency chest compression may be considered a cost-effective alternative to chest physiotherapy (Hansen et al 1994). In other parts of the world where patients are already using independent airway clearance treatments it is unlikely that the expensive and cumbersome alternative of a mechanical device will be seriously considered.

Incentive spirometry

Incentive spirometers are mechanical devices introduced in an attempt to reduce postoperative pulmonary complications. The patient takes a slow deep breath in, with his lips sealed around the mouthpiece (Fig. 8.37) and is motivated by visual feedback, for example a ball rising to a preset marker. The patient aims to generate a predetermined flow or to achieve a preset volume and he is encouraged to hold his breath for 2–3 seconds at full inspiration. A short, sharp inspiration can activate the flow-generated incentive spirometry devices with little increase in tidal volume, but with a volume-dependent device an increase in tidal volume must be achieved before the preset level can be reached.

The pattern of breathing while using an incentive spirometer is important. Expansion of the lower chest should be emphasized rather than the use of the accessory muscles of respiration

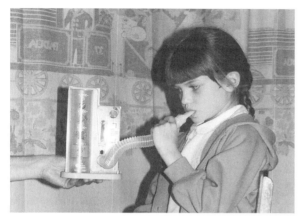

Fig. 8.37 Use of the 'Coach' incentive spirometer.

which would encourage expansion of the upper chest.

Diaphragmatic movement (Chuter et al 1990) is thought to be an important factor in the prevention of postoperative pulmonary complications. Incentive spirometry has been shown to increase abdominal movement in normal subjects, but not in subjects following abdominal surgery (Chuter et al 1989). Postoperatively, an increase in diaphragmatic movement has been observed by encouraging an increase in lung volume while using the pattern of breathing control without the resistive loading of an incentive spirometer (Chuter et al 1990). This may help to reduce postoperative pulmonary complications by increasing ventilation to the dependent parts of the lungs.

Incentive spirometry has been compared with intermittent positive pressure breathing (Oikkonen et al 1991), continuous positive airway pressure (Stock et al 1985) and chest physiotherapy (Hall et al 1991, Gosselink et al 1997) in patients following surgery. Few differences between the regimens have been reported.

There may be a place for the use of incentive spirometry in children and in some adolescents to provide motivation to increase lung volume following surgery, but the use of breathing control and thoracic expansion exercises with an inspiratory hold should be encouraged, and combined with ambulation may be more effective in the prevention of postoperative pulmonary complications

Glossopharyngeal breathing

Glossopharyngeal breathing (GPB) is a technique useful in patients with a reduced vital capacity owing to respiratory muscle paralysis, for example following poliomyelitis or in tetraplegics. It is a trick movement that was first described by Dail (1951) when patients with poliomyelitis were observed to be gulping air into their lungs. It was this gulping action that gave the technique the name 'frog breathing'.

GPB is a form of positive pressure ventilation produced by the patient's voluntary muscles where boluses of air are forced into the lungs. Paralysed patients dependent on a mechanical ventilator may be able to use GPB continuously, other than during sleep, to substitute the mechanical ventilation. The most common use of GPB is in patients who are able to breathe spontaneously but whose power to cough and clear secretions is inadequate. The technique may enable these patients to shout to attract attention and it may help to maintain or improve lung and chest wall compliance (Dail et al 1955).

To breathe in, a series of pumping strokes is produced by action of the lips, tongue, soft palate, pharynx and larynx. Air is held in the chest by the larynx which acts as a valve as the mouth is opened for the next gulp.

Before starting to teach a patient GPB it is helpful for him to inflate his chest using an intermittent positive pressure ventilator with a mouthpiece. He can practise holding the breath while removing the mouthpiece and avoiding escape of air through the larynx or nose. The most important step in learning GPB is the up and down movement of the cricoid cartilage while keeping the jaw still. The patient can practise by watching the movement in a mirror and feeling the cartilage with his fingers.

When this movement has been achieved a cycle of three steps is practised:

1. The mouth and pharynx are filled with air by depressing the cricoid cartilage and tongue (Fig. 8.38a).

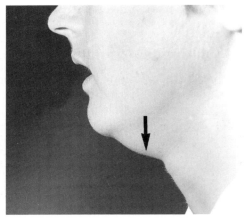

a

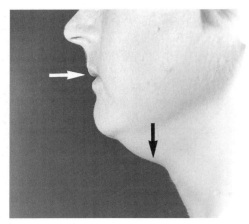

b

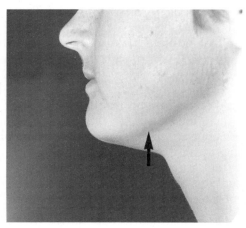

c

Fig. 8.38 The stages of glossopharyngeal breathing.

2. While maintaining this position the lips are closed, trapping the air (Fig. 8.38b).
3. The floor of the mouth and cricoid cartilage are allowed to rise to their normal position while air is pumped through the larynx into the trachea (Fig. 8.38c).

This sequence should be practised slowly at first and then gradually speeded up until the movement flows. A leak of air may occur through the nose and, until it is prevented by the soft palate, a nose clip may be required.

The next stage is to take a maximum breath in and, while holding this breath, to add several glossopharyngeal gulps, to augment the vital capacity. When correct, the patient will feel his chest filling with air, and the physiotherapist can test the 'GPB vital capacity' by putting a mouthpiece attached to the expiratory limb of a Wright's respirometer in the patient's mouth before he exhales.

The respirometer can be used to measure the volume per gulp; the patient will require less effort and reach his maximum capacity more quickly if he develops a bigger volume per gulp. A study by Kelleher & Parida (1957) reported a group of patients in whom the average volume per gulp varied from 25–120 ml, and when teaching GPB an attempt should be made to achieve at least 60 ml per gulp. When used for clearance of secretions, 10–20 gulps may be required to obtain a maximal vital capacity, but if GPB is being used continuously as a substitute for normal tidal breathing approximately 6–8 gulps may be taken before breathing out.

GPB would normally be taught with the patient in a comfortable sitting position, but when mastered should be practised in positions useful for the patient to clear his bronchial secretions. After filling his chest to capacity he signals to the physiotherapist who compresses his chest as he lets the air out. The patient may have sufficient muscle power to apply compression himself or carers can be taught to give assistance.

GPB is learnt easily by some patients, but others need time and patience to acquire this skill and must be motivated to practise frequently during the learning period. It is a valuable technique to consider when treating tetraplegic or poliomyelitis patients with a vital capacity of less than 2 litres. Instruction can begin when the patient has reached a stable condition, but it is inappropriate in the acute phase or during an acute chest infection. When successfully learnt it is invaluable during a period of chest infection to assist in the clearance of secretions. For a patient with a chest infection nursed in a 'tank' ventilator ('iron lung'), assisted coughing (Higgens 1966) may be more effective if the patient uses GPB to augment the inspiratory volume received from the ventilator before chest compression is applied.

It is possible to teach GPB to patients with an uncuffed tracheostomy tube, provided there is an effective seal round the tube to avoid air leaks.

GPB should not be attempted in patients with neuromuscular disorders affecting swallowing, and, in patients with a progressive disorder, intermittent positive pressure breathing (IPPB) may be more appropriate than GPB. The technique is contraindicated in patients with airflow obstruction or pulmonary disease.

Manual hyperinflation

The technique of manual hyperinflation may be indicated to mobilize and assist clearance of excess bronchial secretions and to reinflate areas of lung collapse in the intubated patient. It is described in Chapter 11 (p. 285).

Airway suction

Airway suction is usually necessary to clear secretions from the intubated patient with an endotracheal tube, tracheostomy, minitracheostomy or the patient with an 'airway'. For adults this is described in Chapter 11 (p. 287). For children including the non-intubated infant and small child, see Chapter 13, page 338.

Suction is required occasionally in the non-intubated adult who has retained secretions. The vacuum pressure should be kept as low as possible, and usually in the range 60–150 mmHg (8.0–20 kPa), but this will vary with the viscosity of the mucus. A built-in finger tip control or Y-connector is recommended to allow a more gradual build-up of suction pressure than is possible by the release of a kinked catheter tube.

Before any suction procedure it is important to give an explanation to the patient.

Nasotracheal suction is a means of stimulating a cough, but is an unpleasant procedure for the patient and should only be performed when absolutely necessary. The indication for suction is the inability to cough effectively and expectorate when secretions are retained. It may be necessary, for example, when an acute exacerbation of chronic bronchitis has led to carbon dioxide narcosis and respiratory failure, in neurological disorders, postoperative complications or laryngeal dysfunction. It is contraindicated when there is stridor or severe bronchospasm.

Airway suction causes damage to the tracheal epithelium and this can be minimized by the appropriate choice of catheter and technique. A flexible catheter of suitable size, usually 12 FG in adults, is lubricated with a water-soluble jelly and gently passed through the nasal passage so that it curves down into the pharynx. Occasionally a cough may be stimulated when the catheter reaches the pharynx, suction can then be applied, the secretions aspirated and the catheter withdrawn. More often it is necessary to pass the catheter between the vocal cords and into the trachea to stimulate coughing. The catheter is less likely to enter the oesophagus if the patient's neck is extended, and if he is able to cooperate it is often helpful if he can put his tongue out. The catheter should be inserted during the inspiratory phase and if it passes into the trachea will stimulate vigorous coughing.

Oxygen should always be available during the suction procedure and the patient observed for signs of hypoxia. If it has been difficult to insert the catheter and the patient looks cyanosed, instead of withdrawing the catheter from the trachea, suction should be stopped and oxygen administered until the patient's colour has improved. Suction can then be restarted.

Adults nursed in the sitting position can be suctioned in that position, but comatose patients should be suctioned in side lying to avoid the possibility of aspiration if vomiting occurs.

Using the technique of nasotracheal suction it is important to be aware of the possibility of causing laryngeal spasm (Sykes et al 1976) or vagal nerve stimulation which may lead to cardiac arrhythmias (Jacob 1990). Provided that suction is carried out carefully and oxygen is always available it is a valuable technique and may avoid the need for the more invasive treatments of bronchoscopy, endotracheal intubation or minitracheotomy. However, it should not be undertaken until every attempt to achieve effective coughing has failed.

Suction via the nose is contraindicated in patients with head injuries where there is a leak of cerebrospinal fluid into the nasal passages. *Oropharyngeal suction* through an airway would be an alternative method. An oropharyngeal airway is a plastic tube shaped to fit the curved palate. It is inserted with its tip directed towards the roof of the mouth and is then rotated so that the tip lies over the back of the tongue.

Although retention of secretions may be a problem in patients with respiratory muscle paralysis there is no benefit in using suction in an attempt to stimulate an effective cough. It is the lack of volume of air that prevents clearance of secretions in these patients and it is the combination of gravity-assisted drainage positions, chest compression and intermittent positive pressure breathing or glossopharyngeal breathing (p. 159) which should provide an effective means of clearance.

Portable suction units are available for domiciliary use and for patients in transit. They may be powered manually, by mains electricity, or by battery, e.g. from a car cigarette lighter adapter.

Minitracheotomy

A minitracheotomy (Fig. 8.39) may be considered when a spontaneously breathing patient is retaining bronchial secretions. It has been used successfully in surgical and medical patients (Preston et al 1986). Nasotracheal suction may have been successful in clearing some secretions

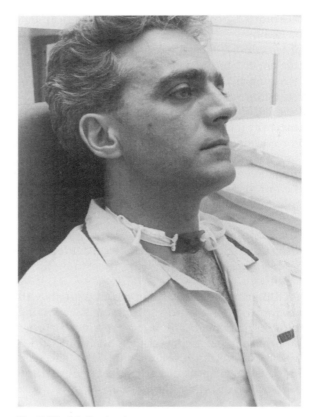

Fig. 8.39 Minitracheotomy.

but is unpleasant and traumatic for the patient if it needs to be repeated frequently. A minitracheotomy is a means of clearing secretions more easily while avoiding the more invasive techniques of bronchoscopy, endotracheal intubation or tracheostomy (Ryan 1990). It would not provide an adequate airway for ventilation and it offers no airway protection.

A cannula with an internal diameter of 4 mm is inserted into the trachea through the cricothyroid membrane (Matthews & Hopkinson 1984). The procedure can be carried out under local anaesthesia and the minitracheotomy allows tracheal suction as often as necessary.

With the small tube in position the patient is able to breathe normally through the mouth and nose and the inspired air is humidified as it passes through the nasal passages. The patient can talk, eat and drink normally and the tube does not prevent him from coughing effectively. Oxygen can be administered by a face mask or nasal cannulae if required.

With a minitracheotomy a size 10 FG suction catheter is the maximum size that can be used. Size 8 FG is usually too narrow to clear secretions effectively. Normal saline solution (1–2 ml) is instilled via the minitracheotomy before suction to assist in maintaining patency of the tube. The catheter is gently inserted either until a cough is stimulated or the carina is reached and suction is applied when starting to withdraw it. There may be copious secretions which will take longer to clear using this small catheter, but the patient is able to breathe with the narrow tracheal tube in situ and the procedure should not be distressing.

As soon as the patient is capable of clearing his secretions effectively without becoming exhausted the minitracheotomy is removed and the small incision heals quickly.

The size of the minitracheotomy was designed for the adult trachea and is not recommended for children under the age of 12 years (Preston et al 1986).

Management of stress incontinence

Many patients with chronic cough and requiring airway clearance techniques, suffer from stress incontinence which often causes them embarrassment. The physiotherapist, during assessment (p. 9), should include questions to identify if this is a problem. Instruction in pelvic floor exercises will probably be helpful, but referral to an expert physiotherapist would ensure the best treatment programme and advice.

NEUROPHYSIOLOGICAL FACILITATION OF RESPIRATION

Neurophysiological facilitation of respiration is the terminology used to describe externally applied proprioceptive and tactile stimuli that produce reflex respiratory movement responses and that appear to alter the rate and depth of breathing.

The chest care of unconscious persons is particularly challenging because of their inability to participate in the more traditional treatment approaches which require a large component of voluntary effort. Although these patients may tolerate chest percussion and vibrations, for a variety of reasons it may not be possible to place them in optimum positions for postural drainage. In order to minimize cerebral oedema it may be necessary to keep the head elevated. Instrumentation to monitor cranial pressure, intubation and external ventilation are some of the factors that must be taken into account.

Inadequate ventilation due to shallow and/or monotonous respiration poses a particular danger to this patient population. Monotonous respiration is a major factor in the development of atelectasis. The normal adult ventilatory pattern includes spontaneous deep breaths every 5–10 minutes. In experiments to study the development of atelectasis, alteration of this pattern to shallow monotonous tidal volume without deep breaths resulted in gradual alveolar collapse beginning within 1 hour in normal volunteers, patients and experimental animals (Bartlett et al 1973). Inadequate ventilation leads to the retention of secretions and in the unconscious patient this creates a need for frequent suctioning. Deranged mechanical respiratory function is another complication frequently encountered. This may be associated with trauma, but often lack of muscle tone and instability of the chest wall is the only apparent cause. It is also possible to be presented with a 'stiff' chest exhibiting little respiratory movement. This may be a result of disease (lack of costal movement) or increased tone in the intercostal muscles may be implicated. Experiments with decerebrate rigidity in cats have demonstrated that the increased muscle tonus also involves the intercostal muscles, proving that the respiratory muscles also obey brain stem mechanisms (Frankstein 1970).

The observed responses to these *facilitatory stimuli* have been remarkably consistent in unconscious patients, normal subjects and laboratory animals observed under fluoroscopy. Application of these procedures results in:

visible deeper respirations – larger expansion of the ribs and increased epigastric excursion; increased visible and often palpable tone in abdominal muscles; change in respiratory rate (usually slower); involuntary coughing; more normal respiratory pattern; rapid return of mechanical stability; changes in breath sounds on auscultation; retention of improved respiratory pattern after the treatment period and apparent increase in the level of consciousness (Bethune 1976).

The responses are most pronounced in the most deeply unconscious. The changes noted during treatment are frequently dramatic. The stimuli used in treatment have been designated as follows (Bethune 1975):

- Perioral pressure
- Intercostal stretch
- Vertebral pressure to the upper thoracic spine
- Vertebral pressure to the lower thoracic spine
- Anterior stretch-lifting of the posterior basal area
- Maintained manual pressure.

Perioral pressure

Perioral stimulation is provided by applying firm maintained pressure to the patient's upper lip. Pressure is maintained for the length of time that the therapist wishes the patient to breathe in the activated pattern. (As a precautionary measure the use of surgical gloves is advised to avoid picking up a contaminant and/or carrying contaminants from one patient to another.) The response to this stimulus is a brief (approximately 5 seconds) period of apnoea followed by increased epigastric excursions. The initial response may frequently be observed as a large maintained epigastric swell. As the stimulus is maintained the epigastric excursions may increase so that movement is transmitted to the upper thorax and the patient appears to be 'deep breathing'. The patient may sigh on initiation of the procedure or sometime after the response has become established.

Margaret Rood taught perioral pressure as a procedure to reduce spastic muscle tone. She considered it a prerequisite to her method of initiating movement by using light moving tactile stimuli. She taught that perioral pressure would inhibit hypertonus and that if the patient's mouth was open the pressure would cause it to close. If the mouth should remain open, then facilitatory touch stimuli around the face were deemed contraindicated.

Perioral pressure was reviewed by Rood (1973) as a stimulus that produced generalized relaxation. In her terminology it produced a 'parasympathetic' bias as opposed to sympathetic influences. This 'parasympathetic' bias she saw as a desirable background for many facilitatory procedures. Conscious patients can and often do apply their own perioral pressure. Many therapists use the stimulus as a method of relaxation. The fact that Rood did not become aware of the respiratory effects of perioral stimulation was probably due to her treatment focus and her patient population.

If in the unconscious patient the mouth is open, perioral pressure often causes the mandible to be drawn up. The mouth may close. Swallowing is noted and sucking movements are often evident even in the presence of oral airways. Swallowing and sucking may not always be demonstrated in initial treatments, but may appear in the most deeply unconscious after repeated stimulation. Occasionally a deeply unconscious patient has been observed to push pursed lips forward in a 'mouth phenomenon' or 'lip phenomenon'. This mouth or lip phenomenon has been observed by several investigators and reported by Peiper (1963) as a reflex response to gentle tapping on the upper lip, noted in young normal infants and in adults with severe cerebral disorders.

Peiper studied the neurology of respiration and the neurology of food intake including the relationship between sucking, swallowing and breathing in infants. The movement of the lips, sucking, swallowing and chewing have been reported on stroking the lips of comatose adults. They are thought to be related to infantile rooting reflexes.

'During the infant's food intake three centrally directed rhythmic movements arise; sucking, breathing and swallowing' (Peiper 1963). Earlier experiments on young animals established the presence of a sucking centre located bilaterally in the medulla. Peiper established that the sucking centre took precedence. The initiation of sucking at once disturbed respiration. There occurred a lowering of the diaphragm for 5 seconds or more before respirations resumed at a new rhythm (led by the sucking centre). Peiper also documented that after sucking movements ceased, the respiratory movements maintained, for a period, the new (in this case, faster) rhythm.

The similarities between Peiper's observations and those in response to perioral stimuli are lowering of the diaphragm (maintained for 5 seconds or more), a new respiratory rhythm and maintenance of that rhythm for a time after removal of the stimulus. This implies that Peiper's recorded phenomena and perioral stimuli are related. Perioral pressure seems to elicit reflex respiratory responses related to early feeding reflexes.

Intercostal stretch

Intercostal stretch is provided by applying pressure to the upper border of a rib in order to stretch the intercostal muscle in a downward (not inward) direction. The stretch position is then maintained while the patient continues to breathe in his/her usual manner. This procedure can be performed unilaterally or bilaterally on any rib with the exception of the floating ribs. Care must be taken to avoid sensitive mammary tissue in female patients.

The response to this stimulus is a gradual increase in respiratory movements in the area under and around the stretch. This procedure appears to be effective in restoring respiratory movement patterns when performed over areas of instability, for example when paradoxical movement of the upper ribs is present (fractured ribs excepted) or over areas of decreased mobility. Epigastric excursions can be observed if intercostal stretch is performed bilaterally over the lower ribs, but above the floating ribs.

The first effect appears to be the response of intercostal muscle spindles to stretch. The latter effect of epigastric excursion on bilateral stimuli to the lower ribs may represent the reflex control of the diaphragm via the intercostal afferents that innervate its margins.

Vertebral pressure

Very firm manual pressure applied with the open hand directly over the uppermost thoracic vertebrae results in increased epigastric excursions via the presence of a mainly relaxed abdominal wall. Pressure applied in the same manner directly over the lower thoracic vertebrae results in increased respiratory movements of the apical thorax. Because of the problem of stabilizing a patient in a side lying position, these procedures are best performed in a supine lying position with patients who are confined to bed.

Dorsal root section has provided a tool for the study of segmental proprioceptive respiratory control. Observations of augmented diaphragmatic activity in response to high thoracic vertebral stimulation and facilitated apical respiratory activity following pressure over the lower thoracic vertebrae seem to correlate with the observations of Helen Coombs. Coombs (1918) demonstrated that section of thoracic dorsal roots diminished costal respiration in cats. Abdominal respiration remained unaltered. In a later study (Coombs & Pike 1930) with kittens she found that dorsal root section of the thoracic nerves almost abolished costal respiration. If the thoracic nerves were left intact and dorsal root section performed at a higher level – the cervical level – movements of the diaphragm were much diminished.

Co-contraction of the abdomen

Co-contraction of the abdomen is a procedure that Margaret Rood (1973) taught to facilitate respiration. It increased the tone in the abdominal muscles. Rood thought that abdominal co-contraction also activated the diaphragm. This procedure is performed by the therapist placing one hand on the patient's lower ribs and one on the pelvis on the same side and pushing with moderate pressure so that force is applied at right angles to the patient. Rood thought that this procedure produced stretch on the abdominal muscles, first on the contralateral side. This would activate the muscle spindles and they in turn would cause their homonymous extrafusal muscles to contract. The contraction of these muscles would in turn stretch the abdominal muscles on the other side (the side nearest the therapist's hands). The stretch would activate the spindles in these muscles which in turn would activate their own extrafusal muscle. A contraction would result and muscles on the other side would again be stretched. Alternating activation was thought to occur as the pressure was maintained.

In practice it does not appear that the side contralateral to the applied pressure is always activated first. The level of pre-existing tone appears to be an important factor. In obese abdomens and sometimes in postoperative abdomens the amount of stretch in the procedure does not seem sufficient to activate the opposite side first and the muscles on the side where the pressure is applied may be the first to react. Abdominal co-contractions must be done on both sides of the abdomen and are usually performed with pressures maintained for some seconds and applied alternately to first one side then to the other and repeated as necessary to obtain the response and maintain it for the time period desired.

This is an effective procedure. Increasing tone in the abdomen can both be seen (by increased muscle definition) and palpated. Increased epigastric excursions occur. If retained secretions are present abdominal co-contraction may produce coughing more readily than other procedures; however, as ventilation increases, coughing may occur with any procedure. The preceding observations are supported by the hypothesis that action of the diaphragm may be enhanced by an increase in abdominal pressure and that lower intercostal afferents may exert reflex control over diaphragmatic activity.

Anterior-stretch basal lift

This procedure is performed by placing the hands under the posterior ribs of the supine patient and lifting gently upwards. The lift is maintained and provides a maintained stretch and pressure posteriorly and stretch anteriorly as well. This may be performed bilaterally if the patient is small enough. Should this not be possible or necessary, it can be done as a unilateral treatment. As the lift stretch is maintained, increasing movements of the ribs in lateral and posterior directions can be seen and felt. Increased epigastric movements also often become obvious.

Maintained manual pressure

It would probably be more correct to call this procedure maintained manual contact since the tendency of most therapists is to press too firmly. Mild pressure of the open hand(s) is maintained over the area in which expansion is desired. Gradual increasing excursion of the ribs under contact will be felt. This is a useful procedure to obtain expansion in painful situations, in the presence of chest tubes for example, or following cardiac surgery which may have required splitting of the sternum. Manual contact is also useful when applied over the posterior chest wall of patients with chronic obstructive lung disease. Such patients may sit leaning forward with their arms supported high on pillows and their head resting on their arms for comfort.

Sumi (1963) in studies of hair, tactile and pressure receptors has reported cutaneous fields for both inspiratory and expiratory motor neurons in cats. He was of the opinion that because the excitatory skin fields for the inspiratory motor neurons were more extensive than those of expiratory motor neurons, more inspiratory than expiratory motor neurons can be excited by a single skin stimulus. Thus, local cutaneous stimulation of the thoracic region would tend to reflexly provoke an inspiratory position of the thorax. Eklund et al (1964) are among other investigators who have demonstrated reflex effects on intercostal motor activity in response to stimulation of afferents from the overlying skin (Table 8.2).

Application to patients

In utilizing these procedures in the hospital setting chest auscultation and the usual assessment procedures should be completed before and after treatment. The patient should also

Table 8.2 Neurophysiological facilitation for the chest

Procedure	Method	Observations	Suggested mechanism
Perioral stimulation	Pressure is applied to the patient's top lip by the therapist's finger – and maintained	• Increased epigastric excursion • 'Deep breathing' • Sighing • Mouth closure • Swallowing • 'Snout phenomena'	Primitive reflex response related to sucking
Vertebral pressure – high	Manual pressure to thoracic vertebrae in region of T_2–T_5	• Increased epigastric excursions • 'Deep breathing'	Dorsal-root-mediated intersegmental reflex
Vertebral pressure – low	Manual pressure to thoracic vertebrae in region of T_7–T_{10}	Increased respiratory movements of apical thorax	
Anterior stretch – lifting posterior basal area	• Patient supine • Hands under lower ribs • Ribs lifted upward	• Expansion posterior basal area • Increased epigastric movements	• Dorsal root as above • Stretch receptors in intercostals, back muscles
Co-contraction – abdomen	• Pressure laterally over lower ribs and pelvis • Alternate right and left sides	• Increased epigastric movements • Increased muscle contraction (rectus abdominus) • Decreased girth in obese • Increased firmness to palpation • Depression of umbilicus	Stretch receptors in abdominal muscles ?intercostal to phrenic reflex
Intercostal stretch	Stretch on expiratory phase maintained	Increased movement of area being stretched	Intercostal stretch receptors
Moderate manual pressure	Moderate pressure open palm	Gradually increased excursion of area under contact	Cutaneous afferents

be assessed during treatment to gauge response and help determine treatment duration. It is essential to note the patient's respiratory movement pattern. Is simultaneous and equal thoracic movement present or is there chest lag on one side? Are there any paradoxical movements between the chest and abdomen? Are there any areas of indrawing on inspiration? The therapist needs to know how patterns of ventilation are changing. The patient's response determines the duration of the treatment which is why assessment is critical. A procedure is continued until the therapist's assessment indicates that the desired effect has been achieved (increased breath sounds, increased respiratory movements, cough).

Changes in breath sounds, as determined by auscultation, have been noted with all the procedures. Breath sounds often become evident in areas that previously appeared silent. Many patients may raise secretions by coughing, but the unconscious are unable to expectorate. Suctioning to remove secretions in these patients may not be required as frequently and may be more effective as secretions are more accessible.

Some unconscious patients appear to become less deeply unconscious during respiratory facilitation. Responses such as fluttering eyelids, head movements, spontaneous movements, opening of the eyes and mumbling have been noted. Sometimes such a patient will push the therapist's hands away. This is a good sign as such patients are frequently considered to be unresponsive. An occasional patient will initially turn his head away from the perioral stimulus but accept it with further application. It is difficult to determine whether these reactions are due to increased ventilation, to the stimulation that handling provides or to both.

It is important to remember that these reactions are responses to stimuli. Every patient will not necessarily demonstrate the same level of responsiveness to each procedure. Response seems to be related to the patient's pre-existing muscle tone, level of consciousness and perhaps other factors such as the adequacy of ventilation. For example, some obese persons may take longer to respond to abdominal co-contractions than to perioral pressure. A certain decerebrate patient had so much muscle tonus in his torso that abdominal co-contractions applied to him while he was in a supine position caused him to begin to elevate into a sitting position. Since this was not desired other procedures were used. It is imperative to observe a patient's response and to modify treatment appropriately. It is not necessary to perform every procedure with every patient.

Conscious medical patients (following cerebral vascular accident, Guillain–Barré syndrome) often appreciate the relaxation and lack of the sense of effort when respiratory facilitation is used in their chest care.

RESPIRATORY MUSCLE TRAINING

Respiratory muscle training devices have been used to increase strength and endurance in the muscles of either inspiration or expiration (Pardy et al 1981, Pardy et al 1988). Whether this 'training' affects exercise ability, activities of daily living, morbidity or mortality has yet to be determined and once training ceases the effect of conditioning declines (Pardy et al 1990, Smith et al 1992). See also Chapter 14, page 380.

The patient breathes through a mouthpiece or a face mask with a resistance applied to either the inspiratory or expiratory limb of a valve. The valve may be 'flow resistive' or 'threshold loading'. With a flow resistive device the patient breathes in and out through an aperture. Alteration in the size of the aperture alters the load on the respiratory muscles, provided the frequency of breathing, tidal volume and inspiratory or expiratory time are kept constant. The load is increased by decreasing the size of the aperture. If the patient breathes more slowly and deeply the pressure exerted on the respiratory muscles will be less than if he breathes more quickly and not as deeply (Pardy et al 1990).

A threshold loading device requires a pre-determined pressure to initiate either inspiration or expiration and this is dependent on the magnitude of the threshold load. When inspiration or expiration has been initiated the pressure required to keep the valve open is constant and independent of the flow rate. To provide a maximal training effect, inspiratory or expiratory time and the frequency of breathing should be controlled (Pardy et al 1990). Threshold loading devices will increase the pressure generated by the inspiratory or expiratory muscles and are more reliable and reproducible as training devices (Flynn et al 1989, Morrison et al 1989, Gosselink et al 1996).

On assessment the appropriate resistance is selected for an individual patient. By increasing the length of time for treatment, endurance may be improved and by increasing the resistance, muscle strength may be increased.

The studies by Flynn et al (1989) and Morrison et al (1989) were undertaken in patients with chronic airflow limitation. In patients with severe respiratory disease it is possible that they will already have 'trained' their respiratory muscles as a result of the increased load created by the increased work of breathing, and further respiratory muscle training would be of limited value (Pardy et al 1990, Moxham 1991).

In conditions of respiratory muscle weakness the underlying cause of the weakness should be treated, for example myasthenia gravis, malnutrition and electrolyte imbalance (Moxham 1991). Disuse atrophy may result from resting the respiratory muscles during prolonged assisted ventilation. Many factors will contribute to improvement in muscle strength and endurance, such as nutrition, and the treatment of infection and other underlying disease processes. It is possible that inspiratory muscle training may assist the weaning process in these subjects (Abelson & Brewer 1987, Aldrich et al 1989).

In cervical and high thoracic spinal injuries, progressive resistive exercises are recommended for increasing respiratory muscle strength and endurance (Gross et al 1980, Morgan et al 1986). McCool & Tzelepis (1995) have reviewed the use of inspiratory muscle training in patients with neuromuscular disease and conclude that the most severely affected patients are least likely to benefit from treatment, but in the early stages it may improve respiratory muscle function.

The response to treatment can be monitored by measuring maximal inspiratory mouth pressures (PiMax) or maximal expiratory mouth pressures (PeMax). Further rigorous clinical trials are necessary to identify the place of respiratory muscle training. Does it significantly improve respiratory muscle strength, endurance and exercise performance, and if so in which patient groups?

INTERMITTENT POSITIVE PRESSURE BREATHING AND PERIODIC CONTINUOUS POSITIVE AIRWAY PRESSURE

Intermittent positive pressure breathing

Intermittent positive pressure breathing (IPPB) is the maintenance of a positive airway pressure throughout inspiration, with airway pressure returning to atmospheric pressure during expiration. The Bird Mark 7 ventilator (Fig. 8.40) is a pressure cycled device convenient to use for providing IPPB as an adjunct to physiotherapy in the spontaneously breathing patient.

IPPB has been shown to augment tidal volume (Sukumalchantra et al 1965), and using an IPPB device in the completely relaxed subject the work of breathing during inspiration approaches zero (Ayres et al 1963). These two effects support the use of IPPB to help in the clearance of bronchial secretions when more simple airway clearance techniques alone are not maximally effective, for example in the semicomatose patient with chronic bronchitis and sputum retention (Pavia et al 1988), or in a patient with neuromuscular disease and a chest infection. The reduction in the work of breathing can be used with effect in the acute severe exhausted asthmatic, but there is no evidence that the effect of bronchodilators delivered by IPPB is greater than from a nebulizer alone (Webber et al 1974).

An ideal IPPB device for use with physiotherapy should be portable and have simple controls. Other important features are:

Positive pressure. The range of pressures is likely to be from 0–35 cmH$_2$O.

Sensitivity. The patient should be able to 'trigger' the inspiratory phase with minimal effort. Fully automatic control is unpleasant for most patients and unnecessary for physiotherapy. A hand triggering device is useful to test the ventilator and nebulizer.

Flow control. With ventilators such as the Bird Mark 7 the inspiratory gas is delivered at

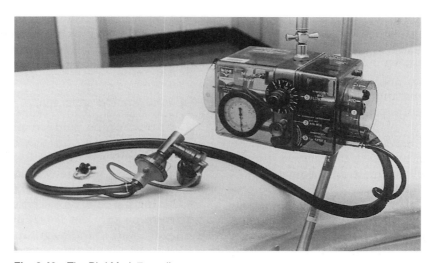

Fig. 8.40   The Bird Mark 7 ventilator.

a flow rate which can be preset by means of a control knob. Optimal distribution of gas to the more peripheral airways is achieved at relatively slow flow rates, but if the patient is very short of breath and has a fast respiratory rate, a slow inspiratory phase may be unacceptable. It is often useful to alter the flow control several times during a single treatment session, providing slow breaths during the periods attempting to mobilize peripheral secretions and a faster flow rate when a patient is recovering his breath after expectoration. The Bennett PR-1 and AP-5 (which are no longer available to purchase in the UK, but may be available within a hospital for use) do not require flow rate adjustment because automatic variable flow is provided with each breath. This feature is known as 'flow sensitivity' and means that the flow of the inspired gas adapts to the resistance of the individual's airways.

Nebulizer. An efficient nebulizer in the circuit is necessary to humidify the driving gas and, when appropriate, to deliver bronchodilator drugs. The nebulizer in the Bird circuit is driven automatically with the inspiratory phase of the ventilator, but the Bennett has a separate control knob for the nebulizer.

Air-mix control. When driven by oxygen, air must be entrained by the apparatus to provide an air/oxygen mixture for the patient. Some Bird devices have a control which should be set to give a mixture, while others have no control but automatically entrain air. The use of 100% oxygen for a patient is very rare, and when it is indicated an IPPB device with an air-mix control will be needed. When air is not entrained through the apparatus the flow rate control must be regulated to provide an adequate flow to the patient.

When IPPB is driven by oxygen and the air-mix control is in use, the percentage of oxygen delivered to the patient is approximately 45% (Starke et al 1979). This percentage will be considerably higher than the controlled percentage delivered by an appropriate venturi mask, for example to a patient with chronic bronchitis. This higher percentage is rarely dangerous during treatment because the patient's ventilation is assisted and the removal of secretions as a result of treatment is likely to lead subsequently to an improvement in arterial blood gas tensions (Gormezano & Branthwaite 1972).

It has been suggested that a few patients become more drowsy during or after IPPB as a result of the high percentage of oxygen received. Starke et al (1979) showed that increased drowsiness caused by hypercapnia occurred whether oxygen or air was the driving gas for IPPB and that the deterioration was dependent on inappropriate settings of the ventilator. The pressure and flow controls must be set to provide an adequate tidal volume, this being particularly important when treating patients with a rigid thoracic cage (Starke et al 1979).

Occasionally, IPPB may be powered by Entonox (p. 300) and in this case the air-mix control would need to be in the position to provide 100% of the driving gas with no additional air entrained.

Breathing circuit. To prevent cross-infection it is essential for each patient to have his own breathing circuit which consists of tubing, nebulizer, exhalation valve and a mouthpiece or mask. The majority of patients prefer to use a mouthpiece, but a face mask is required when treating confused patients. A flange mouthpiece (Fig. 8.41) is useful for patients who have difficulty making an airtight seal around the mouthpiece.

The type of breathing circuit used will depend on the local means of sterilization. They can be autoclavable, non-disposable but non-autoclavable, or disposable.

Preparation of the apparatus

1. Normal saline solution or a combination of a bronchodilator drug and normal saline (3–4 ml in total) is inserted into the nebulizer.

2. The breathing circuit is connected to the IPPB ventilator, and the ventilator connected to the driving gas source. It can be used from an oxygen or air cylinder if piped compressed gas is unavailable.

3. If there is an air-mix control, this should be in the position for entrainment of air.

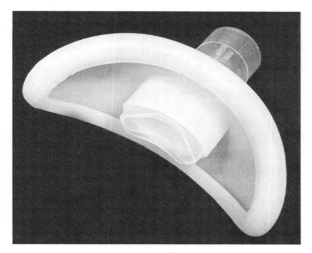

Fig. 8.41 Flange mouthpiece for use with IPPB.

4. If there is an automatic control (expiratory timer) this should be turned off to allow the patient to 'trigger' the machine at his desired rate.

5. The sensitivity, flow and pressure controls are set appropriately for the individual. With the Bird Mark 7 the sensitivity control is usually adjusted to a low number (5–7) where minimal inspiratory effort is required. The pressure and flow controls are adjusted to provide regular assisted ventilation without discomfort. A patient with a rigid rib cage will require a higher pressure setting to obtain an adequate tidal volume than someone with a more mobile rib cage.

When adjusting the settings for a new patient it may be easiest to start with a pressure at approximately 12 cmH$_2$O and the flow at about 10, then gradually increase the pressure and reduce the flow until the pattern of breathing is the most appropriate for the individual. Some IPPB devices do not have numbered markings, but after finding the most effective settings for a patient during one treatment, it is useful to note the positions of the controls in order to use these as a starting point at the next treatment. The controls to be set on the Bennett PR-1 are the nebulizer, sensitivity and pressure.

6. Before starting a treatment the hand triggering device is operated to check that there are no leaks in the breathing circuit and that the nebulizer is functioning well.

Treatment of the patient

The position in which IPPB is used depends on the indication for treatment. It may be used in side lying (Fig. 8.42), high side lying (Fig. 8.43) or in the sitting position. The patient should be positioned comfortably and encouraged to relax the upper chest and shoulder girdle.

After the purpose of the IPPB treatment has been explained, the patient is asked to close his lips firmly around the mouthpiece and then to make a slight inspiratory effort which will trigger the device into inspiratory flow. He should then relax throughout inspiration allowing his lungs to be inflated. When the preset pressure is reached at the mouth the ventilator cycles into expiration; the patient should remain relaxed and let the air out quietly.

If the patient attempts to assist inspiration there will be a delay in reaching the cycling pressure. A delay will also occur if there is a leak around the mouthpiece, at any of the circuit connections, or from the patient's nose. A nose clip may be required until he becomes familiar with the technique.

The physiotherapist will find it useful to watch the manometer on the ventilator in order to detect any faults in the patient's technique. At the start of inspiration the needle should swing minimally to a negative pressure and then swing smoothly up to the positive pressure set, before cutting out into expiration and returning to zero. A larger negative swing at the beginning of inspiration shows that the patient is making an unnecessary effort in triggering the device. If the patient makes an active effort throughout inspiration the needle will rise very slowly to the inspiratory set pressure, and if he attempts to start expiration before the preset pressure is reached the needle will rise sharply above the set pressure and then cut out into expiration.

When IPPB is taught correctly the work of breathing is relieved, but if the patient is allowed

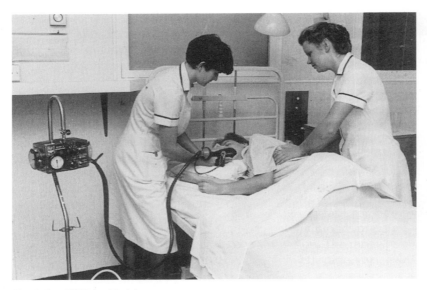

Fig. 8.42 IPPB in side lying.

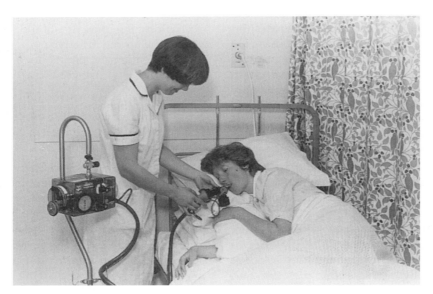

Fig. 8.43 IPPB to reduce the work of breathing during inhalation of nebulized bronchodilator.

to assist either inspiration or expiration there will be an increase in the work of breathing.

The patient should pause momentarily after expiration, before the next inspiration to avoid hyperventilation and possible dizziness. Occasionally children using IPPB tend to swallow air during treatment. It is important to observe the size of the abdomen before and during IPPB to recognize signs of abdominal distension and discontinue IPPB if this occurs.

When IPPB is used to relieve the work of breathing while delivering bronchodilator drugs, e.g. in the acute severe asthmatic patient, it is often helpful for the physiotherapist to hold the breathing circuit to allow the patient to relax his shoulders and arms as much as possible (Fig. 8.43).

A face mask for IPPB is used in the drowsy or confused patient, and in those with facial weakness unable to make an airtight seal at the mouth. When using IPPB to assist in mobilizing secretions the patient would be positioned to assist drainage of secretions, for example in side lying. The patient's jaw should be elevated and the mask held firmly over the face ensuring an airtight fit. Chest shaking during the expiratory phase may be used to assist in mobilizing secretions (Fig. 8.42). In a drowsy patient it may be necessary to stimulate coughing using naso-tracheal suction (p. 161) if spontaneous coughing is not stimulated by IPPB and chest shaking.

In medical patients with retained secretions and poor respiratory reserve IPPB may be useful both to mobilize secretions, and to relieve the effort of breathing following expectoration. The flow control on a Bird ventilator should be adjusted to give a slow but comfortable breath to mobilize secretions, but the patient's increased respiratory requirements following the exertion of expectoration necessitate increasing the flow and possibly reducing the pressure until he has returned to his normal breathing pattern.

IPPB may be used in patients with chest wall deformity, for example kyphoscoliosis, when they have difficulty clearing secretions during an infective episode. To achieve an adequate increase in ventilation in patients with a rigid rib cage, the pressure setting needs to be higher than for a more mobile rib cage.

Occasionally, in postoperative patients, IPPB is the adjunct of choice when the patient is unable to augment his tidal volume adequately during treatment. In these patients in contrast to the relaxed technique normally used with IPPB, thoracic expansion may be actively encouraged during the inspiratory phase.

Bott et al (1992) have reviewed the literature on IPPB and concluded that IPPB is an important adjunct to chest physiotherapy.

Periodic continuous positive airway pressure

Continuous positive airway pressure (CPAP) is the maintenance of a positive pressure throughout inspiration and expiration during spontaneous breathing. Periodic continuous positive airway pressure (PCPAP) is the application of this on a periodic or intermittent basis.

One way of producing CPAP is to use a commercially available high flow (50–80 l/min) generator. Wide-bore tubing transmits the high flow to the patient who breathes in and out using a mouthpiece and nose clip (Fig. 8.44) or a mask (Fig. 8.45). On the expiratory limb of the circuit is a threshold resistor valve and in clinical practice a resistance of 5–10 cmH$_2$O is used. Both fixed inspired oxygen (FiO$_2$) generators and variable FiO$_2$ generators are available. Care must be taken when a fixed FiO$_2$ generator (providing approximately 33% oxygen) is used in a hypercapnic patient. It may be necessary to drive the high flow generator from an air supply with added oxygen entrained through the air supply inlet to provide the appropriate FiO$_2$. As large volumes of room air are entrained, additional humidification is only occasionally required with PCPAP. If humidification is indicated, as in a patient with very tenacious secretions, a large

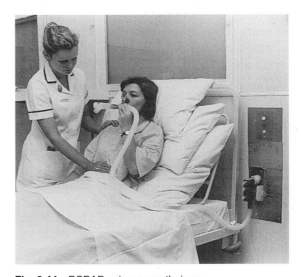

Fig. 8.44   PCPAP using a mouthpiece.

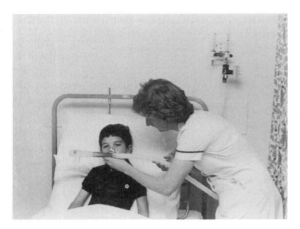

Fig. 8.45 PCPAP using a mask.

volume vapour humidifier is recommended to humidify the high flow adequately (Fig. 8.57, p. 189).

In order to maintain a positive pressure within the airways throughout inspiration and expiration, the patient's peak inspiratory flow rate must be exceeded at all times. This can be detected by a continuous flow of air through the expiratory resistor and can either be felt or monitored using a respirometer or other flow-sensitive device.

PCPAP has been shown to increase functional residual capacity (FRC) (Gherini et al 1979, Stock et al 1985, Lindner et al 1987) and to reduce the work of breathing (Gherini et al 1979). The reduction in the work of breathing is probably due to an increase in lung compliance with the patient breathing at a higher lung volume (Hinds & Watson 1996). These two effects support the use of PCPAP in restrictive lung problems, for example in the treatment of postoperative subsegmental lung collapse.

In normal lungs the resistance to collateral flow via the interalveolar pores of Kohn, bronchiole–alveolar channels of Lambert, and probably the interbronchiolar channels of Martin, is high (Menkes & Traystman 1977) but this alters in disease and may also change at high lung volumes. Andersen et al (1980) have proposed that CPAP increases collateral flow to poorly ventilated or non-ventilated air spaces to aid the

resolution of lung collapse. Interdependence (Mead et al 1970) may also be important and Menkes & Britt (1980) state that an increase in lung volume is the simplest and most effective way of reducing the resistance within the airways.

There are as yet no guidelines for treatment based on rigorous clinical studies. This is probably because there are so many variables to consider – the underlying pathology, the optimal pressure within the airways, the optimal time for treatment and the position of the patient. In addition CPAP has become increasingly used as a means of ventilatory support.

A treatment regimen may be outlined as follows: after positioning the patient, a period of approximately 15 minutes' PCPAP is followed by the appropriate breathing techniques for airway clearance. Treatment sessions are repeated as indicated.

When deciding on the position of the patient during PCPAP, consideration should be given to the optimal position for increasing FRC (i.e. sitting upright) and the effect of gravity on bronchial secretions (which may indicate a tipped position). More than one position may be appropriate; for example, with a left lower lobe collapse, sitting upright should improve FRC (Hinds & Watson 1996) and right side lying with the foot of the bed raised should assist drainage of secretions from the left lower lobe.

When PCPAP is used in children it is important to observe the size of the abdomen before and during PCPAP. Some children swallow air during treatment which may cause abdominal distension and PCPAP should be discontinued if this occurs.

Contraindications for IPPB and PCPAP

- Pneumothorax.
- Large bullae.
- Lung abscess as the size of the air space may increase.
- Severe haemoptysis as treatment is inappropriate until the bleeding has lessened.
- Postoperative air leak unless the advantages

of IPPB or PCPAP will outweigh the possibility of increasing the air leak during treatment.

• Bronchial tumour in the proximal airways would contraindicate the use of IPPB or PCPAP to assist in the clearance of secretions. (Air may flow past the tumour during inspiration and may be trapped on expiration as the airways narrow. There would be no contraindication if the tumour were situated peripherally.)

IPPB or PCPAP?

The effects of IPPB and PCPAP are outlined in Table 8.3. In clinical practice the decision of when to use IPPB and when to use PCPAP is often not straightforward.

The drowsy postoperative patient unable to cooperate with thoracic expansion exercises and huffing will benefit from IPPB to augment tidal volume and to assist in mobilizing secretions. In the more cooperative postoperative patient with subsegmental lung collapse, the increase in FRC produced by PCPAP would be more effective in re-expanding lung tissue than IPPB.

The patient with asthma (an obstructive lung problem) who is exhausted may benefit from IPPB to reduce the work of breathing while receiving nebulized bronchodilators, and in the presence of hyperinflation it would be disadvantageous to consider a modality which would increase FRC. The patient with controlled asthma and subsegmental lung collapse presents with a predominantly restrictive problem and PCPAP would be the modality of choice to aid re-expansion of the lung collapse.

The patient with steroid rib fractures complicating cystic fibrosis presents with a predomi-nantly obstructive problem. PCPAP would not augment tidal volume, but would assist in the mobilization of bronchial secretions probably by increasing collateral ventilation owing to an increase in lung volume. An augmented tidal volume would cause an unnecessary increase in chest wall discomfort.

An adjunct to treatment should be considered when a maximal effect is not being achieved by simpler means. Conversely, when an equivalent effect can be achieved without an adjunct its use should be discontinued.

INHALATION: DRUGS AND HUMIDIFICATION

As the knowledge base of inhalation therapy has increased it has become more complex, and the advantages and disadvantages of the different systems and patient preferences need to be considered (Pedersen 1996). An understanding of the aerosol particle and its pattern of deposition within the airways is essential when considering the delivery of drugs by the inhaled route. A suspension of fine liquid or solid particles in air is known as an 'aerosol'. The pattern of deposition of aerosol particles within the bronchial tree depends on particle size, method of inhalation and on the degree of airflow obstruction (Newman et al 1986).

Large particles in the size range 5–10 μm deposit by impaction in the oropharynx and upper airways where the cross-sectional diameter of the airway is small and the airflow high. The total cross-section of the airway increases rapidly beyond the tenth generation of bronchi, airflow slows significantly and particles of 0.5–5 μm,

Table 8.3 The effects of IPPB and PCPAP (with acknowledgement to Heather Argyle, Physiotherapist, Christchurch, New Zealand)

IPPB	PCPAP
10–20 cmH$_2$O pressure during inspiration	5–10 cmH$_2$O pressure during inspiration and expiration
No change in FRC	Increase in FRC
Reduction in work of breathing	Reduction in work of breathing
Augmented tidal volume	No change in tidal volume
Increase in collateral ventilation(?)	Increase in collateral ventilation(?)

known as the 'respirable particles', deposit in the small airways and alveoli by gravitational sedimentation. It is the particles of less than 2 μm that reach the alveoli. Gravitational sedimentation is time dependent and enhanced by breath holding. A more central patchy deposition is seen in patients with airflow obstruction (Clarke 1988).

The topical deposition of a drug by inhalation allows a smaller dose to be given than when other routes are used, the onset of action is often more rapid, and with minimal systemic absorption the side-effects are lessened.

Metered-dose inhaler (MDI) and dry powder inhalers

Numerous devices are available for the inhalation of drugs, ranging from the simple MDI or powder inhalers to a variety of nebulizers. The physiotherapist should be aware of the range of possibilities to enable the patient to gain maximum benefit from the prescribed drugs. The choice of device will depend on the patient's age, coordination and dexterity, severity of the respiratory condition and patient preference. The propellant of the MDI which contained chlorofluorocarbon (CFC) is being replaced by one which is environmentally acceptable.

Practice with placebo inhalers may be necessary to perfect the technique. Even if a patient has been using an inhalation device for a long time, it is always worth observing his technique as it may not be effective.

To gain maximum effect from an MDI it should first be shaken to ensure that the drug is evenly distributed in the propellant gases. The inhaler is held upright and the cap is removed. The patient breathes out gently, but not fully, and then with the mouth around the mouthpiece of the inhaler, the device is pressed to release the drug as soon as inspiration has begun. The breath in should be slow and deep and inspiration should be held for 10 seconds, if possible, before breathing out gently through the nose (Burge 1986, Clarke 1988). Effective technique is essential as it is known that only about 10% of the drug reaches the lungs (Clarke 1988).

Frequently, the prescribed dose will involve the inhalation of more than one 'puff'. It is recommended that puffs be taken one after the other. If the inhalation technique described above is used, the length of time between inhalations is likely to be 15–20 seconds which allows sufficient time to overcome the problem of cooling of the metering chamber as the gas evaporates. Compliance is improved when doses are taken one after the other (Burge 1986).

Patients with arthritic hands may find the 'Haleraid' (Fig. 8.46) a useful gadget. By altering the direction of pressure required for releasing the drug it becomes an easier action to perform.

Large volume spacers (Fig. 13.14, p. 362) can be used to improve the deposition of the drug in the lungs to approximately 15% (Clarke 1988) and to reduce the deposition in the oropharynx as the larger particles drop out in the spacer

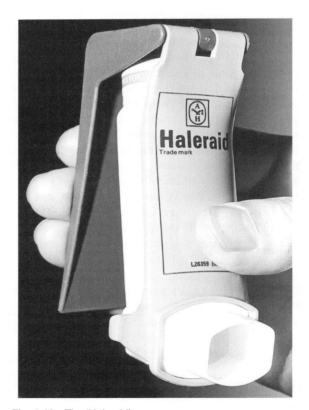

Fig. 8.46 The 'Haleraid'.

rather than the oropharynx. This helps to minimize any adverse effects.

Spacers may be cone or pear shaped, the shape of a 'puff' from an MDI. The patient is encouraged to take a slow deep breath with a hold, but if this is difficult tidal breathing can be used. Gleeson & Price (1988) showed that a bronchodilator was equally effective when a child breathed several times at tidal volume through a spacer when compared with a deep breath and inspiratory hold.

In patients with a good MDI technique there may be no additional advantage in using a spacer, but in patients with a poor technique, in severely breathless patients and in those with candidiasis or dysphonia from inhaled steroids a spacer should be considered (Clarke 1988, Keeley 1992). The addition of a piece of corrugated tubing (approximately 15 cm in length) attached to the mouthpiece of an MDI may act as a cheap and effective spacer. Oral candidiasis can be minimized by rinsing the mouth thoroughly following inhalation.

For people with poor coordination a breath-actuated MDI may be considered (Newman et al 1991) or a dry powder device. The dry powder inhalers are also breath actuated, releasing the drugs on inspiration, and require a faster inspiratory flow rate than a pressurized (MDI) inhaler. The inspiratory flow required depends on the resistance within the device.

It is not only important that the patient can use the device effectively, but also that the patient or parent can easily recall whether a dose of the drug has been taken, and many devices incorporate a monitoring system.

For inhalation therapy to be effective in infants and children, the appropriate device for the age and ability of the child (p. 362) must be selected (British Thoracic Society et al 1997). It may be necessary to use a domiciliary nebulizer system in early childhood.

For each inhalation device the individual instructions should be carefully read and followed.

Nebulizers

A nebulizer may be used for the inhalation of drugs if a more simple method cannot produce the optimal effect. A nebulizer converts a solution into aerosol particles (fine droplets) which are suspended in a stream of gas. The aim of nebulizer therapy (Nebuliser Project Group of the BTS 1997) is to deliver a therapeutic dose of a prescribed drug as an aerosol in the form of respirable particles (particles < 5 μm in diameter) in an acceptable period of time, approximately 5–10 minutes. There are two types of nebulizers – jet nebulizers and ultrasonic nebulizers.

Jet nebulizers

With the jet nebulizer a driving gas (electric air compressor or compressed air or oxygen from a hospital line or cylinder) is forced through a narrow orifice. The negative pressure created around the orifice draws the drug solution up the feed tube from the liquid reservoir and the jet of gas fragments the liquid into droplets. A screening baffle allows the smaller particles in the form of a mist to be available for inhalation by the patient and the larger particles to drop back into the reservoir to be recycled (Medic-Aid Ltd 1996).

Ultrasonic nebulizers

An aerosol can also be created by high-frequency (1–2 MHz) sound waves. An electric current applied to a piezo-electric crystal causes ultrasonic vibrations. The sound waves will travel through a liquid to the surface where they produce an aerosol. The particle size is influenced by the frequency of oscillation of the crystal. Ultrasonic nebulizers can produce a higher output than jet nebulizers. An advantage of ultrasonic nebulizers is that they operate quietly. A small volume of drug can be nebulized in a large volume ultrasonic nebulizer by the insertion of a drug chamber.

The majority of ultrasonic nebulizers are fan assisted (Fig. 21.2, p. 490), but a few models require the patient to breathe in actively to open a valve to the nebulizing chamber. Patients with very poor respiratory reserve, and children, may find this additional effort difficult.

Nebulizer performance

The performance of a nebulizer can be measured by its *respirable output*. The respirable output is the mass of *respirable particles* (particles less than 5 µm in diameter) produced per minute, i.e.:

aerosol output (mg/min) × respirable fraction.

The *respirable fraction* is the percentage of respirable particles within the aerosol output. It is recommended that a nebulizer should provide a respirable fraction of at least 50% at its recommended driving gas flow (British Standards Institution 1994) and a number of nebulizers exceed this level.

The performance of an individual nebulizer has often been described by the mass median aerodynamic diameter (MMAD) of the particles. The MMAD indicates the range of size of particles leaving the nebulizer. Half of the aerosol mass from the nebulizer is of particles smaller than the MMAD and half of the aerosol mass is of particles larger than the MMAD. This is a less useful measurement of nebulizer performance as it is not related to the mass of drug.

It is important to consider an air compressor and nebulizer system as a unit. They should be matched to provide an acceptable output (Kendrick et al 1995).

Factors which affect individual nebulizer performance include (Nebuliser Project Group of the BTS 1997):

Driving gas. Most jet nebulizers operate efficiently with a flow rate of 6–8 l/min. For patients in hospital it is often convenient to use the piped oxygen supply and in hypoxic patients without carbon dioxide retention, oxygen should be used. For patients retaining carbon dioxide who are dependent on their hypoxic drive to stimulate breathing, compressed air should be the driving gas (Gunawardena et al 1984). Occasionally it may be appropriate to increase the inspired oxygen concentration by entraining a low flow of oxygen.

Nebulizer chamber design. With a *'conventional'* nebulizer the output flow (from the nebulizer, towards the patient) is equal to the input flow (from the driving gas source) and nebulization is continuous. With a *'venturi'* nebulizer the output flow is greater than the input flow due to the presence of an open vent, but the output flow does not change with the patient's breathing pattern. With an *'active venturi'* nebulizer the output flow is breath assisted and is increased during inspiration. There is therefore less wastage of the drug during expiration.

When selecting a nebulizer the age of the patient must be considered. The inspiratory flow of an infant will probably be less than the output from a venturi nebulizer. The concentration of the aerosolized drug may be increased as there will be little or no air entrainment, but the total dose of the drug may be reduced (Collis et al 1990).

Consideration should also be given to the optimal particle size of the drug to be delivered. Inhaled pentamidine or antibiotics need to be delivered to the more peripheral airways (requiring a high percentage of particles of less than 2 µm), whereas bronchodilator drugs probably have their effect in the more central airways.

Residual volume. This is the volume of solution which remains in the nebulizer after nebulization has stopped. The Nebuliser Project Group of the BTS (1997) recommends that a fill volume of 2–2.5 ml may be adequate if the residual volume is less than 1 ml, but nebulizers with a higher residual volume will probably require a fill volume of 4 ml. The patient should be encouraged to tap the side of the nebulizer to allow as much as possible to be delivered (Everard et al 1994).

Fill volume. For effective nebulization it is important not to exceed the manufacturer's recommended fill volume.

Physical properties of drug solution or suspension. Most bronchodilator solutions when nebulized have a similar volume output to normal (0.9%) sodium chloride, but solutions with a higher viscosity or a high surface tension (e.g. carbenicillin) are slow to nebulize.

Breathing pattern of the patient. The optimal pattern of breathing has not yet been ascertained, but a recommended one is to intersperse one or two slow deep breaths with breathing at tidal volume. The deep breathing may increase peripheral deposition of the drug and the periods of breathing control will prevent hyperventilation. When inhaling from a nebulizer the patient should be in a comfortable and well-supported position.

Other points for consideration

The dose of a prescribed nebulized bronchodilator may seem large compared with that from a pressurized aerosol, but only 10–20% of the initial dose is received by the patient and only 50% of this reaches the lungs. The drug which does not reach the patient is lost in the equipment and exhaled gas (Lewis & Fleming 1985).

A face mask is necessary for the infant and child (Fig. 8.47), but as soon as the child will cooperate a mouthpiece should be used to minimize deposition of the drug on the face and in the nasal passages (Wolfsdorf et al 1969). Other disadvantages of a mask are facial skin irritation from nebulized antibiotics and steroids, and nebulized ipratropium bromide and salbutamol by mask have been associated with glaucoma in a group of adults with chronic airflow limitation (Shah et al 1992).

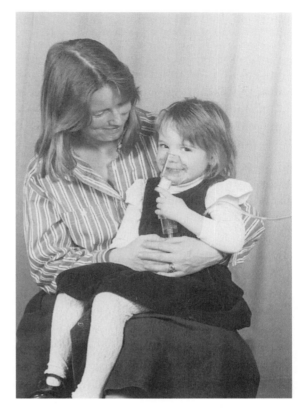

Fig. 8.47 Child using nebulizer with face mask.

Indications for the use of nebulizers

Bronchodilator drugs. Infants and children not yet able to manage the more simple inhalation devices benefit from nebulized bronchodilators, but it has been shown that parents need written instruction in addition to verbal instruction to act appropriately in an acute situation (Bendefy 1991).

Some patients demonstrate a more significant response to nebulized bronchodilators, e.g. β_2 agonists such as salbutamol (Ventolin) and anticholinergics such as ipratropium bromide (Atrovent), than to bronchodilators via a simple inhaler. They include those with asthma and chronic airflow limitation. Patients admitted to hospital with an acute attack of asthma and a few severe asthmatic patients who have life-threatening falls in peak expiratory flow in the night or early morning when at home, may

respond better to nebulized bronchodilator drugs (Fig. 8.48) than to other methods of delivery during these episodes. If nebulized bronchodilators are not producing their usual effect the patient must seek medical advice, as further treatment is probably indicated. A common side-effect associated with β_2 agonists is muscle tremor, especially of the hands.

Corticosteroids. Nebulized corticosteroids are occasionally used in the treatment of airflow obstruction. These drugs are usually in suspension and are more difficult to nebulize than drugs in solution (Nikander 1994). An active venturi jet nebulizer will probably provide a higher output of drug aerosol than either conventional or venturi nebulizers (Nikander & Wunderlich 1996).

Prophylactic drugs. The incidence of attacks of asthma may be reduced by the inhalation

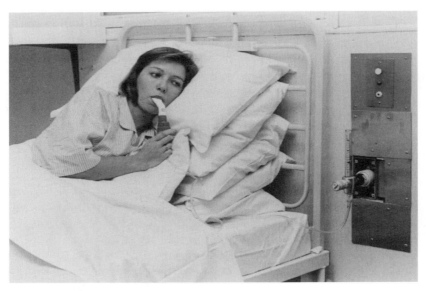

Fig. 8.48 Inhalation of nebulized bronchodilator.

of sodium cromoglycate and related drugs. They are not of value in the treatment of acute attacks of asthma and may be more effective in children than in adults (British Thoracic Society 1997).

Antibiotics, antifungal drugs and pentamidine. Nebulized antibiotic drugs are often used in patients with persistent pseudomonal infections and deteriorating lung function (Mukhopadhyay et al 1996) and may be used prophylactically in an attempt to avoid chronic colonization with *Pseudomonas* (Valerius et al 1991). The nebulizer should have a one-way valve system and either wide-bore tubing to allow the exhaled gas to be vented out through a window (Fig. 8.49) or an effective filter (Fig. 8.50). This is necessary to prevent small quantities of antibiotics from remaining in the atmosphere which could lead to patients, family members and medical personnel in the vicinity receiving a subtherapeutic dose (Smaldone et al 1991) and to environmental organisms becoming resistant to the antibiotic (Sanderson 1984). A nose clip is necessary if the patient is breathing partially through the nose.

Occasionally, inhaled antibiotics are prescribed for a pseudomonal infection in the upper re-

spiratory tract, for example a patient with cystic fibrosis following lung transplantation. For treatment of the upper respiratory tract a nebulizer producing large particles is necessary (Webb et al 1996). A mask should be used and the patient encouraged to breathe through his nose.

More than one antibiotic may be prescribed. A few antibiotics are compatible when mixed, but others must be inhaled separately. Either normal saline or sterile water is used to reconstitute a powdered antibiotic or to make a prescribed solution up to the necessary volume for nebulization. Information on the advisability of mixing drugs should be obtained from a pharmacist.

Nebulized antibiotics may be isotonic, hypo- or hypertonic solutions and may cause airflow obstruction (Dodd et al 1997). The first dose of a nebulized antibiotic should be monitored by recording the FEV_1 and FVC before, immediately after, 15 minutes after and, if evidence of airflow obstruction persists, 30 minutes after the inhalation (Maddison et al 1994). Individual patients respond differently and this response will vary with different drugs. Airflow obstruction can usually be controlled by the inhalation of a bronchodilator taken before physiotherapy

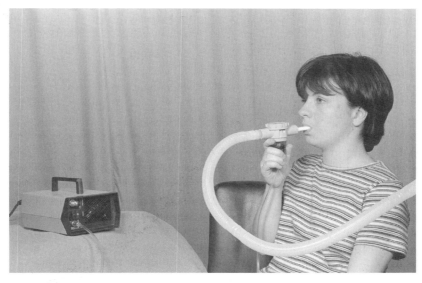

Fig. 8.49   Inhalation of antibiotics using an active venturi nebulizer (Ventstream) and air compressor (CR50) (Medic-Aid Ltd).

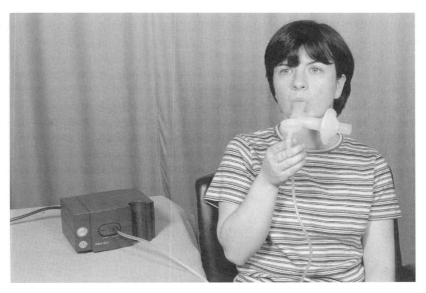

Fig. 8.50   Inhalation of antibiotics using an active venturi nebulizer (LC STAR) and air compressor (PARI TurboBOY) (PARI Medical Ltd).

for the clearance of secretions, preceding the inhalation of the antibiotic.

Antifungal agents are occasionally inhaled in the treatment of pulmonary fungal infections. There is no evidence of resistance to these drugs, but individual drugs may require a one-way valve system to protect health care workers from inhalation. It is important to adhere to local health and safety policies.

Pentamidine isothianate is an antiprotozoal

drug and is sometimes used in the treatment of *Pneumocystis carinii* pneumonia (p. 491). A one-way valve system is necessary (Smaldone et al 1991).

Local anaesthetics and opioids. These drugs have been used in palliative care with some individual patients benefiting (Ahmedzai & Davis 1997). Clinically, morphine has been shown to relieve the breathlessness associated with cancer and severe chronic lung disease in a few patients. Marcain and lignocaine (Howard et al 1977) can be inhaled by nebulizer in the treatment of intractable cough which may occur after a viral infection or with other conditions, e.g. lymphangitis. The analgesic effect of Marcain may be of longer duration and it is usually used in preference to lignocaine. A 3–4 ml dose of 0.5% Marcain is inhaled up to three times per day. The patient should not eat or drink for 1 hour after the inhalation.

Mucolytic agents. Hypertonic saline (3–7%) (Pavia et al 1978, Eng et al 1996) may assist in the clearance of secretions if it is inhaled before physiotherapy. It may also be used in sputum induction (p. 490), but its mode of action is unclear. Hypertonic saline (Schoeffel et al 1981) may cause an increase in airflow obstruction and a test dose using spirometry is necessary.

Acetylcysteine should be used with caution. A reduction in sputum viscosity does not necessarily produce an increase in expectoration of sputum and bronchospasm may be induced. A test dose using spirometry is also necessary with this drug. Acetylcysteine is inactivated by oxygen and, if nebulized, the driving gas should be air.

Recombinant human deoxyribonuclease (DNase) is a mucolytic agent which acts on the deoxyribonucleic acid (DNA) in purulent lung secretions and has been shown to be effective in cystic fibrosis (pp. 472 and 477).

Domiciliary nebulization

If there is an indication for domiciliary nebulization in either children or adults, careful instructions are essential, both verbal and written,

and equipment should be appropriately selected. Ideally, the air compressor should be portable, lightweight and quiet when in operation and the air compressor/nebulizer system should be suitable for the drug prescribed.

Practical and written instructions in the care and cleaning of the equipment must be given in accordance with local infection control policies. A spare jet nebulizer should be available and an inlet filter for the air compressor if necessary. The nebulizer must be washed and dried thoroughly after each treatment to reduce the possibility of bacterial infection (Hutchinson et al 1996) and to keep the jets clear. The transducer of an ultrasonic nebulizer should be cleaned regularly with acetic acid (white vinegar) to maintain its efficiency. An annual check of output, and general and electrical safety should be undertaken, and there should be provision for servicing as required (Dodd et al 1995).

The standard flow head supplied for the domiciliary use of oxygen is unsuitable for driving a nebulizer as the maximum output is only 4 l/min. Flow meters capable of providing higher flows of oxygen could be used, but this system is less economic and more restricting to the patient's lifestyle than a portable compressor. An oxygen concentrator does not produce a high enough flow to drive a nebulizer.

Some patients may benefit from a compressor that can be used when travelling, either by using a 12 volt adaptor in a socket in the car, 'crocodile clips' fitted on to a battery, or more conveniently a compact battery pack supplied with the compressor (Fig. 8.51). Those travelling to a country using a different voltage may require a transformer or a dual-voltage compressor. Some compressors incorporate a universal power pack which adapts to voltages throughout the world. An international travel plug adaptor is an accessory required for all who travel abroad. A foot pump may be useful to power a nebulizer where no electricity is available, but it requires considerable energy to operate. It is advisable to take a letter from a doctor explaining the need to travel with drugs, and possibly syringes and needles, when travelling abroad.

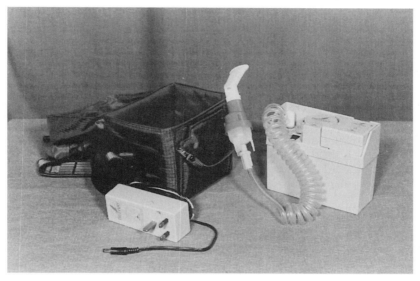

Fig. 8.51   Portable air compressor with battery pack (Freeway Lite, Medic-Aid Ltd).

Bronchodilator response studies

The value of bronchodilator response studies in the assessment of patients for nebulized bronchodilators is controversial (Mestitz et al 1989, O'Driscoll et al 1990, Goldman et al 1992). Short-term responses may not reflect a long-term response. A peak flow meter (Fig. 8.52) is often used to assess bronchodilator response. This will be suitable in a patient with asthma, but will not detect the more subtle response of a change in FVC which can occur in those with more irreversible airflow obstruction (Fig. 8.53). For these patients the response to a bronchodilator, detected by a change in FVC, may lead to an increase in exercise ability and improved quality of life.

The unnecessary use of nebulized bronchodilators can restrict activities of daily living. A nebulizer and air compressor system should only be prescribed if a simple device used correctly is not as effective.

Objective measurements of bronchodilator response can be made by serial recordings of FEV_1 and FVC. Preceding the study the drugs to be tested should be withheld for 4–6 hours, but all other drugs should be continued as prescribed.

Stable baseline readings, with correct technique, must first be obtained. The best result of two or three attempts is taken, allowing a pause of at least 30 seconds between each attempt. Baseline readings are repeated at 5 min intervals until the maximum pretreatment level is known. Some patients will continue to improve over several minutes, while others will soon reach a plateau or decrease their FEV_1 or FVC.

Having ensured a correct technique, the bronchodilator is then inhaled and spirometry is repeated at the appropriate time interval for the particular drug. After salbutamol (Ventolin), or

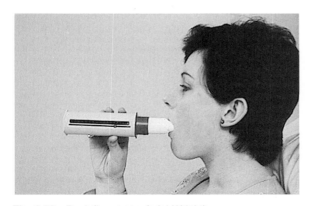

Fig. 8.52   Peak flow meter (mini-Wright).

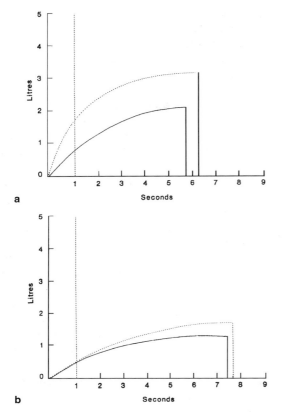

Fig. 8.53 **a** Increase in FEV$_1$ and FVC. **b** Increase in FVC only. Spirometry before bronchodilator ————; spirometry after bronchodilator .....

terbutaline (Bricanyl), readings can be made at 15 and 30 min intervals (Ruffin et al 1977), whereas with the slower acting ipratropium bromide (Atrovent), recordings are made 40 and 60 min from the time of inhalation (Loddenkemper 1975). In each case recordings should be continued until the maximum response is achieved, for example if the response to salbutamol is greater at 30 min than at 15 min the spirometry is repeated at 10 min intervals until a plateau or fall in FEV$_1$ or FVC is recorded. If time is limited, this outline can be modified, recordings being taken at the expected times of maximal improvement (30 min following Ventolin and Bricanyl and 60 min following Atrovent).

The same principle can be applied when comparing different methods of delivery of the same drug or when comparing the response to two different bronchodilators. If comparing the response of a patient to Ventolin by an MDI (or other simple device) and a nebulized solution of Ventolin, measurements are made until maximum response is reached after inhalation by MDI and then the nebulized solution is given immediately. Any additional response is determined by the post-nebulizer recordings. If response to one method of delivery is determined on one occasion and to the other method on a separate occasion, the results are unlikely to be comparable because the baseline readings and other factors such as the time of testing and dose of steroid drugs may be different. Similarly, when comparing the response to two different drugs (for example, Ventolin and Atrovent) the second should be given as soon as maximum response has been achieved with the first (Webber 1988).

McGavin et al (1976) demonstrated that the inhalation of a bronchodilator preceding exercise can improve exercise tolerance, but the improvement does not correlate with changes in FEV$_1$ and FVC.

O'Driscoll et al (1990) in their study on home nebulizers could not demonstrate a correlation between formal lung function testing and the domiciliary use of a nebulizer system. They recommended that patients who are referred for consideration of home nebulizer therapy be given the equipment to try under supervision for several weeks at home and that the patient's subjective assessment should be considered.

In assessing bronchodilator treatment Vora et al (1995) concluded that a quality of life measure (Breathing Problems Questionnaire; Ch. 3, p. 64) and shuttle walking test appeared to be sensitive outcome measures.

An objective study which demonstrates to the patient a positive response to a simple inhalation device with no further response to nebulized drugs, often relieves the patient who has felt that a compressor system would be necessary.

Many patients with asthma keep a diary card at home which will include recordings of peak expiratory flow before and after bronchodilator drugs. These will only be valid if the technique when using the meter is correct. Points to emphasize are:

• The patient should take a maximum breath in (in his haste to carry out the manoeuvre the patient may not take a full deep breath).

• Expiration should be short and sharp.

• Sufficient rests (at least 15 seconds) should be allowed between 'blows' to prevent any increase in airflow obstruction with the forced expiratory manoeuvre.

- The same position, sitting or standing, should be used for taking the readings.

Oxygen therapy

Oxygen therapy is indicated for many patients with hypoxaemia. The physiotherapist frequently treats patients requiring added inspired oxygen and may be involved with the setting up of oxygen therapy equipment. Oxygen is a drug and should be prescribed by a medical practitioner and monitored using arterial blood gas analysis or oxygen saturation (SaO_2) recordings. When using SaO_2 recordings only, it must be remembered that the arterial carbon dioxide could be rising. If a patient is on continuous oxygen therapy the mask should be removed only briefly for expectoration, eating and drinking, and sometimes during these periods oxygen therapy may be continued using nasal cannulae.

Devices for administering oxygen therapy may be divided into fixed and variable performance devices (Hinds & Watson 1996). A *variable performance device* supplies a flow of oxygen which is less than the patient's minute volume. The inspired oxygen concentration (FiO_2) will vary with the rate and volume of breath, and considerable variations between and within subjects have been demonstrated (Bazuaye et al 1992). Commonly used variable performance devices are the simple face mask (Fig. 8.54a) and nasal cannulae (Fig. 8.54b). Nasal cannulae are often preferred as the patient can eat, drink and speak more comfortably and often finds them less claustrophobic than a mask. Although high flows of oxygen can be delivered to nasal cannulae, 1–4 l/min (approximately 24–36%) is the range for patient comfort, as higher flows tend to irritate and dry the nasal mucosa. Nasal cannulae should be used with caution with very breathless hypoxic patients as they are likely to be breathing through the mouth and not benefiting from the nasal oxygen.

Effective humidification cannot be provided by narrow-bore tubing, and if additional humidification is required the mask should be attached via wide-bore tubing to a humidifier or nebulizer. The bubble-through humidifier often attached to nasal cannulae does not provide effective humidification (Campbell et al 1988).

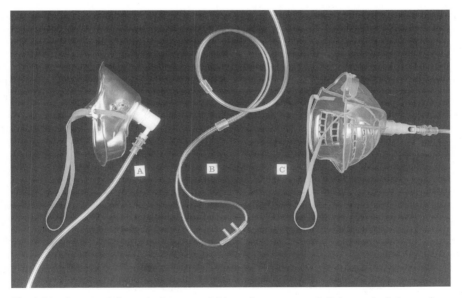

Fig. 8.54 Oxygen delivery devices: **a** variable performance mask (Intersurgical); **b** nasal cannulae (Intersurgical); **c** fixed performance venturi mask (Flexicare Medical).

When accurate delivery of oxygen is required, especially at low concentrations, a fixed performance device is essential because wide variations in inspired oxygen concentration have been shown to be produced by variable performance devices, even with the recommended flows (Jeffrey & Warren 1992).

A *fixed performance device* will deliver a known inspired oxygen concentration (FiO_2), by providing a sufficiently high flow of premixed gas which should exceed the patient's peak inspiratory flow rate. A venturi system allows a relatively low flow of oxygen to entrain a large volume of air and the mixed gas is conveyed to the face mask (Fig. 8.54c). With a 24% venturi mask the usual setting of 2 l/min flow of oxygen will entrain approximately 50 l/min of air giving a total flow of approximately 52 l/min. An extremely breathless patient, with a greatly increased work of breathing and high peak inspiratory flow rate, may find this flow too low and then it is necessary to increase the flow to exceed the inspiratory flow of the patient (Hill et al 1984). The manufacturer should provide information for each mask (e.g. a 24% mask run at 3 l/min may augment the total flow to 78 l/min without changing the oxygen concentration). It is not possible to measure the critically ill patient's peak inspiratory flow, but by careful observation the physiotherapist will be able to tell if the total flow is sufficient. If the face mask is being sucked inwards towards the face during inspiration the flow is inadequate, but if gas can be felt flowing out through the holes and around the edges of the mask the flow will be exceeding the patient's requirements.

For most patients using a venturi mask the entrained room air provides sufficient humidification, but occasionally additional humidification is indicated (p. 191). A bubble-through humidifier attached to the narrow-bore tubing of a ventimask is inappropriate as the flow of oxygen is likely to be reduced by the back pressure from the humidifier device and by condensation blocking the narrow-bore tubing.

When high concentrations of oxygen, at high flows, are required a *high flow variable FiO₂ generator* can be used. The gas flows along wide-bore tubing from the generator across an appropriate heated humidifier to the face mask. It is essential to have an oxygen analyser in the circuit. Oxygen concentrations between 35% and 100% can be delivered at flows of up to 130 l/min. High flow oxygen therapy has been recommended for the acute severe asthmatic patient (Nebuliser Project Group of the BTS 1997).

Nebulizers for the delivery of drugs in hospital are frequently powered by piped oxygen, but in the patient dependent on his hypoxic drive to breathe, air should be used as the driving gas. Occasionally, in the severely hypoxic patient, who is also hypercapnic and dependent on a controlled 24% oxygen mask, the patient should not be deprived of this added oxygen while using a nebulizer. 1 to 2 litres of oxygen can be added through a T-piece into the tubing connecting the air compressor to the nebulizer. The level of oxygen entrained to maintain the baseline oxygen saturation can be monitored using an oximeter.

For most patients an *intermittent positive pressure breathing device* (IPPB) should be driven by compressed oxygen. Starke et al (1979) demonstrated that in hypercapnic patients oxygen can be used as the driving gas (p. 170). In hypoxic patients without hypercapnia, for example in acute asthma, oxygen is required and it is dangerous to use air alone as the driving gas for IPPB.

Long-term oxygen therapy (LTOT) has been shown to improve the length and quality of life in selected patients with severe chronic airflow limitation (Nocturnal Oxygen Therapy Trial Group 1980, Medical Research Council Working Party 1981). The expected gradual progression of pulmonary hypertension associated with this condition is slowed down by the use of long-term oxygen therapy. This benefit will not occur unless oxygen is used at a low flow for a minimum of 15 hours/day and should be prescribed only for carefully selected patients. The value of LTOT in asymptomatic but hypoxaemic patients and the value of alternative techniques, for example non-invasive ventilation (NIV), in improving arterial oxygenation, need further evaluation (Leach & Bateman 1994).

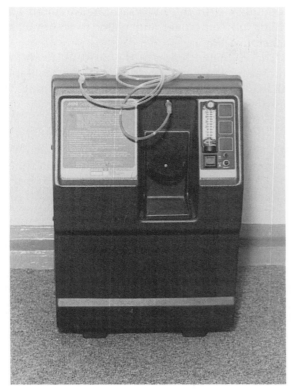

Fig. 8.55 An oxygen concentrator (DeVilbiss Health Care).

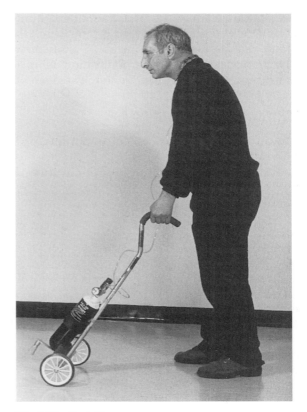

Fig. 8.56 Portable oxygen.

An *oxygen concentrator* (Fig. 8.55) is a convenient and efficient means of providing long-term oxygen therapy in the home, and the oxygen tubing can be fitted in areas of the home to allow for mobility. An oxygen cylinder is necessary for emergency use. Humidifiers are sometimes fitted to oxygen concentrators but care must be taken as these are a potential source of infection (Pendleton et al 1991).

Small *portable oxygen cylinders* can be used for short trips outside the home. These may be transported on a lightweight trolley (Fig. 8.56) or carried over the shoulder. Portable cylinders can be refilled from a larger oxygen cylinder using a special adaptor, but they cannot be refilled from an oxygen concentrator. Careful instruction must be given in refilling the portable cylinder, as this can be a frightening and difficult procedure until the patient or his carer is familiar with it.

In an attempt to give patients who are dependent on oxygen greater mobility and the opportunity to participate in activities outside the home, an *inspiratory phased delivery system* or *oxygen by transtracheal catheter*, may be considered (Shneerson 1992). A microcatheter inserted into the trachea will reduce the dead space and decrease the requirement for oxygen. Some patients find this more cosmetically acceptable than nasal cannulae, but there is the increased possibility of infection.

Liquid oxygen systems are used in some parts of the world. These are portable, lightweight and convenient, and have been shown to improve compliance with treatment and to increase the time spent outside the home (Lock et al 1992).

The physiotherapist may be involved in *assessing* patients who may benefit from portable oxygen. Repeated walking tests, for example the shuttle walking test, with the patient 'blind' to whether he is using oxygen or air during the walk, can be used as a means of assessment. The measurement of oxygen saturation using an oximeter may also be included in the assessment.

Entonox

The inhalation of Entonox (50% nitrous oxide and 50% oxygen) has an analgesic effect which is easily and rapidly induced. See Chapter 12, page 300.

Heliox

A mixture of helium (79%) and oxygen (21%) is sometimes used on a temporary basis to relieve respiratory distress in patients with upper airways obstruction, for example a tumour causing partial obstruction of the trachea. Helium is lighter than the nitrogen in air and the mixture passes more easily through the narrowed airway requiring less effort from the patient (Vater et al 1983). A side-effect of heliox is an alteration in the pitch of the voice, due to its effect on the vocal cords. This is only temporary, but should be explained to the patient before use of heliox to avoid unnecessary concern.

Humidification

A device to provide humidification of the airways may be considered if either the normal means of humidifying the airways or the mucociliary escalator are not functioning effectively.

The mucous membranes of the upper airways normally provide warmth and humidification of the inspired air. The temperature and humidity of the inspired air vary, but the gas in the alveoli is fully saturated with water vapour at body temperature. There is a temperature and humidity gradient from the nose to the point where the gas reaches 37°C and 100% relative humidity (Shelly et al 1988). This point is normally just below the carina in the adult, but varies depending on the temperature and water content of the inspired gas, and the tidal volume. The upper airways act as a heat and moisture

exchanger with the fully saturated expired gas giving up some heat and water to the mucosa (Chatburn 1987).

The epithelial lining of the airways, from the trachea to the respiratory bronchioles, contains ciliated cells which are responsible for moving mucus and particulate matter proximally to the level of the larynx.

The optimal temperature for cilial activity is normal body temperature with reduced activity occurring below 20°C and above 40°C (Wanner 1977). The cilia beat within a watery fluid, the 'periciliary' or 'sol' layer. A mucus layer 'gel' covers the periciliary layer and interacts with the tips of the cilia.

The efficiency of mucus transport is dependent on correctly functioning cilia, and the composition of the periciliary and mucus layers. If the periciliary layer becomes too shallow, as with dehydration, the cilia become enmeshed in the viscous mucus layer and cannot function effectively. If the periciliary layer is too deep the tips of the cilia are not in contact with the mucus layer and propulsion of the mucus is inefficient.

The viscosity of mucus is increased during bacterial infection owing to an increase in the DNA content of the mucus (Wilson & Cole 1988). With hypersecretory disorders of, for example, bronchiectasis, cystic fibrosis and chronic airflow limitation, there is an increase in both quantity and viscosity of mucus secretions. Bacteria directly affect cilial beating and coordination, disrupt the epithelium, stimulate mucus secretion and alter periciliary fluid composition (Cole 1995). Humidification has been shown to enhance tracheobronchial clearance when used as an adjunct to physiotherapy in a group of patients with bronchiectasis (Conway et al 1992). There is some evidence to suggest that there may be an increase in mucociliary clearance with the inhalation of normal saline compared with water (Cole & Wills, personal communication, 1997).

Clarke (1995) has suggested that the efficiency of cough increases with a decrease in viscosity of mucus and an increase in the periciliary layer of the airway. Conway (1992) hypothesizes that humidification by water or saline aerosol produces an increase in depth of the periciliary and mucus layers, thereby decreasing viscosity and enhancing the shearing of secretions by huffing or coughing.

Humidification may be indicated to assist clearance of secretions when the clearance mechanism is not optimally effective or when the normal heat and moisture exchange system of the upper airways is bypassed by an endotracheal or tracheostomy tube. Patients with a long-term tracheostomy may develop metaplasia of the tracheal epithelium. While adequate humidification of the inspired gas occurs normally, additional humidification may be required during an episode of respiratory infection (Oh 1990).

Methods of humidification

Systemic hydration

Adequate humidification may be obtained by increasing the oral or intravenous fluid intake of a patient. Breathless patients find drinking fluids an effort, but need encouragement to avoid dehydration. Patients should be reminded to maintain an adequate fluid intake as this may help to prevent secretions from becoming more tenacious. During periods of infection and fever a higher fluid intake is required.

Heated water bath humidifiers

Gas is blown over a reservoir of heated sterile water and absorbs water vapour which is then inhaled by the patient (Fig. 8.57). If the delivery tube is cold there is a temperature drop as the gas passes along the tube and condensation occurs. The humidifier should be positioned below the level of the patient's airway to avoid flooding of the airway by condensed water. Sealed (to prevent contamination) water traps should be included in the circuit to allow regular emptying without interrupting ventilation. A heated delivery tube eliminates the problem of condensation and allows the gas to be delivered at a desired temperature of 32–36° with a water content of 33–43 g/m^3 (Hinds & Watson 1996). Sterile water must be used in these devices. If saline is used, it is the water only which

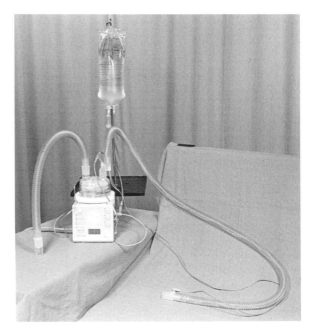

Fig. 8.57 Heated humidifier (Fisher & Paykel).

vaporizes and the sodium chloride crystallizes out.

Humidifiers can be used for the spontaneously breathing patient or can be incorporated into ventilator circuits including continuous positive airway pressure and non-invasive ventilation (Fig. 6.5, p. 115). In some patients using 'high continuous flow CPAP systems' it may be necessary to use two humidifiers in series to increase the humidification (Harrison et al 1993).

Heat and moisture exchangers (HME)

A heat and moisture exchanger or the 'Swedish nose' are lightweight disposable devices and may be used in the intubated patient either mechanically ventilated or breathing spontaneously. In the spontaneously breathing patient it is important to be aware of the slight resistance that will increase the work of breathing. The humidifier acts in a similar way to the nasopharynx. The heat and moisture of the exhaled gas are retained either by condensation (condenser humidifier) or by absorption, and returned in the inhaled gas as it passes through the device.

A variety of hygroscopic materials and chemicals are used for absorption within heat and moisture exchangers.

Heat and moisture exchangers are inefficient if there is a large air leak around an uncuffed tracheostomy tube (Tilling & Hayes 1987) and do not provide adequate humidification for infants. If the secretions of a patient using a heat and moisture exchanger become tenacious, a more effective form of humidification will be required (Bransen et al 1993). The humidifier must be changed at least every 24 hours and immediately if it becomes soiled with secretions.

Nebulizers

A nebulizer for humidification may be a jet nebulizer (Fig. 8.58) or ultrasonic nebulizer (Fig. 21.2, p. 490). Nebulizers produce an aerosol mist of droplets. Some jet nebulizers have a heater incorporated in the system. This increased temperature raises the relative humidity, is less irritative for patients with hyperreactive airways and is less likely to increase airflow obstruction than cold humidification. When a jet nebulizer is powered by oxygen the amount of air entrained by the nebulizer will be determined by the oxygen concentration required. If the concentration of oxygen is not important, consideration should be given to the optimal density of mist and flow produced by the specific device.

The mist particles delivered with a venturi closed (98% setting) appear more dense, but the total flow (approximately 10 l/min) will be insufficient to meet the patient's inspiratory requirement and additional room air will be entrained through the holes in a face mask or mouthpiece, effectively reducing the degree of humidification. A 35% setting on a venturi system will produce a flow of approximately 40 l/min. This would provide a higher degree of humidification as it would meet the inspiratory demand of the patient most of the time.

Many ultrasonic nebulizers do not have a heater, but the mist is at ambient temperature, and warmer than that produced from a jet nebulizer powered from compressed piped gas. There is often an airflow control valve in addition to a control for the density of the mist. By regulating these two controls a density of mist can be obtained that the patient can inhale comfortably.

Sterile normal saline (0.9%) is an isotonic solution and probably the most acceptable to patients inhaling from a nebulizer. Sterile water can be used if saline is unavailable, but has been shown to cause bronchoconstriction in patients with hyperreactive airways (Schoeffel et al 1981).

Bubble-through humidifiers

A device containing cold water, through which the inspired gas is bubbled, is not an effective means of humidification. If connected to an oxygen mask with narrow-bore tubing it may alter the oxygen concentration as water condenses in the tubing. A bubble-through humidifier is often connected to nasal cannulae, but there are neither objective nor subjective benefits from this form of humidification (Campbell et al 1988).

Steam inhalations

Inhalation of steam may be useful in patients

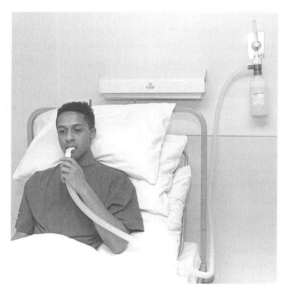

Fig. 8.58 Humidification by nebulization (Quattro nebulizing humidifier) (Medic-Aid Ltd).

with postoperative sputum retention if they are encouraged to breathe deeply. Precautions must be taken to avoid spilling the hot water.

Delivery to the patient

Patients with retained secretions postoperatively or those with excess viscous secretions due to a chronic bronchopulmonary infection may benefit from a period of 10–20 minutes' humidification before physiotherapy to assist the clearance of secretions. If the concentration of oxygen required by the patient is not critical, a *mouthpiece* with a hole for entrainment of additional air is simple and comfortable to use (Fig. 8.58). Deep breathing interspersed with tidal volume breathing may encourage peripheral deposition of an aerosol, while avoiding hyperventilation.

If a patient requires an oxygen concentration of 28% or more, a *face mask* can be connected by wide-bore tubing to a nebulizer and the venturi of the nebulizer should be set to the appropriate concentration.

Patients requiring an inspired oxygen concentration of 24% will probably wear a venturi mask connected to the oxygen by narrow-bore tubing. It is impossible to give high humidification through a narrow-bore tube owing to condensation within the tubing. Effective humidification can be obtained by using a *humidity adaptor* which allows the air entrained by the mask to be humidified. It is a cuff fitted over the air-entraining holes of the mask and connected by wide-bore humidity tubing to a humidifier powered by an air source. This can be piped compressed air if it is available, or an air cylinder or an electric air compressor capable of continuous use ('continuously rated') (Fig. 8.59). An ultrasonic nebulizer, set at a high flow, can be used and is quieter than a jet nebulizer system. A humidity adaptor can be used to give humidification to ventimasks delivering accurate higher concentrations of oxygen (e.g. 28% or 35%), but is unsatisfactory with a 60% ventimask because the air-entraining holes are too small to entrain the humidity.

If a patient is breathing spontaneously through a tracheostomy, a *tracheostomy mask* may be

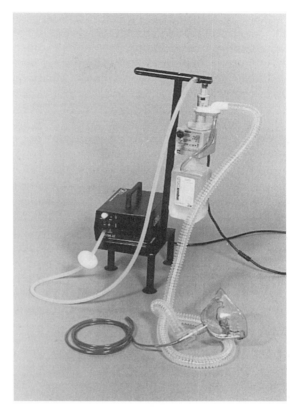

Fig. 8.59 Heated humidification of 24% oxygen using a humidity adaptor (Vickers, Kendall, Medic-Aid).

attached to a humidifier or nebulizer via wide-bore tubing. Alternatively a 'Swedish nose' or a 'laryngectomy-permanent tracheostomy protector' (tracheostomy 'bib') may be used.

Humidification through a *head box* (Fig. 13.6, p. 341) is often used in the treatment of spontaneously breathing infants. With the narrow airways of an infant the risk of mucus plugging is higher than in adults. Humidity to a head box may be either from a heated water bath humidifier or a heated nebulizer system.

Hazards of humidification

Inhalation of cold mist or water (a hypotonic solution) may cause bronchoconstriction in patients with hyperreactive airways (Schoeffel et al 1981). Heated humidification and normal saline solution are less likely to cause this problem. It may be appropriate to take peak flow or spirometry recordings before and immediately after the first treatment.

Water reservoirs may become infected with *Pseudomonas* and other organisms, many of which multiply rapidly at 45°C. A particularly vulnerable site is the catheter mount of the ventilator circuit in the intubated patient. Some control of infection can be obtained by using an operating temperature of 60°C (Oh 1990). Regular disposal, disinfection or sterilization of all humidification equipment is essential to prevent infection and local infection control policies must be observed.

MUSCULOSKELETAL DYSFUNCTION

The patient with chronic hyperinflation typically develops a barrel-shaped chest with an increase in the anteroposterior diameter of the chest,

elevation of the shoulder girdle and protraction of the scapulae (Fig. 8.60). The sternocleidomastoid muscles and the scalenes shorten and draw the head and neck forwards, causing an increase in the upper thoracic kyphosis and the mid-cervical lordosis. The upper cervical spine then hyperextends as the head tilts upward to maintain a vertical orientation of the face. The long thoracic extensors and the deep upper cervical flexors lengthen and lose their endurance capacity, becoming less able to sustain the upright posture. The increased thoracic kyphosis, tight pectoralis minor and major and weak middle and lower fibres of trapezius lead to an elevated, protracted, downwardly rotated and anteriorly tilted position of the scapulae. Overactivity of the upper trapezius and levator scapulae muscles during shoulder flexion accentuates shortening of these muscle groups.

Muscle fatigue related to the excess work of

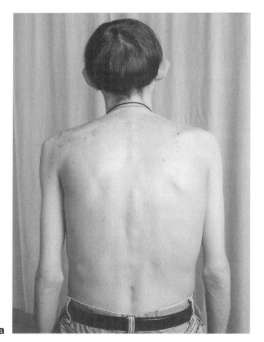 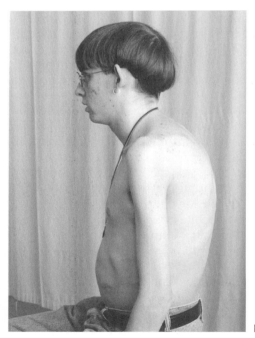

a   b

Fig. 8.60 CJ age 16, cystic fibrosis. **a** Relaxed sitting posture (posterior view). *Note:* Forward head position, tight suboccipital and mid-cervical extensors, tight upper and middle fibres of trapezius, asymmetry and abducted and protracted position of the scapulae, increased thoracic kyphosis, reduced upper lumbar lordosis, posterior rotation of pelvis. **b** Relaxed sitting posture (side view). *Note:* Forward head position, increased sternocleidomastoid activity, increased low cervical lordosis and thoracic kyphosis, abducted and protracted scapulae, anterior position of humerus in glenoid fossa, internal rotation of humerus, lax abdominal muscles.

breathing may further contribute to poor posture in patients with moderate to severe chronic lung disease. In a study of 143 patients with cystic fibrosis, Henderson & Specter (1994) found 77% of females and 36% of males over 15 years of age had a kyphosis greater than 40° (the upper limit of normal). Additionally, both males and females with cystic fibrosis have been found to have low bone mineral density (Bachrach et al 1994, Henderson & Madsen 1996). Whether these musculoskeletal complications can be prevented or minimized by an early intervention programme of mobilizing exercises for the thoracic spine and ribs, and strengthening exercises for the scapular and thoracic extensor muscle groups, has not been reported in the literature.

Individuals with chronic respiratory disease may complain of acute or chronic cervical, thoracic or rib joint pain which may decrease their chest expansion as measured by a reduction in vital capacity (VC). Loss of endurance of the deep upper cervical flexor muscles, associated with a forward head posture, has been linked to cervicogenic headache (Watson & Trott 1993). The kyphotic thoracic spine and abnormal posture of the neck, shoulder girdle and first rib, combined with chronic overuse of the accessory muscles of respiration, may limit the range of movement available in the cervical spine. Tensioning of the neural tissues may also occur in some individuals (Butler 1991).

Tightness in anterior deltoid, teres major and latissimus dorsi muscles will decrease the range of external rotation and flexion available at the glenohumeral joint. Reduced range of thoracic extension will contribute to loss of the final 30° of shoulder flexion and abduction. Additionally, over-stretching of infraspinatus and teres minor, associated with the internally rotated position of the humerus, will lead to poor stability of the humerus in the glenoid fossa. In patients who regularly swim, or are involved in throwing sports, shoulder impingement problems may result.

Subjective assessment

The area of pain reported by the patient can be recorded on a body chart, and the intensity quantified using an absolute visual analogue scale (AVAS) (Zusman 1986). The impact of any pain or movement restriction on activities of daily living may be assessed using a functional disability scale (e.g. Northwick Park Neck Pain questionnaire (Leak et al 1994) or the Modified Roland–Morris questionnaire (Binkley et al 1996)). In the dyspnoeic patient, it may be of help to quantify dyspnoea intensity using an AVAS or Borg scale prior to any postural correction or treatment.

The patient should be questioned specifically regarding the presence of cervicogenic headache, shoulder pain and any upper limb pain or paraesthesia. Aggravating activities may involve either sustained end-range postures of the neck or thoracic spine, shoulder elevation, or movements which require a reversal of the thoracic kyphosis. Pain may also be aggravated by coughing which loads the costotransverse joints. The behaviour of pain at night and in the morning will help clarify the degree of inflammation involved.

Physical assessment

During assessment and treatment of the patient with chronic respiratory disease the physiotherapist should keep in mind the possibility of reduced bone density and fragile skin tissue as a result of long-term use of systemic steroids or increased age. Firm overpressures should be used with caution, while manipulation of the thoracic spine is contraindicated.

The musculoskeletal assessment should proceed in a systematic manner from evaluation of posture, to assessment of joint mobility, muscle recruitment patterns, muscle length and strength, and endurance. Pain, dyspnoea and fatigue will need to be observed concurrently and the assessment adjusted as necessary. The presence of wound and drain sites in the post-surgical patient may require modified assessment positions.

The resting posture of the cervical, thoracic and lumbar spine, the scapulae and arms should be observed posteriorly and laterally with the patient positioned in relaxed sitting. In particular the degree of lumbar and thoracic kyphosis, and the degree of mid- and upper cervical lordosis should be noted. The flexibility or permanence of any increase in these curves may be assessed by assisting the patient to roll the pelvis anteriorly (lumbosacral extension) and noting the ability to reverse the lumbar and thoracic kyphosis. There should also be an automatic reduction in the mid-cervical lordosis and protracted position of the head (Fig. 8.61). If the slumped posture is severe and the thoracic extensors very weak, the patient may require passive assistance to reduce the thoracic kyphosis. The degree of rigidity of the kyphosis will then be more obvious. Equally, the cervical spine and the head may need to be guided into a less protracted position to assess the reversibility of the resting posture. The ability of the patient to then maintain this corrected position will indicate the extent of loss of endurance of the postural muscles.

Any change in symptoms during assessment of spinal and shoulder range of movement should be noted. Gentle overpressure applied at end-range will assist determination of the quality of restriction. Stiffness in the upper thoracic spine may be noted by an inability to reverse the kyphosis during cervical extension and shoulder abduction. In the mid-thoracic region, a flattened or lordotic area usually indicates hypomobility (Boyling & Palastanga 1994). The major portion of thoracic rotation normally occurs in the middle thoracic spine (T6 to T8) (Gregersen & Lucas 1967) with lateral flexion occurring as a conjunct movement (Gregersen & Lucas 1967, White & Panjabi 1990). Normal thoracic rotation has a springy end feel due to limitation by ligamentous tissue and joint capsules. During lateral flexion the ribs should flare and spread

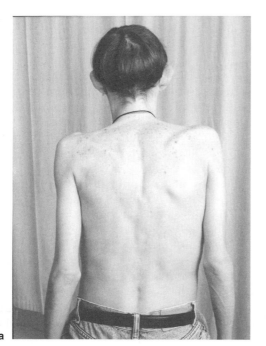 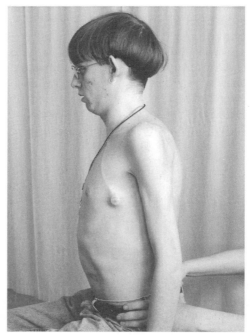

Fig. 8.61 **a** Sitting posture (posterior view) following active assisted anterior rotation of pelvis. *Note:* Decreased mid-cervical lordosis, improved position of scapulae, reduced thoracic kyphosis, neutral rotation of pelvis and improved lumbar lordosis. **b** Sitting posture (side view) following active assisted anterior rotation of pelvis. *Note:* Less forward head position, activation of deep cervical flexors, reduced sternocleidomastoid activity, improved scapulae and humeral position and thoracic kyphosis.

on the contralateral side and approximate on the ipsilateral side (Boyling & Palastanga 1994). Range is dependent on the mobility of the apophyseal, costotransverse, and costovertebral joints, mobility of the ribs, and the extensibility of the intercostal muscles and latissmus dorsi.

During flexion the inferior facets of the apophyseal joint of the superior vertebra glide supero-anteriorly on the facets of the inferior vertebra. In extension the reverse movement occurs. Although the initial limitation is from the anterior ligaments, the anterior annulus and the posterior longitudinal ligament, the normal end feel is one of bony impingement as the inferior articular facets contact the lamina of the caudad vertebrae (White & Panjabi 1990).

The mobility of the upper and middle ribs may be assessed by palpating bilaterally anteriorly and posteriorly during a deep inspiration, while the lower ribs are assessed by palpating laterally. Age changes at the costovertebral joints may restrict rib motion (Nathan 1962).

The range of glenohumeral rotation will depend on tightness of the anterior and posterior shoulder muscles, while the range of bilateral shoulder flexion and abduction will in part be determined by the range of thoracic extension. Any restriction in the range of thoracic lateral flexion and rotation will limit the range of unilateral shoulder elevation (Boyling & Palastanga 1994). Abnormal patterns of muscle recruitment may be noted during shoulder elevation. The upper trapezius and levator scapulae muscles, sternocleidomastoid and the scalenes tend to be overactive, and the deep upper cervical and scapular stabilizers underactive (Fig. 8.62). Abnormal scapulohumeral rhythm is usually most obvious as shoulder movement is initiated and towards the end of range. The excursion, strength and endurance of specific muscle groups identified as overactive or underactive need to be examined individually. While this assessment is ideally performed in supine and prone, examination of dyspnoeic patients may need to be conducted in semi-supine, sitting or high side lying.

Neural tissue provocation tests (Butler 1991) and tests for reflexes, power and sensation

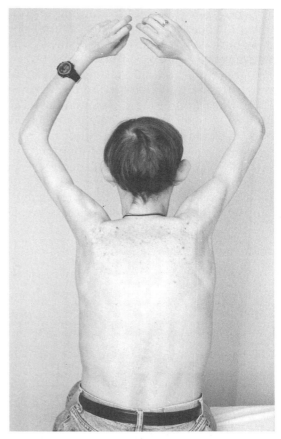

Fig. 8.62 Shoulder abduction. *Note:* Overactivity of upper trapezius, poor reversal of thoracic kyphosis, abducted, protracted and rotated scapulae, shortened teres major and latissimus dorsi and absence of lower trapezius activity.

should be performed if any arm pain or paraesthesia is reported.

Physiotherapy management

The patient's main problems need to be prioritized before treatment can be started. Joint restriction may be treated with passive mobilization techniques, active assisted exercises or active exercises. Posture may be improved by educating awareness of positioning and more efficient movement patterns using visual, auditory and sensory feedback. There are many techniques available to lengthen shortened muscles and to strengthen and improve the endurance of lengthened muscles. Motor learning involves training the holding ability of the postural stabilizers while avoiding substitution by the stronger prime movers (White & Sahrmann 1994).

Postural correction may change the patient's breathing pattern and intensity of dyspnoea; therefore these factors need to be monitored carefully during treatment. As the patient becomes familiar with the gentle effort required to activate the correct muscles, oxygen consumption may be reduced. Compliance with a home exercise programme will be improved if a direct link can be demonstrated between improvement in posture and relief of pain or shortness of breath.

Mobilization techniques

Physiotherapy management of joint restriction and pain may include passive mobilizations of cervical and thoracic apophyseal joints, the costotransverse, costochondral and sternochondral joints (Vibekk 1991, Bray 1994). The patient's position during treatment will need to be carefully selected as many patients will not be able to lie prone or supine because of dyspnoea or pain. General techniques to the upper, mid- or lower regions of the spine or localized techniques to a specific vertebral level or rib can be performed in sitting, forward lean sitting, or in high side lying (Figs 8.63 and 8.64). The focus will usually be on improving the range and quality of thoracic extension and rotation and on increasing the mobility of the ribs.

In forward lean sitting with the head and arms

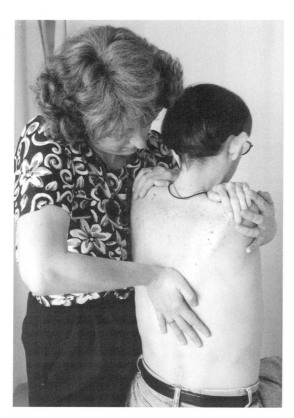

Fig. 8.63 Mobilization of thoracic extension. Passive or active assisted, with fulcrum at T8.

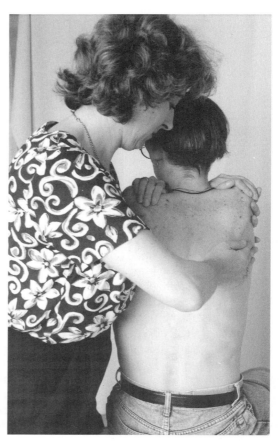

Fig. 8.64 Mobilization of thoracic rotation. Passive, or active assisted, with postero-anterior pressure on ribs 7 and 8.

supported on pillows, the rib cage will be free to move during mobilization techniques. Mobilization of the ribs may also be performed in side lying with the upper arm elevated to stretch the intercostal muscles, or in sitting using active shoulder abduction combined with lateral flexion. Bilateral arm flexion and spine extension may be combined with deep inspiration and expiration to improve rib mobility. In sitting, the patient may perform active extension or rotation while the therapist assists the movement to encourage an increase in range. Self-mobilizations can be performed over the back of a chair, in four-point kneel or leaning against a wall (Fig. 8.65a–e). Home mobilization exercises will be necessary

if the respiratory condition is chronic and the musculoskeletal dysfunction long term.

For patients following sternotomy or thoracotomy, specific gentle passive mobilizations of the sternocostal joints or costotransverse joints may be required if localized painful limitation of shoulder or thoracic movement is present. Bilateral arm movements are preferred in the early stage, initially avoiding abduction and external rotation. Following thoracotomy, patients may tend to immobilize the arm on the side of the incision and need to be encouraged to move within pain limits as early as possible to reduce the risk of frozen shoulder. The scapula may be taken through its range of protraction,

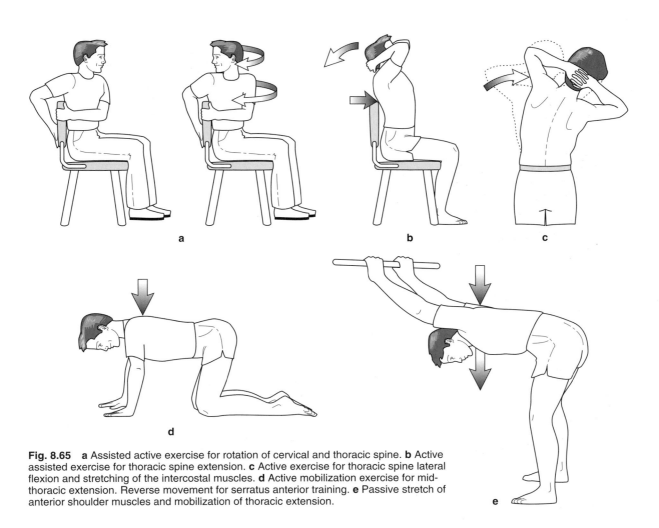

Fig. 8.65   **a** Assisted active exercise for rotation of cervical and thoracic spine. **b** Active assisted exercise for thoracic spine extension. **c** Active exercise for thoracic spine lateral flexion and stretching of the intercostal muscles. **d** Active mobilization exercise for mid-thoracic extension. Reverse movement for serratus anterior training. **e** Passive stretch of anterior shoulder muscles and mobilization of thoracic extension.

retraction, elevation and depression while the patient is in side lying.

The long-term ventilated patient may also develop musculoskeletal problems. Routine passive mobilization of the shoulder through its full range of flexion, external rotation and abduction should be mandatory. Lateral flexion and extension of the thoracic spine can be performed via arm elevation when the patient is in side lying. Gentle passive rotation of the thoracic spine can also be performed in this position with the upper arm resting on the lateral chest wall.

Muscle lengthening techniques

Stretching of tight muscle groups should precede or accompany endurance training of the lengthened muscle groups (Janda 1994). Stretching of the anterior deltoid and pectoralis major muscles using a proprioceptive neuromuscular facilitation hold–relax technique has been shown to increase VC and shoulder range of movement (Putt & Paratz 1996). Other muscles which may

require stretching are: sternocleidomastoid, the scalenes, upper and middle fibres of trapezius, levator scapulae, pectoralis minor, teres major, latissimus dorsi, subscapularis and the upper cervical extensors (Table 8.4). Sustained stretches may be facilitated by conscious or reflex relaxation of the muscle during exhalation, while hold–relax techniques using the agonist, or contract–relax techniques using the antagonist of the shortened muscle (White & Sahrmann 1994), may augment sustained stretches and myofascial release massage along the line of the muscle fibres. Where possible patients should be taught to perform their own stretches and mobilizations.

Postural retraining

Postural exercises are important and should be performed regularly throughout the day if improvement is to be gained and maintained. The initial focus should be on correcting any posterior pelvic rotation in sitting and on re-

Table 8.4 Assessment of muscle length

Muscle	Observation if muscle tight	Length testing position
Pectoralis major	Internal rotation and anterior translation of the humerus	Horizontal extension and abduction to 140°
Pectoralis minor	Anterior and inferior position of coracoid process and elevation of ribs 3–5	Retraction and depression of scapula
Upper cervical extensors	Forward position of head on neck, increased upper cervical lordosis	Flexion of the head on the upper cervical spine
Upper trapezius	Elevation of scapula, palpable anterior border of trapezius (occiput to distal clavicle)	Cervical flexion with contralateral lateral flexion and ipsilateral rotation
Levator scapula	Increased muscle bulk anterior to upper trapezius and posterior to sternocleidomastoid from C2–4 to superior angle of scapula	Cervical flexion, contralateral lateral flexion and contralateral rotation keeping the medial superior scapula border depressed
Sternocleidomastoid	Forward position of head on neck, elevated 1st rib and prominence at the clavicular insertion of sternocleidomastoid	Upper cervical flexion with lower cervical extension
Anterior scalenes	Elevation of ribs 1–3, ipsilateral lateral flexion of head on neck	Exhalation with depression of ribs 1–3 and upper cervical flexion
Latissimus dorsi	Internal rotation of humerus	Elevation of shoulder in external rotation with posterior pelvic tilt
Teres major	Medial rotation of humerus, protracted and upward rotation of scapula	Flex shoulder while sustaining scapular retraction and depression
Diaphragm	Flexed thorax and localized lordosis at the thoracolumbar junction	Relaxed diaphragmatic breathing

ducing the lumbar and thoracic kyphosis to bring the head back over the trunk. A small pillow or lumbar roll may then be used to maintain this position. Further reduction of the thoracic kyphosis may need to be assisted until the holding capacity of the thoracic extensors and lower fibres of trapezius has been improved. Strapping tape, applied with the patient in corrected sitting, may give proprioceptive feedback in the early stages of retraining. A long piece of tape starting anteriorly above the clavicle and crossing the mid-fibres of trapezius is thought to inhibit overactivity of this muscle. The tape is then crossed over at the peak of the thoracic kyphosis and extended down to the lumbar spine. It should not be so firm that pain is produced.

Postural correction can also be commenced in standing, semi-supine or high side lying and then incorporated into maintenance of corrected posture during specific activities. Training of scapular retraction and depression using middle and lower fibres of trapezius is important to complement any gain in range of thoracic extension and to improve scapular stability (Fig. 8.66a–c). The holding capacity of the deep upper cervical flexors and cervicothoracic exten-

sors will need to be trained to reduce the degree of forward head posture and to assist relaxation of sternocleidomastoid and the scalene muscles (Table 8.5). The longus colli and rectus capitus anterior major may be trained initially in high sitting then progressed to supine if shortness of breath allows (Fig. 8.67). Alternatively, gentle nodding of the head on neck against slight resistance can be taught in sitting. Serratus anterior can be retrained to hold the scapula against the chest wall using a half push-up action against a wall (taking care that upper trapezius is not overactive).

A gym ball may be useful for encouraging a more upright sitting posture in younger patients. Prone positions over the ball may be used to stimulate the antigravity muscles. Side lying over the ball will assist with rib mobility and stretching of the intercostal muscles if mobility and shortness of breath allow.

Neural tissue

The primary aim of treatment when neural tissue provocation tests reveal irritation or restriction is to mobilize the tight adjacent structures and improve posture while monitoring the effect

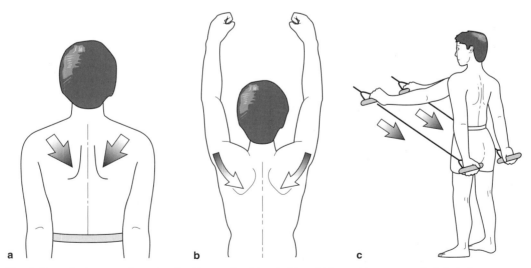

Fig. 8.66   **a** Active scapulae retraction/depression (rhomboids, middle and lower trapezius). **b** Active scapulae retraction/depression in shoulder elevation. **c** Active scapulae retraction/depression in shoulder extension.

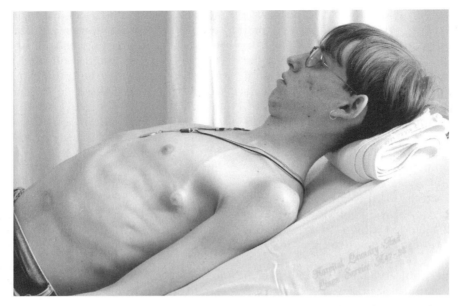

Fig. 8.67 Position for training activation of deep upper cervical flexors and lower trapezius and for stretching of upper cervical extensors and pectoralis minor and major.

Table 8.5 Assessment of holding capacity of lengthened muscles

Muscle	Test position
Deep upper cervical flexors	Half supine, nodding of head on neck. Test holding ability
Middle and lower trapezius	With patient prone (or sitting if SOB), test holding ability by placing scapula in retraction and depression and asking patient to hold
Serratus anterior	Note ability to maintain scapula against chest wall during a partial push up against a wall
Infraspinatus	Test strength of external rotation

on the neural system. If progress is inadequate gentle mobilization (not stretch) of the neural tissues at the site of restriction may be required.

TRANSCUTANEOUS ELECTRICAL NERVE STIMULATION

Transcutaneous electrical nerve stimulation (TENS) is the passing of an electrical current, across the skin, in the therapeutic treatment of pain. Thorough assessment to identify the cause of pain should always be carried out before the application of TENS. Adequate pain control will facilitate the use of other physio-

therapy techniques, e.g. ambulation, huffing and coughing.

There are many TENS units on the market, and each consists of a pulse generator driven by one or two batteries. The unit may be single or dual channel with one or two leads attached to the electrodes. Electrical current is passed across the skin through the electrode pads via a layer of electroconductive gel (Frampton 1994).

The hypothesis for the effectiveness of TENS in the relief of pain is the pain gate theory. It was believed that the gating mechanism lay simply in the substantia gelatinosa, but it is a highly complex area receiving and interpreting inhibitory and excitatory interneuronal information (Melzack & Wall 1984). Briefly the 'opening' and 'closing' of the gate is dependent on activity from large diameter (A-beta) and small diameter (A-delta and C) fibres. A-beta afferent fibres carry impulses rapidly to the dorsal horn, closing the gate to the slower A-delta and C nociceptor fibres and the transmission of pain is presynaptically inhibited. Nociceptive input is also influenced by descending inhibitory systems within the substantia gelatinosa involving complex chemical substances. It is thought that the pain gate modulation is more to do with a balance in the large and small diameter nerve fibre activity, and that the input from the afferent C fibres liberates peptides intraspinally giving rise to neuronal excitation in the dorsal horn (Baldry 1993).

There are four modes of TENS used for the treatment of pain (Mannheimer 1985):

High frequency, low intensity is the most common and usually called conventional TENS. It produces high-frequency impulses at about 50–100 Hz, of short pulse duration, e.g. 30–75 μs at low intensity. It stimulates the larger diameter myelinated afferent nerve fibres. The patient feels a comfortable paraesthesia with a fairly rapid onset. The after effects are relatively short lived – about 60 minutes after stimulation. It is, however, effective for acute pain.

Low frequency, high intensity is another commonly used mode often called 'acupuncture-like TENS'. Impulses are of low frequency (1–4 Hz) and long pulse duration (150–250 μs) at high intensity. This type of stimulation produces muscle contraction without paraesthesia, exciting the small diameter unmyelinated C fibres, and releasing endogenous opioids. This mode is suited to deep, achy, chronic pain and relief may take 30 minutes to occur, but the after effect is long lasting, sometimes several hours.

Burst stimulation/pulse train combines both high and low frequencies and can be delivered at high or low intensity. High-frequency pulses are delivered in low-frequency trains. Patients who do not like the constant tingly/paraesthesia obtained with conventional TENS may prefer this where the pulse is interrupted twice every second. This mode can also be used at high intensity to stimulate a muscle contraction.

Brief intense is the strongest and least comfortable mode of TENS. High frequency at high intensity, produces a strong paraesthesia with possibly muscle tetany or fasciculation. It recruits the full range of motor and sensory nerve fibres producing a response that is rapid but short lived on cessation of stimulation. This may be used for short periods of analgesia for procedures such as skin debridement.

Accommodation may occur with TENS stimulation, particularly the conventional mode where nerve endings are no longer receptive to the stimulation produced by the TENS. This may cause pain to break through or the patient to become hypersensitive to the TENS stimulation. Some TENS units have a modulation mode whereby the unit alters the pulse duration or intensity rhythmically so that tolerance to the more painful stimulation mode may be achieved or accommodation to the mild continuous stimuli may decrease.

Indications are numerous but may include (Lockwood 1996):

* Acute pain, e.g. acute trauma, postoperative pain such as thoracotomy
* Musculoskeletal pain
* Joint pain
* Peripheral nerve disorders, e.g. phantom limb pain, post-herpetic neuralgia, neuropathic pain from scars.

Placement of the electrodes should follow these guidelines employing one or more positions (Frampton 1994, Lockwood 1996):

* over the peripheral nerve proximal to the site of pain
* over the affected dermatome
* above and below the painful area
* over the spinal nerve root
* over acupuncture or trigger points.

If the unit has leads of two colours, the black denotes the cathode and should be placed closest to the spinal column for setting off an electropotential at the nerve root. Electrodes should not be placed within 3 cm of each other to prevent arcing.

For optimal results the area should first be washed and dried to remove lipids and prevent impedance across the skin. The main side-effect from TENS is an allergic reaction to the adhesive tape or conductive gel, and therefore patients should be taught how to assess the skin condition and change electrode pads and/or position frequently. Similarly, they may receive a small burn under the electrode due to lack of conductive gel or a current too intense for a therapeutic technique.

Depending on the mode of TENS used, a treatment period of 30 minutes for assessment should be employed and then increased if necessary for subsequent treatments. Between treatments the unit should be switched off to allow a resting potential to return and prevent accommodation. The literature appears confusing as to the optimal length of treatment time, with some patients responding to 1 hour four times a day and weaning from treatment, while others may use it for 8 hours daily for many months or even years. A trial period is advisable, but the patient should not sleep with the electrodes in situ as they may become displaced or dry out causing a minor burn due to convergence of current. The skin should be examined on a daily basis.

Contraindications include (Mannheimer 1985, Frampton 1994):

- Patients with demand-type pacemakers. The electrical impulse may interfere with the action of the pacemaker and similarly with some monitoring equipment.
- Placing electrodes near or over the heart. The electrical stimulation produced should not be enough to cause cardiac fibrillation; due care must be taken and a muscle contraction should not be evoked.
- Care should be taken in patients with a history of cerebrovascular accident, transient ischaemic attacks or epilepsy.
- Obstetric TENS has been used during childbirth but electrodes should not be placed over the pregnant uterus.
- It is not recommended to drive a vehicle or operate machinery while wearing a TENS device.

TENS is an effective non-invasive, non-addictive method of pain control. However, to achieve maximal therapeutic effect an understanding of the nociceptive pathways (Walsh 1991) and the properties of the afferent fibres will enable careful evaluation of the modalities available and facilitate selection. Careful instructions must be given to the patient and carers as overstimulation may have the opposite effect.

ACUPUNCTURE

Acupuncture, despite thousands of years of history has only been recognized in the Western World as a pain relief technique for the last 30 years. The exact mechanism of how the analgesic effect is obtained is not yet fully understood. It has been noted that stimulating acupuncture points local to the site of pain has a different physiological effect than stimulating distal points (Baldry 1993). Local points would seem to release enkephalin and dymorphin in the lateral horn which block afferent pain transmission, while distal points would seem to stimulate the midbrain to release enkephalin, activating the raphe descending tract to inhibit pain transmission by the synergistic effect of serotonin and noradrenaline. Pain transmission is also inhibited via the pituitary and hypothalamus by the release of β-endorphin into the circulation and cerebrospinal fluid. It has been demonstrated that naloxone inhibits the analgesic effects of acupuncture (Ellis 1994). Lewith & Kenyon (1984) explain in more depth the neurohumoral mechanisms of acupuncture and also the link between substance P in the endogenous opioid system and the pain gate theory.

Patients who respond well to TENS, and need continued pain control after discharge, should be considered for acupuncture if they are unable to apply the TENS unit independently, or a unit is unavailable for home loan. Similarly patients who are on maximal medical treatment for their pain symptoms, unsuccessful with TENS and have no contraindications, should be considered for acupuncture.

Safety to patient and practitioner must be

paramount when practising acupuncture. Disposable needles may minimize the risk of transfer of infectious diseases. Acupuncture is not recommended in patients who are unable to control their movements or are over-anxious. It is usually not recommended during pregnancy (Alltree 1994). Caution should also be taken in patients with skin disorders, tumours, blood disorders and swellings of unknown cause (Duffin 1985). Patients with diabetes may also experience a decrease in blood sugar levels, and forbidden points of acupuncture should be observed.

Indications for treatment are similar to those for TENS. Needles can be applied 'dry' which would stimulate the nerve endings at a low frequency, or by connecting to an electrostimulator therefore applying electro-acupuncture which produces a higher frequency stimulation. The best results are achieved by obtaining deqi or needling sensation with each needle. Acupuncture can be applied to local points around the area of pain or combined with distal points therefore utilizing both pain-relieving pathways. Ah Chi or tender points also respond to acupuncture stimulation, and points along the opposite limb can also be used.

Pain relief may not be immediate and several treatments may be required to reduce pain noticeably especially if the patient is already established on strong opioid analgesics. The requirement for opioids may reduce before the patient reports a reduction in pain. In some cases the patient may at first report a brief increase before a reduction in pain. Other effects of acupuncture may be an erythema around the needle. On some occasions a slight muscle contraction seems to grasp the needle momentarily and there may be slight bleeding from the needle site. These are fairly common responses. The patient may also experience a vasovagal reaction and feel faint or may be sleepy or euphoric with treatment (Alltree 1994).

Successful pain relief with acupuncture can last for several days or even weeks although this phenomenon is not yet understood. The study of acupuncture is far more complex than the simple pain-relieving properties and must be the subject of future research.

REFERENCES

Abelson H, Brewer K 1987 Inspiratory muscle training in the mechanically ventilated patient. Physiotherapy Canada 39: 305–307

Ahmedzai S, Davis C 1997 Nebulised drugs in palliative care. Thorax 52(suppl 2): S75–S77

Aldrich T K, Karpel J P, Uhrlass R M et al 1989 Weaning from mechanical ventilation: adjunctive use of inspiratory muscle resistive training. Critical Care Medicine 17: 143–147

Alltree J 1994 Acupuncture. In: Wells P E, Frampton V, Bowsher D (eds) Pain management by physiotherapy, 2nd edn. Butterworth-Heinemann, Oxford. ch 13

Andersen J B, Olesen K P, Eikard B, Jansen E, Quist J 1980 Periodic continuous positive airway pressure, CPAP, by mask in the treatment of atelectasis. European Journal of Respiratory Diseases 61: 20–25

Arens R, Gozal D, Omlin K J, Vega J, Boyd K P, Keens T G, Woo M S 1994 Comparison of high frequency chest compression and conventional chest physiotherapy in hospitalized patients with cystic fibrosis. American Journal of Critical Care Medicine 150: 1154–1157

Ayres S M, Kozam R L, Lukas D S 1963 The effects of intermittent positive pressure breathing on intrathoracic pressure, pulmonary mechanics, and the work of breathing. American Review of Respiratory Disease 87: 370–379

Bachrach L K, Loutit C W, Moss R B, Marcus R 1994 Osteopenia in adults with cystic fibrosis. American

Journal of Medicine 96: 27–34

Baldry P E 1993 Acupuncture, trigger points and musculoskeletal pain. 2nd edn. Churchill Livingstone, Edinburgh

Bartlett R, Gazzaniga A B, Geraghty T R 1973 Respiratory maneuvers to prevent postoperative pulmonary complications. Journal of the American Medical Association 224: 1017–1021

Bazuaye E A, Stone T N, Corris P A, Gibson G J 1992 Variability of inspired oxygen concentration with nasal cannulas. Thorax 47: 609–611

Bendefy I M 1991 Home nebulisers in childhood asthma: survey of hospital supervised use. British Medical Journal 302: 1180–1181

Bethune D 1975 Neurophysiological facilitation of respiration in the unconscious adult patient. Physiotherapy Canada 27(5): 241–245

Bethune D 1976 Facilitation of respiration in unconscious adult patients. Respiratory Technology 12(4): 18–21

Bethune D 1991 Neurophysiological facilitation of respiration. In: Pryor J A (ed) Respiratory care. Churchill Livingstone, Edinburgh

Binkley J, Soloman P, Finch E, Gill C, Moreland J 1996 Defining the minimal level of detectable change for the Roland–Morris questionnaire. Physical Therapy 76: 359–365

Bott J, Keilty S E J, Noone L 1992 Intermittent positive pressure breathing – a dying art? Physiotherapy 78: 656–660

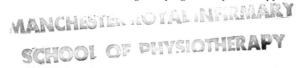
MANCHESTER ROYAL INFIRMARY
SCHOOL OF PHYSIOTHERAPY

Boyling J D, Palastanga N 1994 In: Grieve G P Modern manual therapy of the vertebral column, 2nd edn. Churchill Livingstone, Edinburgh

Bransen R D, Davis K, Campbell R S, Johnson D J, Porembka D T 1993 Humidification in the intensive care unit: prospective study of a new protocol utilizing heated humidification and a hygroscopic condenser humidifier. Chest 104: 1800–1805

Bray C 1994 Thoracic mobilisation in the management of respiratory and cardiac problems. In: The forgotten thoracic spine. Manipulative Physiotherapists Association of Australia Symposium, University of Sydney, Australia

British Standards Institution 1994 Specification for gas powered nebulisers for the delivery of drugs. BS7711 Part 3. British Standards Institution, London

British Thoracic Society, National Asthma Campaign, Royal College of Physicians of London et al 1997 The British guidelines on asthma management – 1995 review and position statement. Thorax 52 (suppl 1): S1–S21

Burge P S 1986 Getting the best out of bronchodilator therapy. Patient Management July: 155–185

Butler D S 1991 Mobilisation of the nervous system. Churchill Livingstone, Melbourne

Campbell A H, O'Connell J M, Wilson F 1975 The effect of chest physiotherapy upon the FEV_1 in chronic bronchitis. Medical Journal of Australia 1: 33–35

Campbell E J, Baker D, Crites-Silver P 1988 Subjective effects of humidification of oxygen for delivery by nasal cannula. Chest 93: 289–293

Carr L, Pryor J A, Hodson M E 1995 Self chest clapping: patients' views and the effects on oxygen saturation. Physiotherapy 81: 753–757

Carr L, Smith R E, Pryor J A, Partridge C 1996 Cystic fibrosis patients' views and beliefs about chest clearance and exercise – a pilot study. Physiotherapy 82: 621–626

Chatburn R L 1987 Physiologic and methodologic issues regarding humidity therapy. Journal of Pediatrics 114: 416–420

Chatham K, Marshall C, Campbell I A, Prescott R J 1993 The Flutter VRPI device in post-thoracotomy patients. Physiotherapy 79: 95–98

Chevaillier J 1995 Autogenic drainage In: Physiotherapy in the treatment of cystic fibrosis, 2nd edn. International Physiotherapy Group for Cystic Fibrosis (IPG/CF), pp 9–12

Chuter T A M, Weissman C, Starker P M, Gump F E 1989 Effect of incentive spirometry on diaphragmatic function after surgery. Surgery 105: 488–493

Chuter T A M, Weissman C, Mathews D M, Starker P M 1990 Diaphragmatic breathing maneuvers and movement of the diaphragm after cholecystectomy. Chest 97: 1110–1114

Clarke S W 1988 Inhaler therapy. Quarterly Journal of Medicine New Series 67(253): 355–368

Clarke S W 1995 Physical defences. In: Brewis R A L, Corrin B, Geddes D M, Gibson G J (eds) Respiratory medicine, 2nd edn. W B Saunders, London, vol 1, ch 3

Cole P 1995 Bronchiectasis. In: Brewis R A L, Corrin B, Geddes D M, Gibson G J (eds) Respiratory medicine, 2nd edn. W B Saunders, London, vol 2, ch 39

Collis G G, Cole C H, Le Souëf P N 1990 Dilution of nebulised aerosols by air entrainment in children. Lancet 336: 341–343

Conway J H 1992 The effects of humidification for patients with chronic airways disease. Physiotherapy 78: 97–101

Conway J H, Fleming J S, Perring S, Holgate S T 1992 Humidification as an adjunct to chest physiotherapy in aiding tracheo-bronchial clearance in patients with bronchiectasis. Respiratory Medicine 86: 109–114

Coombs H C 1918 The relation of the dorsal roots of the spinal nerves and the mesencephalon to the control of respiratory movements. American Journal of Physiology 46: 459–471

Coombs H C, Pike F H 1930 The nervous control of respiration in kittens. American Journal of Physiology 95: 681–693

Currie D C, Munro C, Gaskell D, Cole P J 1986 Practice, problems and compliance with postural drainage: a survey of chronic sputum producers. British Journal of Diseases of the Chest 80: 249–253

Dab I, Alexander F 1979 The mechanism of autogenic drainage studied with flow volume curves. Monographs of Paediatrics 10: 50–53

Dail C W 1951 'Glossopharyngeal breathing' by paralyzed patients. California Medicine 75: 217–218

Dail C W, Affeldt J E, Collier C R 1955 Clinical aspects of glossopharyngeal breathing. Journal of the American Medical Association 158: 445–449

David A 1991 Autogenic drainage – the German approach. In: Pryor J A (ed) Respiratory care. Churchill Livingstone, Edinburgh, pp 65–78

Davidson A G F, Wong L T K, Pirie G E, McIlwaine P M 1992 Long-term comparative trial of conventional percussion and drainage physiotherapy versus autogenic drainage in cystic fibrosis. Pediatric Pulmonology Supplement 8: 298

De Troyer A, Peche R, Yernault J, Estenne M 1994 Neck muscle activity in patients with severe chronic obstructive disease. Journal of Respiratory Care Medicine 150: 41–47

Dean E 1985 Effect of body position on pulmonary function. Physical Therapy 65: 613–618

Dodd M E, Hanley S P, Johnson S C, Webb A K 1995 District nebuliser compressor service: reliability and costs. Thorax 50: 82–84

Dodd M E, Abbott J, Maddison J, Moorcroft A J, Webb A K 1997 Effect of tonicity of nebulised colistin on chest tightness and pulmonary function in adults with cystic fibrosis. Thorax 52: 656–658

Duffin D 1985 Acupuncture and acupressure. In: Michel T H (ed) Pain. Churchill Livingstone, Edinburgh, ch 5

Editorial 1988 Nebulisers and paradoxical bronchoconstriction. Lancet ii: 202

Eklund G, von Euler C, Rutkowski S 1964 Spontaneous and reflex activity of intercostal gamma motoneurones. Journal of Physiology 171: 139–163

Ellis N 1994 Acupuncture in clinical practice. A guide for health professionals. Chapman & Hall, London

Eng P A, Morton J, Douglass J A, Riedler J, Wilson J, Robertson C F 1996 Short-term efficacy of ultrasonically nebulized hypertonic saline in cystic fibrosis. Pediatric Pulmonology 21: 77–83

Everard M L, Evans M, Milner A D 1994 Is tapping jet nebulisers worthwhile? Archives of Disease in Childhood 70: 538–539

Falk M, Andersen J B 1991 Positive expiratory pressure (PEP) mask. In: Pryor J A (ed) Respiratory care. Churchill Livingstone, Edinburgh, pp 51–63

Falk M, Kelstrup M, Andersen J B, Kinoshita T, Falk P, Støvring S, Gøthgen I 1984 Improving the ketchup bottle method with positive expiratory pressure, PEP, in cystic fibrosis. European Journal of Respiratory Diseases 65: 423–432

Flower K A, Eden R I, Lomax L, Mann N M, Burgess J 1979

New mechanical aid to physiotherapy in cystic fibrosis. British Medical Journal 2: 630–631

Flynn M G, Barter C E, Nosworthy J C et al 1989 Threshold pressure training, breathing pattern, and exercise performance in chronic airflow obstruction. Chest 95: 535–540

Frampton V 1994 Transcutaneous nerve stimulation and chronic pain. In: Wells P E, Frampton V, Bowsher D (eds) Pain management by physiotherapy, 2nd edn. Butterworth-Heinemann, Oxford, ch 14

Frankstein S I 1970 Neural control of respiration in breathing. In: Porter R (ed) Breathing: Hering-Breuer Centenary Symposium, Ciba Symposium. J & A Churchill, London

Freitag L, Bremme J, Schroer M 1989 High frequency oscillation for respiratory physiotherapy. British Journal of Anaesthesia 63: 44S–46S

Gallon A 1991 Evaluation of chest percussion in the treatment of patients with copious sputum production. Respiratory Medicine 85: 45–51

George R J D, Johnson M A, Pavia D, Agnew J E, Clarke S W, Geddes D M 1985 Increase in mucociliary clearance in normal man induced by oral high frequency oscillation. Thorax 40: 433–437

Gherini S, Peters R M, Virgilio R W 1979 Mechanical work on the lungs and work of breathing with positive end-expiratory pressure and continuous positive airway pressure. Chest 76: 251–256

Gleeson J G, Price J F 1988 Nebuliser technique. British Journal of Diseases of the Chest 82: 172–174

Goldman J M, Teale C, Muers M F 1992 Simplifying the assessment of patients with chronic airflow limitation for home nebulizer therapy. Respiratory Medicine 86: 33–38

Goodwin M J 1994 Mechanical chest stimulation as a physiotherapy aid. Medical Engineering and Physics 16: 267–272

Gormezano J, Branthwaite M A 1972 Pulmonary physiotherapy with assisted ventilation. Anaesthesia 27: 249–257

Gosselink R, Wagenaar R C, Decramer M 1996 Reliability of a commercially available threshold loading device in healthy subjects and in patients with chronic obstructive pulmonary disease. Thorax 51: 601–605

Gosselink R, De Leyn P, Troosters T, Deneffe G, Lerut A, Decramer M 1997 Incentive spirometry does not affect recovery after thoracic surgery. European Respiratory Journal 10: (Suppl. 25): 72S

Green M, Moxham J 1985 The respiratory muscles. Clinical Science 68: 1–10

Gregersen G G, Lucas D L 1967 An in vivo study of the axial rotation of the human thoraco-lumbar spine. Journal of Bone and Joint Surgery 49-A: 247–262

Gross D, Ladd H W, Riley E J, Macklem P T, Grassino A 1980 The effect of training on strength and endurance of the diaphragm in quadriplegia. American Journal of Medicine 68: 27–35

Gunawardena K A, Patel B, Campbell I A, Macdonald J B, Smith A P 1984 Oxygen as a driving gas for nebulisers: safe or dangerous? British Medical Journal 288: 272–274

Hall J C, Tarala R, Harris J, Tapper J, Christiansen K 1991 Incentive spirometry versus routine chest physiotherapy for prevention of pulmonary complications after abdominal surgery. Lancet 337: 953–956

Hansen L G, Warwick W J, Hansen K L 1994 Mucus transport mechanisms in relation to the effect of high frequency chest compression (HFCC) on mucus clearance. Pediatric Pulmonology 17: 113–118

Harrison D A, Breen D P, Harris N D, Gerrish S P 1993 The performance of two intensive care humidifiers at high gas flows. Anaesthesia 48: 902–905

Hasani A, Pavia D, Agnew J E, Clarke S W 1994 Regional lung clearance during cough and forced expiration technique (FET): effects of flow and viscoelasticity. Thorax 49: 557–561

Henderson R C, Madsen C D 1996 Bone density in children and adolescents with cystic fibrosis. Journal of Paediatrics 128: 28–34

Henderson R C, Specter B B 1994 Kyphosis and fractures in children and young adults with cystic fibrosis. Journal of Paediatrics 125: 208–212

Higgens J M 1966 The management in cabinet respirators of patients with acute or residual respiratory muscle paralysis. Physiotherapy 52: 425–430

Hill S L, Barnes P K, Hollway T, Tennant R 1984 Fixed performance oxygen masks: an evaluation. British Medical Journal 288: 1261–1263

Hinds C J, Watson D 1996 Intensive care, 2nd edn. Saunders, London, pp 33, 175

Hofmeyr J L, Webber B A, Hodson M E 1986 Evaluation of positive expiratory pressure as an adjunct to chest physiotherapy in the treatment of cystic fibrosis. Thorax 41: 951–954

Howard P, Cayton R M, Brennan S R, Anderson P B 1977 Lignocaine aerosol and persistent cough. British Journal of Diseases of the Chest 71: 19–24

Hutchinson G R, Parker S, Pryor J A et al 1996 Home-use nebulizers: a potential source of *Burkholderia cepacia* and other colistin-resistant, gram-negative bacteria in patients with cystic fibrosis. Journal of Clinical Microbiology 34: 584–587

Jacob W 1990 Physiotherapy in the ICU. In: Oh T E (ed) Intensive care manual, 3rd edn. Butterworths, Sydney, ch 4, p 24

Janda V 1994 Muscles and motor control in cervicogenic disorders: assessment and management physical therapy for the cervical and thoracic spine. In: Grant R (ed) Clinics in physical therapy, 2nd edn. Churchill Livingstone, USA

Jeffrey A A, Warren P M 1992 Should we judge a mask by its cover? Thorax 47: 543–546

Jenkins S C, Soutar S A, Moxham J 1988 The effects of posture on lung volumes in normal subjects and in patients pre- and post-coronary artery surgery. Physiotherapy 74: 492–496

Keeley D 1992 Large volume plastic spacers in asthma. British Medical Journal 305: 598–599

Kelleher W H, Parida R K 1957 Glossopharyngeal breathing. British Medical Journal 2: 740–743

Kendrick A H, Smith E C, Denyer J 1995 Nebulizers – fill volume, residual volume and matching of nebulizer to compressor. Respiratory Medicine 89: 157–159

Kieselmann R 1995 Modified AD. In: Physiotherapy in the treatment of cystic fibrosis, 2nd edn. International Physiotherapy Group for Cystic Fibrosis (IPG/CF), pp 13–14

Konstan M H, Stern R C, Doershuk C F 1994 Efficacy of the Flutter device for airway mucus clearance in patients with cystic fibrosis. Journal of Pediatrics 124: 689–693

Langlands J 1967 The dynamics of cough in health and in chronic bronchitis. Thorax 22: 88–96

Leach R M, Bateman N T 1994 Domiciliary oxygen therapy.

British Journal of Hospital Medicine 51: 47–54

Leak A M, Cooper J, Dyer S, Williams K, Turner-Stokes L, Frank O A 1994 The Northwick Park neck pain questionnaire, devised to measure neck pain and disability. British Journal of Rheumatology 33: 474–496

Lewis R A, Fleming J S 1985 Fractional deposition from a jet nebuliser: how it differs from a metered dose inhaler. British Journal of Diseases of the Chest 79: 361–367

Lewith G T, Kenyon J N 1984 Physiological and psychological explanations for the mechanism of acupuncture as a treatment for chronic pain. Social Science and Medicine 19: 1367–1378

Lindemann H 1992 The value of physical therapy with VRP1 Desitin ("Flutter"). Pneumologie 46(12): 626–630

Lindner K H, Lotz P, Ahnefeld F W 1987 Continuous positive airway pressure effect on functional residual capacity, vital capacity and its subdivisions. Chest 92: 66–70

Lock S H, Blower G, Prynne M, Wedzicha J A 1992 Comparison of liquid and gaseous oxygen for domiciliary portable use. Thorax 47: 98–100

Lockwood S 1996 The variable parameters of transcutaneous electrical nerve stimulation (TENS) and their clinical use. New Zealand Journal of Physiotherapy. 24(1): 7–10

Loddenkemper R 1975 Dose- and time-response of Sch 1000 MDI on total (R_t) and expiratory (R_e) airways resistance in patients with chronic bronchitis and emphysema. Postgraduate Medical Journal 51(suppl 7): 97

Lopez-Vidriero M T, Reid L 1978 Bronchial mucus in health and disease. British Medical Bulletin 34(1): 63–74

McCool F D, Tzelepis G E 1995 Inspiratory muscle training in the patient with neuromuscular disease. Physical Therapy 75: 1006–1014

McDonnell T, McNicholas W T, FitzGerald M X 1986 Hypoxaemia during chest physiotherapy in patients with cystic fibrosis. Irish Journal of Medical Science 155: 345–348

McGavin C R, Naoe H, McHardy G J R 1976 Does inhalation of salbutamol enable patients with airway obstruction to walk further? Clinical Science and Molecular Medicine 51: 12–13

Macklem P T 1974 Physiology of cough. Transactions of the American Broncho-Esophalogical Association: 150–157

Maddison J, Dodd M, Webb A K 1994 Nebulised colistin causes chest tightness in adults with cystic fibrosis. Respiratory Medicine 88: 145–147

Mannheimer J S 1985 TENS: uses and effectiveness. In: Michel T H (ed) Pain. Churchill Livingstone, Edinburgh, ch 4

Martin C J, Ripley H, Reynolds J, Best F 1976 Chest physiotherapy and the distribution of ventilation. Chest 69: 174–178

Matthews H R, Hopkinson R B 1984 Treatment of sputum retention by minitracheotomy. British Journal of Surgery 71: 147–150

Mead J, Turner J M, Macklem P T, Little J B 1967 Significance of the relationship between lung recoil and maximum expiratory flow. Journal of Applied Physiology 22: 95–108

Mead J, Takishima T, Leith D 1970 Stress distribution in lungs: a model of pulmonary elasticity. Journal of Applied Physiology 28: 596–608

Medic-Aid Ltd 1996 Nebulizer therapy training pack. Medic-Aid Ltd, Heath Place, Bognor Regis, W Sussex, UK

Medical Research Council Working Party 1981 Long term domiciliary oxygen therapy in chronic hypoxic cor pulmonale complicating chronic bronchitis and emphysema. Lancet 1: 681–686

Melzack R, Wall P 1984 The challenge of pain. Penguin Books, Middlesex

Menkes H A, Traystman R J 1977 Collateral ventilation. American Review of Respiratory Disease 116: 287–309

Menkes H, Britt J 1980 Rationale for physical therapy. American Review of Respiratory Disease 122(suppl 2): 127–131

Mestitz H, Copland J M, McDonald C F 1989 Comparison of outpatient nebulized vs metered dose inhaler terbutaline in chronic airflow obstruction. Chest 96: 1237–1240

Morgan M D L, Silver J R, Williams S J 1986 The respiratory system of the spinal cord patient. In: Bloch R F, Basbaum M (eds) Management of spinal cord injuries. Williams & Wilkins, Baltimore, pp 78–115

Morrison N J, Richardson J, Dunn L, Pardy R L 1989 Respiratory muscle performance in normal elderly subjects and patients with COPD. Chest 95: 90–94

Moxham J 1991 Respiratory muscle weakness – its recognition and management. Respiratory Disease in Practice April/May: 12–17

Mukhopadhyay S, Singh M, Cater J I, Ogsten S, Franklin M, Olver R E 1996 Nebulised antipseudomonal antibiotic therapy in cystic fibrosis: a meta-analysis of benefits and risks. Thorax 51: 364–368

Nathan H 1962 Osteophytes of the vertebral column. An anatomical study of their development according to age, race and sex with considerations as to their aetiology and significance. Journal of Bone and Joint Surgery 44A: 243

Nebuliser Project Group of the British Thoracic Society Standards of Care Committee 1997 Current best practice for nebuliser treatment. Thorax 52(suppl 2): S1–S106

Nelson H P 1934 Postural drainage of the lungs. British Medical Journal 2: 251–255

Newman S P, Pellow P G D, Clarke S W 1986 Droplet size distributions of nebulised aerosols for inhalation therapy. Clinical Physics and Physiological Measurement 7: 139–146

Newman S P, Weisz A W B, Talaee N, Clarke S W 1991 Improvement of drug delivery with a breath actuated pressurised aerosol for patients with poor inhaler technique. Thorax 46: 712–716

Nikander K 1994 Drug delivery systems. Journal of Aerosol Medicine 7(suppl 1): S-19–S-24

Nikander K, Wunderlich E 1996 Output of budesonide suspension for nebulization using different Pari jet nebulizer–compressor combinations. ISAM Focus Symposium, Aerosol therapy with small volume nebulizers: laboratory to bedside. 4–5 September, Tours, France

Nocturnal Oxygen Therapy Trial Group 1980 Continuous or nocturnal oxygen therapy in hypoxemic chronic obstructive lung disease: a clinical trial. Annals of Internal Medicine 93: 391–398

O'Driscoll B R, Kay E A, Taylor R J, Bernstein A 1990 Home nebulizers: can optimal therapy be predicted by laboratory studies? Respiratory Medicine 84: 471–477

O'Neill S O, McCarthy D S 1983 Postural relief of dyspnoea in severe chronic airflow limitation: relationship to respiratory muscle strength. Thorax 38: 595–600

Oberwaldner B, Evans J C, Zach M S 1986 Forced expirations against a variable resistance: a new chest physiotherapy method in cystic fibrosis. Pediatric Pulmonology 2: 358–367

Oberwaldner B, Theissl B, Rucker A, Zach M S 1991 Chest physiotherapy in hospitalized patients with cystic fibrosis: a study of lung function effects and sputum production. European Respiratory Journal 4: 152–158

Oh T E 1990 Humidification. In: Oh T E (ed) Intensive care manual, 3rd edn. Butterworths, Sydney, ch 24, pp 169–173

Oikkonen M, Karjalainen K, Kähärä V, Kuosa R, Schavikin L 1991 Comparison of incentive spirometry and intermittent positive pressure breathing after coronary artery bypass graft. Chest 99: 60–65

Pardy R L, Rivington R N, Despas P J, Macklem P T 1981 The effects of inspiratory muscle training on exercise performance in chronic airflow limitation. American Review of Respiratory Disease 123: 426–433

Pardy R L, Reid W D, Belman M J 1988 Respiratory muscle training. Clinics in Chest Medicine 9: 287–296

Pardy R L, Fairbarn M S, Blackie S P 1990 Respiratory muscle training. Problems in Respiratory Care 3: 483–492

Partridge C, Pryor J, Webber B 1989 Characteristics of the forced expiration technique. Physiotherapy 75: 193–194

Pavia D, Thomson M L, Clarke S W 1978 Enhanced clearance of secretions from the human lung after the administration of hypertonic saline aerosol. American Review of Respiratory Disease 117: 199–203

Pavia D, Webber B, Agnew J E, Vora H, Lopez-Vidriero M T, Clarke S W, Branthwaite M A 1988 The role of intermittent positive pressure breathing (IPPB) in bronchial toilet. European Respiratory Journal 1(suppl 2): 250S

Pedersen S 1996 Inhalers and nebulizers: which to choose and why. Respiratory Medicine 90: 69–77

Peiper A 1963 Cerebral function in infancy and childhood. Consultants Bureau, New York

Pendleton N, Cheesbrough J S, Walshaw M J, Hind C R K 1991 Bacterial colonisation of humidifier attachments on oxygen concentrators prescribed for long term oxygen therapy: a district review. Thorax 46: 257–258

Phillips G E, Davies J C, Krainaya J, Reznik B, Rosenthal M 1996 The isolated introduction of the active cycle of breathing techniques (ACBT) in Ukrainian children with cystic fibrosis (CF): acceptability and clinical outcome. Israel Journal of Medical Sciences 32(June)(suppl): S233

Preston I M, Matthews H R, Ready A R 1986 Minitracheotomy. Physiotherapy 72: 494–497

Pryor J A, Webber B A 1979 An evaluation of the forced expiration technique as an adjunct to postural drainage. Physiotherapy 65: 304–307

Pryor J A, Webber B A, Hodson M E, Batten J C 1979 Evaluation of the forced expiration technique as an adjunct to postural drainage in treatment of cystic fibrosis. British Medical Journal 2: 417–418

Pryor J A, Parker R A, Webber B A 1981 A comparison of mechanical and manual percussion as adjuncts to postural drainage in the treatment of cystic fibrosis in adolescents and adults. Physiotherapy 67: 140–141

Pryor J A, Wiggins J, Webber B A, Geddes D M 1989 Oral high frequency oscillation (OHFO) as an aid to physiotherapy in chronic bronchitis with airflow limitation. Thorax 44: 350P

Pryor J A, Webber B A, Hodson M E 1990 Effect of chest physiotherapy on oxygen saturation in patients with cystic fibrosis. Thorax 45: 77

Pryor J A, Webber B A, Hodson M E, Warner J O 1994 The Flutter VRP1 as an adjunct to chest physiotherapy in cystic fibrosis. Respiratory Medicine 88: 677–681

Putt M T, Paratz J D 1996 The effect of stretching pectoralis major and anterior deltoid muscles on the restrictive component of chronic airflow limitation. In: Proceedings of the National Physiotherapy Conference Brisbane Queensland, Australian Physiotherapy Association, Brisbane, Queensland

Reisman J J, Rivington-Law B, Corey M, Marcotte J, Wannamaker E, Harcourt D, Levison H 1988 Role of conventional physiotherapy in cystic fibrosis. Journal of Pediatrics 113: 632–636

Ricksten S E, Bengtsson A, Soderberg C, Thorden M, Kvist H 1986 Effects of periodic positive airway pressure by mask on postoperative pulmonary function. Chest 89: 774–781

Rood M 1973 Unpublished lectures given at the University of Western Ontario. London, Ontario

Ruffin R E, Fitzgerald J D, Rebuck A S 1977 A comparison of the bronchodilator activity of Sch 1000 and salbutamol. Journal of Allergy and Clinical Immunology 59: 136–141

Ryan D W 1990 Minitracheotomy. British Medical Journal 300: 958–959

Sanderson P J 1984 Common bacterial pathogens and resistance to antibiotics. British Medical Journal 289: 638–639

Schoeffel R E, Anderson S D, Altounyan R E C 1981 Bronchial hyperreactivity in response to inhalation of ultrasonically nebulised solutions of distilled water and saline. British Medical Journal 283: 1285–1287

Schöni M H 1989 Autogenic drainage: a modern approach to physiotherapy in cystic fibrosis. Journal of the Royal Society of Medicine 82(suppl 16): 32–37

Shah P, Dhurjon L, Metcalfe T, Gibson J M 1992 Acute angle closure glaucoma associated with nebulised ipratropium bromide and salbutamol. British Medical Journal 304: 40–41

Sharp J T, Drutz W S, Moisan T, Forster J, Machnach W 1980 Postural relief of dyspnea in severe chronic obstructive pulmonary disease. American Review of Respiratory Disease 122: 201–211

Shelly M P, Lloyd G M, Park G R 1988 A review of the mechanisms and methods of humidification of inspired gases. Intensive Care 14: 1–9

Shneerson J 1992 Transtracheal oxygen delivery. Thorax 47: 57–59

Smaldone G C, Vinciguerra C, Marchese J 1991 Detection of inhaled pentamidine in health care workers. The New England Journal of Medicine 325: 891–892

Smith K, Cook D, Guyatt G H, Madhavan J, Oxman A D 1992 Respiratory muscle training in chronic airflow limitation: a meta-analysis. American Review of Respiratory Disease 145: 533–539

Starke I D, Webber B A, Branthwaite M A 1979 IPPB and hypercapnia in respiratory failure: the effect of different concentrations of inspired oxygen on arterial blood gas tensions. Anaesthesia 34: 283–287

Stock M C, Downs J B, Gauer P K, Alster J M, Imrey P B 1985 Prevention of postoperative pulmonary complications with CPAP, incentive spirometry, and conservative therapy. Chest 87: 151–157

Sukumalchantra Y, Park S S, Williams M H 1965 The effect of intermittent positive pressure breathing (IPPB) in acute ventilatory failure. American Review of Respiratory Disease 92: 885–893

Sumi T 1963 The segmental reflex relations of cutaneous afferent inflow to thoracic respiratory motoneurones. Journal of Neurophysiology 26: 478–493

Sutton P P, Parker R A, Webber B A et al 1983 Assessment of

the forced expiration technique, postural drainage and directed coughing in chest physiotherapy. European Journal of Respiratory Diseases 64: 62–68

Sykes M K, McNicol M W, Campbell E J M 1976 Respiratory failure, 2nd edn. Blackwell Scientific, Oxford, p 153

Thompson B 1978 Asthma and your child, 5th edn. Pegasus Press, Christchurch, New Zealand

Thompson B, Thompson H T 1968 Forced expiration exercises in asthma and their effect on FEV_1. New Zealand Journal of Physiotherapy 3: 19–21

Thoracic Society 1950 The nomenclature of bronchopulmonary anatomy. Thorax 5: 222–228

Tilling S E, Hayes B 1987 Heat and moisture exchangers in artificial ventilation. British Journal of Anaesthesia 59: 1181–1188

Valerius N H, Koch C, Høiby N 1991 Prevention of chronic *Pseudomonas aeruginosa* colonisation in cystic fibrosis by early treatment. Lancet 338: 725–726

van der Schans C P, van der Mark Th W, de Vries G et al 1991 Effect of positive expiratory pressure breathing in patients with cystic fibrosis. Thorax 46: 252–256

van Hengstum M, Festen J, Beurskens C, Hankel M, van den Broek W, Corstens F 1990 No effect of oral high frequency oscillation combined with forced expiration manoeuvres on tracheobronchial clearance in chronic bronchitis. European Respiratory Journal 3: 14–18

Vater M, Hurt P G, Aitkenhead A R 1983 Quantitative effects of respired helium and oxygen mixtures on gas flow using conventional oxygen masks. Anaesthesia 38: 879–882

Vibekk P 1991 Chest mobilization and respiratory function. In: Pryor J A (ed) Respiratory care. Churchill Livingstone, Edinburgh, pp 103–119

Vora V A, Vara D D, Walton R, Morgan M D L 1995 The assessment of nebulised bronchodilator treatment in COPD by shuttle walk test and breathing problem questionnaire. Thorax 50(suppl 2): A29

Walsh D 1991 Nociceptive pathways – relevance to the physiotherapist. Physiotherapy 77: 317–321

Wanner A 1977 Clinical aspects of mucociliary transport. American Review of Respiratory Disease 116: 73–125

Ward R J, Danziger F, Bonica J J, Allen G D, Bowes J 1966 An evaluation of postoperative respiratory maneuvers. Surgery, Gynecology and Obstetrics 123: 51–54

Watson D, Trott P 1993 Cervical headache – an investigation of natural head posture and upper cervical flexor muscle performance. Cephalgia 13: 272–284

Webb A K, Egan J J, Dodd M E 1996 Clinical management of cystic fibrosis patients awaiting and immediately following lung transplantation. In: Dodge J A, Brock D J H, Widdicombe J H (eds) Cystic fibrosis – current topics. Wiley, Chichester, vol 3, p 332

Webber B A 1988 The Brompton Hospital guide to chest physiotherapy, 5th edn. Blackwell Scientific, Oxford, p 43

Webber B A 1990 The active cycle of breathing techniques. Cystic Fibrosis News Aug/Sep: 10–11

Webber B A 1991 The role of the physiotherapist in medical chest problems. Respiratory Disease in Practice Feb/Mar: 12–15

Webber B A, Shenfield G M, Paterson J W 1974 A comparison of three different techniques for giving nebulized albuterol to asthmatic patients. American Review of Respiratory Disease 109: 293–295

Webber B A, Parker R, Hofmeyr J, Hodson M 1985 Evaluation of self-percussion during postural drainage using the forced expiration technique. Physiotherapy Practice 1: 42–45

Webber B A, Hofmeyr J L, Morgan M D L, Hodson M E 1986 Effects of postural drainage, incorporating the forced expiration technique, on pulmonary function in cystic fibrosis. British Journal of Diseases of the Chest 80: 353–359

West J B 1992 Pulmonary pathophysiology, 4th edn. Williams & Wilkins, Baltimore

White A A, Panjabi M M 1990 Clinical biomechanics of the spine, 2nd edn. Lippincott, Philadelphia

White S, Sahrmann S 1994 Physical therapy for the cervical and thoracic spine. In: Grant R (ed) Clinics in physical therapy, 2nd edn. Churchill Livingstone, USA

Wilson G E, Baldwin A L, Walshaw M J 1995 A comparison of traditional chest physiotherapy with the active cycle of breathing in patients with chronic suppurative lung disease. European Respiratory Journal 8(suppl 19): 171S

Wilson R, Cole P J 1988 The effect of bacterial products on ciliary function. American Review of Respiratory Disease 138: S49–S53

Wolfsdorf J, Swift D L, Avery M E 1969 Mist therapy reconsidered; an evaluation of the respiratory deposition of labelled water aerosols produced by jet and ultrasonic nebulizers. Pediatrics 43: 799–808

Wollmer P, Ursing K, Midgren B, Eriksson L 1985 Inefficiency of chest percussion in the physical therapy of chronic bronchitis. European Journal of Respiratory Diseases 66: 233–239

Zack M B, Pontoppidan H, Kazemi H 1974 The effect of lateral positions on gas exchange in pulmonary disease. American Review of Respiratory Disease 110: 49–55

Zusman M 1986 The absolute visual analog scale (AVAS): as a measure of pain intensity. Australian Journal of Physiotherapy 32: 244–246

FURTHER READING

Musculoskeletal dysfunction

Biomechanics of the thoracic spine and ribs

Lee D 1994 Manual therapy for the thorax – a biomechanical approach. DOPC, Delta BC

White A A, Panjabi M M 1990 Clinical biomechanics of the spine, 2nd edn. Lippincott, Philadelphia

Disorders of the thoracic spine

Boyling J D, Palastanga N 1994 In: Grieve G P (ed) Modern manual therapy of the vertebral column, 2nd edn. Churchill Livingstone, Edinburgh

Grieve G P 1988 Common vertebral joint problems, 2nd edn. Churchill Livingstone, Edinburgh

Musculoskeletal assessment and treatment techniques

Grieve G P 1991 Mobilisation of the spine – a primary handbook of clinical method, 5th edn. Churchill Livingstone, UK

Janda V 1994 Muscles and motor control in cervicogenic disorders: assessment and management physical therapy for the cervical and thoracic spine. In: Grant R (ed) Clinics in physical therapy, 2nd edn. Churchill Livingstone, USA

Kendal F P, McCreary E 1983 Muscle testing and function, 3rd edn. Williams & Wilkins, Baltimore

Maitland G D 1986 Vertebral manipulation, 5th edn. Butterworth, London

White S, Sahrmann S 1994 Physical therapy for the cervical and thoracic spine. In: Grant R (ed) Clinics in physical therapy, 2nd edn. Churchill Livingstone, USA

9

Interpersonal aspects of care: communication, counselling and health education

Julius Sim

INTRODUCTION

The intent of this chapter is to provide an insight into the part that various features of interpersonal communication can play in the management of patients with cardiac and respiratory problems. In addition to a general account of the role of communication in the therapeutic relationship, particular attention will be given to two specialist applications of communication, namely counselling and health education. Some of the associated ethical issues will also be touched upon. Underlying the discussion in this chapter is the notion that the disability and handicap associated with any illness – and chronic illness especially – occur within a social and interpersonal context, and are not merely the result of a biological process. The effective care and rehabilitation of patients with cardiorespiratory dysfunction must acknowledge this.

In order to examine these aspects of the physiotherapist's work, it is necessary to examine the psychological and social aspects of cardiorespiratory dysfunction. Accordingly, it is to these topics that the first part of this chapter is directed.

THE PSYCHOSOCIAL DIMENSION OF CARDIORESPIRATORY DYSFUNCTION

Like all illnesses, those of cardiorespiratory origin have psychosocial as well as physiological dimensions. Thus, at a general level, social factors play a part in the aetiology of many chronic respiratory diseases and, reflecting a general pattern for morbidity and mortality (DHSS 1980), such patients come disproportionately from the lower social classes (Williams 1989, French 1992) and from areas characterized by industrialization. Psychological factors may be similarly implicated, either as aetiological factors in their own right, or as significant cofactors. Once a cardiac or respiratory disease has become established in a particular individual, it impinges on the person's consciousness. The objective biological fact of dysfunction becomes a subjective experience – a disease becomes an illness (Sim 1990a).

Consequently, a problem-oriented or problem-based assessment of the cardiorespiratory patient should encompass psychosocial as well as physical factors. The problems which are identified in the course of the assessment will consist of those to do with the condition as it is subjectively experienced as well as its physical manifestations. Of course, the same clinical feature will very often represent problems of both types – for example, breathlessness – and there will be an interaction between the physical and the psychological factors. However, it should be noted that the degree to which patients experience subjective problems may only be weakly related to the severity of such objective factors as airflow limitation (Guyatt et al 1987).

Some psychosocial features of cardiorespiratory illness

It will be useful to look briefly at just some of the social and psychological forces that operate in cardiorespiratory illness.

1. *Anxiety* – many of the symptoms experienced by cardiac or respiratory patients are particularly distressing, e.g. breathlessness, palpitations, angina, and bronchospasm. This is not only because of their inherent unpleasantness, but also because their onset is frequently unexpected and unpredictable. The asthmatic patient may be prone to an attack with little warning, and suddenness of onset is perhaps the characteristic most associated with angina. The popular image of conditions such as these tends to exaggerate their more dramatic features; this is likely to have been internalized by the patient and may heighten feelings of anxiety. Stress and anxiety are also associated with the trajectory of the disease. In cystic fibrosis, for example, there is a combination of a poor prospect of cure and uncertainty as to outcome in the shorter term (Waddell 1982). Aspects of treatment and management can also be anxiety producing. Strange environments such as the intensive care unit can give rise to disorientation, loneliness, fear and helplessness (Hough 1996). According to a study by Williams some patients find exercise tests not only distressing and anxiety-provoking, but even 'unethical or punitive' (Williams 1993, p. 37).

2. *Defence mechanisms* – patients may respond to crises, such as a diagnosis of heart disease or bronchial carcinoma, with a variety of responses. These may include maladaptive psychotic mechanisms such as denial, distortion and projection, or less severe neurotic mechanisms such as displacement, intellectualization and repression (Porritt 1990). In cases of cystic fibrosis, where the family impact of the diagnosis is especially great (Dushenko 1981), these reactions may involve parents as well as patients themselves.

3. *Depression* – reactive depression is relatively common in cases of chronic cardiac and respiratory impairment. Indeed, psychiatric morbidity has been reported in 42–50% of patients with chronic bronchitis (Rutter 1977; McSweeny et al 1982).

4. *Stigmatization* – symptoms of cardiorespiratory dysfunction may become a source of stigma, owing to their disruptive effect on smooth social interaction (Sim 1990b). An awareness of others' discomfort at their breathlessness may cause patients with advanced emphysema to curtail social contact (Fagerhaugh 1973). A number of clinical features of cystic

fibrosis are potentially stigmatizing; for example, coughing, expectoration, and flatus. Williams (1993, p. 110) points out that such symptoms 'tend to violate tacit, yet culturally entrenched, social expectations, codes of etiquette and decorum, found deeply embedded within routine social interaction'. In addition, diminutive stature, underweight and delayed development of secondary sex characteristics may adversely affect body image (Norman & Hodson 1983). Perceived lack of attractiveness may reduce social confidence and inhibit sexual and emotional relationships, leading to feelings of reduced self-worth. Most males with cystic fibrosis are infertile, which may undermine feelings of manhood.

5. *Disruption of family relationships* – although in some cases illness can cause a strengthening of family ties, in other cases it can be a source of stress or conflict. The need to look after a disabled spouse, with the resulting toll on financial, personal and emotional resources, can place strain on the marital relationship (Williams 1993). In the case of a child with cystic fibrosis, there may be strong feelings of guilt in the parents, in view of the hereditary nature of the disease, and resentment in the child at the degree of dependency on his or her parents for physiotherapy. Overprotectiveness on the part of the parents may keep the child from normal activities with those of the same age, and lead to a degree of social isolation (Norman & Hodson 1983). Adolescence is a time when family relationships may be especially strained (Dushenko 1981). Clearly, an assessment of the patient which focuses solely on the individual, and neglects his or her family and social context, will necessarily be incomplete.

These, then, are some of the psychosocial features of cardiorespiratory dysfunction. An awareness of these aspects of the individual's illness is crucial to the success of subsequent management and treatment (Williams 1993). However, these are processes which have their own important psychosocial dimension, and these too should be understood.

PSYCHOSOCIAL ASPECTS OF CARE AND TREATMENT

There are certain features of the physiotherapist–patient relationship that have an important bearing on issues to do with communication. Above all, it tends to be an unequal relationship, with a differential distribution of power. The physiotherapist has specialized knowledge which the patient usually lacks, thereby creating a competency gap which is reinforced by the fact that, in hospital settings at least, the physiotherapist is on home ground whereas the patient is in an unfamiliar environment.

Coupled with this competency gap in many cases is a status gap. One of the key features of the doctor–patient relationship is the difference in social status that usually exists between the doctor and the patient (Navarro 1978); the same obtains, although to a less marked degree, in the case of the physiotherapist and the patient. When this status gap exists, the professional can use superior social status to enhance his or her status as 'expert' to exert leverage on the client (Friedson 1962); again, physiotherapists are not immune from such tendencies (Hugman 1991). In the process, patients or clients are likely to be inhibited in initiating or discussing their own agenda of topics or concerns (Cartwright & O'Brien 1976, Tuckett et al 1985), and 'the transmission of information is likely to be halting and imperfect' (Thompson 1984, p. 89).

There is also a tendency (perhaps more in hospital and acute-care settings than in community health care) for the physiotherapist to act as an 'active initiator', leading the interaction and setting the agenda for treatment, while the patient assumes the role of 'passive responder'. As a result, the physiotherapist will tend to set the agenda for the encounter, and direct the flow and pattern of communication. There may therefore be a neglect of issues which are of concern to the patient, but which the physiotherapist is unaware of or unconcerned with.

Finally, an element of professional distance or detachment characterizes the practitioner's role. This is reinforced by such factors as the wearing of uniform, the avoidance of certain kinds of informality, and simple physical distance. There are, however, certain features of the physiotherapist's role which tend to reduce professional distance. Physiotherapists are generally in frequent and prolonged contact with their patients, which may allow a certain degree of informality to develop between them. In addition, they are almost always in a position of close physical proximity, with varying degrees of direct physical contact. The determinants of professional distance can therefore be adjusted when appropriate in order to facilitate the communication process.

Categories of intervention

The physiotherapist's role with respect to the cardiorespiratory patient can be roughly divided into three forms of involvement:

1. *Physical treatment* – this involves the direct use of various physical modalities, such as breathing exercises, postural drainage, chest shaking.
2. *Psychological care* – given that most respiratory conditions have little prospect of ultimate cure, assisting the patient in coming to terms with the impact of respiratory impairment is an important part of the therapist's role. This may involve some form of counselling.
3. *Education* – by various forms of health education, the physiotherapist can help the patient adapt to the functional constraints imposed by cardiorespiratory impairment, and can encourage preventive strategies which may limit further deterioration.

There is, of course, no real dividing line between these areas of involvement. Physical treatment can have direct psychological benefit, and psychological care can enhance the effectiveness of physical treatment by lessening anxiety and increasing compliance. Similarly, by fostering a sense of purpose, self-confidence and empowerment, health education can provide the patient with psychological support. Above all, these facets of the therapist's role have in common the need for effective communication, and it is to this that we will now turn.

COMMUNICATION
A model of the communication process

Communication is a complex process, involving both verbal and nonverbal elements. Verbal communication can be either oral or written. Nonverbal communication incorporates such factors as facial expression, body language, spatial factors such as the relative position of the participants, and ecological factors relating to the environment in which communication occurs, with its various visual, olfactory and other exteroceptive stimuli. Verbal and nonverbal elements of communication exist in a mutual relationship, such that they can either reinforce or counteract one another. Northouse and Northouse (1992, p. 118) suggest four reasons why nonverbal elements of communication may be particularly important in the context of health care:

1. To lessen feelings of uncertainty and anxiety, patients become particularly sensitive to nonverbal cues from health professionals.
2. Patients may not wholly trust or believe the explicit information given to them by health care staff, and may seek to discern the 'true' message from nonverbal communication on the part of the professional.
3. Patients may rely on nonverbal cues for information before any verbal interaction has occurred.
4. If a practitioner seems to be busy or unapproachable, patients may rely heavily on nonverbal messages.

For a single communication act, there will be an *initiator*, who encodes the intended meaning into a message of a certain form (e.g. a sentence with a certain grammatical structure) which is then transferred by means of a *medium* (e.g. the spoken word) to a *recipient*, who decodes the message. This process is subject to slippage at virtually any point: the process of encoding can distort the intended message; the medium can lend changes in emphasis or undertones of meaning (e.g. tone of voice, or its absence in the case of written communication); there can be further distortion as the recipient decodes the message (e.g. words may be taken to have a different meaning or connotation from that intended, or may even be unintelligible); or nonverbal behaviour can be taken as a gloss on the message which may or may not accord with the desired meaning.

Moreover, just as the recipient responds to the message, so the initiator monitors and reacts to the recipient's response in an ongoing feedback process (e.g. signs of non-comprehension are likely to prompt elaboration, whereas apparent understanding will probably encourage the initiator to encode a fresh message). Although it is helpful for the purposes of analysis to look at single communication acts, they are of course not discrete events, like shots in a game of tennis. There is, rather, a constant interplay within as well as between communication acts – the initiator relies on constant feedback from the recipient during the process of encoding, while the recipient similarly relies on various cues from the initiator while decoding. The roles of initiator and recipient are held simultaneously, not sequentially.

For purposes of clarity, the communication process so far has been seen in essentially dyadic terms; needless to say, the intricacy and essential vulnerability of the process increase when more than two participants are involved. The complexity of the communication process suggests:

- that it is likely to take different forms in different contexts and to serve different purposes
- that it requires a considerable degree of skill in the participants if it is to be effective
- that there are a large number of diverse factors which are capable of enhancing or detracting from the process.

It is in the context of these considerations that we now pass on to some more specific aspects of communication.

Purposes of communication

In a therapeutic setting, there are many possible purposes of communication, of which perhaps the foremost are:

- To pass on information
- To gain or extract information
- To establish interpersonal relationships
- To influence another's attitudes, opinions or behaviour
- To express feelings or emotions
- To gain an understanding of others' feelings, emotions, attitudes, etc.
- To create or maintain personal identity.

Any of these purposes can, of course, be held by either physiotherapist or patient, and can exist in virtually any combination. Moreover, they can be held either consciously or subconsciously. They can also be characterized as predominantly either instrumental or expressive. Instrumental communication is that which aims to secure a particular outcome or accomplish a specific task, such as when a physiotherapist asks a patient to take a deep breath, or requests a specific item of factual information. Expressive communication has to do with the communication of emotions or states of mind and does not require (though of course it often obtains) a response from the other participant. Expressive communication is often referred to as 'consummatory', in that 'the goal is achieved by the act of communicating' (Dickson et al 1989, p. 10). Expressive and instrumental aspects of communication often come together in a single communication act. Thus, a physiotherapist may smile at a patient to convey a feeling of caring (expressive goal), or to reassure the patient (instrumental goal), or, of course, for both reasons.

Detractors from effective communication

There are a number of factors which can militate against effective physiotherapist–patient communication.

Inappropriate attitudes. As MacWhannell (1992) argues, a prerequisite for effective communication is a willingness to form a relationship and an accompanying quality of 'openness'. The importance of good communication must be appreciated by both parties.

Inadequate skills. A disproportionate focus

on the acquisition of motor skills and manual techniques during their training may cause physiotherapists to overlook the fact that communication is a skill that can be learnt like any other. Listening skills are just as important as those concerned with the delivery of messages (Nelson-Jones 1990). In particular, the therapist should acquire the skills of 'active listening', in which the listener overtly displays the fact that he or she is paying attention to what is being said (Hargie et al 1994).

Language-related factors. As part of the competency gap identified earlier, health professionals are in possession of a specialized vocabulary which is likely to be unfamiliar to most patients. The inappropriate use of jargon fosters 'unshared meanings' and hinders effective communication (Northouse & Northouse 1992); therapists should learn 'when and how to use professional jargon and translate it into lay terms' (Purtilo 1990, p. 124). Syntax is equally important; complex, lengthy sentences may obscure meaning and confuse the recipient. The term 'register' is defined as 'a variety of the use of language as used by a particular speaker or writer in a particular context' (Darbyshire 1967, p. 23); the choice of inappropriate register in a therapeutic context will clearly detract from communication.

Emotional factors. Various emotions on the part of one or both participants may obscure or distort intended meanings. Fear, anxiety, defencelessness, embarrassment, hostility and depression are common emotional responses in health care contexts which may prevent good communication, particularly if they are unacknowledged by one or both parties.

Cultural factors. Certain features of verbal and nonverbal communication carry different meanings from culture to culture. As an example, the degree of touch or eye contact acceptable in Latin cultures is greater than in Western Europe (Hyland & Donaldson 1989). Argyle (1988) notes that, during conversation, Arabs will exhibit a far higher degree of mutual gaze than British or American interlocutors, and that black Americans exhibit less eye contact, during both talking and listening, than white Americans.

If proper allowance is not made for such cultural variations, communication is likely to be misinterpreted.

Noise. The term 'noise' is applied to any form of extraneous interference to the communication process. It may take the form of: visual, auditory or olfactory distractions; impairment of visual cues between participants; concurrent activity which diverts the attention; physical discomfort; unconducive positioning of participants; etc. It is not hard to imagine how all of these could simultaneously detract from communication in a setting such as an intensive care unit.

Facilitators of communication

To a large extent, factors which facilitate communication are the obverse of those that detract from it. Thus, the appropriate choice of register, judicious selection of vocabulary, absence of 'noise', and the appropriate attitudes will all make for good communication. However, there are also some more specific considerations which will allow positive steps to be taken to improve communication.

Positioning. It is important to consider the appropriate use of physical distance. The anthropologist Edward Hall (1966) has defined four basic distances for social interaction, ranging from 'intimate distance' (from direct contact to 18 inches between participants) to 'public distance' (12–25 feet or more between participants). It is clear that many of the physiotherapist's activities will bring him or her into the intimate distance, with the risk of invading the patient's personal space. At times, such as when implicit permission has not been gained, such intimacy may be a barrier to communication. On other occasions, when more expressive purposes are concerned, such proximity can instil confidence and a sense of caring, and thereby enhance communication; use of public distance in such a case would be clearly inappropriate. Exaggerated physical distance from a patient who is expectorating can easily convey a sense of discomfort or distaste. The relative height of participants is also important. MacWhannell (1992) points out that an action such as sitting on the patient's bed facilitates eye contact and promotes a feeling of equality. It also counteracts the feeling of hurriedness that can often seem to characterize therapeutic activities.

Posture and gestures. For the purposes of analysing communication, there are two fundamental types of bodily posture. A closed posture is one which indicates that social interaction is not desired, whereas an open posture signals a willingness to interact (Hyland & Donaldson 1989). Sitting back in a chair with legs closely crossed and arms folded defensively would be a typical closed posture. Gestures, used appropriately, can illustrate meaning and be used as a form of emphasis. Excessive gesturing can constitute a source of 'noise'.

Facial expression and eye contact. Appropriate use of facial expression and eye contact can reinforce communication. Signs of attentiveness on the part of the physiotherapist provide positive feedback and encourage the patient to communicate more openly. The phenomenon of 'turn-taking' in conversation is partially governed by the participants' control of eye contact (Hargie et al 1994). Although in some situations it can connote hostility, eye contact is often a sign of affinity between individuals, and can therefore be used by the therapist to create empathy. It can also be used to counteract various emotional detractors from communication. Avoiding eye contact can help to eliminate inappropriate levels of arousal, and thus defuse aggression and hostility (Hyland & Donaldson 1989). When engaged in intimate procedures which might cause embarrassment to the patient, minimizing eye contact can help to define the procedure as instrumental rather than expressive, and thus reduce embarrassment. Argyle (1983) notes that excessive eye contact, in the form of 'mutual gaze', can be distracting.

Touch. Judicious use of touch can convey liking and a sense of caring. Porritt (1990, p. 8) notes that the 'laying on of hands has always been synonymous with healing, and these days is an important counter-balance to the technology of health care'. However, bodily touching can carry powerful emotional, sexual and cultural undertones (Lawler 1991). There is, therefore, a risk that touch may be perceived as inappropriate. Purtilo (1990, p. 145) notes that the health professional, who is accustomed to touching patients, 'probably has so firm a concept of his or her good intentions that the question of inappropriateness or improper familiarity never arises'. Accordingly, Hargie et al (1994) point out the necessity of ensuring that touch on the part of health professionals is not misinterpreted. Hyland & Donaldson (1989) point out that touching often connotes dependency on the part of the person touched, and that this may not be welcomed. Hargie et al (1994) note that certain groups of individuals, such as elderly people with no close relatives or those who have been widowed (categories which are likely to include many patients with chronic respiratory illness), may rarely experience touch from others, and to this extent are deprived of a certain degree of emotional fulfilment. They point out that health professionals, by the appropriate use of touch, can help to redress this deficiency.

Memory

An important feature of effective communication is the ability of participants to retain information that is imparted. Although it is crucial that communication in the physiotherapist–patient relationship should be a two-way process, specific problems of recall seem to occur most often on the part of the patient. Reflecting this concern, extensive research has been conducted within health care on factors that may either hinder or facilitate memory and thus determine the degree of subsequent compliance (Ley 1988). Table 9.1 summarizes some of the principal steps that can be taken to maximize the information that patients will retain and recall; further discussion of these and other factors can be found in Ley (1988) and Hill (1992). Baddeley (1997) provides a comprehensive coverage of this topic. It is important to stress that such techniques, useful though they are, should not be seen as a substitute for the less tangible interpersonal skills and attitudes that help to create the sort of relationship with the patient that is a prerequisite for good communication.

Table 9.1 Strategies to facilitate memory

Utilizing primacy and recency effects	Information given either at the beginning or the end of the encounter tends to be best retained
Limiting the number of items of information given	Too many items can lead to 'overcrowding' of the short-term memory
Emphasizing the key points	This can be done by using repetition or by explicitly highlighting items
Categorization	Information is placed into separate categories, which are explicitly identified to the patient
Simplification	Short words and sentences are generally better, and jargon should be avoided; the content of information should also be simple; whilst patients may comprehend complex ideas, they are likely not to retain them
Being specific	Instructions in particular should be specific rather than general
Providing feedback	This can be either positive or negative
Using written reinforcement	This gives the patient a source of subsequent reference
Making use of 'dual encoding'	The use of both concrete and abstract concepts brings into play both hemispheres of the brain when the information is processed by the listener
Contextualization	Information or instructions should be conveyed in the context in which they need to be recalled; alternatively, a variety of contexts should be used if information needs to be generalized
Cueing	Especially when behaviour has to be remembered (e.g. exercises or postural drainage), specific regular cues for recall, such as a radio programme or a meal, can be suggested

The importance of communication

As Thompson (1984, p. 88) points out, 'dissatisfaction with medical communications remains the most prominent of patient complaints and a major factor in the move to alternative medicine'. Moreover, it is not merely a question of patients' perceptions; ever since Egbert and colleagues' seminal study (Egbert et al 1964), the direct therapeutic value of good communication has repeatedly been demonstrated. It is, moreover, important not to take too restricted a view of the role of communication in health care:

First and foremost, all health professionals need to enlarge their repertoire of communication skills. In some circumstances 'controlling' and 'managerial' communication may be required and appropriate, particularly in a crisis, but the other more sensitive communication skills, associated with 'counselling' and 'helping' patients to sort out their own problems and take their own decisions, require quite different training and the development of quite different skills. (Thompson et al 1988, p. 161)

These authors go on to argue that traditional forms of education and training for health professionals do little to instil these additional skills.

Therefore, good communication on the part of physiotherapists is not only a means of securing patient satisfaction, but is also an essential component of effective care and treatment. The quality of communication is at a particularly high premium in two specialist areas of the cardio-respiratory physiotherapist's work (counselling and health education) to which we will shortly turn. Before doing so, however, it is important to emphasize that communication also has moral significance. Good communication is required not only for the *effectiveness* of the relationship between therapist and patient, but also for the *ethics* of this relationship. In the course of caring for a patient, therapists may come into possession of information which, they may feel, the patient has a right to know (Sim 1986a). For example, a man with unexplained unilateral pneumonia may be found to be suffering from previously undiagnosed bronchial carcinoma, and it may be felt that this should be made known to him. Alternatively, a young woman with cryptogenic fibrosing alveolitis may seem to have unrealistic beliefs as to the prospects of cure. Should she be given a more accurate picture of her future?

Ethical issues also surround consent. Informed

consent can be defined as 'the voluntary and revocable agreement of a competent individual to participate in a therapeutic or research procedure, based on an adequate understanding of its nature, purpose, and implications' (Sim 1986b, p. 584). In some instances, gaining consent to treatment procedures can be accomplished fairly straightforwardly. However, in the case of nasopharyngeal suction, the patient may not be in a state of consciousness that permits explicit consent. Alternatively, the patient may seem to be withholding consent, and a decision must be made whether or not to proceed nonetheless, on the grounds that the patient is expressing a wish that is not fully autonomous, or perhaps on the basis that the therapeutic benefits likely to accrue justify disregarding a lack of consent. Presumably with this latter argument in mind, Hough (1996, p. 140) argues that '[f]orcible suction is unethical, usually illegal and acceptable only in life-threatening situations'.

COUNSELLING

Henry is a middle-aged man with emphysema who is suffering increasing restriction on his activities due to breathlessness, to the extent that he is unable to participate fully in running the family business. He is experiencing feelings of inadequacy and guilt, and finds that he is losing what he perceives to be his role within the family.

Karla, an 18-year-old woman with cystic fibrosis, recently discovered that another patient of the same age, whom she has got to know very well during the course of several shared inpatient admissions, has died of the disease. The sense of purpose and hopefulness with which Karla previously pursued her treatment now seems to be weakening, and she is becoming increasingly fatalistic about her future.

Gary is a young man with asthma who is subject to acute attacks of moderate severity. He is increasingly unwilling to engage in social activities, anticipating the disruption and alarm that a sudden attack may cause, and fearful of straying from the support of his family, who 'know what to do'.

Each of these vignettes demonstrates the way in which the psychosocial features of respiratory disease may affect the patient. They equally show how the physiotherapist will require skills other than those of direct physical treatment in order to help. The focus here is on the second category of intervention that we identified earlier (psychological care) and in order to accomplish this the physiotherapist may feel the need to assume the role of counsellor in situations such as these. However, it is important first of all to be clear what counselling is, and what it is not. It has been defined thus:

Counselling is a technique concerned to help people help themselves by the development of a special relationship which leads a client into a greater depth of self-understanding, clarifies the identity of problems and conflicts and mobilises personal coping abilities. (Nichols 1984, p. 142)

Counselling is not just being a passive receptacle for people's anxieties, fears, emotions, problems, etc. Equally, it does not consist in providing specific pieces of advice, guidance or reassurance; indeed, in his classification of helping strategies, Griffiths (1981) explicitly separates counselling from strategies such as 'giving information', 'teaching', and 'giving advice'. Rather, it is a process whereby the patient (or 'client' in counselling parlance) is assisted towards insight and an understanding of his or her own emotional, attitudinal and social situation. Emotions are not suppressed by the counsellor, nor are they permitted to flow in a totally free and unrestrained manner – they are clarified. Instead of providing ready-made strategies, the counsellor helps the client in setting his or her own goals. The counsellor frequently acts as a catalyst (Nichols 1984).

This all requires specific communication skills, which are as much to do with listening as with talking. Physiotherapists must assess carefully the extent to which they possess such skills. While some sort of counselling role is well within the capabilities of most, if not all, physiotherapists, it is important to recognize the limit of one's expertise, and to refer patients to a more fully trained counsellor, or even to a clinical psychologist, when the case demands.

Essential elements in counselling

Naturally, it is not possible to provide here a practical account of the skills required in counselling. However, it is perhaps worth looking briefly at some of what are generally agreed to be the essential ingredients of effective counselling. It should be remembered that there are many different approaches to counselling, and each approach will tend to attach varying importance to the different factors.

Genuineness. Genuineness, or authenticity, has been defined as '[t]he degree to which we are freely and deeply ourselves, and are able to relate to people in a sincere and undefensive manner' (Stewart 1992, p. 100). This quality is important in encouraging trust and disclosure on the part of the client.

Positive regard. The counsellor should show some degree of detachment. On the one hand, there should be no signs of disapproval, censure or blame. The counsellor should display 'unconditional positive regard' for the client (Burnard 1989), i.e. positive feelings towards the client which do not need to be 'earned', will not be affected by what the client may say or may have done, and which the client should not necessarily feel obliged to reciprocate. Without such openness, acceptance and apparent liking, the client is unlikely to be forthcoming and confide in the counsellor. In the case of Gary, for example, any suggestion by the therapist that his anxieties are inappropriate or exaggerated would be likely to inhibit a counselling relationship. On the other hand, undue sympathy or emotional closeness should be avoided. Explicit emotional identification ('I know just how you feel') may threaten the essential privacy and uniqueness of the client's state of being, and may accordingly be resented.

Non-possessiveness. A young female physiotherapist may be able to identify strongly with a patient such as Karla, and feel that she understands the emotions which she is experiencing. As a result of this powerful sense of empathy, she may experience an intense desire to help. However, the counsellor should not become possessive with regard to the client. Undue sympathy for the client may cause the helper to seek to impose what he or she sees as the optimum solution to the individual's problems, without due regard for what the client would regard as optimum. Dickson et al (1989) see

altruism as an essential attribute for the counsellor, and one result of this is that it is all too easy for the counsellor to become paternalistic. Just because the client has permitted access to what are often private and sensitive aspects of his or her life, does not mean that the client has in any way surrendered personal control. The professional has to balance feelings of benevolence and a desire to help against respect for the client's autonomy. Above all, the therapist should be wary of what Swain (1995) calls exploitation; a process whereby the counselling relationship is used more to serve the counsellor's psychological needs and emotional interests than those of the client.

Willingness to yield control. The counsellor should not control the encounter excessively. Indeed, many counsellors adopt a 'non-directive' approach, and try to ensure that the course taken by the consultation is, as far as possible, in the control of the client. At the same time, skilful use of probing questions can facilitate this process, and confrontation techniques may be required if the consultation seems to have reached an impasse, with the client 'going over the same ground without any new insights' (Brearley & Birchley 1994, p. 8). What are termed 'prescriptive interventions' do have a part to play in counselling, but Burnard (1989) warns that they can very easily be overused. Specific practical advice might seem to be useful in the case of someone like Henry. However, it is often only of short-term usefulness, and may encourage dependency. Moreover, if a suggested strategy does not work, the counsellor may be blamed and the relationship may be broken, depriving the counsellor of the opportunity to help further.

Orientation to action. Greater self-understanding on the part of the client is an important aim of counselling, but this is only of value if it in turn leads to a solution (whether partial or total) of the individual's problems (Munro et al 1989). According to Burnard (1989), immediacy is an essential quality in the counselling relationship; that is, the counsellor should have a concern with the here-and-now, and should discourage the client from undue reminiscing about the past, which may remove the focus from issues of immediate practical concern. Accordingly, many counsellors feel that the client should always leave a consultation with some definite course of action to pursue, however minimal it may appear to be.

Establishing a contract. It is important to clarify mutual expectations. The counsellor should make it understood what sort of help is likely to be forthcoming, so that the client does not bring unrealistic hopes to the relationship (Brearley & Birchley 1994). Similarly, boundaries should be set. The client should understand that, whilst help is freely given, this can only be for a certain period of time, and that the counsellor may not necessarily be available at unarranged times between sessions. Setting a time limit to the session assists both counsellor and client (Brearley & Birchley 1994). As part of an effective working relationship, the client will be expected to confide information relating to often private and intimate aspects of his or her life. The client can only be expected to do so with an assurance of confidentiality on the part of the counsellor – indeed it is unlikely that information will be freely disclosed otherwise (Sim 1996). Indeed, a degree of privacy is surrendered on the understanding of an implicit assurance of discretion and confidentiality on the part of the counsellor. If it is felt that other professionals need to be consulted in order adequately to help the client, the counsellor will need to explain this to the client and obtain consent for information to be revealed to another party. In such a case, the benevolent aim of helping the client does not override the ethical requirement to respect privacy. It should also be remembered that patients may have legal redress in certain cases of breach of confidentiality (Mason & McCall Smith 1994).

Assuming the counselling role

It is fair to say that not all physiotherapists take readily to the role of counsellor. In common with many other practitioners, they may often be 'reluctant to deal with emotional and psychological dimensions of patients' problems' (Dickson et al 1989, p. 126). There may be an unwillingness to explore aspects of patients' lives to do with such areas as intensely felt emotions, their personal fears, and feelings related to their sexuality.

More specifically, the predominant accent within physiotherapy training and education on physical treatment strategies may cause physiotherapists to feel, albeit unconsciously, that they are not performing their proper role if they are apparently 'just talking' to patients. It should be accepted that the process of 'problem solving' is likely to take a very different form in psychological care from that undertaken in physical treatment. The strategies adopted will often be far less tangible, and may involve, in comparison, little active participation by the physiotherapist. Frequently, the therapist engaged in psychological care will not be providing specific, concrete interventions, but will be involved in a more passive, facilitatory role, involving considerably more response than initiation. Any action to be taken is generally for the client rather than the therapist. Thus, Griffiths describes counselling as 'helping someone to explore a problem, clarify conflicting issues and discover alternative ways of dealing with it, so that they can decide what to do about it; that is, helping people to help themselves' (Griffiths 1981, p. 267).

In a similar way, the sort of dialogue which is likely to be engaged in may often appear to be less purposeful than those to which physiotherapists have become accustomed in the course of physical treatment. Pauses, and even considerable periods of silence, are often not only acceptable but positively beneficial in counselling and other forms of psychological care (Bendix 1982); however, they may initially be a source of unease to therapists who are used to more 'business-like' exchanges with their patients.

Counselling, if it is to be effective, involves a new set of skills for many physiotherapists and, just as important, a new perspective on their professional role. However, appropriate training in counselling skills, and a fuller understanding of the psychosocial dynamics of cardiorespiratory illness, will reveal a wider and more holistic approach to the management of these patients.

HEALTH EDUCATION

Health education and health promotion

The terms 'health education' and 'health promotion' are sometimes used almost interchangeably. However, a valuable distinction can be drawn between them. 'Health promotion' is used to cover a broad spectrum of activities that seek to improve or restore health. The term has been defined by Downie et al (1996, p. 60) as follows: 'Health promotion comprises efforts to enhance positive health and reduce the risk of ill-health, through the overlapping spheres of health education, prevention, and health protection.'

This model of health promotion incorporates three key elements, earlier identified by Tannahill (1985). One of these is *health education*, which we will return to in due course. The notion of *prevention* concerns activities which are designed to reduce the incidence or risk of occurrence of any undesirable health-related state of being – whether this is physical illness, mental illness, physical injury, physical disability, or handicap. Traditionally, prevention has been classified into three types (Farmer & Miller 1991). Primary prevention seeks to prevent the disease process from starting, while secondary prevention aims to detect disease at an early stage and forestall further progression. Tertiary prevention, meanwhile, 'aims at "damage limitation" in persons with manifest disease by modifying continuing risk factors such as smoking and the implementation of effective programmes of rehabilitation' (Farmer & Miller 1991, p. 111).

Downie et al (1996) criticize this typology for being unduly centred in the narrow concept of disease, and for identifying prevention with the idea of treatment. They also note the lack of unanimity with which these three phases are used by various commentators. Downie et al (1996, p. 51) propose, instead, what they call 'four foci of prevention', which give a rather fuller idea of the potentialities of prevention:

- Prevention of the onset or first manifestation of a disease process, or some other first occurrence, through risk reduction

- Prevention of the progression of a disease process or other unwanted state, through early detection when this favourably affects outcome
- Prevention of avoidable complications of an irreversible, manifest disease or some other unwanted state
- Prevention of the recurrence of an illness or other unwanted phenomenon.

The third key element in health promotion is that of *health protection*. This comprises various legal controls, policy initiatives, codes of practice, and other regulatory mechanisms which are designed to improve or restore health.

Health education is therefore just one of the ways in which the goals of health promotion can be pursued. There is, of course, a large degree of interrelation between the three elements; for example, a considerable proportion of health education may concern itself with prevention.

The scope of health education

Downie et al (1996, p. 28) define health education as: 'communication activity aimed at enhancing positive health and preventing or diminishing ill-health in individuals and groups, through influencing the beliefs, attitudes, and behaviour of those with power and of the community at large.'

Thus, health education, like education in other contexts, has three main targets – beliefs (or knowledge), attitudes and behaviour. By seeking to influence one or more of these factors, the health educator hopes to enhance or restore health. Ewles & Simnett (1995) use these factors to construct, respectively, 'knowing', 'feeling' and 'doing' objectives in health education. 'Knowing' objectives are 'concerned with giving information, explaining it, ensuring that the client understands it, and thus increasing the client's knowledge', while objectives about 'feeling' are 'concerned with clarifying, forming or changing attitudes, beliefs, values or opinions'. Objectives about 'doing' have to do with the client's skills and actions (Ewles & Simnett 1995, pp. 100–101). In seeking to achieve these objectives, the health educator is not restricted to activities centred on individuals. Ewles & Simnett (1995, p. 38) describe a 'societal change approach' which aims to 'effect changes on the physical, social and economic environment in order to make it more conducive to good health', and Kiger (1995) draws attention to the role of political action within health promotion and education (which may involve the physiotherapist taking such action or encouraging and empowering the patient to do so for him- or herself). Thus, although physiotherapists may spend most of their time dealing with individual patients, they should not neglect opportunities to take a broader approach to health. For example, in the case of children with cystic fibrosis, health education may extend to advising schools of the need for treatment facilities or special diets. In the case of persons with acquired immune deficiency syndrome (AIDS), it may involve attempts to dispel misconceptions and to foster more tolerant attitudes in the wider community (Sim & Purtilo 1991). Furthermore, it is not only important that the wider community should be educated about health-related matters; patients themselves need to know about the broader context into which their health (or lack of it) fits.

Draper et al (1980) emphasize this wider remit for health education in their description of three types of health education:

The first and most common is education about the body and how to look after it …. The second is about health services – information about available services and the 'sensible' use of health care resources. But the third, about the wider environment within which health choices are made, is relatively neglected. It is concerned with education about national, regional, and local policies, which are too often devised and implemented without taking account of their consequences for health.

They argue that health education that is restricted to the first two types is 'partial to the point of being socially irresponsible'.

At the heart of health education is the notion of empowerment. 'True health education should work to enable people to understand better what they are, what they believe, and what they know' (Seedhouse 1986, p. 91). Of equal, and related, importance is the idea of partnership between patient and health professional; effective health education cannot be a unilateral activity. 'The key to full partnership is continual patient/ health professional communication' (Lorig 1996, p. xiv).

Health education and the physiotherapist

The question now arises as to how, and to what extent, the physiotherapist should incorporate the role of health educator in the management of patients with cardiac and respiratory conditions. There would seem to be a number of factors which suggest that this is a highly appropriate role. First, it must be recognized that, with some exceptions (e.g. acute lobar pneumonia, hyperventilation syndrome), most of these conditions are not amenable to cure. There is, therefore, a need for a programme of long-term management, in addition to any short-term treatment. Second, any physical treatment that is administered is generally only beneficial for these conditions if it is continued between periods of direct contact with the therapist and, in addition, is augmented by self-care strategies on the part of the patient. Effective management of these patients consists therefore as much in what takes place in the patient's personal, domestic and social life as in what occurs in the health care setting. Third, cardiorespiratory disease offers full scope for prevention, under each of the four foci identified by Downie et al (1996), and health education is an important means of implementing preventive health measures. Finally, there are many areas of the individual's life in which changes in behaviour can have a beneficial effect on cardiorespiratory dysfunction, e.g. dietary adjustments, avoidance of possible sources of infection or allergic reaction, the taking of exercise, etc. Here, too, health education has a clear contribution to make.

Accordingly, the physiotherapist involved in the care of patients with cardiorespiratory problems can fulfil the role of health educator in a wide variety of ways, of which just some are:

- by explaining the underlying pathological

processes and the significance of these in terms of prevention and treatment

- by advising on means by which general health may be maintained (e.g. adequate nutrition, appropriate balance of rest and activity)
- by teaching treatment modalities which can be carried out independently, such as the active cycle of breathing techniques, and strategies for coping with the physiological demands of the disease, such as breathing control
- by instructing patients in the use of items of equipment, such as air compressors, nebulizers and oxygen concentrators
- by providing information on appropriate health and social services available, including information on patients' statutory rights
- by putting patients in contact with self-help groups and patients' organizations such as those that exist in many countries for patients with cystic fibrosis
- by helping to create attitudes of confidence, self-worth and confidence, thereby empowering patients in their efforts to cope with disability.

In order to achieve such goals, the physiotherapist will need highly developed communication skills, and an awareness of the factors identified previously which may either enhance or detract from the communication process. There are, however, some specific points which should be considered. The first is that health education should not consist of unilateral giving of instruction and advice. It is essential that goals are mutually negotiated, otherwise the patient will not see him- or herself as a partner in the overall process, and will be poorly motivated to carry through recommended courses of action. Second, the therapist must gain a sound insight into the patient's psychological profile and social environment. Patients with a primarily internal locus of control (i.e. those who broadly regard themselves as capable of determining their own destiny) will respond to different forms of goal setting compared with patients who have an external locus of control (i.e. those who see themselves as subject to more fatalistic, external influences). Similarly, ignorance of the patient's social situation may lead the therapist to advocate

inappropriate strategies that are incompatible with the individual's lifestyle. In the light of this, talk of 'non-compliant' patients is singularly unhelpful. Locating failures of compliance in the patient is to overlook the fact that compliance is the property of a relationship, not of an individual. If compliance is not achieved, the relevant shortcomings reside in the rapport and understanding that exist (or perhaps do not exist) between therapist and patient. Such rapport and understanding are a shared responsibility. Patients and professionals may have very different notions of what compliance is, or should be (Coy 1989, Roberson 1992); these should be explored carefully and sensitively.

The third important consideration is that effective health education, like all areas of health work, relies on sound liaison and teamwork. It is important that messages are echoed and reinforced by all those with whom the patient comes into contact. Above all, it should be remembered that team members each have their own agenda, and some sort of compromise must be effected in order that a shared set of priorities can be drawn up. Needless to say, the patient has his or her own agenda, and this should be given full consideration in the process.

This leads us to the final consideration, which concerns a respect for the individual's autonomy. In many instances, the physiotherapist's expertise may allow him or her to identify authoritatively the best means of achieving a certain health-related goal. However, this does not mean that the therapist is in a privileged position to identify this as a valuable goal in the first instance. Such goals only have value in the context of the person's total state of being, and the ultimate authority on what matters to a given individual is, necessarily, that individual. The patient's values and priorities may differ from the therapist's. If health education goals are defined disproportionately by the therapist, with insufficient regard for the desires of the patient, and then imposed unilaterally, the recipient's self-determination is likely to be overridden. The physiotherapist must recognize the dividing line between education and indoctrination (Campbell 1990).

CONCLUSION

This chapter has attempted to highlight the role that communication can play in the management of patients with cardiorespiratory problems. Communication skills are fundamental to the three main categories of intervention – physical treatment, psychological care, and health education – and, like other professional skills, can be learnt and further developed in order to improve the quality of patient care.

REFERENCES

Argyle M 1983 The psychology of interpersonal behaviour, 4th edn. Penguin, Harmondsworth

Argyle M 1988 Bodily communication, 2nd edn. Methuen, London

Baddeley A D 1997 Human memory: theory and practice, 2nd edn. Psychology Press, Hove

Bendix T 1982 The anxious patient: the therapeutic dialogue in clinical practice. Churchill Livingstone, Edinburgh

Brearley G, Birchley P 1994 Counselling in disability and illness, 2nd edn. Mosby, London

Burnard P 1989 Counselling skills for health professionals. Chapman & Hall, London

Campbell A V 1990 Education or indoctrination? The issue of autonomy in health education. In: Doxiadis S (ed) Ethics in health education. Wiley, Chichester

Cartwright A, O'Brien M 1976 Social class variations in health care and the nature of general practitioner consultations. In: Stacey M (ed) The sociology of the National Health Service. Sociological review monograph 22. University of Keele, Keele

Coy J A 1989 Philosophic aspects of patient noncompliance: a critical analysis. Topics in Geriatric Rehabilitation 4: 52–60

Darbyshire A E 1967 A description of English. Edward Arnold, London

DHSS 1980 Inequalities in health: report of a research working group (Black Report). HMSO, London

Dickson D A, Hargie O, Morrow N C 1989 Communication skills training for health professionals: an instructor's handbook. Chapman & Hall, London

Downie R S, Tannahill C, Tannahill A 1996 Health promotion: models and values, 2nd edn. Oxford University Press, Oxford

Draper P, Griffiths J, Dennis J, Popay J 1980 Three types of health education. British Medical Journal 281: 493–495

Dushenko T W 1981 Cystic fibrosis: a medical overview and critique of the psychological literature. Social Science and Medicine 15E: 43–56

Egbert L D, Battit G E, Welsh C E, Bartlett M K 1964 Reduction of postoperative pain by encouragement and instruction of patients. New England Journal of Medicine 270: 825–827

Ewles L, Simnett I 1995 Promoting health: a practical guide, 3rd edn. Scutari Press, London

Fagerhaugh S Y 1973 Getting around with emphysema. American Journal of Nursing 73: 94–99

Farmer R, Miller D 1991 Lecture notes on epidemiology and public health medicine, 3rd edn. Blackwell Scientific Publications, Oxford

French S 1992 Inequalities in health. In: French S (ed) Physiotherapy: a psychosocial approach. Butterworth-Heinemann, Oxford

Friedson E 1962 Dilemmas in the doctor–patient relationship. In: Rose A M (ed) Human behavior and social processes: an interactionist approach. Routledge & Kegan Paul, London

Griffiths D 1981 Psychology and medicine. British Psychological Society / Macmillan, London

Guyatt G H, Townsend M, Berman L B, Pugsley S O 1987 Quality of life in patients with chronic airflow limitation. British Journal of Diseases of the Chest 81: 45–54

Hall E T 1966 The hidden dimension: man's use of space in public and private. Bodley Head, London

Hargie O, Saunders C, Dickson D 1994 Social skills in interpersonal communication, 3rd edn. Routledge, London

Hill P 1992 Communication in physiotherapy practice (2). In: French S (ed) Physiotherapy: a psychosocial approach. Butterworth-Heinemann, Oxford

Hough A 1996 Physiotherapy in respiratory care: a problem-solving approach to respiratory and cardiac management, 2nd edn. Chapman & Hall, London

Hugman R 1991 Power in caring professions. Macmillan, London

Hyland M E, Donaldson M L 1989 Psychological care in nursing practice. Scutari Press, Harrow

Kiger A M 1995 Teaching for health, 2nd edn. Churchill Livingstone, Edinburgh

Lawler J 1991 Behind the screens: nursing, somology and the problem of the body. Churchill Livingstone, Melbourne

Ley P 1988 Communicating with patients: improving communication, satisfaction and compliance. Chapman & Hall, London

Lorig K 1996 Patient education: a practical approach. Sage Publications, Thousand Oaks

McSweeny A J, Grant I, Heaton R K, Adams K M, Timms R M 1982 Life quality of patients with chronic obstructive pulmonary disease. Archives of Internal Medicine 142: 473–478

MacWhannell D E 1992 Communication in physiotherapy practice (1). In: French S (ed) Physiotherapy: a psychosocial approach. Butterworth-Heinemann, Oxford

Mason J K, McCall Smith R A 1994 Law and medical ethics, 4th edn. Butterworths, London

Munro A, Manthel B, Small J 1989 Counselling: the skills of problem-solving. Routledge, London

Navarro V 1978 Class struggle, the state and medicine: an historical and contemporary analysis of the medical sector in Great Britain. Martin Robertson, Oxford

Nelson-Jones R 1990 Human relationship skills: training and self-help, 2nd edn. Cassell, London

Nichols K A 1984 Psychological care in physical illness. Croom Helm, London

Norman A P, Hodson M E 1983 Emotional and social aspects

of treatment. In: Hodson M E, Norman A P, Batten J C (eds) Cystic fibrosis. Baillière Tindall, London

Northouse P G, Northouse L L 1992 Health communication: strategies for health professionals, 2nd edn. Appleton & Lange, Norwalk

Porritt L 1990 Interaction strategies: an introduction for health professionals. Churchill Livingstone, Melbourne

Purtilo R B 1990 Health professional and patient interaction, 4th edn. W B Saunders, Philadelphia

Roberson M H B 1992 The meaning of compliance: patient perspectives. Qualitative Health Research 2: 7–26

Rutter B M 1977 Some psychological concomitants of chronic bronchitis. Psychological Medicine 7: 459–464

Seedhouse D 1986 Health: the foundations for achievement. Wiley, Chichester

Sim J 1986a Truthfulness in the therapeutic relationship. Physiotherapy Practice 2: 121–127

Sim J 1986b Informed consent: ethical implications for physiotherapy. Physiotherapy 72: 584–587

Sim J 1990a The concept of health. Physiotherapy 76: 423–428

Sim J 1990b Stigma, physical disability and rehabilitation. Physiotherapy Canada 42: 232–238

Sim J 1996 Client confidentiality: ethical issues in occupational therapy. British Journal of Occupational Therapy 59: 56–61

Sim J, Purtilo R B 1991 An ethical analysis of physical therapists' duty to treat persons with AIDS: homosexual patients as a test case. Physical Therapy 71: 650–655

Stewart W 1992 An A–Z of counselling theory and practice. Chapman & Hall, London

Swain J 1995 The use of counselling skills: a guide for therapists. Butterworth-Heinemann, Oxford

Tannahill A 1985 What is health promotion? Health Education Journal 44: 167–168

Thompson I E, Melia K M, Boyd K M 1988 Nursing ethics, 2nd edn. Churchill Livingstone, Edinburgh

Thompson J 1984 Communicating with patients. In: Fitzpatrick R, Hinton J, Newman S, Scambler G, Thompson J (eds) The experience of illness. Tavistock Publications, London

Tuckett D, Boulton M, Olson C, Williams A 1985 Meetings between experts: an approach to sharing ideas in medical consultations. Tavistock Publications, London

Waddell C 1982 The process of neutralisation and the uncertainties of cystic fibrosis. Sociology of Health and Illness 4: 210–220

Williams S J 1989 Chronic respiratory illness and disability: a critical review of the psychosocial literature. Social Science and Medicine 28: 791–803

Williams S J 1993 Chronic respiratory illness. Routledge, London

10

Patients' problems, management and outcomes

Sue Jenkins   Beatrice Tucker

INTRODUCTION

This chapter discusses the problems commonly encountered by the physiotherapist when working with adult patients who have respiratory or cardiovascular dysfunction. These problems are identified by the analysis and interpretation of data obtained during patient assessment (see Chapter 1). The presence of pathology affecting the respiratory and cardiovascular systems affects normal physiological functioning and the signs and symptoms produced are the clinical manifestations of this pathophysiology. The physiotherapist therefore requires a thorough knowledge of normal physiology as well as the pathology and pathophysiology of the respiratory and cardiovascular systems.

The problem-oriented approach to patient management not only assists with the identification of existing problems but also enables recognition of potential patient problems. For example, a high-risk surgical patient may develop problems of impaired airway clearance or reduced lung volume but, if preventive treatment is started during the at-risk period, these problems may not develop. Often patients will have more than one problem; however, physiotherapy management may be similar for the different problems. Further, some problems are not amenable to physiotherapy intervention or physiotherapy intervention may be detrimental. For the patient with more than one problem, it is essential to prioritize the problem list and to establish the short- and long-term goals for each problem. Some problems may only be short term, for example when a patient is incorrectly using a metered-dose inhaler. Developing and prioritizing the problem list, and developing the goals should whenever possible take place in consultation with the patient. For example, an individual who is considered to be at risk of developing ischaemic heart disease (IHD) may seek physiotherapy assistance to develop an exercise programme designed to decrease the likelihood of IHD. Such a programme would be very different from one aimed at achieving and maintaining high levels of physical fitness.

Having identified the goals, the next stage is to identify the means of achieving these goals through physiotherapy intervention and the time frame over which they are to be achieved. The appropriate intervention requires selecting the optimal physiotherapy management strategy based where possible on research findings. When a patient has several physiotherapy problems, the physiotherapy techniques selected should ideally address more than one of the high-priority problems. When selecting a treatment approach, the potential risks to the patient (e.g. the possibility of causing adverse physiological responses) and methods to minimize such risks must be taken into consideration. Patient assessment will also identify the presence of any important factors which must be considered when applying the principles of physiotherapy management for a particular problem to an individual patient. Such factors may include: coexisting conditions or diseases, for example diabetes mellitus, pain, raised intracranial pressure or osteoporosis. Other factors to be considered include ensuring that the intervention is acceptable to the specific cultural group, is appropriate for the patient's age, ability and level of motivation, and the presence of any psychosocial factors which may interfere with the treatment approach (e.g. anxiety or depression). It is also important to determine the patient's likes and dislikes, for example patient preferences for types of activities are vital considerations when developing an exercise training programme. Common to the management of most problems is the education of the patient

by the physiotherapist. This is essential to ensure that patients take responsibility for their own treatment and become actively involved in the management of their problem and the prevention of associated problems. Patient education is covered in Chapter 9.

The key to effective physiotherapy management of a patient is accurate assessment which leads to identification of the patient's problems. If the problem is amenable to physiotherapy, treatment should be commenced. With some problems, a stage will be reached when the natural rate of recovery will no longer be augmented by physiotherapy intervention, and treatment should be discontinued.

In this chapter the problems commonly encountered are discussed. The problems are:

- Dyspnoea
- Decreased exercise tolerance
- Impaired airway clearance
- Airflow limitation
- Respiratory muscle dysfunction
- Reduced lung volume
- Impaired gas exchange
- Abnormal breathing pattern
- Pain
- Musculoskeletal dysfunction – postural abnormalities, decreased compliance, or deformity of the chest wall.

OUTCOME MEASURES

The selection and use of appropriate outcome measures is fundamental to the evaluation of physiotherapy intervention. Demonstrating the effects of physiotherapy intervention, using instruments which have high reliability and validity, is increasingly being required by health care fund holders. Other parties which require outcome data include the patient, caregivers, employers of physiotherapists, clinicians, groups and associations of patients with particular conditions (e.g. cystic fibrosis), members of professions and insurers (Pashkow 1996). Thus when selecting which outcome data to monitor it is important to take into account for whom the data are needed.

Broadly, outcome measures can be grouped into three domains – health, clinical and behavioural (Pashkow 1996). The health outcome domain comprises measures of mortality and morbidity (e.g. symptoms) and quality of life (QOL). Of these, measurement of QOL is very important to the evaluation of physiotherapy intervention as in some instances there is only a weak correlation between physiological measures and QOL (e.g. the relationship between pulmonary function indices and QOL in chronic lung disease). Quality of life scales measure the effect of an illness and its management upon a patient as perceived by the patient. A number of both generic and disease-specific QOL scales are available which allow data to be gathered principally by self-report questionnaires or interview. Quality of life scales available for assessment of patients with respiratory or cardiovascular disease are reviewed elsewhere (Aaronson 1989, Mayou & Bryant 1993, Curtis et al 1994, Pashkow et al 1995, Kinney et al 1996). The choice of a QOL measure requires an evaluation of QOL scales with respect to their reliability, validity, responsiveness and appropriateness (Aaronson 1989).

The clinical outcome domain can be subdivided into four categories (Pashkow 1996): (1) physical measures (e.g. body weight, blood pressure (BP)), symptoms (e.g. angina, cough, dyspnoea), oxygenation, pulmonary function, exercise tolerance; (2) psychological measures (e.g. anxiety, depression, hostility); (3) social measures (interpersonal relationships, social functioning, vocational status, sexual functioning); and (4) medical utilization measures (e.g. time lost from work/studies, number of periods of hospitalization, number of general practitioner consultations).

Finally, the behavioural outcome domain is important because lifestyle changes are frequently an important part of the management of patients with chronic conditions. Behaviourally based interventions include smoking cessation, stress management and interventions aimed at improving adherence with exercise, physiotherapy, diet and medication. Assessment of behavioural outcomes is usually by diary, interview or questionnaire. Measurement of self-efficacy (the judgement by an individual of his capabilities of achieving designated performances) may also be useful to evaluate physiotherapy intervention and has been fairly widely used in the management of patients with cardiovascular disease. Self-efficacy measures can be used for predicting health behaviours (i.e. to identify individuals at greater risk of demonstrating unhealthy behaviour) and to evaluate lifestyle interventions such as dietary control, weight reduction and smoking cessation (Henderson & Cole 1992). Benefits from exercise training in patients with cardiovascular disease (e.g. improvements in an individual's self-confidence in his ability to perform specific physical activities) may be demonstrated using measures of self-efficacy (Stewart et al 1994, Vidmar & Rubinson 1994, Foster et al 1995).

Given the range of outcome measures available, the physiotherapist is required to select for an individual patient (or group of patients) those measures that are the most valid and reproducible, have high patient acceptability, are efficient in terms of the time and equipment needed, and are inexpensive. Selection should include measures from more than one domain where possible. The physiotherapist should possess the required expertise to use the outcome measures selected.

This chapter includes a discussion of the underlying pathophysiology, the clinical features and physiotherapy assessment for each of the problems. The medical and physiotherapy management is discussed alongside each problem. The discussion of each problem concludes with guidelines for the choice of clinical outcome measures (in particular the physical measures) to be used to evaluate physiotherapy intervention.

PROBLEM – DYSPNOEA

Dyspnoea (from the Greek *dys*, painful, difficult, disordered, and *pnoia*, breathing) is a sensation perceived by an individual and is the awareness of increased respiratory effort which is unpleasant and recognized as inappropriate (Brewis 1991, Stulbarg & Adams 1994). Clinically, the terms breathlessness and dyspnoea are used interchangeably. Dyspnoea is one of the most common and distressing symptoms experienced by patients with chronic respiratory disease. In addition to limiting physical and social functioning, the sensation of dyspnoea is often accompanied by fear and anxiety, and, in some patients, may be perceived as life threatening (Dudley et al 1980, Kaplan et al 1985, Eakin et al 1993). Dyspnoea is not tachypnoea (increased rate of breathing), hyperventilation (breathing in excess of metabolic needs) or hyperpnoea (increased breathing). These three terms all describe ventilation in response to different stimuli. Although a decrease in the partial pressure of oxygen in the arterial blood (PaO_2) and an increase in the partial pressure of carbon dioxide in arterial blood ($PaCO_2$) may give rise to increased ventilation, it is unclear whether the altered chemoreceptor stimulation can be directly perceived (Tobin 1990). The sensation of dyspnoea may arise from the ventilatory response rather than from the stimulus itself (Nunn 1987, Tobin 1990).

Breathlessness is a frequent presenting complaint in patients seeking medical help. On occasions, it may be difficult to distinguish from the patient's account whether the symptoms are of respiratory or cardiovascular origin as in both situations the patient may complain of breathlessness on exertion, when lying down (orthopnoea, due to the increased work of breathing (WOB) in supine), breathlessness waking the patient at night (paroxysmal nocturnal dyspnoea) and of acute episodes of breathlessness at rest.

Although it can be readily appreciated how dyspnoea leads to decreased exercise tolerance and poor QOL, the understanding of the mechanisms responsible for the sensation of dyspnoea and dealing with its management pose considerable difficulties.

Different terms used by patients to describe their breathlessness include 'difficulty in breathing', 'chest tightness', 'heavy breathing', 'feeling of suffocation' and 'difficulty in filling the lungs' and it is likely that the term 'breathlessness' embraces several types of sensation (Howell 1990, Manning & Schwartzstein 1995).

There is only a weak correlation between dyspnoea and objective measures of pulmonary function (Eakin et al 1993, O'Donnell 1994). A moderately strong positive correlation exists between dyspnoea and level of physical function as measured by walking tests (Eakin et al 1993). The finding that the level of dyspnoea experienced for a given level of functional impairment varies considerably among patients, may be due to the fact that dyspnoea is a subjective sensation and thus dependent on a variety of stimuli including behavioural influences and the ability of the patient to describe the unpleasant sensation of dyspnoea (Tobin 1990).

Clinically dyspnoea results from several different pathophysiological mechanisms and in some patients more than one mechanism will be responsible (Table 10.1) (Burns & Howell 1969, Gift et al 1986, Tobin 1990, McCarren 1992, Zadai & Irwin 1992, Cheitlin et al 1993, Gardner 1996).

Clinical features and assessment

The time course for the onset of dyspnoea gives important information as to the likely aetiology and will be elicited from the subjective assessment. The patient's account will often reveal that exercise tolerance is limited by breathlessness unless the patient has a chronic hyperventilation disorder in which case dyspnoea usually occurs at rest and is often accompanied by an excessive frequency of sighs (see Ch. 19 on hyperventilation disorders). Careful questioning should also ascertain whether the patient experiences any problems with bladder and bowel function (see Special case, below).

The patient will usually display an altered breathing pattern (see Problem – abnormal breathing pattern, p. 254). This may include the use of the accessory muscles of respiration (including an increase in abdominal effort during expiration) and, in patients with chronic airflow limitation (CAL), paradoxical breathing and pursed lip breathing may be present. The rate and depth of breathing should be observed, as well as the symmetry of chest movements and the inspiratory to expiratory ratio. Characteristically, expiratory time will be prolonged in the

Table 10.1 Pathophysiological basis for dyspnoea in respiratory and cardiovascular disease and clinical examples

Pathophysiological basis	Clinical examples
Added load on mechanics of breathing imposed by: 1. Increase in elastic WOB owing to: a. Decrease in C_L	Increases the inspiratory muscle work required to overcome the elastic recoil of the lungs. This work increases with increases in $\dot{V}_E$ which is achieved with a low V_T and high respiratory rate, e.g. fibrotic lung diseases, breathing at low lung volumes, pulmonary congestion
b. Decrease in C_T and/or compliance of the abdominal compartment	Increases the WOB, e.g. obesity, kyphoscoliosis, ankylosing spondylitis
2. Increase in airways resistance	Requires increased work on inspiration and expiration to effect airflow through narrowed airways. $\dot{V}_E$ requirements met with increased V_T and slowed flow rate in order to minimize the flow-resistive WOB
Weakness or fatigue of the respiratory muscles	See Problem – respiratory muscle dysfunction
Increase in ventilatory requirements	Increase in metabolic rate due to fever or exercise Hypoxaemia
Low CO/ischaemia	Inadequate CO causes reflex medullary ventilatory stimulation when oxygen supply to exercising muscle is inadequate to meet metabolic needs, e.g. in IHD, heart failure or in the presence of ventricular arrhythmias, valvular problems or cardiomyopathy
Decrease in oxygen-carrying capacity of arterial blood	Anaemia Carboxyhaemoglobin Carbon monoxide poisoning
Cardiovascular and respiratory deconditioning	May lead to dyspnoea with low-intensity exercise
Acute changes in permeability of pulmonary capillaries	Pulmonary oedema resulting from heroin overdose, exposure to toxic fumes
Perfusion limitation	The presence of a large $\dot{V}/\dot{Q}$ mismatch or shunt invariably causes dyspnoea, e.g. pulmonary embolus, pulmonary infarction, cyanotic heart disease, pulmonary congestion
Psychosocial factors	Anxiety and depression may heighten perception of breathlessness
Psychogenic factors	May contribute to the aetiology of hyperventilation disorders

Abbreviations: WOB, work of breathing; C_L, lung compliance; $\dot{V}_E$, minute ventilation; V_T, tidal volume; C_T, thoracic compliance; CO, cardiac output; IHD, ischaemic heart disease; $\dot{V}/\dot{Q}$, ventilation/perfusion ratio.

presence of airflow limitation. The patient may complain of feeling hot and appear sweaty if the WOB is excessive. Assessment may reveal signs and symptoms of other problems, in particular airflow limitation, impaired airway clearance, impaired gas exchange or, in the case of cardiac disease, angina may accompany dyspnoea. If respiratory muscle weakness is known or suspected, maximum inspiratory and expiratory mouth pressures (PiMax and PeMax) should be measured. The chest radiograph may show signs of pleural involvement (e.g. effusion, pneumothorax), pulmonary oedema, lung hyperinflation, areas of collapse or consolidation and in some patients may be normal (e.g. chronic hyper-

ventilation disorder, dyspnoea associated with angina). Arterial PO_2 and arterial oxygen saturation (SaO_2) may be low or normal. Arterial CO_2 may be raised, normal or low. A graded exercise test may be useful to differentiate between dyspnoea from cardiovascular and respiratory origin.

Measurement of dyspnoea is useful to classify the severity of a patient's functional impairment due to dyspnoea, individualize rehabilitation programmes and monitor a patient's condition and response to therapy (Weiser et al 1993). Quantification of a sensation such as dyspnoea is difficult. The methods available include dyspnoea threshold scales, dyspnoea intensity scales and multidimensional scales (Weiser et al 1993). Dyspnoea threshold scales require the patient to rate the activity that is the threshold for provoking dyspnoea. Examples include the British Medical Research Council Scale (MRC), American Thoracic Society Scale for dyspnoea and the Oxygen Cost Diagram (OCD) (Eakin et al 1993, Weiser et al 1993, Stulbarg & Adams 1994). The visual analogue scale (VAS) and the modified Borg rating scale are examples of dyspnoea intensity scales which can be used to rate the intensity of dyspnoea at a particular moment in time, for example during or following physical activity (Mahler 1987, Eakin et al 1993, Weiser et al 1993, Stulbarg & Adams 1994). Multidimensional scales were developed to offer a more comprehensive description of dyspnoea and of other symptoms which are highly related. Some multidimensional scales are specific dyspnoea scales, for example the Baseline and Transition Dyspnoea Indexes (BDI and TDI) (Weiser et al 1993, Stulbarg & Adams 1994), the Modified Dyspnoea Index (Eakin et al 1993) and the Breathing Problems Questionnaire (Hyland et al 1994). Two widely used multidimensional scales for assessing QOL in patients with CAL – the St. George's Respiratory Questionnaire (Jones et al 1991, Jones et al 1992) and the Chronic Respiratory Disease Questionnaire (Guyatt et al 1987) – assess the impact of dyspnoea and other symptoms on QOL. In patients with heart disease, the New York Heart Association scale (p. 393) may be used to grade the degree of exertion which causes dyspnoea (Walker & Tan 1994). A specific scale is available for measuring dyspnoea and fatigue in patients with heart failure (Feinstein et al 1989).

Special case – problems with bladder and bowel function

Problems with continence arise in the patient who is breathless and/or has a decrease in exercise tolerance. Such patients often have a reduced appetite and fluid intake, and difficulty with food preparation leading to inadequate soluble fibre intake which may result in constipation. Added to this, the breathless patient who is also constipated may have difficulty breath-holding and assuming an adequate position which causes difficulty in defaecation (Markwell & Sapsford 1995). Reduced fluid intake and frequent or 'just in case' toileting to prevent stress or urge urinary incontinence can result in the bladder becoming accustomed to accommodating smaller volumes of urine. This results in an increased frequency of voiding, which requires more effort for the individual who is breathless. In the patient with respiratory disease, dyspnoea is exacerbated during functional tasks requiring the upper limbs, such as undressing, and this may make the symptom of urgency worse or even result in incontinence.

Incontinence may be due to a reduction in exercise tolerance because the patient is unable to reach the toilet in time.

Medical management

Identification and management of the underlying cause of dyspnoea (e.g. airflow limitation, hypoxaemia, heart failure) and any associated problems are essential. By optimizing nutritional support using a high protein, low carbohydrate diet, respiratory muscle strength should be enhanced and the intensity of dyspnoea may be diminished (Fernandez et al 1993a, Weiser et al 1993). Resting the respiratory muscles using negative pressure ventilation or non-invasive positive pressure ventilation (NIPPV) may enhance respiratory muscle function and decrease dyspnoea.

Psychotropic drugs including opiates and anxiolytics may be useful in anxious or depressed patients with chronic lung disease. Psychoemotional support is essential.

Physiotherapy management

As dyspnoea is one of the manifestations of associated problems including impaired gas exchange, respiratory muscle dysfunction, airflow limitation and reduced lung volumes, treatment strategies should be directed towards the underlying pathophysiology. The following strategies are used in the patient with dyspnoea.

Breathing control and positioning are used to decrease the WOB and eliminate unnecessary muscular activity (O'Neill & McCarthy 1983, McCarren 1992). Pursed-lip breathing and assisted ventilation (e.g. NIPPV, continuous positive airway pressure (CPAP), bi-level positive airway pressure (BiPAP)) may decrease dyspnoea. Relaxation techniques which do not involve breath-holding or the contraction of large muscle groups are particularly useful for patients who are anxious (Hough 1996). Symptomatic relief may be achieved by increasing the movement of cold air onto the patient's face (e.g. sitting by an open window, use of a fan) (Weiser et al 1993). Extremes of temperature and humidity should be avoided (Weiser et al 1993). Vibration (100 hertz) on the chest wall may decrease dyspnoea and alter breathing to a slower and deeper pattern in patients with severe chronic respiratory disease (Sibuya et al 1994).

Patients should be educated on the conservation of energy during activities of daily living. When ambulating, recovery from dyspnoea can be achieved by interspersing physical activity with positioning and breathing control. The application of ventilatory support (e.g. BiPAP, CPAP) during exercise may improve exercise capacity and decrease dyspnoea following exercise (Keilty et al 1994). Oxygen is used in patients who desaturate during exercise. Walking aids can result in an improved ability to exercise and may reduce hypoxaemia and dyspnoea (Honeyman et al 1996). The mechanisms by which strength and endurance training of the respiratory muscles and general exercise training of the upper and lower limbs may improve dyspnoea are complex (Stulbarg & Adams 1994). Conditioning may occur in patients who are able to exercise beyond their anaerobic threshold. The majority of patients will demonstrate improvement of coordination and performance of a physical activity, become accustomed to the sensation of dyspnoea and become more confident in performing tasks (as measured using self-efficacy scales).

The use of high-frequency oscillation and external chest wall compression to relieve dyspnoea are experimental (George et al 1985).

Clinical outcomes

Medical management of the underlying problem, for example pulmonary oedema and pneumothorax, will often result in a rapid reduction in dyspnoea as measured using a dyspnoea intensity scale. Involvement in an exercise programme may improve exercise endurance and decrease dyspnoea because of improvements in coordination, a reduced fear of dyspnoea, improved confidence, motivation and emotional state, and a greater tolerance to the sensation of dyspnoea as measured using a dyspnoea threshold or multidimensional scale (Stulbarg & Adams 1994). These changes should be reflected in an improved QOL.

PROBLEM – DECREASED EXERCISE TOLERANCE

Exercise capacity in patients with respiratory or cardiovascular disease is usually limited by dyspnoea, pain (chest or legs) or fatigue (general or local). This section outlines the pathophysiological basis for exercise limitation occurring in commonly encountered respiratory and cardiovascular conditions.

Many patients with chronic respiratory or cardiovascular disease avoid exercise and become physically deconditioned (Hamilton et al 1995). In a deconditioned individual, the oxygen cost of exercise is higher at any given exercise intensity than in an individual who is physically fit. This is due to central and peripheral mechanisms which include an increased heart rate (HR) response to exercise, increase in cardiac afterload and a decrease in muscle capacity for aerobic exercise. In addition, failure to exercise may decrease the skill and efficiency of physical movements. Physical activities which were commonplace may, in the deconditioned individual, require a much higher level of cognitive function. These processes give rise to an increase in the oxygen cost of exercise.

A number of patients with chronic respiratory or cardiovascular disease are elderly. In addition to the age-related decline in physical work capacity these patients may have orthopaedic, neurological or musculoskeletal factors that impair the ability to exercise. Depression and anxiety often accompany chronic disease and further limit exercise capacity and decrease the motivation to exercise.

Respiratory disease

Patients with respiratory disease terminate exercise because of dyspnoea and fail to reach maximal heart rates. In a proportion of patients leg fatigue is also a limiting factor (O'Donnell et al 1995).

A respiratory impairment to exercise may be due to dysfunction of any or all components of the respiratory system. Normally, the ventilation requirements for exercise are met by an increase in both the tidal volume (V_T) and respiratory rate. Physiological abnormalities present in respiratory disease limit the ability to increase V_T during exercise and thus minute ventilation ($\dot{V}_E$) is met by a disproportionate increase in respiratory rate. This occurs in CAL, restrictive lung disease, chest wall defects and respiratory muscle weakness. The excessive increase in respiratory rate is very costly in terms of the oxygen required by the respiratory muscles because of the much larger number of muscle contractions and the increase in wasted ventilation. In effect, the respiratory muscles use oxygen at the expense of the other skeletal muscles. Under resting conditions, healthy individuals use only about 1–2% of total body oxygen consumption ($\dot{V}O_2$) for the task of respiration, increasing to 10–20% at maximal exercise. In contrast, patients with CAL, at rest, may require about 15% of the total body $\dot{V}O_2$ for respiration increasing to an estimated 35–40% of total body $\dot{V}O_2$ during moderate exercise (Levison & Cherniack 1968, Pardy et al 1984). Airflow limitation reduces the ability to breathe as deeply and rapidly as required during exercise. The decrease in expiratory time, as a consequence of the increased respiratory rate, limits expiration and so functional residual capacity (FRC) rises. The associated lung hyperinflation serves to improve ventilation by decreasing airway resistance and increasing expiratory flow rates.

However, the main disadvantage of this compensatory mechanism is the altered dynamics of the respiratory muscles and the increase in the elastic WOB. There is also a relative increase in dead space and a reduction in alveolar ventilation.

With interstitial lung disease, the reduction in peak $\dot{V}O_2$ has been shown to be due to abnormalities of the pulmonary circulation with accompanying gas exchange impairment (Hansen & Wasserman 1996).

The presence of fibrosis severely limits inspiratory capacity. Thus, the extent to which V_T can be increased with exercise is reduced and the patient has to breathe at a much higher rate in order to meet the ventilatory requirements. An excessive increase in respiratory rate during exercise also occurs in the presence of reduced thoracic compliance (Wasserman et al 1987).

In patients with respiratory muscle weakness, there is a decreased ability to generate the maximal intrapleural pressures needed to expand the lungs during exercise; therefore V_T fails to increase normally with increasing workloads.

Exercise capacity may be limited by bronchoconstriction in patients with asthma and exercise-induced asthma (EIA) may be the only symptom in young patients with mild disease. The bronchoconstriction occurs within 5–10 minutes following cessation of exercise. The mechanism responsible is thought to be due to the increase in ventilation during exercise which causes a loss of water from the respiratory mucosa. The resultant hypertonicity of airway fluid and decreased temperature in the respiratory tract causes the release of mediators from the mast cells and consequent bronchoconstriction and bronchial oedema (Alison & Ellis 1992). Following exercise, there is a refractory period lasting 1–2 hours. When exercise is performed in this refractory period the exercise-induced bronchoconstriction is much less severe (Wardlaw 1993).

One of the major problems experienced by many patients with moderate to severe respiratory disease is marked dyspnoea when performing activities of daily living which involve use of the upper limbs, especially when the upper limbs are unsupported (e.g. teeth cleaning, shaving, washing and hair combing). Patients with severe ventilatory limitation often fix their shoulder girdle so that accessory muscles can exert an expanding force on the rib cage in an effort to shift more air in and out of the lungs. Activities involving the upper limbs may mean loss of these shoulder girdle muscles as muscles of elevation thereby reducing their contribution to the generation of the intrapleural pressure needed for inspiration. The breathing pattern during unsupported upper limb exercise is often noticed to be rapid and irregular, and dysynchronous thoracoabdominal movements may be observed (Celli 1994). A further stress is imposed when exercise involves raising the arms above the head. Lactate accumulates in the blood immediately with the onset of upper limb exercise. This leads to an increase in CO_2 production and thus ventilation.

Gas exchange may be abnormal during exercise and this may contribute to a decrease in exercise capacity. In CAL, different patterns of arterial blood gas changes occur with exercise and it is difficult to accurately identify patients likely to exhibit arterial desaturation. Patients with a less severe reduction in forced expiratory volume in one second (FEV_1) and diffusing capacity tend not to have a fall in PaO_2 or SaO_2 with exercise (Moss & Make 1993). In restrictive lung diseases, hypoxaemia often occurs on exercise and is thought to be due to an increase in ventilation perfusion ($\dot{V}/\dot{Q}$) mismatching and a loss of the alveolar-capillary surface area required for effective gas transfer (Wasserman et al 1987).

Cardiovascular impairment

In cardiac disease (e.g. IHD, valvular heart disease, heart failure and cardiomyopathy) the increase in stroke volume and cardiac output with exercise is limited. This results in inadequate oxygen being supplied to the exercising muscles leading to an increased production of lactic acid by the ischaemic muscles and is thought to account for the fatigue. In some patients, metabolic acidosis develops at low levels of exercise and may even be present at rest. In order to rid the body of the excess CO_2 produced, breathing is stimulated and this may contribute to the sensation of dyspnoea. Chronic metabolic acidosis occurs in persistent heart failure and for a given workload the ventilation is relatively high.

In patients with peripheral vascular disease, the oxygen supply to the working muscles is decreased. This leads to a build-up of lactic acid and pain occurs during low intensity exercise.

Other disorders

Obesity is present in many individuals with cardiovascular disease and is a risk factor for IHD. Obesity decreases exercise capacity owing to the increase in resting metabolic requirements and the greater respiratory and cardiac work required by an obese individual when exercising. Another risk factor for IHD is diabetes mellitus, which, if poorly controlled, leads to chronic metabolic acidosis causing an increase in ventilation at any given workload. Cigarette smoking increases the level of carboxyhaemoglobin, thus reducing the oxygen-carrying capacity of the haemoglobin. When exercise is performed immediately after smoking a cigarette, cardiac work is increased owing to the smoking-related rise in HR and BP.

Fatigue may be present in many acute and chronic conditions and is an important limiting factor to exercise. Fatigue may be cardiovascular (low cardiac output, anaemia), pulmonary (excessive WOB), metabolic (hyperglycaemia, hypothyroidism), neurological, muscular (local muscle glycogen depletion, lactate accumulation in muscle and blood) or psychogenic in origin (anxiety, depression), or simply due to poor patient motivation.

Clinical features and assessment

A graded exercise test, including measurements of relevant subjective and physiological measures before, during and following the test, is essential (see chapters on assessment, cardiac rehabilitation and pulmonary rehabilitation).

These measures may include HR, pulse, BP, rate pressure product (RPP), electrocardiograph, breathing pattern including respiratory rate and SaO_2. Peak expiratory flow rate or FEV_1 should be measured in patients with suspected EIA. Rating of perceived exertion and dyspnoea scales should also be used. For patients with angina or peripheral vascular disease, severity of pain should be assessed (see Problem – pain, p. 256). It is important to assess the effect of physical functioning on QOL.

Medical management

Identification and management of the underlying cause of reduced exercise tolerance (e.g. CAL, IHD, valvular heart disease, heart failure, cardiomyopathy, metabolic abnormality) are essential. Optimizing management of associated conditions (e.g. diabetes mellitus, peripheral vascular disease) is necessary for patients to achieve their maximum exercise capacity.

Oxygen therapy is used to prevent a significant decrease in PaO_2, to maintain the metabolic needs, reduce dyspnoea and to prevent the compensatory effects of chronic hypoxaemia.

Respiratory muscle strength is enhanced by ensuring that nutrition is optimal for patients who are malnourished (Fernandez et al 1993a, Weiser et al 1993). Weight reduction will reduce the increased load on the respiratory muscles which results from obesity (Alison & Ellis 1992). Resting the respiratory muscles using negative pressure ventilation or NIPPV may enhance respiratory muscle function, decrease dyspnoea and improve exercise tolerance. Suppression of the associated psychoemotional problems such as anxiety and depression using psychotropic drugs (e.g. opiates, anxiolytics) may allow patients with chronic lung disease to increase their exercise capacity.

Physiotherapy management

An exercise programme should be designed to meet the specific requirements of the patient. The mode, intensity, duration and frequency of exercise should be individually selected for each patient based on assessment findings and established goals. The programme should consist of a warm-up, stretches, an aerobic component, resistive training (when appropriate) and a cool-down. Postural correction is also important (see Problem – musculoskeletal dysfunction – postural abnormalities, decreased compliance, or deformity of the chest wall, p. 259). The programme should include upper limb and lower limb activities, including both supported and unsupported upper limb exercises (Celli 1994). Although it is recognized that endurance training is beneficial for most patients, it may be more important for some patients to improve their speed of movement over a short distance (e.g. to improve their ability to reach the toilet because of urinary or faecal urgency) rather than focusing on improving the distance the patient can walk.

Interval training is useful to improve the exercise endurance of patients who are severely deconditioned, fatigued or have intermittent claudication. Oxygen, rest, energy conservation, positioning and breathing control, and ventilatory support (e.g. NIPPV, CPAP, BiPAP) may improve exercise tolerance (see Problem – dyspnoea, p. 229). Breathing strategies used to relieve dyspnoea (e.g. pursed lip breathing, exhale with effort, paced breathing) may be useful to improve exercise tolerance. Specific respiratory muscle training, however, results in an increased strength and capacity of these muscles to meet a respiratory load; improvement in exercise performance is still debated (Celli 1994) (see chapter on pulmonary rehabilitation). Exercise testing and prescription for special cases, such as patients with diabetes mellitus, is covered elsewhere (Skinner 1993).

Patients with hyper-reactive airways should, when possible, exercise in an appropriate environment. Cold dry conditions, airborne irritants and pollutants should be avoided. Patients should be encouraged to stay indoors during extreme conditions.

Coached training with appropriate emotional support and encouragement is beneficial for patients with fatigue, dyspnoea or anxiety.

Special case – exercise-induced asthma

Exercise training is beneficial to patients with EIA for several reasons. At a given workload, ventilation is reduced by training thereby reducing the prime trigger for EIA. Patients are thus able to train at a higher workload before symptoms occur. The increases in respiratory muscle endurance may benefit patients during a prolonged asthma attack (Alison & Ellis 1992). Patients with symptoms may be reluctant to exercise and should be encouraged to participate in regular physical exercise to prevent deconditioning and gain psychological benefits. Symptoms of EIA may be reduced by: (1) administering an aerosol beta$_2$-adrenoceptor agonist or sodium cromoglycate prior to exercise; (2) adequately warming up prior to exercise and including interval training to provide and make use of the refractory period; and (3) exercising in an appropriate environment. Cold dry environments should be avoided (e.g. by avoiding early morning or late night activity). Swimming is beneficial as a choice of exercise because of the humidity provided by the water.

Clinical outcomes

Improved cardiorespiratory fitness should be expected in patients who are able to participate in an endurance training programme. A true training effect may occur in patients who are able to exercise above their anaerobic threshold (Stulbarg & Adams 1994). The physiological benefits of endurance training include a reduction in cardiac and respiratory workload at a given intensity of submaximal exercise. This should be associated with a reduction in HR and RPP at rest and with submaximal exercise. Oxygen consumption, stroke volume, cardiac output, peripheral vascular resistance, muscle blood flow and oxygen extraction are all increased at maximal exercise. Following training, HR, BP and respiratory rate should return more rapidly to pre-exercise levels. Additional benefits may include an increase in muscle mass and loss of adipose tissue, and an improved sense of well-being. In patients with more severe

disease who are unable to exercise at a sufficient intensity to obtain a true training effect, exercise training is still beneficial and should be associated with an increase in walking distance and a decrease in dyspnoea. Such patients may report an increased ease with which activities of daily living are able to be performed. The patient may score lower on the rating of perceived exertion scale.

Following an endurance exercise training programme, patients with IHD may be able to exercise at a higher RPP before the onset of angina (Laslett et al 1987). Improved physical functioning should be reflected in improvements in QOL.

The benefits from participation in cardiac or pulmonary rehabilitation programmes are discussed in detail in the chapters relating to pulmonary and cardiac rehabilitation.

PROBLEM – IMPAIRED AIRWAY CLEARANCE

Impaired airway clearance is an important physiotherapy problem because of the potential for the patient to develop an overwhelming infection, major atelectasis and other associated problems such as impaired gas exchange and airflow limitation.

In the healthy lung approximately 100 ml of mucus is produced each day (Moxham & Costello 1994). Mucus is produced from four main sources of which the first two are by far the most important (Clarke 1990):

1. The submucosal glands located chiefly in the cartilaginous airways
2. The goblet cells lining the trachea, bronchi and bronchioles
3. Clara cells (non-ciliated bronchiolar cells) found in the small bronchi, bronchioles and terminal bronchioles
4. Tissue fluid transudate.

The composition of mucus in health is 95% water, 5% glycoproteins, carbohydrates, lipids, deoxyribonucleic acid, some cellular debris and foreign particles (Des Jardins 1990).

Mucus is carried upwards on the mucociliary

blanket, the major mechanism for clearing particles from the airways, and eventually swallowed. In situations where mucus secretion is greatly increased (e.g. very dusty environments), clearance of secretions is augmented by cough and expectoration. Absorptive mechanisms operating at the alveolar level are responsible for clearing some of the peripheral secretions. When the volume of mucus reaching the larynx and pharynx has increased to the extent that an individual becomes conscious of its presence on coughing or 'clearing the throat' then the mucus is defined as sputum; the presence of sputum is abnormal.

One of the most important causes of impaired airway clearance is the absence of an effective cough. Reflex coughing is initiated by the stimulation of irritant receptors. The most sensitive sites for initiating a cough are the larynx and tracheobronchial tree, especially at the carina and at bifurcations. Receptors in the terminal bronchioles and alveoli respond to chemical stimuli, for example noxious gases. Receptors in both sites show some adaptation when subjected to continuous stimulation as in the smoker who only coughs after the first cigarette of the day. There is a decreased sensitivity of the receptors during sleep and in elderly individuals (Hara & Shepard 1990). Afferent impulses from the receptors travel mainly in the vagus nerve to the medulla from where an automatic sequence of events (the cough reflex) is triggered (Flenley 1990, Irwin & Widdicombe 1994).

The inspiratory phase of coughing consists of an inspiration, through a widely opened glottis. The inspired volume varies greatly from a VC breath to a much smaller volume. This phase may be absent when cough is initiated by stimulation of mechanical receptors in the larynx. The glottis then closes and the expiratory muscles contract rapidly raising the intrapleural and intra-alveolar pressures to as high as 300 mmHg (40 kPa) and intra-abdominal pressure to 50–100 mmHg (Flenley 1990, Irwin & Widdicombe 1994). This compressive phase lasts only about 200 milliseconds (Irwin & Widdicombe 1994).

The expulsive phase begins with the glottis suddenly opening so that the air under pressure

is rapidly expelled (the rate of this may exceed 12 litres per second in health). The trachea narrows to one-sixth of its normal diameter and the rapid flow, combined with the dynamic compression of the airways, increases the explosive force of the expelled air. This has the effect of dislodging mucus and foreign particles and bringing them to the pharynx.

Table 10.2. lists the pathophysiological basis of impaired airway clearance and includes clinical examples (Johnson & Pierson 1986, Foltz & Benumof 1987, Clarke 1990, Irwin & Widdicombe 1994, Judson & Sahn 1994).

Infection develops when there is retention of mucus. Once infection occurs, mucus retention is aggravated by oedema of the airway walls, bronchoconstriction due to irritation of the mucous membrane, extrinsic compression of the bronchial airways by secondary lymph node enlargement and an increase in mucus viscosity. The marked inflammatory response to infection is characterized by the persistent influx of neutrophils which further contributes to the increase in mucus viscosity and mucus retention. Destruction of bronchial airways may occur with chronic infection owing to the production of toxic inflammatory mediators such as leukotrienes, proteases and elastases (Hardy 1994). The problem of mucus retention is compounded by the increased mucus produced by the abnormal airways (Hardy 1994). The pathophysiological effects of mucus retention are given in Table 10.3.

Clinical features and assessment

The clinical features are usually those resulting from mucus retention. These include an abnormal breathing pattern due to increased WOB, hypoxaemia, and on occasions hypercapnia. The presence of infection may produce fever and tachycardia. When the secretions cause marked airflow limitation, wheezing may be audible with the unaided ear (see Problem – airflow limitation, p. 242). Auscultatory findings may include diminished or absent breath sounds, bronchial breath sounds, crackles and wheezes.

The following features of cough should be

Table 10.2   Pathophysiological basis of impaired airway clearance

Pathophysiological basis	Comment and clinical examples
Increase or altered composition of mucus: 1. Increase in production	Chronic bronchitis, asthma, cystic fibrosis, bronchiectasis, presence of an artificial airway Tracheal intubation may provoke reflex mucus secretion
2. Colonization of mucus, e.g. viral, bacterial and fungal organisms	Chest infection Bypassing of upper respiratory tract — cuffed tube mechanically blocks mucociliary escalator and may lead to pooling and stagnation of secretions promoting colonization and infection
3. Systemic dehydration	Leads to viscous secretions which are difficult to mobilize and expectorate May occur postoperatively especially if fluid restriction is imposed
Abnormalities in cilia structure or function	Primary ciliary dyskinesia Endobronchial suctioning may lead to mucosal haemorrhage and erosions in the tracheobronchial tree, slowing mucociliary transport by damaging ciliated epithelium
Impaired mucociliary clearance: 1. Age 2. Sleep 3. Environmental pollutants 4. Drugs 5. High inspired oxygen 6. Hypoxia and hypercapnia 7. Social factors	Rate of mucociliary clearance is decreased by as much as 60% in the elderly Reduces mucociliary clearance These may disturb clearance. The effects sometimes depend on dose Some general anaesthetics, morphine and other narcotics depress mucociliary transport May produce acute tracheobronchitis leading to loss of ciliated epithelium, mucus retention and slowed transport of mucus Slow mucociliary clearance Failure to expectorate, owing to embarrassment
Abnormal cough reflex: 1. Decreased	Decreased level of consciousness, general anaesthesia, narcotic analgesics Inhibition due to pain, e.g. following surgery, pleurisy, chest wall trauma Damage to the vagal or glossopharyngeal nerves Laryngectomy Paralysed vocal cords Denervated lungs (lung, heart–lung transplant)
2. Increased	Occurs especially in patients with poorly controlled asthma Cause uncertain but not thought merely to be due to bronchial hyperreactivity. Viral infections also increase sensitivity
Ineffective cough due to the inability to generate sufficient expiratory airflow	Severe reduction in vital capacity Expiratory muscle weakness decreases the cough-induced dynamic compression of the airways Airflow limitation may cause the cough to be weak and/or ineffective Cough is ineffective in the presence of bronchiectatic segments because of lack of airflow through these segments
Abnormal cough: 1. Post-nasal drip syndrome 2. Gastro-oesophageal reflux	Cough results from the stimulation of the cough reflex May lead to chronic cough and aspiration of gastric contents May be associated with complaints of heartburn, sour taste, regurgitation

assessed: precipitating factors; the severity; the pattern of occurrence; sound of the cough; and presence of accompanying sounds or complaints such as wheeze, stridor or hoarseness. Smoking history and occupational history are important in the assessment of a patient with impaired airway clearance. The quality of the cough should be assessed (e.g. dry, hacking, effectiveness). Assessment should identify the presence of any adverse effects associated with cough. The adverse effects of cough which are commonly encountered are increase in airflow limitation, fatigue, arterial oxygen desaturation, cough syncope and cardiac rhythm disturbances. The

Table 10.3 Pathophysiological effects of mucus retention

Pathophysiological effect	Cause
Increase in airways resistance	Partial or complete airway obstruction from mucus in airway lumen. This may lead to atelectasis from absorption of gas (complete obstruction) or to air trapping and regional over-distension (partial obstruction)
Hypoxaemia	$\dot{V}/\dot{Q}$ mismatch due to premature airway closure in dependent lung regions and atelectasis Intrapulmonary shunting may occur with lobar collapse
Hypercapnia	May occur especially if sputum retention occurs in chronic bronchitis

Abbreviations: $\dot{V}/\dot{Q}$, ventilation/perfusion ratio.

adverse musculoskeletal effects include chest wall pain, hernia, vertebral disc herniation and fractured ribs. Although not widely reported in the literature, stress incontinence is a frequent occurrence with chronic cough.

The examination of any sputum produced is important. In a patient with a chronic disease, assessment should include the pattern of daily sputum production, amount, type and consistency of the sputum, and a review of the patient's physiotherapy regimen. Ease of sputum expectoration can be measured using a Likert scale or a VAS. Measurement of $PeMax$ may be helpful with low values frequently being associated with difficulty in moving the secretions proximally.

Arterial blood gas analysis may show a lowered PaO_2 and SaO_2. Arterial PCO_2 may be normal, increased or lowered (e.g. due to hyperventilation in the early stages of acute asthma). The chest radiograph may show signs of lung collapse, consolidation or hyperinflation. Other chest radiograph abnormalities may reflect the underlying condition, for example cystic fibrosis. Pulmonary function tests may reveal signs of airflow limitation, gas trapping or reduced lung volumes.

Assessment may also reveal signs of associated problems, for example dyspnoea, decreased exercise tolerance, airflow limitation, abnormal breathing pattern, respiratory muscle dysfunction and impaired gas exchange.

Medical management

Recognition and management of the underlying cause of impaired airway clearance are essen-tial. The most common causes of chronic cough are post-nasal drip syndrome, asthma, gastro-oesophageal reflux, chronic bronchitis, bronchiectasis and, less commonly, the administration of angiotensinogen-converting enzyme inhibitors (Irwin & Widdicombe 1994).

Antihistamines and decongestants administered orally or via a nasal spray are useful in post-nasal drip syndrome. When inflammation is present a corticosteroid nasal spray may be used. Impaired cough due to pain is treated by analgesic drugs. Cough expectorants and mucolytics such as hypertonic saline and acetylcysteine may be used to decrease the viscosity of tenacious secretions. Inhaled beta$_2$-adrenoceptor agonists and mucolytics such as recombinant human deoxyribonuclease (DNase), hypertonic saline and acetylcysteine have been shown to increase mucociliary clearance (Barnes 1994). Chronic, irritating, non-productive cough may be treated by non-specific antitussives such as ipratropium bromide (Irwin & Widdicombe 1994).

Infection (bronchial or nasal) is treated using appropriate antibiotic, antifungal or antiprotozoal therapy. Adequate fluid intake is essential. Patients who are at risk of developing recurrent infections should be immunized annually. All patients should be counselled to cease tobacco use. Avoidance of irritants or allergic precipitating factors is encouraged wherever possible.

Appropriate drug management combined with dietary control and head-up positioning during sleep is beneficial for the majority of patients with gastro-oesophageal reflux (Irwin & Widdicombe 1994).

Intubation, tracheostomy or minitracheostomy, and humidification may be required, for example following depression of the central nervous system, damage to the glossopharyngeal or vagal nerves, or surgical excision of the larynx.

Physiotherapy management

Physiotherapy has an important place in the management of impaired airway clearance; however, bronchial secretions only become a physiotherapy problem when they are excessive, retained or difficult to eliminate. Physiotherapy may also have a place in the management of problems associated with impaired airway clearance. Many patients expectorate a small amount of foul-smelling, tenacious sputum postoperatively but this is not a problem if the patient is conscious, able to huff or cough effectively and self-ambulating.

Patients should be educated on the avoidance of environmental factors such as cigarette smoke and cold wet environments as these may trigger cough and predispose to infection. Education to enable early recognition of chest infection and treatment strategies to initiate early management are important.

A large range of airway clearance techniques are available (see Ch. 8). Factors for consideration when selecting airway clearance techniques are listed in Box 10.1. Humidification is especially important when the upper airway is bypassed,

when high concentrations of inspired oxygen are being delivered and in patients who have thick and tenacious secretions. Administration of nebulizers containing saline (normal or hypertonic), water or mucolytics are used to liquefy secretions, enhance mucociliary clearance and increase sputum yield prior to airway clearance techniques (Conway et al 1992). Bronchodilators may be given to reduce airflow limitation and may improve mucociliary transport.

Mobilization of secretions may be achieved using ambulation which enhances mucociliary clearance by spontaneous increases in V_T and flow rates (Wolff et al 1977). Breathing techniques such as the active cycle of breathing techniques and autogenic drainage, body positioning including gravity assisted drainage positions and continuous lateral rotation therapy, and manual techniques including percussion, shaking and vibrations are used to mobilize secretions. Pressure devices such as the positive expiratory pressure mask and intermittent positive pressure breathing are used for the mobilization of secretions as are devices using the principle of oscillations such as oral high-frequency oscillation, high-frequency chest wall compression and the Flutter. Manual hyperinflation may be required in some intubated patients. These techniques are discussed in the chapter on physiotherapy skills and techniques.

Removal of secretions can be facilitated using the forced expiration technique, high lung volume huff or cough with support where necessary and suctioning. Spontaneous cough may be elicited by physical activity. The cough reflex may be elicited using a tracheal rub or suctioning. Strengthening of the abdominal muscles and assisted cough techniques (e.g. abdominal support with an upward pressure) may be helpful for patients with impaired cough due to weakness of the abdominal muscles. Assisted cough techniques may also be necessary when treating the intellectually impaired patient with retained secretions.

For patients with pain, relief of pain is essential prior to airway clearance techniques (see Problem – pain, p. 256).

Patients who have stress incontinence or

Box 10.1 Factors for consideration when selecting airway clearance techniques (adapted from Hardy 1994, p. 449)

- Patient motivation
- Patient's goals
- Physiotherapist's/physician's goals
- Patient preferences
- Effectiveness of considered technique
- Limitations of technique
- Patient's age and ability to concentrate and learn technique
- Ease of teaching/learning technique
- Skill of physiotherapist with particular techniques
- Need for equipment and/or assistants
- Time necessary to use technique
- Desirability of combining techniques

excess flatus, should be encouraged to contract their pelvic floor muscles prior to, and during, forced expiratory manoeuvres.

Clinical outcomes

Short-term benefits should be observed by an increase in sputum expectorated, as measured by weight, volume or rate of expectoration. Pulmonary function tests may show an improvement in measures of airflow limitation, for example FEV_1 and peak expiratory flow rate (PEFR). With acute conditions, resolution of chest radiograph abnormalities may be seen. Removal of excess bronchial secretions may improve or eliminate the associated problems such as impaired gas exchange and dyspnoea.

Long-term benefits in patients with chronic lung disease may include a reduction in the number of exacerbations per year, fewer courses of antibiotics, fewer and shorter periods of hospitalization and a reduction in the number of days lost from studies or work. Such benefits will also be demonstrated by cost savings. Measurable improvements in QOL should also be seen.

In the high-risk postoperative patient with excess bronchial secretions, benefits from physiotherapy intervention may be measured by the prevention of chest infection.

Improved cough or huff technique may be associated with a reduction in associated problems such as fatigue, dyspnoea, syncope, arterial oxygen desaturation or stress incontinence.

PROBLEM – AIRFLOW LIMITATION

Airflow limitation generally occurs in conjunction with other physiotherapy problems, such as dyspnoea, decreased exercise tolerance, impaired airway clearance and abnormal cough. The pathophysiological basis for airflow limitation is given in Table 10.4.

Special case – lung hyperinflation in chronic airflow limitation

Lung hyperinflation is a compensatory mechanism aimed at overcoming the increase in expiratory airflow resistance. In order to achieve adequate ventilation, most patients with CAL breathe with a smaller V_T and increased rate

Table 10.4 Pathophysiological basis of airflow limitation and clinical examples (West 1992, Wardlaw 1993)

Pathophysiological basis	Clinical examples
Changes in the airway wall:	
1. Smooth muscle contraction	Asthma
2. Smooth muscle hypertrophy and hyperplasia	Asthma
3. Inflammation of the mucosa	Asthma
4. Hypertrophy of mucous glands	Chronic bronchitis
5. Thickening of the bronchial wall	Chronic bronchitis, asthma
6. Dilatation and destruction of airway walls	Cystic fibrosis, bronchiectasis
7. Infiltration of the bronchial mucosa with eosinophils and mononuclear cells	Asthma
8. Changes in osmolarity of normal airway fluid produced by cooling	EIA. FEV_1 falls rapidly after cessation of exercise. EIA is exacerbated by exercise in cold, dry atmospheres
Factors outside the airway:	
1. Loss of radial traction due to a decrease in elastic recoil secondary to increases in lung compliance	Emphysema
2. Compression	Enlarged lymph node, neoplasm, peribronchial oedema as occurs with pulmonary oedema
Partial or total occlusion of airway lumen	Mucus, e.g. in chronic bronchitis, cystic fibrosis, bronchiectasis, asthma Inhaled foreign body

Abbreviations: EIA, exercise-induced asthma; FEV_1, forced expiratory volume in 1 second.

when compared to healthy individuals. The increased rate reduces expiratory time and may lead to the development of intrinsic positive end-expiratory pressure (PEEP). In order to initiate inspiratory airflow, the inspiratory muscles are required to generate a pleural pressure in excess of the intrinsic PEEP. The excessive lowering of the intrapleural pressure required to ventilate the lungs may cause indrawing of the intercostal spaces and supraclavicular fossae on inspiration. The WOB on inspiration is also increased due to the decrease in lung compliance that occurs with lung hyperinflation. The fibres of the diaphragm are shortened and the altered length–tension relationship may decrease its ability to generate muscle tension and inspiratory pressure. In extreme cases, the diaphragm contracts isometrically (i.e. as a fixator) and at high lung volumes the function of the inspiratory intercostal muscles is markedly reduced. When acting as a fixator, the main effect of the diaphragm is to prevent transmission of the negative intrapleural pressure to the abdomen thereby preventing suction of the diaphragm into the thorax. Lung hyperinflation reduces the zone of apposition of the diaphragm. The net effect of this is a decreased ability of the diaphragm to elevate the lower rib cage. When hyperinflation is severe, the zone of apposition is lost and the diaphragm fibres are realigned in a horizontal direction. In this instance, contraction of the diaphragm pulls the lower rib cage inwards (Hoover's sign). At rest, the ribs are in a more horizontal position and, when the parasternal and intercostal muscles contract, there is little elevation of the ribs (McCarren 1992, Ferguson 1993). Some patients with severe hyperinflation, especially during exercise, may use the abdominal release mechanism to decrease the work of the diaphragm while still maintaining its output. To effect this mechanism, the patient contracts the abdominal muscles at the end of expiration thus pushing the contents of the abdomen up against the diaphragm and improving its length–tension relationship. The increase in lung volume during the subsequent inspiration occurs by a sudden release of the abdominal pressure which acts to passively pull the diaphragm downwards. Normally, expiration is passive, but with a decrease in expiratory airflow the patient may recruit the abdominal muscles and other expiratory muscles in an attempt to augment expiration.

Clinical features and assessment

The patient with airflow limitation may complain of chest tightness, cough and breathlessness. Exercise tolerance is often limited. In asthma, cough and dyspnoea may be particularly evident at night and may lead to poor sleep patterns. Wheezing may be audible with the unaided ear. With long-standing disease, examination of the chest may reveal signs of hyperinflation. Signs include a barrel-shaped chest with an increase in the anteroposterior diameter, use of accessory muscles and a raised shoulder girdle. Indrawing of the intercostal spaces and supraclavicular fossae may be visible. Pursed lip breathing is seen in some patients with moderate to severe airflow limitation. Hoover's sign may also be present. Auscultatory findings associated with hyperinflation include reduced breath sounds and the percussion note may be hyper-resonant. Wheezes heard on auscultation in patients with airflow limitation are often multiple, polyphonic and widespread.

The chest radiograph may show signs of hyperinflation as well as signs consistent with the underlying condition, for example, the presence of emphysematous bullae or bronchiectatic changes.

Abnormalities in pulmonary function indicative of airflow limitation consist of a reduction in FEV_1, FEV_1/forced vital capacity (FVC), PEFR and forced expiratory flow over the middle half of the FVC manoeuvre ($FEF_{25-75\%}$). Characteristic patterns can be seen in the flow–volume loop and may help with identifying the cause and site of the airflow limitation. Functional residual capacity, residual volume (RV) and total lung capacity (TLC) are often increased. An absolute increase in TLC reflects hyperinflation whereas air trapping is the term used to describe increases in FRC and RV (Ruppel 1994). Gas exchange abnormalities may include hypoxaemia due to $\dot{V}/\dot{Q}$ mismatching. Arterial PCO_2 is often normal, especially in patients with predominant emphysema and is generally raised in all patients with severe chronic lung disease. It may be lowered in the early stages of an asthma attack.

Medical management

Education of patients by health professionals includes explaining in simple terms the mechanism of airflow limitation, the importance of avoiding trigger factors including cigarette smoke, use and effects of medication and a self-management plan (e.g. the use of a peak flow meter for patients with variable airflow limitation and management of symptoms including a plan of action in the event of progressive symptoms).

This involves management of the underlying cause of airflow limitation. If airflow limitation is reversible, management consists of:

1. Pharmacological therapy
2. Control of environmental allergens and irritants in some patients
3. Appropriate monitoring
4. Patient education (Bone 1996).

Bronchodilators and anti-inflammatory drugs are used to relieve the reversible elements of airflow limitation and to reduce mucus production in some patients. Patients who manifest mild symptoms of airflow limitation on rare occasions may only require symptomatic relief using short-acting inhaled bronchodilators. However, when patients begin to use inhaled bronchodilators on a regular basis, anti-inflammatory agents such as inhaled corticosteroids are also required. Prophylactic drugs such as sodium cromoglycate may also be used. If airflow limitation is severe, oral or intravenous drugs are required. Bronchodilators and sodium cromoglycate are also used in the prevention of EIA (British Thoracic Society, National Asthma Campaign, Royal College of Physicians of London et al 1997).

Inhaled foreign bodies are generally removed by bronchoscopy. Surgical intervention, laser treatment, chemotherapy and/or radiotherapy may be indicated for the management of neoplasms compressing or occluding airways.

Physiotherapy management

Patient education is essential for optimal management and should include the factors outlined in the section on medical management.

Effective delivery of bronchodilators prior to airway clearance techniques or exercise is essential. A number of devices are available for the delivery of aerosols including nebulizers, metered-dose inhalers and dry powder inhalers (see Ch. 8). The doctor and physiotherapist should choose a delivery device suitable for the patient and educate the patient in its use including the appropriate breathing pattern necessary to ensure maximum penetration and deposition of the drug (Pedersen 1996).

Airway clearance techniques should be adapted to ensure that no increase in airflow limitation occurs (see Ch. 8).

For management of EIA see page 237.

Clinical outcomes

These may include a reduction in symptoms such as chest tightness, wheeze, cough, dyspnoea and an increase in exercise tolerance. With reversibility or improvement of airflow limitation, the abnormal findings observed in the breathing pattern may disappear (e.g. following recovery from an acute attack of asthma) or be reduced. Lung function and gas exchange abnormalities may be reversible depending on the underlying aetiology. Improved nocturnal control of asthma should lead to improved QOL.

PROBLEM – RESPIRATORY MUSCLE DYSFUNCTION

Weakness (the inability of rested muscles to generate the expected maximum force) and fatigue (the inability of muscle to sustain a given level of work or a loss in the capacity of a muscle to develop a force due to loaded muscle activity that is reversible by rest) of the respiratory muscles may occur in a wide range of conditions

(National Heart, Lung, and Blood Institute Workshop Summary 1990). Mild forms of dysfunction are often difficult to detect clinically and, in some patients, both weakness and fatigue may be present. Assessment of the respiratory muscles is important because:

- Dyspnoea in patients with no respiratory or cardiovascular disease may be due to respiratory muscle weakness
- There may be few clinical signs of dysfunction even in patients with moderate to severe weakness
- Respiratory muscle weakness is invariably present in patients with significant generalized neuromuscular disease and can be a compounding factor in many conditions, for example steroid myopathy and malnutrition (Polkey et al 1995)
- Respiratory muscle weakness may be the cause of ineffective cough.

The factors which predispose to respiratory muscle dysfunction can broadly be divided into three groups (Reid & Dechman 1995). The first group comprises factors which decrease the force-generating ability of the respiratory muscles, for example neuromuscular disorders, myopathies, connective tissue disorders and systemic abnormalities (endocrine disorders or metabolic abnormalities, including hypoxia, hypercapnia and metabolic acidosis). Factors which increase respiratory muscle work by increasing the WOB (e.g. changes in lung compliance or an increase in airway resistance) comprise the second group. The third group consists of factors which decrease the efficiency of the respiratory muscles (e.g. lung hyperinflation, flail chest). All these factors lead to respiratory muscle overload and predispose to fatigue (Reid & Dechman 1995).

Clinical features and assessment

The main features associated with respiratory muscle dysfunction are dyspnoea, a decrease in exercise tolerance and, in patients with more severe disease, type II respiratory failure (Reid & Dechman 1995). The patient may report breathlessness, especially when supine or when standing in water up to the chest, for example when entering the sea or a swimming pool (Mier et al 1986). The weight of water causes pressure on the abdominal wall and thus descent of the diaphragm is impeded. Daytime somnolence, early morning headaches and impaired mental function may be present if arterial desaturation and hypercapnia occur during sleep. In the dyspnoeic patient, the abnormalities in breathing pattern may include increased respiratory rate, decreased V_T, reduced chest expansion, use of accessory muscles, respiratory alternans (periods of breathing using only chest wall muscles alternating with periods of breathing using the diaphragm) and paradoxical movement of the rib cage or abdomen (Mier 1990, Wilkins et al 1990). Profound diaphragm weakness or paralysis gives rise to paradoxical inward abdominal movement occurring during inspiration and is most easily seen with the patient in supine (Laroche et al 1988). This occurs because of the passive transmission of the negative intrapleural pressure generated by the other inspiratory muscles which causes the abdominal contents to be pulled upwards, unresisted by the ineffectual diaphragm (Macklem 1982). When upright, recruitment of the abdominal muscles may occur during expiration in order to elevate the diaphragm so that gravity can assist diaphragm descent during inspiration (Gibson 1989). However, these clinical signs are often not present unless the diaphragm is paralysed or diaphragm strength is reduced to approximately 25% of normal (Mier-Jedrzejowicz et al 1988). The patient may have a weak cough which may be due to inadequate inspiration and/or weakness of the expiratory muscles. Weakness of the bulbar muscles may contribute to the impaired cough and may also contribute to aspiration. Physical examination may reveal signs of generalized muscle weakness and there may be marked weight loss.

The plain chest radiograph and fluoroscopic screening of the diaphragm during sniffing are useful diagnostic tools in hemidiaphragm weakness. The affected side is raised and moves paradoxically upwards on sniffing. Radiography and fluoroscopy are less useful when the problem is bilateral (Green & Laroche 1990). Movement of the diaphragm can also be assessed using ultrasonography (Polkey et al 1995). Chest radiographs may show a reduction in lung volume with elevated hemidiaphragms.

Lung function

Lung function may be normal in the absence of marked weakness. The characteristic abnormalities of inspiratory muscle weakness are a reduced VC and TLC. In the presence of severe bilateral diaphragm weakness, the VC is low when the patient is upright and typically falls by more than 50% when supine (Moxham 1995). This fall in VC is due to the weight of the abdominal contents in supine which push up against the diaphragm (Green & Laroche 1990). Measurement of VC is especially useful in the management of progressive disorders such as Guillain–Barré syndrome. Residual volume will be normal unless the expiratory muscles are also involved. The RV/TLC ratio is therefore normal or high but, in contrast to diseases characterized by airflow limitation, the FEV_1/FVC is not reduced. Carbon monoxide transfer coefficient is normal or raised (Green & Laroche 1990). Functional residual capacity is decreased due to the loss of end-expiratory tone in the muscles that hold the chest wall out. Muscle weakness occurring acutely has no effect on lung compliance but with persistent weakness both lung and chest wall compliance are reduced (Mier 1990, Polkey et al 1995). Global respiratory muscle strength can be assessed by measuring PiMax and PeMax but for quantification of diaphragmatic weakness the transdiaphragmatic pressure must be measured (see Ch. 3). Since respiratory muscle weakness is often associated with generalized muscle weakness, it is useful to obtain an indication of limb muscle strength, for example by measuring hand grip strength. Respiratory muscle endurance can be assessed by measuring the maximal voluntary ventilation and the maximum sustained ventilation or by assessing the ventilatory response to added inspiratory loads (Ferguson 1993, Clanton & Diaz 1995). Exercise

tolerance and QOL should also be assessed, when appropriate. The PaO_2 and the SaO_2 may be low due to microatelectasis and $\dot{V}/\dot{Q}$ mismatching (Mier 1990). Hypercapnia, in the absence of coexistent lung disease, is uncommon until VC has fallen to 50% of normal or the PiMax is reduced to 30% predicted (Moxham 1995).

Nocturnal blood gas abnormalities

In the patient with severe weakness of the respiratory muscles, hypercapnia often develops insidiously at night. When healthy subjects sleep, a degree of hypoventilation occurs which results in an increase in $PaCO_2$ of 0.3–1 kilopascals (kPa) (2–8 mmHg) and a fall in PaO_2 and SaO_2 of 0.4–1.3 kPa (3–10 mmHg) and 2–3% respectively (Hara & Shepard 1990). In the elderly, periods of apnoea, hypopnoea and desaturation frequently occur during sleep (Phillips et al 1992). Tidal volume is decreased by 15–25% and is shallower during rapid eye movement (REM) than non-REM sleep. In addition, hypercapnic and hypoxic ventilatory responses are depressed (Hara & Shepard 1990). Further problems occur during REM sleep in patients with diaphragm dysfunction because a reduction in the tone of the intercostal and accessory muscles increases the work of the diaphragm (Des Jardins 1990). Nocturnal desaturation in patients with respiratory muscle weakness is mainly due to hypoventilation. An additional mechanism in some patients might be increased $\dot{V}/\dot{Q}$ mismatching arising from the small fall in FRC which occurs during sleep (Hudgel & Devadatta 1984). With progressive hypoventilation, signs of type II respiratory failure develop.

Medical management

Patients with neurological dysfunction may recover spontaneously (e.g. Guillain–Barré syndrome) or may require periods of mechanical ventilation. For patients with a chronic disorder, assisted ventilation may be useful at night to rest the respiratory muscles and increase long-term survival and QOL. If the diaphragm is intact, pacing of the phrenic nerve may sustain ventilation. Adequate nutrition is essential for malnourished patients as is weight loss for obese patients (Fernandez et al 1993a). Correction of metabolic and electrolyte imbalance is necessary to reduce muscle weakness. Attempts have been made to improve respiratory muscle function with drugs. Methylxanthines may have a very small inotropic action and may be used in patients with impending respiratory failure (Fernandez et al 1993b, Jenne 1993).

Physiotherapy management

Respiratory muscle strength and endurance training may be achieved by resistive loading, hyperpnoeic loading or intensive upper limb exercise (see Ch. 14, p. 379, and Alison & Ellis 1992). Intensive upper limb exercise is probably more beneficial in patients who are able to sustain high levels of ventilation thus achieving a training effect of the ventilatory muscles. Patients with CAL may be unable to tolerate the high intensity of upper or lower limb exercise necessary to train the ventilatory muscles and are more likely to benefit from specific resistive loading of the respiratory muscles (Alison & Ellis 1992). Patients may also benefit from general exercise training to enhance oxygen transport (Dean & Ross 1992).

The presence of fatigue, for example in a patient who is acutely unwell, will necessitate that treatments are short and interspersed with sufficient rest periods.

Clinical outcomes

These depend on the aetiology. Benefits may be seen fairly rapidly if the underlying cause is a metabolic abnormality which is easily corrected. In selected patients, the benefits from resting the respiratory muscles using assisted nocturnal ventilation include physiological benefits of improved daytime blood gas tensions, respiratory muscle function and restoration of normal sleep pattern (Rochester 1993). Functional benefits are reflected by an increased work capacity and increased ability to participate in rehabilitation

programmes. Exercise training, incorporating intensive upper limb training and, in some patients inspiratory muscle training, may improve tolerance of dyspnoea, increase respiratory muscle strength and improve QOL.

In some patients, the underlying cause of respiratory muscle dysfunction is progressive and benefit from physiotherapy may largely be seen by the successful management of associated and potential problems, such as impaired airway clearance and prevention of chest infection.

PROBLEM – REDUCED LUNG VOLUME

Reduced lung volumes occur in a variety of situations and may be short-lived (e.g. following major surgery) or chronic (e.g. fibrotic lung disease). On occasions the cause is a disease process affecting the lung parenchyma but in many situations the reduction in lung volume arises from processes affecting other structures, such as the respiratory muscles or the pleura. Reduced lung volume is an almost universal finding following upper abdominal surgery or cardiothoracic surgery. The physiotherapist does not always have a role in the management of the problem, for example when the cause is abdominal ascites or pregnancy unassociated with respiratory disease. The pathophysiological basis for a reduction in lung volume, clinical examples, and examples of medical intervention are given in Table 10.5.

The main consequences of a decrease in lung volume are:

- Atelectasis in dependent lung regions.
- Impaired oxygenation due to $\dot{V}/\dot{Q}$ mismatching and, in some cases, intra-pulmonary shunting. This occurs because the small airways in the dependent lung regions may close during quiet breathing. With acute lobar atelectasis, hypoxaemia may be absent or minimal if there is an accompanying decrease in perfusion to the affected area (i.e. if hypoxic pulmonary vasoconstriction occurs). Low tidal volume breathing may be associated with a failure to clear the anatomical dead space.

Table 10.5 Pathophysiological basis for reduced lung volume, clinical examples and examples of medical intervention (Johnson & Pierson 1986)

Pathophysiological basis	Clinical examples	Examples of medical interventions
Atelectasis:	Normal consequence of UAS and CT surgery due to the anaesthetic, operation and changes occurring in the postoperative period including a lack of periodic deep breaths	CPAP
1. Reduced function of surfactant	ARDS, smoke inhalation, high FiO_2	Mechanical ventilation (e.g. PPV)
2. Airway obstruction	Foreign body, mucus plugging	Removal of foreign body/mucus by bronchoscopy
	Hilar adenopathy, mediastinal masses	Surgical removal, laser treatment, radiotherapy, chemotherapy
3. Negative airway pressure	Endobronchial suctioning	
Compression of lung tissue: 1. Pleural space encroachment	Effusion, empyema	Insertion of ICC; antibiotics or surgical decortication for empyema
2. Mediastinal structures	Tension pneumothorax causing mediastinal shift and compression of the contralateral lung	Insertion of ICC
3. Cardiomegaly	Decreases ventilation to left lower lobe when supine, e.g. left ventricular failure, IHD	Management of cause of cardiac failure
4. Abdominal distension	Obesity, ascites, following surgery, running-in phase of peritoneal dialysis, pregnancy	Dietary advice for the obese patient; drainage of ascites or peritoneal dialysis
Decrease in compliance: 1. Lung	Restrictive diseases, e.g. pulmonary fibrosis	Corticosteroids or immunosuppressants for some restrictive lung diseases Mechanical ventilation or support using BiPAP, NIPPV or NPV
2. Thorax	Kyphoscoliosis, ankylosing spondylitis; disruption to the integrity of the chest wall because of trauma, e.g. rib fractures	Surgical correction; PPV for patients with fractured ribs
Decreased ability of respiratory muscles to generate sufficient negative pressure	Respiratory muscle dysfunction (see Problem – respiratory muscle dysfunction)	Mechanical ventilation or support using BiPAP, NIPPV or NPV
Posture	Supine position associated with a low resting lung volume owing to increased thoracic blood volume	
Pain	May cause patient to take shallower breaths with the absence of sighs. Absence of sighs leads to atelectasis in dependent lung regions, reduces surfactant activity and decreases lung compliance	Pain control using analgesics administered orally, intramuscularly, intravenously, regional nerve blocks (epidural, intercostal nerve block), acupuncture/acupressure or hypnosis

Abbreviations: UAS, upper abdominal surgery; CT, cardiothoracic; CPAP, continuous positive airway pressure; ARDS, acute respiratory distress syndrome; FiO_2, fraction of inspired oxygen; PPV, positive pressure ventilation; ICC, intercostal catheter; IHD, ischaemic heart disease; BiPAP, bi-level positive airway pressure; NIPPV, non-invasive positive pressure ventilation; NPV, negative pressure ventilation.

• Inefficient cough due to the reduction in VC which reduces the ability to generate an adequate expiratory airflow.
• Increased WOB as airway resistance is increased and lung compliance is reduced.
• Decreased exercise tolerance due to the inability to meet the ventilatory demands of exercise.

Special case – the surgical patient

Following upper abdominal or cardiothoracic

surgery, a restrictive ventilatory defect and arterial hypoxaemia occur. The changes in lung function are most severe within the first 24–72 hours after surgery and are followed by a gradual return to preoperative levels. This may take up to 7 days after upper abdominal surgery and several weeks after cardiac surgery (Meyers et al 1975, Morran et al 1983, Jenkins et al 1990, Locke et al 1990). A rise in $PaCO_2$ is unusual unless marked respiratory depression occurs, for example following high doses of narcotic analgesics. However, in many patients lung function abnormalities will resolve spontaneously with normal postoperative care. Some patients have an increased risk of developing a postoperative chest infection or clinically significant atelectasis and it is important for the physiotherapist to be able to identify such patients. The following section discusses the factors which increase the likelihood of a patient developing a clinically significant postoperative pulmonary complication.

Studies show that chest infection occurs in approximately 15–20% of patients after abdominal surgery (Celli et al 1984, Hall et al 1991) and in no more than 10% of patients following cardiac surgery (Stock et al 1984, Jenkins et al 1989, Stiller et al 1994). These values assume that preoperative lung function is within the normal range. The risk of developing a chest infection is significantly increased in patients who smoke cigarettes or who have only recently ceased to smoke (Morran et al 1983, Warner et al 1989, Jenkins et al 1990, Dilworth & White 1992). The mechanisms responsible include mucus hypersecretion, impaired tracheobronchial clearance, bronchial hyperreactivity and impairment of the immune system (Pearce & Jones 1984, Fairshter & Williams 1987). The presence of chronic respiratory disease, in particular airflow limitation, increases the risk of respiratory infection in the postoperative period (Dilworth & White 1992).

Severe malnutrition significantly increases the chance of developing a postoperative chest infection (Garibaldi et al 1981, Windsor & Hill 1988). The factors responsible in malnourished patients are ineffective cough secondary to expiratory muscle weakness and impaired function of the immune system (Arora & Gal 1981, Arora & Rochester 1982, Rochester & Esau 1984, Branson & Hurst 1988).

An increased risk of postoperative pulmonary complications has been demonstrated in some studies of obese patients (Latimer et al 1971, Garibaldi et al 1981, Celli et al 1984). Obesity, even when mild, increases the WOB, lung volumes are reduced and gas exchange is impaired (Jenkins & Moxham 1991). The compliance of the respiratory system, particularly that of the chest wall, is decreased and excursion of the diaphragm is restricted (Naimark & Cherniack 1960, Farebrother 1979). Functional residual capacity is decreased leading to closure of small airways in dependent lung regions. These regions are therefore relatively overperfused and an increase in $\dot{V}/\dot{Q}$ mismatching is responsible for the reduction in PaO_2. The majority of obese and grossly obese subjects maintain a normal $PaCO_2$ (Farebrother 1979). Sleep apnoea is more common in obese patients and will be exacerbated by narcotics and benzodiazepines.

The evidence of advanced age as a risk factor is controversial (Celli et al 1984, Roukema et al 1988, Windsor & Hill 1988, Dilworth & White 1992). There appears, however, to be no absolute threshold of preoperative pulmonary function for predicting the occurrence of postoperative pulmonary complications; such information, when available, assists clinical decision making in the postoperative period (Tisi 1979, Gass & Olsen 1986). In patients with CAL, the most useful predictors of the need for prolonged assisted ventilation after surgery are the preoperative PaO_2 and whether the patient is breathless at rest, and not the FEV_1/FVC (Nunn et al 1988).

There is evidence that a nasogastric tube present for more than 24 hours postoperatively is associated with an increased frequency of postoperative pulmonary complications (Mitchell et al 1982, Dilworth & White 1992).

Other factors which have not been studied extensively but which are considered to increase the risk include emergency surgery, systemic dehydration and patient motivation. High levels of neuroticism or trait-anxiety are thought to slow the recovery from surgery (Mathews & Ridgeway 1981).

Clinical features and assessment

Many patients with reduced lung volumes present with the problems of dyspnoea, decreased exercise tolerance or mucus retention due to an ineffective cough. Orthopnoea may also be present.

In general there will be an abnormal breathing pattern characterized by a small V_T and increased rate. In the presence of pain, or fear of pain (e.g. in the patient with a surgical incision or pleuritic pain) there will be absence of periodic deep breaths. Chest expansion will be reduced and this may be a localized finding, for example in the area overlying a collapsed lobe.

The cough will be weak, owing mainly to the inability to generate adequate expiratory airflow because of the low V_T. Pain will inhibit effective coughing in some patients.

Symptoms resulting from acute lobar collapse depend on the extent of the collapse, the abruptness of onset and the underlying respiratory impairment. A slowly developing segmental or lobar collapse may produce few symptoms if the patient has otherwise normal lungs. If the same degree of collapse occurs suddenly in a patient with chronic lung disease, severe respiratory distress may develop.

On auscultation there will be absent, diminished or bronchial breath sounds. Over the area of a pneumothorax, the percussion note will be hyper-resonant.

Lung function testing will show a decrease in VC and all other lung volumes except when the expiratory muscles are weak, in which case the RV is raised. Peak inspiratory and expiratory mouth pressures may be reduced if there is weakness of the respiratory muscles. Hypoxaemia may be present primarily as a result of $\dot{V}/\dot{Q}$ mismatch resulting from changes in the FRC/closing volume relationship. Hypercapnia is often absent but will occur if there is associated hypoventilation.

Chest radiograph findings may be very helpful in identifying the cause of the reduction in lung volumes such as a pleural disorder, effusion, lobar or lung collapse.

Medical management

Medical management involves the management of the underlying cause of reduced lung volume. Examples of medical interventions are listed in Table 10.5.

Physiotherapy management

Patients with a high risk of developing a clinically significant postoperative pulmonary complication should be identified by the physiotherapist so that prophylactic treatment can be commenced.

Optimization of lung volumes is achieved by upright positioning. As upright positions increase FRC, high sitting, sitting out of bed and ambulation are encouraged. The side lying position is preferred to slumped or supine positions and may be modified by tilting the patient towards prone to further decrease compression on lung tissue. This is especially so in patients with abdominal distension (Jenkins et al 1988).

Tidal volume is increased using breathing exercises (e.g. thoracic expansion exercises, sustained maximal inspirations with or without the use of an incentive spirometer, intermittent positive pressure breathing) and manual hyperinflation. Ambulation increases $\dot{V}_E$ and is useful to assist with the re-expansion of lung tissue in patients with pleural disease or atelectasis. Functional residual capacity may be increased with the use of CPAP or BiPAP. In patients with pain, treatment should be performed when pain management is optimal (see Problem – pain, p. 256).

Obese patients may benefit from exercise programmes designed to achieve weight reduction provided that exercise is accompanied by dietary control.

Clinical outcomes

In the high-risk surgical patient, the main outcome should be the prevention of chest infection/clinically significant atelectasis.

Physiological improvements from physiotherapy intervention may include an increase in lung volumes, for example VC, and a rise in PaO_2 and SaO_2. Peak inspiratory and expiratory mouth pressures may increase if the cause is reversible weakness of the respiratory muscles. The physiological changes may be associated with an improvement in breathing pattern, a reduction in dyspnoea and an increase in exercise tolerance. Auscultation may reveal improved breath sounds to the affected area(s). Chest radiograph changes are not always a good indication of clinical progress, for example following coronary artery surgery small pleural effusions may persist for a considerable time after the patient has recovered clinically.

In the obese individual, the abnormal physiological changes will be reversed with weight loss (Thomas et al 1989).

PROBLEM – IMPAIRED GAS EXCHANGE

Impaired gas exchange is common in patients with respiratory or cardiovascular disease. In some patients, abnormalities may only become evident when increased demands are imposed on the respiratory and cardiovascular systems such as during exercise, with an infective exacerbation, or when changes in ventilation occur as a normal consequence of sleep. Gas exchange abnormalities rarely occur in the absence of one or more of the other problems discussed in this chapter. Although changes in ventilation arise in response to hypoxia and hypercapnia, dyspnoea is not necessarily present. An example of this is seen in the patient with interstitial oedema who has a low PaO_2 but in whom dyspnoea is due to the increased WOB caused by a reduction in lung compliance and not as a result of the hypoxaemia per se. The physiotherapist does not always have a role in the management of impaired gas exchange, for example in the patient with acute pulmonary embolus, or in the postoperative patient who has minimal hypoxaemia but is self-ambulating and has no other problems which are amenable to physiotherapy intervention.

The following section outlines the pathophysiology, clinical features and assessment of hypoxaemia, hypercapnia and hypocapnia (West 1990, Vas Fragoso 1993).

Hypoxaemia

This is seen in a wide range of conditions. The pathophysiological basis and clinical examples of hypoxaemia are given in Table 10.6.

Hypercapnia

A raised $PaCO_2$ is the hallmark of type II respiratory failure and accompanies a decrease in PaO_2. The pathophysiological basis of hypercapnia and clinical examples are given in Table 10.7.

Hypocapnia

In clinical practice, a low $PaCO_2$ is a far less common occurrence than a raised $PaCO_2$. An increase in rate or depth of breathing is not necessarily associated with hypocapnia. For example, a large V_T in conjunction with a slow rate may not reduce $PaCO_2$ below normal levels. Conversely, a low V_T and high rate, such as when panting, may not lower $PaCO_2$ or may even raise $PaCO_2$ if the V_T fails to clear the anatomic dead space (Gardner 1996). The pathophysiology of hyperventilation disorders is reviewed in detail by Gardner (1996).

Clinical features and assessment

Hypercapnia is a powerful respiratory stimulant and, under normal conditions, $PaCO_2$ is an important factor in the chemical control of ventilation. When the $PaCO_2$ is normal, there is little increase in ventilation until PaO_2 has fallen below 8 kPa (60 mmHg) (Weil et al 1975). When hypercapnia is present, the ventilatory response to hypoxia is enhanced (West 1990). The ventilatory response to hypoxia and hypercapnia varies considerably among subjects and is reduced with advanced age and during sleep (Hara & Shepard 1990, West 1990). In some patients with severe CAL, the ventilatory response to $PaCO_2$ is significantly decreased (West 1992). Patients may adapt to gradual changes in arterial

Table 10.6 Pathophysiological basis of hypoxaemia and clinical examples

Pathophysiological basis	Comment	Clinical examples
Hypoventilation	Site of abnormality:	
	1. Respiratory centre	Hypoxic and hypercapnic ventilatory drives depressed by drugs, anaesthesia and as a normal consequence of sleep
	2. Medulla	Trauma, neoplasm
	3. Spinal cord	Trauma, neoplasm
	4. Anterior horn cell	Poliomyelitis
	5. Innervation of the respiratory muscles	Phrenic nerve paralysis
	6. Disease of the myoneural junction	Myasthenia gravis
	7. Respiratory muscles	Weakness or fatigue from many causes (see Problem – respiratory muscle dysfunction)
	8. Upper airway obstruction	Foreign body, during sleep apnoea syndrome
	9. Excessive WOB	Variety of causes including added load on the mechanics of breathing such as in the patient with acute severe asthma who is exhausted
$\dot{V}/\dot{Q}$ mismatch	Low $\dot{V}/\dot{Q}$ ratio is the commonest cause of hypoxaemia in respiratory disease $\dot{V}/\dot{Q}$ mismatch arises owing to abnormalities in FRC/CV relationship, e.g.:	
	1. Decrease in FRC	Reduced lung volumes secondary to UAS or CT surgery, obesity, ascites, atelectasis, supine position, restrictive lung disease
	2. Increase in CV	Small airway closure due to AL, cigarette smoking, pulmonary oedema, increased age
	Perfusion limitation	Pulmonary embolus Pulmonary infarction
	Intrapulmonary shunt	Atelectasis, pneumonia, pulmonary oedema, ARDS
	Cardiac shunt	ASD, VSD
Diffusion limitation	Decrease in alveolar–capillary surface area	Emphysema
	Decrease in diffusion gradient	Low FiO_2 as occurs at high altitude
	Increased thickness of alveolar–capillary membrane	Scarring or fluid in the interstitial space, e.g. fibrotic lung disease, pulmonary oedema
	Decreased transit time of RBC in pulmonary capillary	May cause hypoxaemia on exercise in the presence of another cause of diffusion limitation
Decrease in FiO_2	High altitude	
	Malfunctioning of respiratory equipment	Disconnection of gas supply
	Endobronchial suctioning	
Mixed causes	Combination of $\dot{V}/\dot{Q}$ mismatch, diffusion limitation, shunt and hypoventilation	Seen in severe chronic lung disease
Imbalance between $\dot{V}O_2$ and DO_2	This causes a reduction in PvO_2 which reflects greater oxygen extraction to compensate for inadequate DO_2 relative to $\dot{V}O_2$. Low PvO_2 magnifies the effects of $\dot{V}/\dot{Q}$ mismatch and shunt on a patient's level of oxygenation	Low cardiac output states, severe anaemia, severe hypoxaemia

Abbreviations: WOB, work of breathing; $\dot{V}/\dot{Q}$, ventilation perfusion ratio; FRC, functional residual capacity; CV, closing volume; UAS, upper abdominal surgery; CT, cardiothoracic; AL, airflow limitation; ARDS, acute respiratory distress syndrome; ASD, atrial septal defect; VSD, ventricular septal defect; FiO_2, fraction of inspired oxygen; RBC, red blood cell; $\dot{V}O_2$, oxygen consumption; DO_2, oxygen delivery; PvO_2, mixed venous oxygen tension.

Table 10.7 Pathophysiological basis of hypercapnia and clinical examples (Vas Fragoso 1993)

Pathophysiological basis	Clinical examples
Hypoventilation: 1. Reduced central drive	Obesity–hypoventilation syndrome, depression of the respiratory centre due to unconsciousness, anaesthesia, narcotics, barbiturates
2. Respiratory muscle dysfunction	Variety of causes, e.g. neuromuscular disorders (see Problem – respiratory muscle dysfunction)
3. Added load on the mechanics of breathing	Changes in compliance of the lung or chest wall, e.g. chest wall trauma, pulmonary oedema, large pleural effusion, fibrotic lung disease Increase in airways resistance, e.g. severe CAL
Increased $\dot{V}CO_2$	Increased metabolism, e.g. fever, sepsis, trauma, burns, exercise Metabolic acidosis Nutritional supplements with excessive carbohydrate
Increased dead space as a fraction of V_T	CAL, pulmonary embolus, low lung volume breathing, e.g. with pain, respiratory muscle weakness

Abbreviations: CAL, chronic airflow limitation; $\dot{V}CO_2$, carbon dioxide production; V_T, tidal volume.

blood gas tensions whereas acute hypoxia and hypercapnia are less well tolerated.

There are few clinical features noticed with mild hypoxaemia. The features of moderate to severe hypoxaemia which develops acutely are restlessness, confusion, sweating, tachycardia, hypertension, skin pallor and cyanosis. As hypoxaemia worsens, pulmonary hypertension may develop and with severe hypoxaemia the cardiovascular system may respond with bradycardia and hypotension. Circulatory failure and shock occur when the PaO_2 falls to profoundly low levels (West 1992, Youtsey 1994). Hypoxaemia exacerbates cardiac arrhythmias and angina in patients with IHD and may predispose to heart failure. The long-term cardiovascular consequences of hypoxaemia are pulmonary hypertension and cor pulmonale. Raised levels of CO_2 in arterial blood cause vasodilatation. The patient has warm peripheries and the greatly increased cerebral blood flow is responsible for headache, raised cerebrospinal fluid pressure and sometimes papilloedema. A raised $PaCO_2$ may be associated with a flapping tremor of the outstretched hands (asterixis). The clinical features which result from a combination of hypoxia and hypercapnia on the central nervous system are restlessness, confusion, slurred speech and fluctuations of mood. High levels of $PaCO_2$ cause clouding of consciousness.

The signs and symptoms of hypocapnia are many and varied (Gardner 1996). They include tetany, and paraesthesia in the hands, face and trunk. A reduction in central nervous system and cerebral blood flow may be responsible for dizziness, loss of consciousness, visual disturbances, headache, tinnitus, ataxia and tremor. With acute hypocapnia, arterial BP falls and HR increases. Peripheral vasoconstriction is thought to be responsible for the complaint of cold hands. Hyperventilation is a cause of atypical chest pain. Hyperventilation may be associated, but is not synonymous, with dyspnoea. The physiotherapy assessment of the patient with a hyperventilation disorder is detailed in the chapter on hyperventilation disorders (Ch. 19).

Assessment must include measures of oxygenation, commonly the PaO_2 or SaO_2, the $PaCO_2$ and the arterial hydrogen ion concentration. These can be measured by intermittent arterial blood sampling or monitored continuously using a pulse oximeter for SpO_2 and a transcutaneous electrode for $PaCO_2$. Nocturnal monitoring of SaO_2 and $PaCO_2$ may provide important information. For patients with a suspected hyperventilation disorder, measurement of expired CO_2 is useful.

The age of the patient is an important consideration in the interpretation of PaO_2 values. Average values for PaO_2 range from 11.2–13.9 kPa (84–104 mmHg) in individuals aged 25 years and from 9.5–12.1 kPa (71–91 mmHg) for those aged 65 years (Nunn 1987). In addition, obesity decreases PaO_2 because of an increase in $\dot{V}/\dot{Q}$ mismatching unless there is coexisting obstructive sleep apnoea (Jenkins & Moxham 1991). Inter-observer reliability for the detection of central cyanosis is poor when SaO_2 is above 85%. Anaemia impairs the detection of central cyanosis, whereas it is more easily diagnosed if polycythaemia is present (Flenley 1990).

Medical management

The recognition and management of the underlying cause of hypoxaemia are essential. Oxygen therapy is indicated whenever tissue oxygenation is impaired, in order to allow essential metabolic reactions to occur, and to prevent complications attributed to hypoxaemia (Oh 1990).

Nocturnal and ambulatory oxygen are useful in patients who desaturate during sleep or during physical activity and may prevent/reverse the consequences of chronic hypoxaemia. Mechanical support such as CPAP, BiPAP, NIPPV or positive pressure ventilation may be required.

Impaired perfusion due to pulmonary emboli may only require thrombolytic therapy or surgical intervention.

Physiotherapy management

It is essential that the pathophysiological cause(s) is identified. Gas exchange may be optimized by patient positioning. In adult patients with unilateral lung pathology, during spontaneous breathing $\dot{V}/\dot{Q}$ matching may be improved by positioning in lying with the unaffected lung dependent. Hypoxaemia due to hypoventilation may be worsened by positioning in lying.

The use of breathing techniques (e.g. breathing control, pursed lip breathing) and assisted breathing devices (e.g. CPAP, BiPAP, NIPPV) may improve gas exchange. Physical activity may improve gas exchange by improving oxygen transport or may result in desaturation in some patients with severe cardiopulmonary dysfunction. Hypoxaemia is avoided by the correct application of techniques such as suctioning and can be avoided during periods of increased $\dot{V}O_2$

by using the correct oxygen therapy device and its correct application.

Clinical outcomes

As restoration of blood gas tensions and arterial hydrogen ion concentration to normal levels occurs there should be a measurable improvement in mental state. Depending on the presence of associated problems, there may be a reduction in dyspnoea and an increase in exercise tolerance. Long-term domiciliary oxygen therapy has been shown to improve survival and QOL in patients with cor pulmonale by ameliorating the adverse cardiovascular effects of chronic hypoxaemia.

PROBLEM – ABNORMAL BREATHING PATTERN

This rarely occurs alone and is more usually associated with other problems many of which are amenable to physiotherapy intervention. Such associated problems include airflow limitation, reduced lung volumes, impaired airway clearance and impaired gas exchange. Many patients who have an abnormal breathing pattern will complain of breathlessness. The pathophysiological basis of an abnormal breathing pattern and clinical examples are given in Table 10.8.

Clinical features and assessment

These include abnormalities in rate, depth, including excessive sighing or breath-holding, and changes in the inspiratory to expiratory ratio. Observation and palpation may reveal limited or asymmetrical chest wall movement, asynchronous movements or respiratory alternans. The patient may use the accessory muscles of inspiration and fix the shoulder girdle in order to maximize accessory muscle function. Abdominal movement may be absent or significantly reduced and, on palpation, the anterior abdominal wall may be splinted. Increased abdominal effort during expiration may be present owing to recruitment of the accessory expiratory muscles.

Table 10.8 Pathophysiological basis of abnormal breathing pattern and clinical examples (MacIntyre 1990, Tobin 1990)

Pathophysiological basis	Clinical examples
Increase in elastic or resistive WOB due to abnormalities of the lung or thorax	Decrease in C_L or C_T, e.g. pulmonary fibrosis, kyphoscoliosis, ankylosing spondylitis, obesity Any factor causing airflow limitation (see Problem – airflow limitation)
Impaired ventilatory pump	Respiratory muscle dysfunction from a variety of causes (see Problem – respiratory muscle dysfunction)
Abnormal respiratory centre control	Depression of the respiratory centre due to loss of consciousness, anaesthesia, narcotics, barbiturates
CNS disorders	Ataxic (Biot's) breathing Irregular pattern. Variable V_T with periods of apnoea
Brain stem disorders	Apneustic breathing – slow rate, large V_T followed by apnoea, irregular rhythm
Cerobrovascular disorders	Cheyne–Stokes respiration – cyclical pattern of periods of deep breathing becoming progressively more shallow and then periods of apnoea. Seen in severe neurological disorders and occasionally in LVF, uraemia, drug-induced respiratory depression
Chemical control of breathing	Hypoxia, hypercapnia and acid–base disturbances (raised H^+) increase ventilation
Renal acidosis, diabetic ketoacidosis	Kussmaul breathing – large V_T, fast, normal or slow rate, high $\dot{V}_E$
Stimulation from intrapulmonary receptors	Irritant receptors (rapidly adapting) respond to chemical or physical stimuli Pulmonary stretch receptors (slowly adapting) respond to marked increases in lung volume C-fibre receptors deep within lung parenchyma (J receptors) and in bronchi respond to vascular engorgement and congestion, chemical stimuli and less so to mechanical stimuli
Voluntary factors	Inhibition of sighs owing to pain from abdominal or thoracic incisions, pleural disorders, e.g. pleurisy, pneumothorax
Anxiety	May be associated with a variety of abnormal patterns including excessive sighing, rapid breathing, small V_T, breath-holding

Abbreviations: WOB, work of breathing; C_L, lung compliance; C_T, thoracic compliance; CNS, central nervous system; V_T, tidal volume; LVF, left ventricular failure; H^+, hydrogen ions; $\dot{V}_E$, minute ventilation.

If WOB is markedly increased, the patient's posture may show the characteristic features of a fixed shoulder girdle and dilatation of the nares may be evident. Pursed-lip breathing may be seen if the cause of the abnormal breathing pattern is moderate to severe airflow limitation. Assessment may reveal signs of chronic lung hyperinflation (see Problem – airflow limitation, p. 242). Arterial blood gas analysis, pulmonary function test results, auscultatory and chest radiograph findings may demonstrate abnormalities consistent with an underlying problem.

Medical management

Recognition of the underlying cause and amelioration where possible are essential. Management is mainly directed at reducing the WOB.

Disorders of the brain stem or central nervous system may resolve spontaneously or as a result of interventions aimed at decreasing intracranial pressure (e.g. corticosteroids, paralysis and positive pressure ventilation).

Physiotherapy management

Physiotherapy management of associated problems such as airflow limitation, reduced lung volume, impaired airway clearance and impaired gas exchange may reduce the WOB. In some patients, abnormal breathing patterns such as pursed lip breathing and fixation of the shoulder girdle are necessary to optimize gas exchange (Breslin 1995). Breathing patterns should not be altered in these patients and breathing strategies such as pursed-lip breathing are often encouraged. The excessive use of muscle activity should be discouraged and positioning used to relieve dyspnoea and reduce $\dot{V}O_2$. Breathing strategies used to relieve dyspnoea (e.g. breathing control, exhale with effort, paced breathing) may be useful to improve breathing patterns during activity and rest. When an abnormal breathing pattern results from anxiety, strategies such as relaxation and breathing control are encouraged (see Ch. 19).

Neurophysiological facilitation techniques may be used to alter rate and depth of breathing in some patients (Ch. 8, p. 163).

Clinical outcomes

These will be evaluated by assessment of the presenting breathing pattern and changes in the pattern in response to physiotherapy. Benefits from physiotherapy intervention may include associated improvements in exercise tolerance and QOL, and a reduction in dyspnoea.

PROBLEM – PAIN

This section discusses pain of respiratory and cardiovascular origin as well as other causes of pain located in the chest.

Patients tend not to ignore chest pain unless it has a familiar and recurrent pattern. Thus, patients may be more likely to seek medical advice for chest pain than for chronic cough and sputum production, especially when cough and sputum occur in a patient who smokes cigarettes.

Chest pain of respiratory origin

Pain of respiratory origin arises from the parietal pleura and from stimulation of the mucosa of the trachea and main bronchus. The lung parenchyma and visceral pleura are insensitive to pain. However, inflammatory processes in peripheral regions of the lung that involve the overlying visceral pleura often lead to pain from involvement of the adjacent parietal pleura. The origin and characteristic features of pain of respiratory origin, together with clinical examples, are given in Table 10.9.

Chest pain of cardiovascular origin

Table 10.10 outlines the main causes and characteristic features of pain of cardiovascular origin.

Clinical features and assessment

Clinical features are outlined in Tables 10.9. and 10.10. Associated with the pain may be signs

Table 10.9 Site and characteristic features of chest pain of respiratory origin (Murray & Basbaum 1994)

Origin	Characteristic features	Stimulus	Clinical examples
Pleura Tends to be limited to the affected region but may be referred to the ipsilateral neck or shoulder tip or to the upper abdomen or lower back	Sharp stabbing pain due to inflammation or stretching of the parietal pleura Described as sharp, dull, ache, burning or a catching pain	Exacerbated by deep inspiration, coughing, and sneezing May be associated with dyspnoea	Pneumonia, carcinoma, pulmonary tuberculosis, pneumothorax, pleurisy, pulmonary infarction
Chest wall pain Commonly due to strain, inflammation, malposition of, or injury to, muscles, ligaments, cartilage or bone	Usually localized to affected area May be a dull ache or sharper pain	Usually increased on respiratory movements, including deep inspiration and cough Also exacerbated by trunk and shoulder movements	Often seen in patients with chronic cough or dyspnoea Post-ICC insertion, CT surgery, fractured ribs, musculoskeletal disorders Tumours involving ribs or soft tissues
Tracheobronchial tree	Generally described as a raw, retrosternal discomfort or a dull ache	Deep inspiration, coughing	Usually acute inflammation from infection or from inhalation of irritant fumes May occur with oxygen therapy

Abbreviations: ICC, intercostal catheter; CT, cardiothoracic.

Table 10.10   Causes and characteristic features of chest pain of cardiovascular origin

Cause	Characteristic features	Stimuli
Myocardial ischaemia: 1. Stable angina pectoris	Myocardial ischaemia does not always cause pain Described as severe pressure, squeezing, ache, tightness or retrosternal burning Maximal intensity is retrosternal or to the left of the sternum but may radiate to the neck, jaw, shoulder or down the inner aspects of the arms, more commonly the left Often associated with dyspnoea	Physical exertion – often occurs at the same RPP Emotional stimuli Heavy meal Inhalation of cigarette smoke With rest, the pain tends to subside within 2–10 minutes Relieved by nitroglycerin
2. Unstable angina pectoris	As for stable angina	Unpredictable pattern and may occur at rest
3. Myocardial infarction	Pain is similar to that of angina but is much more severe and of longer duration	Usually requires large doses of opiates to control the pain
Pain mimicking angina is common in patients with aortic stenosis and occurs in some patients with mitral valve prolapse, myocarditis and hypertrophic cardiomyopathy		
Pericarditis due to inflammation of parietal pericardium from a variety of causes – bacterial, viral, neoplasm, post-MI	Sharp stabbing pain, central or left side of chest and left arm and may radiate to neck, back and upper abdomen May be associated with friction rub in the absence of effusion	Deep inspiration, supine and left side lying positions Sitting and leaning forwards may decrease pain
Diseases of the aorta: 1. Aortic stenosis 2. Dissection of the aorta	Produces angina-like pain on exertion Searing severe pain of sudden onset May present in upper back and may radiate to neck and face	
Peripheral vascular disease	Cramp-like pain in the calves, thighs and buttocks May be accompanied by profound weakness in the legs	In the early stages pain occurs on exercise (intermittent claudication) and is relieved by rest With severe ischaemia, rest pain and paraesthesia occur, especially when in bed

Abbreviations: RPP, rate pressure product (systolic blood pressure × heart rate); MI, myocardial infarction.

of an abnormal breathing pattern and systemic signs such as sweating, pallor and tachycardia. In addition to the subjective history, pain scales, for example VAS, or pain questionnaires should be used to quantify pain and its effects on function. Several scales are available to assess the severity of angina occurring with exercise, for example the American College of Sports Medicine scale (1995):

1+ Light, barely noticeable
2+ Moderate, bothersome
3+ Severe, very uncomfortable
4+ Most severe or intense pain ever experienced.

An alternative scale is provided in the chapter on cardiac rehabilitation (Ch. 15). Measurement of the RPP may be useful in patients with IHD who are undergoing exercise training.

Chest pain which is unrelated to respiratory or cardiovascular disease

Neural, muscular or skeletal pain. Examples of causative factors are disc degeneration, bony metastases, muscle injuries, inflammation of soft tissues and disorders of the costal cartilages.

Oesophageal pain. The causes of pain arising from the oesophagus are:

1. Spasm – when this occurs the pain may last up to 1 hour and there may not be an obvious provoking factor. The pain closely resembles that of unstable angina and is often relieved by nitroglycerin.

2. Oesophageal tear – this may occur in association with prolonged vomiting. The pain is felt centrally.

3. Gastro-oesophageal reflux gives rise to pain felt in the centre of the chest and the epigastrium. The pain is increased when lying down and relieved by sitting upright and by taking antacids. The commonest cause is hiatus hernia.

Peptic ulceration and gallbladder disease. Diseases of the stomach, duodenum or biliary system may give rise to pain felt in the chest although it is more commonly confined to the abdomen. With peptic ulceration the pain is burning in nature, occurs following meals and is relieved by antacids.

The postprandial pain occurring in gastric ulceration may resemble angina following heavy meals.

Pain of biliary origin is usually colicky in nature and felt on the right side of the abdomen, the front and back of the chest. The pain may be related to the ingestion of certain foods.

'Pseudoangina' due to hyperventilation syndrome. Hyperventilation may cause atypical chest pain which may mimic angina in some patients (Gardner 1996).

Medical management

Diagnosis and management of the underlying cause are essential.

Anti-inflammatory agents or analgesics are used for musculoskeletal, pleuritic or pericardial pain. Pain relief may also be achieved using acupuncture/acupressure or hypnosis. Medical management of chest pain for coronary insufficiency is based on reducing myocardial oxygen demand. Management of angina may include pharmacological therapy, angioplasty or coronary artery surgery. Antiarrhythmic drugs and anticoagulants may be indicated in some patients. Management of cardiac dysfunction may include insertion of a pacemaker or heart transplantation.

Methods to reduce risk factors may include education on smoking cessation, the benefits of regular physical exercise, dietary management, and the use of lipid-lowering drugs to reduce hyperlipaemia and body weight, counselling on lifestyle changes and hormone replacement therapy for menopausal women.

Patients and families often require psycho-emotional support especially when pain is of cardiac origin, as such pain is often associated with a fear of impending death.

Management of intermittent claudication includes the use of analgesics. In some patients, hyperbaric oxygen may be indicated. Revascularization procedures for significant stenosis include bypass surgery (e.g. aortofemoral and axillofemoral bypass) or transluminal angioplasty. Amputation may be necessary if repeated attempts at grafting fail and further grafting becomes impossible.

Physiotherapy management

Direct methods of pain management include heat modalities, interferential, transcutaneous electrical nerve stimulation (p. 200), Entonox (p. 300), acupuncture (p. 202) and manual therapy (p. 192). Knowledge of pain management (drugs and their onset/duration of action, route of administration) is required so that treatment can be provided when pain management is optimal.

Education of the patient regarding risk factors for cardiovascular disease (described in the section on medical management), exercise training and exercise for weight reduction are essential for the prevention or progression of disease. For the management of patients with stable angina and patients following myocardial infarction including risk factor modification and exercise training, see chapter on cardiac rehabilitation (Ch. 15).

Special case – intermittent claudication

Exercise training for patients with intermittent claudication as the limiting factor to exercise is important. Aerobic exercise such as walking or cycling is most beneficial. This can take the form of interval training with the patient exercising to the point of pain intolerance. Progression to continuous aerobic activity is necessary to develop a higher mechanical efficiency for performance of the specific activity and a higher anaerobic capacity (tolerance to ischaemic pain and blood lactate). Improvement of leg muscle oxygenation following exercise training may be due to: increased blood flow through collateral vessels and the development of collaterals, higher arterial–venous oxygen difference locally, more local muscle capillary beds and higher levels of oxidative enzymes (Cohen & Michel 1988).

Education on foot care and hygiene for the prevention of gangrene includes the avoidance of minor trauma, poorly fitted footwear and the importance of regular toenail clipping.

Clinical outcomes

These should include a reduction in pain and an increase in function as measured using pain scales and from subjective questioning. There may be a decreased need for analgesics. In the patient with stable angina pectoris, endurance exercise training should be associated with an improved exercise tolerance and the onset of angina at a higher RPP. An increased distance walked before the onset of leg pain and fatigue, and a reduction in symptoms at rest should occur in the patient with intermittent claudication.

PROBLEM – MUSCULOSKELETAL DYSFUNCTION – POSTURAL ABNORMALITIES, DECREASED COMPLIANCE, OR DEFORMITY OF THE CHEST WALL

The risk of developing chest wall stiffness and abnormal posture is greatest in patients with chronic respiratory disease especially when this is associated with lung hyperinflation. Also at risk are patients following sternotomy or thoracotomy and patients who receive mechanical ventilation for long periods. Changes in muscle length, strength and endurance will occur as a result of chest wall and postural abnormalities.

As a number of these patients will be in the older age group they will, in addition, have age-related changes affecting the musculoskeletal system. With increased age, there is a decrease in the range of movement of the costovertebral joints and a decrease in the elasticity of the cartilage in the thoracic spine. These changes increase thoracic kyphosis.

Clinical features and assessment

The patient may present with an abnormal posture, reduced range of movement of the cervical spine, thoracic spine and glenohumeral joint, and may complain of pain or stiffness resulting in decreased function.

The assessment of pain, associated functional limitation, posture, muscle length, strength and endurance, and joint range of movement are covered in detail in the chapter on physiotherapy skills and techniques (Ch. 8).

Medical management

Management of chronic chest wall deformities may include the use of non-steroidal anti-inflammatory agents when pain is an accompanying feature. External bracing or surgical correction may be used to correct deformity (Adams & Hamblen 1995).

Physiotherapy management

Physiotherapy management should include, where appropriate, postural correction, stretching of tight muscles, mobilizations to the cervical spine and thoracic spine, costotransverse, costochondral and sternochondral joints, to the ribs, and to the glenohumeral joint (Vibekk 1991, Bray et al 1995) and muscle strengthening exercises. Postural correction and stretches to improve chest wall mobility should be incorporated into other active exercises and activities of daily living. Where possible, especially when chronic lung disease is present, patients should be taught to perform their own treatment including mobilizations.

The patient's position during treatment will need to be carefully selected as many patients will not be able to lie prone or supine owing to dyspnoea, and mobilizations will have to be performed in sitting or forward lean sitting.

The physiotherapy management of this problem is covered in detail in Chapter 8.

Clinical outcomes

These should include improved posture, an increase in VC and in the range of movement of the cervical spine, thoracic spine and glenohumeral joints. Associated with the increased range of movement should be an improvement in function and a decrease in pain. These changes may be associated with a decrease in dyspnoea. The psychosocial benefits may consist of enhanced self-esteem as a result of improved physical appearance, and improved QOL.

ACKNOWLEDGEMENTS

We wish to thank the following for their assistance with this chapter: Peter Middleton for his advice regarding the contents of the chapter and for editing the sections on medical management; Nola Cecins and Lorna Johnson for reviewing the chapter.

REFERENCES

Aaronson N K 1989 Quality of life assessment in clinical trials: methodologic issues. Controlled Clinical Trials 10: 195S–208S

Adams J C, Hamblen D L 1995 Outline of orthopaedics, 12th edn. Churchill Livingstone, Edinburgh, ch 10

Alison J, Ellis, E 1992 Pulmonary limitations to exercise performance. In: Ellis E, Alison J (eds) Key issues in cardiorespiratory physiotherapy. Butterworth-Heinemann, Oxford, ch 7

American College of Sports Medicine 1995 ACSM's guidelines for exercise testing and prescription, 5th edn. Williams & Wilkins, Baltimore, pp 99–100

Arora N S, Gal T J 1981 Cough dynamics during progressive expiratory muscle weakness in healthy curarized subjects. Journal of Applied Physiology 5(3): 494–498

Arora N S, Rochester D F 1982 Respiratory muscle strength and maximal voluntary ventilation in undernourished patients. American Review of Respiratory Disease 126(2): 5–9

Barnes P J 1994 Airway pharmacology. In: Murray J F, Nadel J A (eds) Respiratory medicine, 2nd edn. W B Saunders, Philadelphia, vol 1, ch 10

Bone R C 1996 Goals of asthma management. A step-care approach. Chest 109(4): 1056–1065

Branson R D, Hurst J M 1988 Nutrition and respiratory function: food for thought. Respiratory Care 33(2): 89–92

Bray C E, Partridge J E, Banks S K 1995 Thoracic mobilisation in the management of respiratory and cardiac patients. Proceedings of the Australian Physiotherapy Association Cardiothoracic Special Group, 4th National Conference, 22–24th April, Melbourne

Breslin E H 1995 Breathing retraining in chronic pulmonary disease. Journal of Cardiopulmonary Rehabilitation 15: 25–33

Brewis R A L 1991 Lecture notes on respiratory disease, 4th edn. Blackwell Scientific Publications, Oxford, p 26

British Thoracic Society, National Asthma Campaign, Royal College of Physicians of London et al 1997 The British guidelines on asthma management – 1995 review and position statement. Thorax 52(suppl 1): S1–S21

Burns B H, Howell J B L 1969 Disproportionately severe breathlessness in chronic bronchitis. Quarterly Journal of Medicine 38: 277–294

Celli B R 1994 Physical reconditioning of patients with respiratory diseases: legs, arms, and breathing retraining. Respiratory Care 39(5): 481–495

Celli B R, Rodriguez K S, Snider G L 1984 A controlled trial of intermittent positive pressure breathing, incentive spirometry, and deep breathing exercises in preventing pulmonary complications after abdominal surgery. American Review of Respiratory Disease 130: 12–15

Cheitlin M D, Sokolow M, McIlroy M B 1993 Clinical cardiology, 6th edn. Prentice Hall, London, pp 39–41

Clanton T L, Diaz P T 1995 Clinical assessment of the respiratory muscles. Physical Therapy 75(11): 983–995

Clarke S 1990 Physical defences. In: Brewis R A L, Gibson G J, Geddes D M (eds) Respiratory medicine. Baillière Tindall, London, pp 176–189

Cohen M, Michel T H 1988 Cardiopulmonary symptoms in physical therapy practice. Churchill Livingstone, New York, pp 207–209

Conway J H, Fleming J S, Perring S, Holgate S T 1992 Humidification as an adjunct to chest physiotherapy in aiding tracheo-bronchial clearance in patients with bronchiectasis. Respiratory Medicine 86(2): 109–114

Curtis J R, Deyo R A, Hudson L D 1994 Health-related quality of life among patients with chronic obstructive pulmonary disease. Thorax 49: 162–170

Dean E, Ross J 1992 Mobilisation and exercise conditioning. In: Zadai C C (ed) Pulmonary management in physical therapy. Churchill Livingstone, New York, ch 8

Des Jardins T 1990 Clinical manifestations of respiratory disease, 2nd edn. Mosby Year Book, St Louis, pp 60–61, 286

Dilworth J P, White R J 1992 Postoperative chest infection after upper abdominal surgery: an important problem for smokers. Respiratory Medicine 86: 205–210

Dudley D L, Glaser E M, Jorgenson B N, Logan D L 1980 Psychosocial concomitants to rehabilitation in chronic obstructive pulmonary disease: Part 1. Psychosocial and psychological considerations. Chest 77(3): 413–420

Eakin E G, Kaplan R M, Ries A L 1993 Measurement of dyspnoea in chronic obstructive pulmonary disease. Quality of Life Research 2: 181–191

Fairshter R D, Williams J H 1987 Pulmonary physiology in the postoperative period. Critical Care Clinics 3(2): 287–306

Farebrother M J B 1979 Respiratory function and cardiorespiratory response to exercise in obesity. British Journal of Diseases of the Chest 73: 211–229

Feinstein A R, Fisher M B, Pigeon J G 1989 Changes in dyspnoea-fatigue ratings as indicators of quality of life in the treatment of congestive heart failure. American Journal of Cardiology 64: 50–55

Fernandez E, Park S, Make B J 1993a Nutritional issues in pulmonary rehabilitation. Seminars in Respiratory Medicine 14(6): 482–494

Fernandez E, Tanchoco-Tan M, Make B J 1993b Methods to improve respiratory muscle function. Seminars in Respiratory Medicine 14(6): 446–465

Ferguson G T 1993 Respiratory muscle function in chronic obstructive pulmonary disease. Seminars in Respiratory Medicine 14(6): 430–445

Flenley D C 1990 Respiratory medicine, 2nd edn. Baillière Tindall, London, p 56

Foltz B D, Benumof J L 1987 Mechanisms of hypoxemia and hypercapnia in the perioperative period. Critical Care Clinics 3(2): 269–286

Foster C, Oldridge N B, Dion W et al 1995 Time course of recovery during cardiac rehabilitation. Journal of Cardiopulmonary Rehabilitation 15(3): 209–215

Gardner W N 1996 The pathophysiology of hyperventilation disorders. Chest 109(2): 516–534

Garibaldi R A, Britt M R, Coleman M L, Reading J C, Pace N L 1981 Risk factors for post-operative pneumonia. The American Journal of Medicine 70: 677–680

Gass G D, Olsen G N 1986 Preoperative pulmonary function testing to predict postoperative morbidity and mortality. Chest 89(1): 127–135

George R J D, Winter R J D, Flockton S J et al 1985 Ventilatory saving by external chest wall compression or oral high frequency oscillation in normal subjects and those with chronic airflow limitation. Clinical Science 69: 349–359

Gibson G 1989 Diaphragmatic paresis: pathophysiology, clinical features and investigation. Thorax 44: 960–970

Gift A G, Plant S M, Jacox A 1986 Psychologic and physiologic factors related to dyspnea in subjects with chronic obstructive pulmonary disease. Heart Lung 15(6): 595–601

Green M, Laroche C M 1990 Respiratory muscle weakness. In: Brewis R A L, Gibson G J, Geddes D M (eds) Respiratory medicine. Baillière Tindall, London, pp 1373–1387

Guyatt G H, Berman L B, Townsend M, Pugsley S O, Chambers L W 1987 A measure of quality of life for clinical trials. Thorax 42: 773–778

Hall J C, Tarala R, Harris J, Tapper J, Christiansen K 1991 Incentive spirometry versus routine chest physiotherapy for prevention of pulmonary complications after abdominal surgery. Lancet 337: 953–956

Hamilton A L, Killian K J, Summers E, Jones N L 1995 Muscle strength, symptom intensity, and exercise capacity

in patients with cardiorespiratory disorders. American Journal of Respiratory and Critical Care Medicine 152: 2021–2031

Hansen J E, Wasserman K 1996 Pathophysiology of activity limitation in patients with interstitial lung disease. Chest 109(6): 1566–1576

Hara K S, Shepard J W 1990 Sleep and critical care medicine. In: Martin R J (ed) Cardiorespiratory disorders during sleep. Futura, Mount Kisco, pp 324–325

Hardy K A 1994 A review of airway clearance: new techniques, indications and recommendations. Respiratory Care 39(5): 440–452

Henderson K, Cole J 1992 The effects of exercise rehabilitation on perceived self-efficacy. Australian Journal of Physiotherapy 38(3): 195–201

Honeyman P, Barr P, Stubbing D G 1996 Effect of a walking aid on disability, oxygenation, and breathlessness in patients with chronic airflow limitation. Journal of Cardiopulmonary Rehabilitation 16: 63–67

Hough A 1996 Physiotherapy in respiratory care. A problem-solving approach to respiratory and cardiac management, 2nd edn. Chapman & Hall, London, pp 164–166

Howell J B L 1990 Breathlessness. In: Brewis R A L, Gibson G J, Geddes D M (eds) Respiratory medicine. Baillière Tindall, London, pp 221–228

Hudgel D W, Devadatta P 1984 Decrease in functional residual capacity during sleep in normal humans. Journal of Applied Physiology 57(5): 1319–1322

Hyland M E, Bott J, Singh S, Kenyon C A P 1994 Domains, constructs and the development of the breathing problems questionnaire. Quality of Life Research 3: 245–256

Irwin R S, Widdicombe J 1994 Cough. In: Murray J F, Nadel J A (eds) Textbook of respiratory medicine, 2nd edn. W B Saunders, Philadelphia, vol 1, ch 20

Jenkins S C, Moxham J 1991 The effects of mild obesity on lung function. Respiratory Medicine 85: 309–311

Jenkins S C, Soutar S A, Moxham J 1988 The effects of posture on lung volumes in normal subjects and in patients pre- and post-coronary artery surgery. Physiotherapy 74(10): 492–496

Jenkins S C, Soutar S A, Loukota J M, Johnson L C, Moxham J 1989 Physiotherapy after coronary artery surgery – are breathing exercises necessary? Thorax 44: 634–639

Jenkins S C, Soutar S A, Loukota J M, Johnson L C, Moxham J 1990 A comparison of breathing exercises, incentive spirometry and mobilisation after coronary artery surgery. Physiotherapy Theory and Practice 6: 117–126

Jenne J W 1993 Pharmacology in the respiratory patient. In: Hodgkin J E, Connors G L, Bell W C (eds) Pulmonary rehabilitation. Guidelines to success, 2nd edn. J B Lippincott, Philadelphia, ch 9

Johnson N T, Pierson D J 1986 The spectrum of pulmonary atelectasis: pathophysiology, diagnosis, and therapy. Respiratory Care 31(11): 1107–1120

Jones P W, Quirk F H, Baveystock C M 1991 The St George's Respiratory Questionnaire. Respiratory Medicine 85(suppl B): 25–31

Jones P W, Quirk F H, Baveystock C M, Littlejohns P 1992 A self-complete measure of health status for chronic airflow limitation. The St. George's respiratory questionnaire. American Review of Respiratory Disease 145: 1321–1327

Judson M A, Sahn S A 1994 Mobilization of secretions in ICU patients. Respiratory Care 39(3): 213–226

Kaplan R M, Reis A, Atkins C J 1985 Behavioural issues in the management of chronic obstructive pulmonary disease. Annals of Behavioural Medicine 7: 5–9

Keilty S E J, Ponte J, Fleming T A, Moxham J 1994 Effect of inspiratory pressure support on exercise tolerance and breathlessness in patients with severe stable chronic obstructive pulmonary disease. Thorax 49: 990–994

Kinney M R, Burfitt S N, Stullenbarger E, Rees B, DeBolt M R 1996 Quality of life in cardiac patient research: a meta-analysis. Nursing Research 45(3): 173–180

Laroche C M, Carroll N, Moxham J, Green M 1988 Clinical significance of severe isolated diaphragm weakness. American Review of Respiratory Disease 138: 862–866

Laslett L, Paumer L, Amsterdam E A 1987 Exercise training in coronary artery disease. Cardiology Clinics 5(2): 211–225

Latimer R G, Dickman M, Day W C, Gunn M L, Schmidt S D 1971 Ventilatory patterns and pulmonary complications after upper abdominal surgery determined by preoperative and postoperative computerized spirometry and blood gas analysis. American Journal of Surgery 122: 622–632

Levison H, Cherniack R M 1968 Ventilatory cost of exercise in chronic obstructive pulmonary disease. Journal of Applied Physiology 25: 21–25

Locke T J, Griffiths T L, Mould H, Gibson G J 1990 Rib cage mechanics after median sternotomy. Thorax 45: 465–468

McCarren B 1992 Dynamic pulmonary hyperinflation. Australian Journal of Physiotherapy 38(3): 175–179

MacIntyre N R 1990 Respiratory monitoring without machinery. Respiratory Care 35(6): 546–553

Macklem P T 1982 The diaphragm in health and disease. Journal of Laboratory and Clinical Medicine 99(5): 601–610

Mahler D A 1987 Dyspnea: Diagnosis and management. Clinics in Chest Medicine 8(2): 215–230

Manning H L, Schwartzstein R M 1995 Pathophysiology of dyspnea. New England Journal of Medicine 333(23): 1547–1553

Markwell S, Sapsford R 1995 Physiotherapy management of obstructed defaecation. Australian Journal of Physiotherapy 41(4): 279–283

Mathews A, Ridgeway V 1981 Personality and surgical recovery: a review. British Journal of Clinical Psychology 20: 243–260

Mayou R, Bryant B 1993 Quality of life in cardiovascular disease. British Heart Journal 69: 460–466

Meyers J R, Lembeck L, O'Kane H, Baue A E 1975 Changes in functional residual capacity of the lung after operation. Archives of Surgery 110: 576–583

Mier A 1990 Respiratory muscle weakness. Respiratory Medicine 84: 351–359

Mier A K, Brophy C, Green M 1986 Out of depth, out of breath. British Medical Journal 292: 1495–1496

Mier-Jedrzejowicz A, Brophy C, Moxham J, Green M 1988 Assessment of diaphragm weakness. American Review of Respiratory Disease 137: 877–883

Mitchell C, Garrahy P, Peake P 1982 Postoperative respiratory morbidity: identification and risk factors. Australian and New Zealand Journal of Surgery 52(2): 203–209

Morran C G, Finlay I G, Mathieson M, McKay A J, Wilson N, McArdle C S 1983 Randomized controlled trial of physiotherapy for post-operative pulmonary complications. British Journal of Anaesthesia 55: 1113–1116

Moss M, Make B J 1993 Pulmonary response to exercise in health and disease. Seminars in Respiratory Medicine 14(2): 106–120

Moxham J 1995 Respiratory muscles. Medicine International 23(9): 376–379

Moxham J, Costello J F 1994 Respiratory disease. In: Souhami R L, Moxham J (eds) Textbook of medicine, 2nd edn. Churchill Livingstone, Edinburgh, pp 444–534

Murray J F, Basbaum A I 1994 Chest pain. In: Murray J F, Nadel J A (eds) Textbook of respiratory medicine, 2nd edn. W B Saunders, Philadelphia, vol 1, ch 21

Naimark A, Cherniack R M 1960 Compliance of the respiratory system and its components in health and obesity. Journal of Applied Physiology 15(3): 377–382

National Heart, Lung, and Blood Institute Workshop Summary 1990 Respiratory muscle fatigue. Report of the respiratory muscle fatigue workshop group. American Review of Respiratory Disease 142: 474–480

Nunn J F 1987 Applied respiratory physiology, 3rd edn. Butterworths, London

Nunn J F, Milledge J S, Chen D, Dore C 1988 Respiratory criteria of fitness for surgery and anaesthesia. Anaesthesia 43: 543–551

O'Donnell D E 1994 Breathlessness in patients with chronic airflow limitation. Mechanisms and management. Chest 106: 904–912

O'Donnell D E, McGuire M, Samis L, Webb K A 1995 The impact of exercise reconditioning on breathlessness in severe chronic airflow limitation. American Journal of Respiratory and Critical Care Medicine 152: 2005–2013

O'Neill S, McCarthy D S 1983 Postural relief of dyspnoea in severe chronic airflow limitation: relationship to respiratory muscle strength. Thorax 38: 595–600

Oh T E 1990 Oxygen therapy. In: Oh T E (ed) Intensive care manual, 3rd edn. Butterworths, Sydney, ch 18

Pardy R L, Hussain S N A, Macklem P T 1984 The ventilatory pump in exercise. Clinics in Chest Medicine 5(1): 35–49

Pashkow P 1996 Outcomes in cardiopulmonary rehabilitation. Physical Therapy 76(6): 643–656

Pashkow P, Ades P A, Emery C F et al 1995 Outcome measurement in cardiac and pulmonary rehabilitation. Journal of Cardiopulmonary Rehabilitation 15(6): 394–405

Pearce A C, Jones R M 1984 Smoking and anaesthesia: preoperative abstinence and perioperative morbidity. Anesthesiology 61: 576–584

Pedersen S 1996 Inhalers and nebulizers: which to choose and why. Respiratory Medicine 90: 69–77

Phillips B A, Berry D T R, Schmitt F A, Magan L K, Gerhardstein D C, Cook Y R 1992 Sleep-disordered breathing in the healthy elderly. Clinically significant? Chest 101(2): 345–349

Polkey M I, Green M, Moxham J 1995 Measurement of respiratory muscle strength. Thorax 50: 1131–1135

Reid W D, Dechman G 1995 Considerations when testing and training the respiratory muscles. Physical Therapy 75(11): 971–982

Rochester D F 1993 Respiratory muscles and ventilatory failure: 1993 perspective. American Journal of Medical Science 305(6): 394–402

Rochester D F, Esau S A 1984 Malnutrition and the respiratory system. Chest 85(3): 411–415

Roukema J A, Carol E J, Prins J G 1988 The prevention of pulmonary complications after upper abdominal surgery in patients with noncompromised pulmonary status. Archives of Surgery 123: 30–34

Ruppel G 1994 Manual of pulmonary function testing, 6th edn. Mosby, St Louis, p 11

Sibuya M, Yamada M, Kanamaru A et al 1994 Effect of chest wall vibration on dyspnea in patients with chronic respiratory disease. American Journal of Critical Care Medicine 149: 1235–1240

Skinner J S 1993 Exercise testing and exercise prescription for special cases: theoretical basis and clinical application, 2nd edn. Lea & Febiger, Philadelphia

Stewart K J, Kelemen M H, Ewart C K 1994 Relationships between self-efficacy and mood before and after exercise training. Journal of Cardiopulmonary Rehabilitation 14(1): 35–42

Stiller K, Montarello J, Wallace M et al 1994 Are breathing and coughing exercises necessary after coronary artery surgery? Physiotherapy Theory and Practice 10: 143–152

Stock M C, Downs J B, Cooper R B et al 1984 Comparison of continuous positive airway pressure, incentive spirometry, and conservative therapy after cardiac operations. Critical Care Medicine 12(11): 969–972

Stulbarg M S, Adams L 1994 Dyspnea. In: Murray J F, Nadel J A (eds) Textbook of respiratory medicine, 2nd edn. W B Saunders, Philadelphia, vol 1, ch 19

Thomas P S, Cowen E R T, Hulands G, Milledge J S 1989 Respiratory function in the morbidly obese before and after weight loss. Thorax 44: 382–386

Tisi G M 1979 Preoperative evaluation of pulmonary function. Validity, indications and benefits. American Review of Respiratory Disease 119: 293–310

Tobin M J 1990 Dyspnea. Pathophysiologic basis, clinical presentation, and management. Archives of Internal Medicine 150: 1604–1613

Vas Fragoso C A 1993 Monitoring in adult critical care. In: Kacmarek R M, Hess D, Stoller J K (eds) Monitoring in respiratory care. Mosby, St Louis, ch 21

Vibekk P 1991 Chest mobilization and respiratory function. In: Pryor J A (eds) Respiratory care. Churchill Livingstone, Edinburgh, pp 103–119

Vidmar P M, Rubinson L 1994 The relationship between self-efficacy and exercise compliance in a cardiac population. Journal of Cardiopulmonary Rehabilitation 14(4): 246–254

Walker J M, Tan L-B 1994 Cardiovascular disease. In: Souhami R L, Moxham J (eds) Textbook of medicine, 2nd edn. Churchill Livingstone, Edinburgh, pp 320–443

Wardlaw A J 1993 Asthma. BIOS Scientific Publishers, Oxford, pp 17–18, 38–42

Warner M A, Offord K P, Warner M E, Lennon R L, Conover M A, Jansson-Schumacher U 1989 Role of preoperative cessation of smoking and other factors in postoperative pulmonary complications: a blinded prospective study of coronary artery bypass patients. Mayo Clinic Proceedings 64: 609–616

Wasserman K, Hansen J E, Sue D Y, Whipp B J 1987 Principles of exercise testing and interpretation. Lea & Febiger, Philadelphia, pp 47–57

Weil J V, McCullough R E, Kline J S, Sodal I E 1975 Diminished ventilatory response to hypoxia and hypercpania after morphine in normal man. New England Journal of Medicine 292: 1103–1106

Weiser P C, Mahler D A, Ryan K P, Hill K L, Greenspon L W 1993 Dyspnea: symptom assessment and management. In: Hodgkin J E, Connors G L, Bell C W (eds) Pulmonary rehabilitation. Guidelines to success, 2nd edn. J B Lippincott, Philadelphia, ch 26

West J B 1990 Respiratory physiology – the essentials, 4th edn. Williams & Wilkins, Baltimore

West J B 1992 Pulmonary pathophysiology – the essentials, 4th edn. Williams & Wilkins, Baltimore

Wilkins R L, Sheldon R L, Krider S J 1990 Clinical assessment in respiratory care, 2nd edn. C V Mosby, St Louis, p 36

Windsor J A, Hill G L 1988 Risk factors for post-operative pneumonia. The importance of protein depletion. Annals of Surgery 208(2): 209–214

Wolff R K, Dolovich M B, Obminski G, Newhouse M T 1977 Effects of exercise and eucapnic hyperventilation on bronchial clearance in man. Journal of Applied Physiology 43(1): 46–50

Youtsey J W 1994 Oxygen and mixed gas therapy. In: Barnes T A (ed) Core textbook of respiratory care practice, 2nd edn. Mosby, St Louis, p 150

Zadai C C, Irwin S 1992 Exercise pathophysiology: pulmonary impairment. In: Zadai C C (ed) Pulmonary management in physical therapy. Churchill Livingstone, New York, ch 3

The needs of specific patients

SECTION CONTENTS

11

Intensive care for the critically ill adult

Fran H. Woodard   Mandy Jones

INTRODUCTION

The intensive care unit (ICU) is perceived as a daunting environment to the undergraduate or newly qualified physiotherapist. The patients present with a complexity of problems which may be multisystem in origin, and the technology used in their treatment is continually being updated and advanced. Illness severity scoring systems such as the Acute Physiology and Chronic Health Evaluation II (APACHE II) are used to quantify the severity of illness, to determine the success of different forms of treatment and to predict mortality (Knaus et al 1985).

The physiotherapist has a vital role to play in the ICU. Once the initial fear has been conquered, this area provides a forum in which skills and knowledge acquired from all the different specialist areas can be utilized. The physiotherapist must consider the general condition of the patient and must remember the possible feelings and fears that he may have in his unnatural surroundings. Areas of concern are an inability to speak and a loss of perception of time. The patient will also probably suffer from chronic sleep deprivation.

There is no place for routine physiotherapy in the ICU. A thorough analytical assessment will highlight physiotherapy problems which may respond to treatment, and associated contraindications.

This chapter attempts to guide the physiotherapist through this assessment and the implications of its findings, the problems associated with mechanical ventilation and patient groups with specific needs. Once all appropriate information has been gathered, the relevant physiotherapy treatment can be selected.

ASSESSMENT OF THE CRITICALLY ILL PATIENT IN THE INTENSIVE CARE UNIT (ICU)

Although the respiratory physiotherapist may be primarily concerned with the patient's respiratory system, an analytical assessment must be conducted on other related systems to allow a full overview of the patient's medical stability and suitability for treatment. This holistic approach must incorporate an understanding of both the implications and use of drug therapy (Pearson & Parr 1993).

Neurological system

The early stages of the management of the acute head injury and the neurosurgical patient involve sedation and frequently paralysis. Adequate sedation and/or paralysis is essential in the maintenance of stable intracranial pressure. Fluctuating intracranial pressures will occur as a result of environmental stimuli, including physiotherapeutic intervention in the poorly sedated patient.

Important factors in assessment

Level of consciousness. The most widely used and accepted scoring system of the neurological patient is the Glasgow Coma Scale (GCS). Neurological centres may use their own scoring system in addition to the GCS (Frisby 1990) (see p. 10).

Pupils
- *Size.* The pupils are graded either numerically or by description ranging from pinprick to dilated. The most significant cause of sudden pupil dilatation is neurological deterioration (e.g. cerebral oedema). Pharmacological treatment can alter pupil size (e.g. reduced or pinprick as a result of opioid use, or dilated after administration of atropine or adrenaline).

- *Reactivity.* The pupils' reaction to light indicates optic and oculomotor nerve function. Fixed dilated pupils may indicate severe neurological impairment, or be caused by drug treatment, hypoxia or biochemical abnormalities.
- *Equality.* Each pupil is tested individually, as inequality may be an important localizing sign.

Cerebral perfusion pressure (CPP). This is the critical pressure required to ensure adequate blood supply to the brain and prevent acidosis, hypoxia and damage. The brain attempts to maintain a constant cerebral blood flow, despite variations in blood pressure, by a process of autoregulation. The range of blood pressure over which it is effective varies with the individual. Autoregulation may be impaired by a severe head injury or other neurological insults.

CPP = mean arterial pressure (MAP) *minus* intracranial pressure (ICP)	
Normal value	> 70 mmHg
Critical value	< 50 mmHg

Intracranial pressure (ICP). The components influencing ICP are the blood, brain and CSF within the rigid skull. The blood component can be influenced by changes in $PaCO_2$ and venous drainage. Rises in ICP from normal levels correlate with a worse outcome (Miller et al 1977). ICP measurement is used as a diagnostic tool and to guide and assess the effectiveness of medical treatment. It can be measured by an extradural, subdural or subarachnoid bolt, intraparenchymal sensor or ventricular drain (Fig. 4.5, p. 79) (German 1994).

Normal value	< 10 mmHg
Critical value	> 25 mmHg

Drugs. See Table 11.1.

Considerations for physiotherapy
- Consistent levels of ICP (below the critical level) suggest a patient may be stable enough to tolerate intervention, whereas a fluctuating ICP indicates neurological instability which may

Table 11.1   Drugs in the ICU: the neurological system

Drug		Action	Considerations for physiotherapy
Hypnovel Versed	midazolam	Sedatives	May need to be increased prior to physiotherapy intervention to prevent acute rises in ICP or BP. Care with manual hyperinflation as sedation can cause a drop in BP. Causes impairment of cough reflex, therefore difficulty in clearing secretions
Chloractil Ormazine	chlorpromazine		
Diprivan	propofol		
Ketalar	ketamine		
Durogesic	fentanyl		
Rapifen Alfenta	alfentanil	Sedatives and analgesics	
MST Astramorph	morphine		
Pavulon	pancuronium	Muscle relaxants	Used by continuous infusion usually reflects either severe respiratory failure with difficulty in ventilation or neurological instability. Care with manual hyperinflation as it may not be tolerated. Absence of cough reflex. Care with positioning as reduced muscle tone leads to joint vulnerability
Tracrium	atracurium		
Norcuron	vecuronium		
Intraval Pentothal	thiopentone	Sedative	Main indication for use is intractable fitting or very unstable ICP. Closely monitor CPP, ICP and MAP during treatment
Nimotop	nimodipine	Specific cerebral artery vasodilator	Usually used in patients whose ICP is raised and/or unstable. If physiotherapy is absolutely essential, monitor parameters carefully throughout treatment
Osmitrol	mannitol	Osmotic diuretic	
Decadron Aerosels–Dex	dexamethasone	Corticosteroid–reduces cerebral oedema	
Epanutin Dilantin	phenytoin	Anticonvulsant	If fitting is well controlled there is no contraindication for treatment

be magnified by any physiotherapeutic intervention. It is worth noting that a sudden rise in ICP (which will reduce CPP) can be caused by hypercapnia secondary to respiratory complications such as atelectasis or sputum retention.

• In situations of increased or unstable ICP it may be necessary to use inotropic support to maintain MAP at a level to preserve CPP.

• The patient's level of sedation needs to be considered. It is well documented that sedation leads to a lowering of blood pressure. Therefore, it is essential that the patient's cardiovascular system is assessed thoroughly and any necessary drugs given before physiotherapy. It is important to note that when sedation is being weaned, the patient may become agitated and self-extubation is a risk.

Cardiovascular system

The cardiovascular stability of the critically ill patient is influenced by many interrelated factors. In some situations physiotherapeutic intervention may be contraindicated. A thorough assessment is therefore essential before any treatment is instigated.

Important factors in assessment

Heart rate (HR) and rhythm. The critically ill patient may develop a multitude of arrhythmias. There are many possible causes (e.g. electrolyte imbalance, action of drugs), but physiotherapy intervention in the unstable patient may precipitate or worsen them. The arrhythmias that may be encountered vary from severe rhythm disturbances causing cardiovascular compromise (e.g. decreased blood pressure potentially leading to reduced urine output), to more benign disturbances, but even ventricular ectopics may be a precursor of more serious arrhythmias (p. 79).

Normal value	50–100 bpm
Bradycardia	< 50 bpm
Tachycardia	> 100 bpm

Arterial blood pressure (BP). Blood pressure is dependent on various parameters. Blood pressure is equal to the rate of blood flow multiplied by the resistance produced by the vessels. Therefore in the cardiovascular system:

Mean BP = Systemic vascular resistance (SVR) × Cardiac output (CO)

CO = Stroke volume (SV) × HR

Therefore:

BP = SVR × SV × HR

Normal values: 95/60–140/90 mmHg

Mean arterial pressure (MAP) = Diastolic + $\dfrac{\text{(Pulse pressure)}}{3}$

Pulse pressure = the difference between systolic and diastolic pressures

The critically ill patient may develop hypotension because of hypovolaemia, sepsis, excessive use of sedative or vasodilatory drugs or a primary cardiac dysfunction. Hypertension may reflect, for example, inadequate sedation and analgesia or a Cushing's response to a raised ICP (Ganong 1995). If uncontrolled, both of these may be a contraindication to physiotherapy. The management of hypotension may require a fluid challenge or inotropic support. Increasing doses of inotropes indicate escalating cardiovascular instability.

Central venous pressure (CVP). In the absence of cardiovascular or pulmonary disease, CVP is a reflection of circulatory volume and therefore has a direct correlation with fluid balance (also see p. 274). It is measured via a central venous catheter situated in a central vein (see p. 76).

Normal value	3–15 cmH$_2$O

Pulmonary artery pressure (PAP) and pulmonary capillary wedge pressure (PCWP). A normal PAP is approximately one-sixth of systemic pressure (West 1995). High PAPs may be seen in severe respiratory disease.

PCWP pressure gives an indirect measurement of left arterial pressure and left ventricular filling pressure. A high PCWP may be caused by poor left ventricular function, fluid overload, mitral valve disease and positive pressure ventilation. A low PCWP may be caused by hypovolaemia.

The pulmonary artery catheter (Swan–Ganz) may be used to derive numerical values for cardiac output, stroke volume and ventricular workload and may guide the use of inotropic support and fluid balance (p. 70).

Normal values:

Mean pulmonary artery pressure (PAP)
           10–20 mmHg (1.3–2.7 kPa)
Pulmonary capillary wedge pressure
(PCWP)   6–15 mmHg (0.8–2 kPa)
Cardiac output (CO)   5 l/min

Drugs. See Table 11.2.

Considerations for physiotherapy

• The presence of arrhythmias must be assessed. Some arrhythmias can be essentially stable (e.g. slow atrial fibrillation). In this situation if the rhythm is normal for the patient, or no cardiovascular compromise is present, physiotherapy may be carried out if indicated. Fast atrial fibrillation and many other supraventricular and ventricular tachycardias are unstable rhythms and therefore physiotherapy is contraindicated.

• A high PAP may indicate high pulmonary vascular resistance which would be exacerbated during manual hyperinflations. Manual hyperinflations must also be used with caution in patients with a low cardiac output (p. 285).

Respiratory system

The patient is assessed for the level of ventilatory support required, i.e. full, assisted or spontaneous ventilation. The presence of an endo-

Table 11.2 Drugs in the ICU: the cardiovascular system

Drug		Action	Considerations for physiotherapy
Inotropes			
Epifrin	adrenaline	↑ Heart rate ↑ Cardiac output	
Levophed	noradrenaline	Peripheral vasoconstriction ↑ Systemic vascular resistance	
Medihaler-Iso	isoprenaline	↑ Heart rate ↑ Cardiac output	
Dobutrex	dobutamine	↑ Myocardial contractility ↑ Heart rate	Inotropes are used to support blood pressure. Evaluation of cardiovascular stability and effect of inotropic support must be noted. Care with hyperinflations as blood pressure may be labile
Intropin	dopamine	Low doses < 5 μ/kg/min ↑ Myocardial contractility ↑ Renal perfusion Higher doses > 5 μ/kg/min ↑ Systemic vascular resistance	
Dopacard	dopexamine	↑ Heart rate ↑ Renal perfusion ↑ Splanchnic perfusion	
Perfan	enoximone	↑ Myocardial contractility ↑ Peripheral dilatation	
Primator	milrinone	↓ Systemic vascular resistance	
Hypertensin	angiotensin	Potent vasoconstriction	Used in some centres in the severely unstable patient
Other relevant cardiac drugs			
Adalat	nifedipine	Vascular smooth muscle relaxant Coronary and peripheral artery dilator Antihypertensive	Used primarily in control of hypertension especially those at risk of myocardial ischaemia. Monitor BP and ECG during treatment
Coro-Nitro Tridil	GTN–glyceryl trinitrate	Vasodilator	
Angeze Imdur	ISMN–isosorbide mononitrate		
Lanoxin	digoxin	Control of supraventricular tachycardia, atrial fibrillation or flutter	
Cordarone	amiodorone		Stable arrhythmias are not a direct contraindication to treatment. Monitor rhythm throughout intervention
Adenocor Adenocord	adenosine		
Berkaten Cordilox	verapamil	Anti-arrhythmic	
Laryng-o-Jet Anestacon	lignocaine		
Calciparine Hep-Lock	heparin		
Marevan Coumadin	warfarin	Anticoagulant	If over-anticoagulated, bleeding is a risk. Care during suction

tracheal or tracheostomy tube, nasal mask or full face mask should be noted.

Important factors in assessment

Mode of ventilation/PEEP/CPAP. See also Chapter 5.

Humidification. The ability to clear secretions effectively must be assessed. If compressed dry air has been given, the need for humidifica-

tion must be assessed. The alternatives are heat moisture exchangers (HME) or heated humidification (p. 188) (Branson et al 1993).

Oxygen therapy. An increase in oxygen requirement may reflect a deteriorating primary respiratory problem or impaired gas exchange as a result of multisystem disorder. The level of therapeutic oxygen available ranges from room air at 21% (FiO_2 0.21) to 100% oxygen (FiO_2 1.0).

Respiratory rate (RR). The respiratory rate

will vary depending on the type and amount of ventilatory support. In a fully ventilated patient, the rate is set and only originates from the ventilator. The rate may be set to achieve a specific goal in the individual patient. For example, a high respiratory rate may be desirable in a neurological patient to lower $PaCO_2$ (and thus ICP), or a lower respiratory rate may be preferred to produce a high normal $PaCO_2$ (permissive hypercapnia) in a patient with chronic airflow limitation (CAL).

In assisted modes, a proportion of the rate is delivered by the ventilator with the patient able to initiate his/her own additional respiratory rate. The ventilator rate may be gradually reduced to encourage weaning (p. 92).

Patients who are breathing spontaneously may have abnormally high respiratory rates because of exhaustion, neurological impairment, anxiety, pain or biochemical abnormalities. The pattern of respiration in the spontaneously breathing patient is also important because it may reflect mechanical obstruction, poor coordination (e.g. residual muscle relaxation) and neurological impairment (e.g. periods of apnoea, p. 15).

Airway pressures. In the ventilated patient, although no pressure is totally safe, barotrauma is unlikely to occur in patients whose peak inspiratory pressure (PIP) is less than 40 cmH$_2$O. Raised PIPs may be indicative of many differing clinical situations, e.g. reduced compliance, fibrosis, acute respiratory distress syndrome (ARDS), pulmonary oedema, sputum plugging or bronchospasm. Both mean and peak airway pressures can be displayed throughout the respiratory cycle on monitors.

Auscultation. In the ventilated patient normal breath sounds tend to be more harsh. This can be attributed to transmitted noises originating from the ventilator itself, or accumulated water in the tubes. During assessment it is important to compare zones on each side of the chest. The bases of a ventilated patient are difficult to access in the supine position but essential to auscultate (p. 17).

Percussion note. This is an extremely useful technique in the assessment of the ICU patient. The information gained from percussion may help to differentiate between pathologies, e.g.

pleural effusion (stony dull), atelectasis or consolidation (dull). In an emergency, percussion can be used to distinguish quickly between a patient who has collapsed a lung (dull) and one who has sustained a pneumothorax (hyper-resonant).

Expansion. Equality of expansion may be felt by palpating a patient's chest. Palpation is also useful as an indicator of any underlyingsecretions, bronchospasm or surgical emphysema.

Chest radiograph (CXR). Chest radiographs are used as an adjunct in the respiratory assessment. In the intensive care setting portable anteroposterior (AP) radiographs are taken. AP films can produce magnification of certain structures such as the heart. Correct interpretation of the chest radiograph can be difficult because optimal positioning of the patient is limited and the film is rarely taken at full inspiration. Accurate day-to-day comparison between films can only be used as a rough guide as portable radiographs are taken at differing distances and exposures. It is important to note that in some conditions such as pneumonia, radiological appearances may lag behind the clinical situation (see Ch. 2).

Arterial blood gases (ABGs). ABG analysis and interpretation is used to ascertain the state of a patient's respiratory and metabolic function and acid–base balance (Table 11.3). It is measured by a blood sample from a line sited in any available artery, or from an arterial stab (pp. 59 and 83). To gain a full picture of a patient's condition, it is beneficial to observe trends or a series of arterial blood gas samples rather than one set of results in isolation.

Normal values:	
pH	7.35–7.45
$PaCO_2$	4.7–6.0 kPa (35–45 mmHg)
PaO_2	10.7–13.3 kPa (80–100 mmHg)
HCO_3^-	22–26 mmol/l
Base excess	−2 to +2

Sputum/haemoptysis. The presence of tenacious secretions which may potentially lead to plugging is an indication for urgent assessment and treatment. The analysis of a sputum specimen can be used as a guide for antibiotic therapy.

Evidence of fresh blood in the respiratory tract

Table 11.3 Arterial blood gases

Imbalance	Indicator	Clinical situation	Compensatory mechanisms
Respiratory acidosis	↓pH ↑$PaCO_2$	Sputum retention Atelectasis Hypoventilation V̇/Q̇ inequalities	↑HCO_3^- ↑H^+ ions excreted
Respiratory alkalosis	↑pH ↓$PaCO_2$	Hyperventilation, e.g. pain, anxiety Mechanical ventilation Neurogenic	↓HCO_3^- via excretion
Metabolic acidosis	↓pH ↓HCO_3^-	Myocardial infarction Sepsis Gastrointestinal bleed Overaggressive diuretic therapy	↑RR → ↓$PaCO_2$
Metabolic alkalosis	↑pH ↑HCO_3^-	Profuse vomiting Profuse diarrhoea	↓RR → ↑$PaCO_2$

Table 11.4 Drugs in the ICU: the respiratory system

Drug	Action	Considerations for physiotherapy
β₂-adrenoceptor agonists Aerolin/Ventolin ⎫ Airet ⎬ salbutamol Bricanyl ⎫ Brethine ⎬ terbutaline	⎫ ⎬ Bronchodilatation ⎭	⎫ ⎬ Assess the degree of bronchospasm by auscultation and airway pressures. May be beneficial to use bronchodilatation therapy pre- and post-physiotherapy intervention
Anticholinergics Atrovent ipratropium bromide		
Smooth muscle relaxants Biophylline+ ⎫ Accurbron ⎬ theophylline Amnivent ⎫ Phyllocontin ⎬ aminophylline	⎫ ⎬ Bronchodilatation ⎭	High doses can lead to arrhythmias
Corticosteroids Anflam+ ⎫ Acticort ⎬ hydrocortisone	Anti-inflammatory	Increased risk of infection. Used in patients with irritable airways
Respiratory stimulants Dopram doxapram	Central respiratory stimulant	Can be used in patients with rising $PaCO_2$. Can produce fatigue such that physiotherapy is not tolerated. Patients may become agitated and uncooperative during treatment

(e.g. pulmonary haemorrhage) may be a direct contraindication to some types of physiotherapy. However, bleeding may occur with some pneumonias and in this situation physiotherapy may be appropriate.

Drugs. See Table 11. 4.

Considerations for physiotherapy
• A full assessment of the respiratory system

will indicate a patient's ability to tolerate physiotherapeutic intervention. It is important to know the cause of raised airway pressures in a patient as some causes are an indication for treatment, whereas in others treatment would be strongly contraindicated. For example, raised airway pressures due to gross sputum retention or plugging can be relieved with appropriate physiotherapeutic intervention. However, acute bronchospasm could be exacerbated by physiotherapy. A sudden increase in airway pressure may be indicative of a sputum plug, gross atelectasis, pneumothorax, airway occlusion, or a kink in the ventilator tubing.

Renal system

The kidneys have a vital role in homeostasis. They are responsible for excretion of waste products of metabolism including drugs, production of hormones, control of the extracellular fluid composition which influences intracellular volume, osmolarity and acid–base status.

Important factors in assessment of fluid balance

- Measures of intravascular volume – HR/MAP/CVP/PCWP
- Urine output
- Assessment of peripheral perfusion and tissue turgor
- Daily weight
- Serum and urinary electrolytes
- Arterial blood gases
- Daily chest radiograph
- Net fluid balance

Acute renal failure (ARF) is associated with a rapidly rising urea and creatinine concentration, usually with a falling urine output. Hyperkalaemia, acidosis and fluid overload are common problems. ARF is often precipitated by hypotension, hypoxia and sepsis in the critically ill patient. Patients whose underlying renal function has already been compromised by diabetes, hypertension and vascular problems are particularly at risk. Renal replacement therapy is usually instigated when measures such as fluid resuscitation, cardiovascular support and the use of diuretics (Table 11.5) fail to improve function (Kirby & Davenport 1996). See Table 11.6.

Haematological/immunological system

The haematological and immunological stability of a patient is often overlooked during the physiotherapy assessment. However, these systems may produce strong contraindications for physiotherapy. Patients with sepsis are often complicated by abnormal coagulation. Prolonged clotting times coupled with low platelet counts may lead to spontaneous bleeding from both mucous membranes and the respiratory tract. Physiotherapy may aggravate bleeding.

Patients who are immunocompromised either through primary disease processes (e.g. malignancy), drug therapy (e.g. use of steroids) or as a complication of sepsis are particularly at risk from nosocomial infections (hospital acquired) and cross-infection.

Considerations for physiotherapy
- Appropriate care must be taken to minimize cross-infection (see Ch. 4) with respect to local health and safety recommendations. Most ICUs advocate the use of a clean apron and gloves for each patient. Masks may be worn if indicated (e.g. open tuberculosis). While suctioning (p. 287), a sterile or second glove should be worn and goggles may be recommended.

Gastrointestinal system

A patient who has sustained a large gastrointestinal bleed may become hypovolaemic due to blood loss. A metabolic acidosis may be evident from arterial blood gas analysis. The patient may adopt an abnormal breathing

Table 11.5 Drugs in the ICU: the renal system

Drug		Action	Considerations for physiotherapy
Inopin	dopamine	See Table 11.2	
Frusid	} frusemide	Loop of Henlé diuretic	} Over-diuresis can cause hypotension and dried secretions. Monitor BP. Hypokalaemia can be a problem. Care with arrhythmias
Lasix			
Osmitrol	mannitol	Osmotic diuretic	

Table 11.6 Types of renal support

Replacement therapy	Applications	Considerations for physiotherapy
Continuous haemofiltration/haemodiafiltration Requires vascular access to divert blood through an extracorporeal circuit, passing the blood continually via a filter (haemofiltration) which can be itself bathed in dialysis fluid (haemodiafiltration)	More effective correction of biochemical abnormalities May require anticoagulation Cardiovascular upset usually avoidable	Use of anticoagulation may cause bleeding, therefore care with suction Good for patients who are relatively unstable Care needs to be taken with large IV lines during changes of position
Intermittent haemodialysis Also requires access to the circulation but the treatment is carried out for only 3–5 hours every 24–48 hours	Large fluid shifts may cause severe cardiovascular disturbance Rapid correction of biochemistry	As above although physiotherapy can continue when patients are not on haemodialysis
Peritoneal dialysis Uses the peritoneum as a dialysis membrane Involves instillation of large volumes of fluid into the abdomen (1–2 litres)	Simple Little cardiovascular disturbance More suitable for chronic use Slow to alter biochemical abnormalities	Good positioning is essential to facilitate breathing as fluid leads to splinting of the abdomen. Ventilator weaning is more difficult because of diaphragmatic splinting

pattern in an attempt to 'blow off' carbon dioxide and therefore reduce overall acidity.

Nutritional support is an important aspect of the care of the critically ill patient. Adequate nutrition is essential to prevent the loss of lean body tissue, provide material for repair and to facilitate recovery. Poor nutritional status, particularly deficits of magnesium and phosphates, may contribute to respiratory muscle weakness and delayed weaning from the ventilator (Rapper & Maynard 1992).

Routes of administration:

- Enteral – tube feeds directly into the gastrointestinal tract, e.g. nasogastric feeds or gastrostomy/jejunostomy
- Parenteral – intravenous feeding via central or peripheral line
- Oral – usually with supplementation.

Considerations for physiotherapy

- Ventilated patients with a reduced level of consciousness and a poor gag reflex may be prone to pulmonary aspiration if the endotracheal tube is uncuffed or the cuff deflated. Overfeeding may result in increased CO_2 production especially in patients with respiratory failure (Browne 1988a).

Musculoskeletal system

It is beneficial to know the patient's state of pre-admission mobility. It is unlikely that a patient who does not have musculoskeletal complications will require regular passive movements but it is important to assess this regularly as the critically ill patient may develop musculoskeletal problems. Patients who have sustained musculoskeletal trauma, have pre-existing pathology or who have been ventilated for a prolonged time will require an in-depth assessment and appropriate treatment.

Positioning. The frequent turning of a patient will not only benefit the musculoskeletal system and aid pressure relief, but will also enhance the respiratory system. A change of position may have several effects, assisting the drainage of secretions, improving ventilation–perfusion relationships, and increasing functional residual capacity.

Beds. A wide variety of specialist beds are available to assist in the turning and positioning of the critically ill patient (Birtwistle 1994). It is essential for any patient, but imperative for the multi-trauma patient, to be assessed adequately for the appropriate specialist bed.

Considerations for physiotherapy
- The unstable patient may not tolerate a change in position.

MECHANICAL VENTILATION – IMPLICATIONS FOR PHYSIOTHERAPY

Mechanical ventilation is used in patients undergoing a general anaesthetic and in most patients requiring intensive care. Modern ventilators provide a wealth of different modalities to cater for patients from the most critically ill, through the weaning process to extubation. At every different stage, a full assessment must be undertaken to identify the presence of any physiotherapy problems. Physiotherapy may need to be modified depending on a patient's ventilatory requirements and during the weaning process.

Intubation

The decision to intubate and ventilate a patient is never taken lightly, as this procedure in itself has an associated level of morbidity and mortality. Endotracheal tubes come in a variety of types and sizes. Most of those routinely used for adults have a high-volume, low-pressure cuff to limit tracheal damage. Paediatric tubes are uncuffed and tracheostomy tubes vary. See Table 11.7.

Considerations for physiotherapy
- When assessing the mechanically ventilated patient, it is important to note the ventilation requirements and to understand their implication. The level of stability of both the cardiovascular and respiratory systems must be established. A patient with an unstable respiratory system requiring high levels of oxygen ($FiO_2 > 0.6$) and/or high levels of PEEP ($> 10\ cmH_2O$) should have an absolute indication for treatment before physiotherapy is undertaken.
- If manual hyperinflations are indicated in a patient requiring a high level of PEEP, a PEEP valve should be used (p. 286).
- The inspiratory : expiratory (I : E) ratio can be altered in mechanical ventilation to meet an individual patient's needs. A prolonged expiratory time or an expiratory pause can be used in patients with chronic airflow limitation. A prolonged inspiratory time (inverse ratio ventilation) improves oxygenation in ARDS. An altered I : E ratio may be vital to maintain good oxygenation. In this situation, manual hyperinflation may not be tolerated.
- When positioning the mechanically ventilated patient it must be remembered that

Table 11.7 Intubation

Site of tube	Indications and advantages	Type of tube
Oral	Most commonly used in adults Used in emergency situations	Endotracheal tube – cuffed (adults) – uncuffed (paediatrics)
Nasal	Used when oral intubation impossible or impractical, e.g. trauma Most commonly used in paediatrics	
Tracheostomy – temporary – permanent	Used for long-term ventilation Improves comfort, reduces need for sedation, facilitates normal eating and drinking Maintains and protects airway where a neurological or anatomical abnormality is present	Portex® – cuffed or uncuffed – single lumen – speaking valve Shiley® – cuffed or uncuffed – fenestration for speech – long-term use – inner cannulae Silver – uncuffed – permanent use – single lumen – phonation tube

the physiological factors affecting ventilation–perfusion matching are altered. The application of positive pressure leads to non-dependent areas of lung being preferentially ventilated. Therefore as perfusion is influenced by gravity some degree of inequality is always present. For example in right side lying, the right lung is dependent and therefore preferentially perfused, whereas the left lung is non-dependent, thus preferentially ventilated. As this mismatching occurs in all positions, frequent changes of position are essential. Use of the prone position has been shown to be of benefit in some patients with severe lung disease (Pappert et al 1994).

• When assessing a patient who requires an unconventional form of ventilation, e.g. high-frequency ventilation and/or nitric oxide (p. 94), and in whom physiotherapy is indicated, it is advantageous to discuss the plan of treatment with the medical staff.

Weaning

Weaning is the process of reducing or removing ventilatory support. As soon as the patient's condition stabilizes, weaning can start.

Influences on the weaning process

Neurological system. A reduced level of consciousness is not a direct contraindication to weaning as airway patency and protection can be maintained with an endotracheal or tracheostomy tube. The patient must be able to sustain adequate spontaneous ventilation. Sedative drugs need to be reduced during the weaning process.

Pathology such as Guillain–Barré syndrome and myasthenia gravis may require weaning to take place during the daytime as fatigue and poor diaphragmatic function may lead to nocturnal hypoventilation.

Cardiovascular system. A stable cardiovascular system is necessary for successful weaning. Reduced cardiac output due to hypovolaemia or arrhythmias may potentially result in respiratory muscle oxygen deprivation.

Respiratory system. The patient must be able to initiate an adequate respiratory drive during each stage of the weaning process. Any primary lung pathology should have resolved significantly to allow for improved respiratory function.

It is necessary that adequate oxygenation can be sustained with reducing levels of oxygen and PEEP. In the final stages of weaning, patients must be able to generate adequate minute volumes to maintain their $PaCO_2$ within the normal range.

Acid–base balance. It should be noted that the weaning process can be complicated in patients with an abnormal acid–base balance, e.g. severe metabolic acidosis will induce a raised respiratory rate, whereas metabolic alkalosis may lead to hypoventilation.

Renal system. Electrolyte balance is imperative to prevent excessive respiratory muscle fatigue. Acute renal failure with fluid overload will make weaning more difficult.

Nutrition. Adequate nutritional support is essential during weaning to help prevent muscle weakness and fatigue.

Infection. Overwhelming sepsis can cause impaired gas exchange with an increased O_2 consumption and CO_2 production which may delay weaning (Browne 1988a).

Methods of weaning

In the uncomplicated postoperative situation the whole process of weaning may only take a short period. As the patient regains consciousness and breathes spontaneously, rapid extubation can take place. In the long-term ventilated patient, the weaning process is started by reducing sedation and positioning for optimal diaphragmatic excursion. Modern ventilators have an extensive range of weaning modalities. The patient is encouraged to self-ventilate on an assisted mode, e.g. synchronized intermittent mandatory ventilation (SIMV), while still receiving additional support for each spontaneous breath, e.g. inspiratory pressure support (IPS) (p. 91).

Gradually the IPS can be reduced together with the number of mandatory breaths. Once the patient can maintain adequate oxygenation and normal $PaCO_2$ levels, progression to either CPAP or a T-piece is achieved. At each stage ABG analysis will indicate whether adequate ventilation is being maintained. Weaning may be very protracted in some patients and the use of individualized programmes will smooth progress and maintain patients' morale (Browne 1988b).

In chronic respiratory patients a tracheostomy tube may aid the weaning process by reducing the anatomical dead space.

The patient who is difficult to wean because of pre-existing chronic lung pathology may benefit from the use of non-invasive positive pressure ventilation (Chapter 6).

Considerations for physiotherapy

• In the weaning phase a patient on assisted ventilation may have a high spontaneous respiratory rate. Manual hyperinflation may cause the patient distress and may be ineffective if only small tidal volumes are achieved. If a primary respiratory problem is causing the high respiratory rate, physiotherapy is indicated. It is important to start manual hyperinflation matching the patient's own respiratory rate and depth. By slowly increasing the tidal volume, the $PaCO_2$ levels can be lowered, temporarily inhibiting the patient's respiratory drive and allowing effective manual hyperinflations.

• When a patient has been weaned on to CPAP, it is important that adequate physiotherapy input continues. Good positioning is essential to maximize further weaning potential. If sputum is present airway clearance techniques should be utilized.

Extubation

Although successful weaning culminates in extubation, the two processes must be assessed independently. Extubation should not be considered until the patient can protect his own airway, and can cough and swallow (Browne 1988b).

Minitracheostomy tube

The sole purpose of the minitracheostomy is access for the removal of excess bronchial secre-

tions. It can also be used in the decannulation process of a tracheostomy tube. It is important to remember that a minitracheostomy offers no airway protection (p. 162).

MUSCULOSKELETAL PROBLEMS

The critically ill patient in ICU will require a musculoskeletal assessment. A short-term ventilated patient with no pre-existing musculoskeletal pathology should require minimal intervention. This should be reviewed regularly. However, any patient will benefit from sitting out of bed during the weaning process (Ciesla 1996) (see p. 124).

A patient requiring long-term ventilation or who presents with pre-existing musculoskeletal or neurological pathologies will require an in-depth assessment and identification of specific problems. Special attention should be given to the following areas: head and neck, shoulder girdle, hip extension and adduction, knee extension and Achilles tendon length. Muscle length and joint range of movement can be maintained by good positioning incorporating joint alignment, passive range of movements and muscle stretches. Liaison with the nursing staff will allow coordination of physiotherapy and nursing intervention especially turning to maximize patient care. A regular change of position will not only relieve pressure, but provide proprioceptive input. Once medical stability has been achieved, and it is appropriate, the patient should be sat out of bed. It may be necessary to use a hoist or an assisted transfer. The progression of sitting in a chair, standing and ultimately walking (Fig. 11.1) is not only of great physiological benefit but also a psychological boost (Sciaky 1994).

Considerations for physiotherapy

• *Multiple trauma.* The injuries sustained during multiple trauma require a detailed assessment as each problem can be unique in presentation. It is important to discuss the management with the relevant medical team. Fixation of unstable joints or fractures may be difficult in the early stages until cardiovascular stability

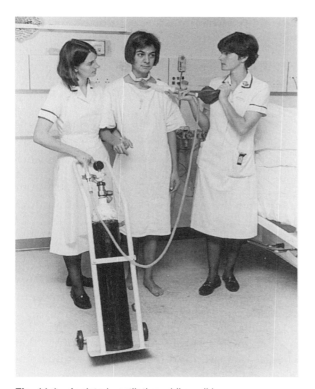

Fig. 11.1 Assisted ventilation while walking.

has been established. Any spinal injury particularly of the cervical spine must be considered unstable until it has been reviewed by a specialist. If external fixators have been applied, it is necessary to maintain range of movement and muscle length to the adjacent areas. The opinion of the relevant physiotherapy specialist should be sought (e.g. orthopaedic or plastics specialist).

• *Acute neurology*. While the patient is neurologically unstable musculoskeletal intervention is not indicated. However, once neurological stability is achieved, early rehabilitation is essential for successful outcomes. It is important to assess the range of joint movement, two-joint muscle lengths, volitional and non-volitional motor activity and the presence of any prevalent patterns. Treatment is aimed at maintenance of passive range of joint movement, two-joint muscle stretches, maintaining anatomical alignment and inhibiting reflex activity by position-

ing. Plaster casting may be indicated to prevent significant shortening of tendons and muscle length and to assist in reduction of tone (Connine et al 1990). A change of position will aid proprioceptive input.

Rehabilitation is progressed to sitting and standing. This will assist in gaining trunk control and pelvic alignment. This can be started while the patient is still requiring ventilatory support. It is advisable to turn a ventricular drain off before moving the patient. Close liaison with the nursing staff and the multidisciplinary team is essential to ensure effective ongoing rehabilitation. Early referral to the specialist physiotherapist and rehabilitation team will maximize potential recovery.

PATIENT GROUPS WITH SPECIFIC NEEDS

The critically ill patient requiring intensive care may develop complications secondary to the primary diagnosis. The nature of these secondary complications may alter or even contraindicate physiotherapeutic intervention. An understanding of the commonly encountered complications is essential for complete assessment of these potentially unstable patients.

Systemic inflammatory response syndrome (SIRS) and sepsis

SIRS

Various insults to the body may lead to an exaggerated, generalized inflammatory response called systemic inflammatory response syndrome (SIRS). This inflammatory response involves highly complex interactions between several cell groups (macrophages, neutrophils, etc.), inflammatory mediators (histamine) and internal regulatory pathways (fibrinolytic, clotting, complement) (Emery & Salmon 1991).

In its worst form there is severe disruption of vascular haemostasis with impairment of the endothelial barriers in many organs. This causes increased capillary permeability often resulting in organ failure. There may be an associated loss of normal vascular tone causing hypotension in the systemic circulation and intrapulmonary shunting in the pulmonary circulation. Breakdown of the normal clotting/fibrinolytic pathways may result in prolonged clotting, intravascular thrombosis and thrombocytopenia.

If this inflammatory response is secondary to an infective cause, it is termed 'sepsis'. Causative organisms implicated in sepsis include bacteria, fungi, rickettsiae and other parasites. Sepsis is the major cause of mortality in the ICU.

SIRS can be defined clinically as the presence of two or more of the following criteria:

Temperature	$> 38°$ or $< 36°C$
Tachycardia	> 90 bpm
Tachypnoea	$> 20/$min or $PaCO_2 < 4.3$ kPa (32.3 mmHg)
WBC	$> 12 \times 10^9/$litre or $< 4 \times 10^9/$litre or $< 10\%$ immature neutrophils

Sepsis

Sepsis can be classified into three groups:

- *Sepsis.* The presence of SIRS, with a documented cultured infection.
- *Severe sepsis.* Sepsis with organ dysfunction, hypotension and hypoperfusion (e.g. hypoxaemia, lactic acidosis, oliguria).
- *Septic shock.* Severe sepsis with hypotension despite fluid resuscitation. The development of secondary abnormalities due to hypotension (e.g. cardiovascular instability, acute renal failure) (Kulkarni & Webster 1996).

Generalized management of SIRS and sepsis

If sepsis is suspected, every attempt should be made to identify the causative organisms. Cultures are taken from blood, urine, line sites and open wounds etc. Imaging may include a chest radiograph and an ultrasound of the abdomen and pelvis. Possible sources of infection such as lines and abscesses must be eliminated. If a causative organism can be identified, appropriate antimicrobials are started. The main-

stay of treatment in severe SIRS or sepsis is supportive.

Cardiovascular system. Fluid resuscitation, inotropes and vasopressors are used to maintain mean arterial blood pressure and adequate tissue perfusion.

Respiratory system. Ventilatory support is used to ensure adequate gaseous exchange.

Renal system. The use of fluids, diuretics and dopamine will support renal function. Haemofiltration or haemodialysis, may become necessary as the septic process advances.

Haematological system. Blood, blood products and clotting factors can be given to assist the correction of abnormalities.

Gastrointestinal system. Adequate nutrition is essential to maintain tissue viability in the septic patient. The risk of stress ulceration can be minimized by the use of hydrogen receptor agonists.

Musculoskeletal system. Pressure area care is essential to prevent further foci of infection. The use of a specialist mattress and/or bed may be advantageous.

Considerations for physiotherapy
- The septic patient will require extensive monitoring of simple parameters such as temperature, blood pressure, urine output and arterial blood gases, as well as haemodynamic factors such as pulmonary artery pressure, pulmonary artery wedge pressure and central venous pressure. Measurements of cardiac output and the calculation of pulmonary vascular resistance can be used to guide medical management. Physiotherapeutic intervention should only be undertaken in a situation where there is a strong indication and the patient is cardiovascularly stable (see p. 269). If manual hyperinflation is indicated, additional inotropic support and increased fluids may be required. Close monitoring of all parameters throughout treatment is essential.

Acute respiratory distress syndrome (ARDS)

ARDS represents the severe end of the spectrum of acute lung injury. This syndrome results from the disruption of the alveolar–capillary membrane, secondary to either local or distant injury. It is characterized by three features:

- Hypoxaemia – this may vary in level of severity
- Diffuse radiographical infiltrates
- Reduced respiratory system compliance.

The acute phase is characterized by increased capillary permeability. This leads to the development of non-cardiogenic oedema. In those patients that survive there is subsequent repair, involving regeneration of the alveolar epithelium, producing varying degrees of lung fibrosis. The aetiology of ARDS is diverse ranging from direct lung trauma (e.g. aspiration, inhalation and near drowning) to systemic disorders (e.g. poisoning, obstetric complications, sepsis, major haemorrhage, etc.) (Murray 1996).

The management of patients with ARDS is essentially supportive. Where possible the identification and treatment of the underlying cause is paramount. Haemodynamic monitoring and support is necessary to maintain an adequate blood pressure and cardiac output, while monitoring and preventing fluid overload in the lungs.

Ventilatory strategies are aimed at improving alveolar recruitment, while avoiding further injury to the lungs. This is currently achieved by using pressure-controlled ventilation, with an inverse ratio of inspiration to expiration, combined with PEEP. Inverse ratio ventilation is sometimes not well tolerated in non-paralysed patients. It should be noted that a high level of PEEP may compromise cardiac output.

More experimental techniques being used are high-frequency jet ventilation, extracorporeal gas exchange systems, inhaled nitric oxide and exogenous surfactant.

Changes of position from supine to prone and/or prone to supine may improve ventilation–perfusion matching as dependent oedema is redistributed (Pappert et al 1994). The use of continuous rotation on a specialist bed (kinetic therapy) may also be beneficial. As yet none of the above have been proven to have a positive effect on outcome (Mulnier & Evans 1995).

Considerations for physiotherapy
- In the early stages of ARDS when the main manifestation is interstitial oedema, physiotherapy has very little to offer. As the syndrome progresses and fibrosis is the most prominent feature, physiotherapy may assist in preventing areas of atelectasis and sputum plugging. Patients with ARDS frequently develop pneumothoraces due to decreased compliance. It should be noted that if several chest drains are in position, manual hyperinflation is of no benefit, as air escapes through the chest drains. In the later stages, if physiotherapy is indicated in a PEEP-dependent patient, a PEEP valve is recommended (p. 286). If nitric oxide is being entrained during ventilation, physiotherapy is contraindicated. When suction is required, a closed-circuit suction system should be used (p. 288).

Disseminated intravascular coagulation (DIC)

DIC is a condition in which there is increased activation of both the normal procoagulant and anticoagulant pathways. It may be triggered by a variety of disorders including infection, trauma, malignancy and vasculitis. The increased activity leads to abnormal consumption of platelets, clotting factors and associated regulating factors. Initially the release of stored platelets and factors may maintain the balance of these two pathways. However, in severe conditions this compensation is lost and the situation is worsened as fibrinolysis produces fibrin degradation products which act as anticoagulants (Kesteven & Saunders 1993).

Also abnormal fibrin formation in the vasculature causes occlusion and is closely related to development of multi-organ failure. Treatment is aimed at eliminating the trigger, arresting intravascular clotting and replacement of clotting factors (Hambley 1995).

Considerations for physiotherapy
- DIC can be mild, moderate or severe. As it is a marker of severe illness, the overall stability of the patient must be assessed. In the mild

situation where bleeding is minimal, physiotherapy can continue. In the severe state, blood loss may be considerable and the patient may become unstable. Any intervention which may exacerbate bleeding, e.g. suction, should be avoided unless it is essential.

Inhalation burns

15–25% of patients who suffer significant burns, will present with respiratory complications. Respiratory failure and infection account for the majority of mortalities associated with burns (Bordow & Landers 1985). Smoke inhalation is suggested by soot around the nostrils and mouth. Initially hypoxia is caused by the high affinity of carbon monoxide for haemoglobin (210–250 times greater than oxygen). The oxygen-dissociation curve shifts to the left (Murray 1976) greatly reducing the oxygen-carrying capacity of haemoglobin and thus reducing oxygen delivery to the tissues. Toxic elements in smoke can cause oedema of the mucosa, bronchospasm, destruction of cilia and loss of surfactant.

Thermal injury can be isolated to the pharynx and upper airway or if steam is inhaled there may be significant alveolar damage. Toxic elements (e.g. noxious gas) and thermal injury contribute to 'on-going' hypoxia.

Considerations for physiotherapy

• Patients with either significant facial burns or inhalation injury will require intubation and ventilation. Following inhalation burns, patients can present with thick tenacious, soot-stained secretions. These will require adequate humidification. Nebulized bronchodilators are essential in the presence of bronchospasm.

• Suction should be carried out with care to prevent further trauma to damaged airways. Careful consideration must be given to soft tissue damage and positioning of the patient (Keilty 1993).

Trauma

Injury in the trauma patient can result from many different mechanisms, ranging from a high-impact insult following a road traffic accident to assault or merely a fall. The patient may sustain multiple injuries which are often complex and interrelated. The scale of these injuries may predispose this group of patients to developing secondary associated problems such as ARDS or DIC (Antonelli et al 1994).

Head injury

Trauma to the head may involve a haemorrhage or contusion which may be focal or diffuse. Diagnosis is assisted by CT scanning. Primary damage sustained at the time of insult cannot be reversed. However, subsequent secondary damage (e.g. hypoxia and hypotension) can be minimized. Surgical intervention may be indicated as first-line management (e.g. evacuation of a clot or insertion of a ventricular drain or shunt). Patients who have undergone extensive surgery and remain critical or unstable will require continued care in the ICU. Patients not suitable for surgical intervention are conservatively managed in the ICU (e.g. gross cerebral oedema). Close monitoring is essential as neurological vital signs can change very suddenly. ICP and CPP valves are used to guide medical management (p. 268).

These patients are sedated and often paralysed in order to prevent fluctuating ICPs rising to critical levels (see Table 11.1). Intubation and ventilation are essential not only for airway protection but to enable manipulation of $PaCO_2$ levels. Carbon dioxide can have vasodilatory effects on blood vessels. By maintaining low carbon dioxide levels with hyperventilation, cerebral vasodilatation may be reduced thus lowering cerebral blood flow so reducing ICP. This approach is only used for the first 48 hours as after this time it is less effective (Eisenhart 1994).

These patients are nursed in 15–30° head elevation with their head in midline (i.e. nose in line with sternum). This will ensure maximal venous drainage from the cerebral circulation.

Inotropic support may be necessary to maintain adequate MAP and therefore CPP. Diuretic therapy such as mannitol is used to assist in the reduction of cerebral oedema. The use of steroids in head-injured patients remains controversial.

In extreme circumstances, when the brain stem is irreversibly damaged, the patient cannot sustain spontaneous ventilation. This is defined as brain stem death. This is assessed by specific tests. Some patients may be suitable for organ donation (Thomas 1991).

Considerations for physiotherapy

• Critically ill patients should always be closely assessed and monitored during any intervention, but this is paramount in the neurologically impaired patient as vital signs can fluctuate rapidly (e.g. ICP, CPP, MAP).

• A thorough assessment will demonstrate an indication for physiotherapy treatment of the acute neurological patient. It is important to distinguish between a neurological cause of deterioration and an underlying respiratory problem.

• Before physiotherapy the patient's level of consciousness and sedation should be reviewed, and a bolus of sedation may be given as appropriate to prevent excessive rises in ICP. If indicated, the patient's position can be altered for treatment purposes. During movement the head must be maintained in the midline position at all times. Direct pressure should not be applied to the bolt, drain or shunt site.

• Ventricular drains should be closed during excessive movement and physiotherapy, but opened immediately after treatment. After a craniotomy, if the bone flap is not replaced, the patient can be repositioned provided that pillows are arranged to prevent direct pressure on the unprotected brain.

• The use of sedation and paralysing agents may result in a poor cough reflex and lead to the retention of secretions or atelectasis. Both these can lead to hypoxia and hypercapnia which in turn will cause cerebral vasodilatation and raised ICP (Garradd & Bullock 1986). Physiotherapy intervention may be essential. If manual hyperinflation is indicated, small rapid breaths should be interspersed between hyperinflations to maintain the low $PaCO_2$. It is important to note that manual hyperinflation may reduce cardiac output and therefore compromise CPP. As the cerebral and thoracic venous systems are in open communication, the increased intrathoracic pressure during manual hyperinflation may increase ICP. The increased intrathoracic pressure may also compromise cerebral venous drainage (Paratz & Burns 1993).

• Suction should only be used when absolutely indicated as it has been well documented to dramatically increase ICP. This is thought to be due to direct tracheal stimulation and increased intrathoracic pressure causing reduced venous return during a cough (Rudy et al 1991). It may be necessary to pre-oxygenate the unstable patient before suction. Excessive stimulation from manual techniques may increase ICP.

• In the early stages patients should be reassessed regularly but treatment should be restricted and of limited duration. It is important to remember that during the initial stages of reducing sedation, the patient may become agitated and self-extubation is a potential hazard. Similarly, in the first 48–72 hours, good positioning is adequate in the absence of tonal change. As soon as the patient is medically stable, intensive rehabilitation should start. Despite ventilatory support the patient can sit or stand as indicated.

• Patients suitable for organ donation will require ongoing physiotherapy assessment and treatment to maintain optimum respiratory function.

Flail chest injury and pulmonary contusion

See Chapter 12, page 316.

Pulmonary emboli. Pulmonary embolism is one of the potential complications of the trauma patient. It is a complication of deep vein thrombosis in which fragments of thrombus enter the pulmonary circulation and cause obstruction.

Considerations for physiotherapy

• Once anticoagulation therapy has been started and the risk of thrombus formation minimized, physiotherapy can continue as indicated. Anticoagulation therapy must be strictly monitored as excess use may lead to bleeding problems, therefore care must be taken with suction.

Fat emboli. Fat embolism is a complication of the multi-trauma patient. The release of fat may be associated with fractures particularly of the pelvis or long bones or entry of fat globules into the venous circulation with massive trauma or extensive burns. These emboli may obstruct the pulmonary and/or cerebral circulation.

Considerations for physiotherapy
• Treatment is supportive and aimed at maximizing oxygen delivery to peripheral tissues. In the acute phase musculoskeletal intervention is contraindicated until any long bone fractures are stabilized. Chest physiotherapy can be complicated by the development of DIC.

Neurological conditions requiring intensive care

Myasthenia gravis

Myasthenia gravis is a disease which is due to a transmission defect at the neuromuscular junction (Scadding 1990). The disease is characterized by fatiguable weakness occurring in striated muscle. This may be local or generalized.

Considerations for physiotherapy
• Severe progression of the disease will necessitate ventilation. Treatment involves the administration of anticholinesterase drugs which help to maximize muscle function. These drugs frequently lead to excess secretions. Where possible, physiotherapy should be timed to occur after administration of the drug. Nocturnal ventilation may be required even after daytime weaning has been successful. A progressive rehabilitation programme should be instigated as soon as possible.

Guillain–Barré syndrome

Guillain–Barré syndrome is an acute demyelinating polyradiculoneuropathy affecting predominantly motor neurons (Tharakan et al 1989,

Hughes & Rees 1994). Although prognosis is excellent for the majority of patients, 10–20% have significant residual disabilities as a result of muscle weakness, contracture, sensory dysfunction and psychological factors (Ferner et al 1987, van-der-Meche & Schmitz 1992, Lennon et al 1993). The course of the disease is divided into three stages (Karni et al 1984, Watson & Wilson 1989): initial acute stage, plateau stage and recovery stage. In the acute stage respiration may be compromised as a result of respiratory muscle weakness and bulbar palsy and mechanical ventilation may be indicated (Ferner et al 1987, Watson & Wilson 1989, Scadding 1990). Plasma exchange and intravenous immunoglobulin therapy are the main treatments available, both resulting in decreased morbidity and improved final outcome (Guillain–Barré Syndrome Study Group 1985, Rees 1993, Hughes & Rees 1994).

Considerations for physiotherapy
• From the onset of paralysis, physiotherapy intervention must be aimed at prevention of atelectasis and chest infection and maintenance of ventilation in addition to maintenance of joint range and soft tissue length (Rees 1993). Treatments for the musculoskeletal system include passive/active-assisted/strengthening exercises, stretches, positioning, splinting, standing using a tilt table or standing frame and provision of suitable seating (Ferner et al 1987, Fowler & Falkner 1992, Edwards 1996). Pain can be quite severe in all stages of the disease. Analgesia such as opiates, non-steroidal anti-inflammatories or Entonox may be administered prior to physiotherapy intervention to provide adequate pain control (Clark 1985, Ferner et al 1987, Fowler & Falkner 1992).
• As muscle function improves, an active weaning programme should be devised. The patient is encouraged to breathe spontaneously for increasing periods during the day, but is often given ventilatory support at night to ensure adequate rest (Ferner et al 1987). Once the patient is off ventilatory support, treatment is usually continued in a multidisciplinary rehabilitation unit.

Tetanus

Tetanus is a disease caused by a neuromuscular toxin produced by spores causing general muscle rigidity and convulsions. The respiratory muscles can be affected and paralysis and mechanical ventilation is necessary (Oh 1990).

Considerations for physiotherapy

• Adequate sedation and muscle relaxants must be given to ensure effective physiotherapy. Rehabilitation should start once the condition is stabilized.

Poliomyelitis

This virus attacks the grey matter of the spinal cord, brain stem and cortex. In particular, damage is sustained by anterior horn cells especially those of the lumbar segments (Macleod et al 1987). The disease varies from influenza-like symptoms to severe paralysis including the respiratory muscles. Intubation and ventilation may be necessary using intermittent positive pressure ventilation, although the use of negative pressure ventilation (iron lung) may still be seen (Higgens 1966), or non-invasive ventilation can be used.

Considerations for physiotherapy

• Irrespective of the method of ventilation, chest physiotherapy will be indicated in the presence of excess bronchial secretions and/or lung collapse. Early instigation of a rehabilitation programme is essential.

PHYSIOTHERAPY TECHNIQUES

Once a thorough assessment has been completed, the findings must be analysed to identify relevant physiotherapeutic problems. For each problem a suitable treatment plan must be formulated taking into consideration any potential influencing factors. Again, it should be emphasized that because of the complex nature of the ICU patient, there is no place for routine chest physiotherapy. It must be remembered that there will be situations when an indication for treatment exists, but the patient's overall instability would result in the treatment having

a negative effect. ICU patients may become 'end-stage' and not for resuscitation, but this does not preclude them from a daily assessment and treatment as indicated (Pearson & Parr 1993).

Despite the fact that the ICU patient is often sedated and paralysed, communication is of paramount importance. As with a conscious patient an introduction must be made together with an explanation of the planned treatment. This not only will ensure that the patient is informed of procedures but will provide an explanation and involve the relatives with the physiotherapy.

Gravity-assisted positioning

These positions use gravity to assist in the drainage of a specific bronchopulmonary segment (p. 151). When positioning the patient, care must be taken with tubes, drains and lines. The patient's cardiovascular stability must be assessed before any change of position. Modified positioning may be indicated.

Ventilation perfusion ratios ($\dot{V}/\dot{Q}$) during mechanical ventilation are not the same as those during spontaneous breathing (p. 124). After physiotherapy the patient can be positioned to optimize $\dot{V}/\dot{Q}$ matching. In the mechanically ventilated patient, where there will always be a $\dot{V}/\dot{Q}$ mismatch patients should be assessed individually to ascertain the most beneficial position (Pearson & Parr 1993).

Manual hyperinflation

'Bagging' can be used as a technique to hand-ventilate a patient or during physiotherapy. When hand ventilating, normal tidal volumes are generally delivered, whereas to facilitate physiotherapy larger breaths or hyperinflations are necessary. Manual hyperinflation can be given either using a Water's bag circuit or an Ambu-bag. A greater range of volume is available with a Water's bag. For an adult a 2 or 3 litre Water's bag, connected to a flow of 10–15 litres of oxygen is commonly used (Fig. 11.2). By altering the expiratory valve, volume and therefore inspiratory pressure can be manipulated. The use of a manometer acts as a guide

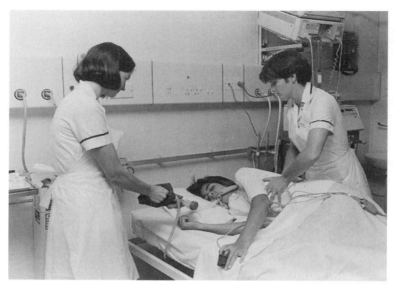

Fig. 11.2 Manual hyperinflation with chest shaking.

to inflation pressures which are recommended to be less than 40 cmH$_2$O (Pearson 1996). If manual hyperinflation is indicated in a PEEP-dependent patient, a PEEP valve must be used to maintain positive end-expiratory pressure during treatment (Jones et al 1992).

Indications (Jones et al 1992, Hodgson et al 1996)

- To aid removal of secretions
- To aid reinflation of atelectatic segments
- To assess lung compliance
- To improve lung compliance.

Therapeutic effects of manual hyperinflation

The most common technique used is a slow inspiration, and inspiratory hold followed by quick expiratory release (Clement & Hübsch 1968). A prolonged inspiratory hold is contra-indicated in a patient who is already hyper-inflated (e.g. emphysema).

Slow deep inspiration:
- Recruits collateral ventilation thus promoting mobilization of secretions
- Enhances interdependence to aid re-expansion of atelectatic segments

- Improves gaseous exchange
- Assesses and potentially improves compliance.

Inspiratory hold (at full inspiration):
- Further utilizes collateral ventilation and interdependence as at higher volume; therefore maximizes pressure distribution.

Fast expiratory release:
- Mimics a forced expiration (huff or cough)
- Stimulates a cough.

Hand-held PEEP:
- By grasping and holding the end of a semi-filled bag throughout inspiration and expiration it is possible to maintain a low level of PEEP.

Hazards of manual hyperinflation

Reduction in blood pressure. During manual hyperinflation the normal mechanism which 'sucks' the remaining blood from the inferior vena cava to the right atrium during negative pressure inspiration is lost. In addition, the positive pressure generated during manual hyper-inflation increases intrathoracic pressure. Both mechanisms compromise venous return. The resultant effect could be a reduction in stroke volume and therefore a drop in blood pressure. This risk is potentially increased when using a PEEP valve, or during prolonged inspiratory holds. It should be noted that if a bolus of sedation is given before treatment, this may lower the blood pressure through vasodilatation (Singer et al 1994).

Considerations for physiotherapy
• If the blood pressure drops during treatment, smaller tidal breaths should be given. If the blood pressure remains compromised the patient should be put back onto the ventilator, positioned appropriately and a medical review requested.

Reduced saturations. Oxygen saturations can be compromised by sputum plugging, collapse, pneumothorax, bronchospasm and $\dot{V}/\dot{Q}$ mismatching.

Considerations for physiotherapy
• Reassessment will highlight the cause. Intermediate measures such as increasing the FiO_2 can be used.

Raised intracranial pressure. The presence of increased levels of $PaCO_2$ in cerebral blood vessels may lead to vasodilatation. The resultant increased cerebral blood flow may increase ICP (Eisenhart 1994).

Considerations for physiotherapy
• To prevent fluctuations in ICP during manual hyperinflation small fast breaths should be interspersed between hyperinflations.

Reduced respiratory drive. $PaCO_2$ levels may be reduced during effective treatment. This may reduce the patient's respiratory drive.

Considerations for physiotherapy
• After finishing manual hyperinflation, the patient's spontaneous respiratory effort should be monitored.

Contraindications to manual hyperinflation

• Undrained pneumothorax (presence of patent intercostal drain – treat as normal)
• Potential bronchospasm
• Severe bronchospasm

• Gross cardiovascular instability inducing arrhythymias and hypovolaemia
• Unexplained haemoptysis
• An absolute indication for treatment should be present before manual hyperinflation is used on patients requiring PEEP levels greater than 15 cmH$_2$O plus maximal ventilatory support, or patients with high peak and mean inspiratory pressures.

Suctioning the intubated patient

Each day the normal person generates an average of 100 ml of bronchial secretions. If the normal mechanisms such as ciliary action are compromised, alveolar ventilation may be impaired. Suction may be indicated to remove these secretions. The suction catheter used must be less than half the diameter of the endotracheal tube. Trauma can be further minimized by the use of a catheter with an atraumatic end and a Y-connector. The vacuum pressure should be as low as possible (e.g. 8–20 kPa, 60–150 mmHg). Suction should never be routine, only when there is an indication. A full explanation of the procedure reduces patient anxiety (Copnell & Fergusson 1995).

Indications

• Inability to cough effectively
• Sputum plugging
• To assess tube patency.

Technique

The technique (Fig. 11.3) should either be sterile or clean, depending on the hospital's infection control policy. Before suctioning, an explanation of the procedure is given to the patient and equipment is made ready. Pre- and post-oxygenation can be used as required. In the majority of patients the depth of insertion is that sufficient to elicit a cough reflex. In the paralysed patient, insertion must be done with great care. Once the end point is reached (e.g. mucosa) the catheter must be withdrawn 1 cm before suction is applied to prevent mucosal

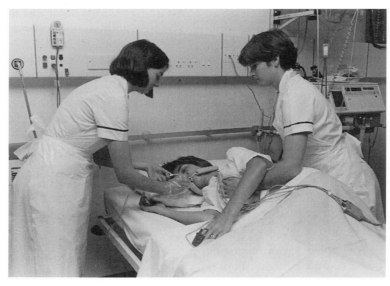

Fig. 11.3 Endotracheal suction (with chest support).

invagination and trauma. The duration in adults should be limited to 10–15 seconds. Suction should be applied constantly while removing the catheter. Intermittent suction should only be used when removing a sticky plug. Saline can be used as an aid in suctioning. The use of a sputum trap to obtain a specimen for microbiological assessment will assist with the correct antibiotic therapy (Ciesla 1996).

Hazards of suctioning

Mucosal trauma. Mucosal trauma is reduced by using an atraumatic catheter, good suctioning technique, and the correct pressures.

Cardiac arrhythymias. Direct tracheal stimulation causing a vasovagal reflex can cause arrhythmias (Young 1984). Pre- and post-oxygenation can minimize this effect. If suction is necessary in patients who demonstrate arrhythmias on suctioning, it is advisable to discuss with medical staff regarding the use of pharmacological agents to prevent arrhythmias (e.g. atropine).

Hypoxia. Hypoxia can be caused by the interruption of ventilation, reflex bronchospasm and the removal of the oxygen supply. Pre- and post-oxygenation can minimize this effect.

Raised intracanial pressure. Suction has been proven to increase ICP dramatically, therefore suction should be used only when indicated (Young 1984).

Contraindications to suctioning the intubated patient

- Frank haemoptysis
- Severe bronchospasm
- Undrained pneumothorax
- Compromised cardiovascular system.

Closed-circuit suction

Closed-circuit suction systems are available and consist of a catheter in a protective closed sheath which remains attached to the endotracheal or tracheostomy tube for 24 hours (Crimlisk et al 1994). The indications for use are: immuno-suppressed patients, actively infectious patients (e.g. open TB) and patients with severe refractory hypoxaemia on high levels of PEEP.

Nasal and oral suction

Sedated and/or paralysed patients with a loss of gag and swallowing reflexes may need nasal and oral suction. A soft catheter (size 12 or 10) can be used for the nose, but a rigid sucker (Yankauer) may be necessary for the mouth, or a catheter passed through an oral airway. To minimize trauma to the nasal passages a nasal airway (nasal trumpet) may be used. For suction of the non-intubated patient, see page 161.

Saline administration

The administration of normal saline as a physiotherapy adjunct is widespread, although the evidence for its efficacy is not established (Raymond 1995). It is usual to use up to 5 ml of normal saline (0.9%), but on occasions it may be necessary to use greater volumes (e.g. removal of a large plug occluding the endotracheal tube). As with any adjunct to physiotherapy the use of normal saline should not be routine. If it is difficult to loosen and clear tenacious secretions on suction, the use of normal saline is indicated. It is important to assess a patient's overall level of hydration as systemically dehydrated patients are at greater risk of plugging. Additional continuous heated humidification may be necessary and reduce the need for normal saline. Normal saline nebulizers can be incorporated into the ventilator circuit when indicated.

Considerations for physiotherapy
• Normal saline can be used to assist the removal of tenacious secretions during physiotherapy and/or used to assess and maintain patency of an endotracheal tube. Normal saline can be administered just prior to treatment to stimulate a cough and to maximize the clearance of secretions. If normal saline is to be introduced at the beginning of a treatment, the use of short sharp hyperinflations can potentially aid dispersal of the fluid and heighten the stimulation of a cough.
• In the event of acute lobar collapse, it can be beneficial to administer normal saline at the beginning of treatment with the patient positioned with the 'collapsed' area in the dependent position. Gravity will then assist the passage of the saline. Once the saline has been administered and a few breaths by manual hyperinflation have been given, the patient should be repositioned in the correct gravity-assisted position. Manual hyperinflation in conjunction with manual techniques will aid in reinflation of the collapsed area.

Manual techniques

These encompass a variety of manual skills. Shaking and vibrations during the expiratory phase increase expiratory flow and aid the removal of secretions. Chest clapping may be indicated to assist in the mobilization of tenacious secretions.

Considerations for physiotherapy
• After assessment, if a patient is considered too unstable to tolerate manual hyperinflation, shaking and/or vibrations can be performed during the expiratory phase of the respiratory cycle in synchrony with the ventilator. This may aid removal of secretions.

Intermittent positive pressure breathing (IPPB)

IPPB can be used in the treatment of an intubated patient. The appropriate catheter mount is used in place of a mouthpiece or mask to connect the circuit to an endotracheal or tracheostomy tube (see p. 169).

Considerations for physiotherapy
• IPPB is extremely useful for physiotherapy in the weaning process. The positive pressure augments tidal volume in an essentially self-ventilating patient with respiratory muscle weakness or fatigue. A patient who has a depressed cough reflex following long-term intubation can be assisted with the use of IPPB. The increased tidal volume utilizes collateral ventilation and assists the mobilization of secretions. These patients often fatigue easily and IPPB reduces the work of breathing.

Box 11.1 Commonly encountered problem situations

Cardiopulmonary arrest
- Alert help immediately
- Follow 'arrest' procedure

Sudden drop in blood pressure
- Stop manual hyperinflations – give tidal breaths
- Check arterial line
  – correct reading
  – correct trace
- Alert help
- Terminate treatment – put patient back on to ventilator
- Put patient supine
- Monitor vital signs

Cardiac arrhythmias
- Check chest leads
  – attached
  – reading accurately
- Alert help
- Terminate treatment immediately and put patient back on to ventilator

Sudden rise in intracranial pressure
- Check ICP tracing
- Alert help
- Give rapid shallow breaths with bag – hyperventilate
- Terminate treatment and put patient back on to ventilator
- Check head and neck alignment and position

Dislodged endotracheal tube
- Alert help immediately
- If effective, continue to hand ventilate with tidal volumes until help arrives
- If ineffective – urgent help imperative
- Monitor vital signs especially saturation

Self-extubation
- Alert help immediately
- Assist ventilation with a resuscitation bag (e.g. Ambu) with face mask
- Closely monitor vital signs especially saturations
NB: If patient appears to be making adequate spontaneous effort with good saturations, administer high level of oxygen via a face mask and monitor closely.

Fully blocked endotracheal or tracheostomy tube
- Alert help immediately
- Check positioning of endotracheal tube
- Attempt suction with saline
- Deflate cuff
- Assist ventilation with a resuscitation bag (e.g. Ambu) with face mask until help arrives
- Monitor vital signs especially saturations

Partially blocked endotracheal or tracheostomy tube
- Notify nursing staff
- Continue manual hyperinflations, saline administration and suction
- If unable to clear – inform medical staff
- Monitor vital signs especially saturations

Accidental removal of chest drain
- Apply immediate constant pressure to drain site occluding the hole
- Alert help immediately
- Terminate treatment immediately and put patient back on to ventilator
- Monitor vital signs
NB: If patient awake and making spontaneous effort, ask patient to exhale prior to applying pressure to drain site.

Sudden desaturation
- Check saturation probe – accurate reading
- Notify nursing staff
- Assess cause (e.g. pneumothorax, 'plugging off', collapse, bronchospasm, cardiovascular instability)
- If physiotherapy will relieve problem – continue treatment
- Monitor vital signs – especially saturation
- Medical problem – alert help immediately
- Terminate treatment and put patient back on to ventilator

Sudden onset no breath sounds one lung
- Assess cause (e.g. collapse, sputum plug, pneumothorax, misplaced tube)
- If physiotherapy will relieve problem – continue treatment
- Monitor vital signs especially saturations and blood pressure
- Medical problem – alert help immediately
- Terminate treatment and put patient back on to ventilator

Sudden reduction in level of consciousness
- Alert help immediately
- Terminate treatment and put patient back on to ventilator
- Monitor vital signs

Accidental removal of vascular catheter or arterial line
- Apply constant pressure to site immediately
- Alert help

Accidental removal or dislodging of CVP line or PA catheter
- Apply constant pressure to site if removed
- If dislodged, prevent further traction on line
- Notify nursing staff

Periodic continuous positive pressure ventilation (PCPAP)

PCPAP is a useful adjunct in patients presenting with reduced lung volumes and/or areas of atelectasis (see p. 173). The circuit can be attached directly to an endotracheal or tracheostomy tube or via a face mask or mouthpiece in an extubated patient.

Considerations for physiotherapy
• PCPAP can be used to maximize functional residual capacity and to aid reinflation of areas of atelectasis immediately following extubation. In the multi-problematic patient CPAP or PCPAP can be used in conjunction with IPPB.

EMERGENCY SITUATIONS

Box 11.1 lists a few commonly encountered problem situations, together with some physiotherapy action guidelines. It must be remembered that whenever faced with an emergency or potential crisis help must be sought immediately. In the intensive care setting help is never far away. The patient's nurse should be alerted immediately. If the situation continues to be problematic, the medical team should be asked to review the patient urgently.

ACKNOWLEDGEMENTS

We would like to acknowledge the assistance of Dr Mark Evans, Dr Jane Howard and Dr Andrew Jones.

REFERENCES

Antonelli M, Moro M L, Capelli O et al 1994 Risk factors for early onset pneumonia in trauma patients. Chest 105: 224–228

Birtwistle J 1994 Pressure sore formation and risk assessment in intensive care. Care of the Critically Ill 10: 154–159

Bordow R A, Landers C F 1985 Pulmonary injury. In: Bordow R A, Moser K M (eds) Manual of clinical problems in pulmonary medicine, 2nd edn. Little Brown, Boston

Branson R D, Davis K, Campbell R S, Johnson D J, Porembka D T 1993 Humidification in the intensive care unit. Prospective study of a new protocol utilizing heated humidification and a hygroscopic condenser humidifier. Chest 104: 1800–1805

Browne D R G 1988a Weaning patients from ventilators 1. Hospital Update July: 1809–1817

Browne D R G 1988b Weaning patients from ventilators 2. Hospital Update August: 1898–1906

Ciesla N D 1996 Chest physical therapy for patients in the intensive care unit. Physical Therapy 76: 609–625

Clark K J 1985 Coping with Guillain–Barré syndrome. Intensive Care Nursing 1: 13–18

Clement A J, Hübsch S K 1968 Chest physiotherapy by the 'bag squeezing' method. Physiotherapy 54: 355–359

Connine T, Sullivan T, Mackie T, Goodman M 1990 Effect of serial casting for the prevention of equinus in patients with acute head injury. Archives of Medical Rehabilitation 71: 310–312

Copnell B, Fergusson D 1995 Endotracheal suctioning: time-worn ritual or timely intervention? American Journal of Critical Care 4: 100–105

Crimlisk J T, Paris R, McGonagle E G, Calcutt J A, Farber H W 1994 The closed tracheal suction system: implications for critical care nursing. Dimensions of Critical Care Nursing 13: 292–300

Edwards S 1996 Neurological physiotherapy, a problem-solving approach. Churchill Livingstone, Edinburgh

Eisenhart K 1994 New perspectives in the management of adults with severe head injury. Critical Care Nursing 17: 1–12

Emery P, Salmon M 1991 Systemic mediators of inflammation. British Journal of Hospital Medicine 45: 164–168

Ferner R, Barnett M, Hughes R A C 1987 Management of Guillain–Barré syndrome. British Journal of Hospital Medicine Dec: 526–530

Fowler R, Falkner T 1992 The use of hypnosis for pain relief for patients with polyradiculoneuritis. Australian Physiotherapy 38: 217–221

Frisby J R 1990 Predicting outcome of critical illness. In: Oh T E (ed) Intensive care manual, 3rd edn. Butterworths, Sydney, ch 2, pp 7–12

Ganong W F 1995 Review of medical physiology, 17th edn. Appleton & Lange, Connecticut, pp 482–496

Garradd J, Bullock M 1986 The effect of respiratory therapy on intracranial pressure in ventilated neurosurgical patients. Australian Journal of Physiotherapy 32: 107–111

German K 1994 Intracranial pressure monitoring in the 1990's. Critical Care Nursing 17: 21–32

Guillain–Barré Syndrome Study Group 1985 Plasmapheresis and acute Guillain–Barré syndrome. Neurology 35: 1096–1104

Hambley H 1995 Coagulation (II) – clinical problems in coagulation disorders. Care of the Critically Ill 11: 203–205

Higgens J M 1966 The management in cabinet respirators of patients with acute or residual respiratory muscle paralysis. Physiotherapy 52: 425–430

Hodgson C, Denehy L, Ntoumenopoulos G, Santamaria J 1996 The acute cardiorespiratory effects of manual lung hyperinflation on ventilated patients. European Respiratory Journal 9(suppl 23): 37s

Hughes R A C, Rees J H 1994 Guillain–Barré syndrome current opinion. Neurology 7: 386–392

Jones A J M, Hutchinson R C, Oh T E 1992 Effects of bagging and percussion on total static compliance of the respiratory system. Physiotherapy 78: 661–666

Karni Y, Archdeacon L, Mills K R, Wiles C M 1984 Clinical assessment and physiotherapy in Guillain–Barré syndrome. Physiotherapy 70: 288–292

Keilty S E J 1993 Inhalation burn injured patients and physiotherapy management. Physiotherapy 79: 87–90

Kesteven P, Saunders P 1993 Disseminated intravascular coagulation. Care of the Critically Ill 9: 22–27

Kirby S, Davenport A 1996 Haemofiltration/dialysis treatment in patients with acute renal failure. Care of the Critically Ill 12: 54–58

Knaus W A, Draper E A, Wagner D P, Zimmerman J E 1985 APACHE II: a severity of disease classification system. Critical Care Medicine 13: 818–829

Kulkarni V, Webster N 1996 Management of sepsis. Care of the Critically Ill 12: 122–127

Lennon S M, Koblar S, Hughes R A C, Goellar J, Riser A C 1993 Reasons for persistent disability in Guillain–Barré syndrome. Clinical Rehabilitation 7: 1–8

Macleod J, Edwards C, Bouchier I (eds) 1987 Davidson's principles and practice of medicine, 15th edn. Churchill Livingstone, Edinburgh, ch 15, p 644

Miller J D, Becker D P, Ward J D et al 1977 Significance of intracranial hypertension in severe head injury. Journal of Neurosurgery 47: 503–516

Murray J F 1996 ARDS introduction and definition. In: Evans T W, Haslett C ARDS acute respiratory distress in adults. Chapman & Hall, London, pp 3–12

Murray J S 1976 The normal lung: the basis of diagnosis and treatment of pulmonary disease. W B Saunders, Philadelphia

Mulnier C, Evans T 1995 Acute respiratory distress in adults (ARDS). Care of the Critically Ill 11: 182–186

Oh T E 1990 Tetanus. In: Oh T E (ed) Intensive care manual, 3rd edn. Butterworths, Sydney, ch 45, pp 305–309

Pappert D, Rossaint R, Salma K, Gruning T, Falke K J 1994 Influence of positioning on ventilation–perfusion relationships in severe adult respiratory distress syndrome. Chest 106: 1511–1516

Paratz J, Burns Y 1993 The effect of respiratory physiotherapy on intracranial pressure, mean arterial pressure, cerebral perfusion pressure and end tidal carbon dioxide in ventilated neurosurgical patients. Physiotherapy Theory and Practice 9: 3–11

Pearson S J 1996 Peak airway pressures exerted during manual hyperinflation by physiotherapists and nursing staff. British Journal of Therapy and Rehabilitation 3: 261–266

Pearson S, Parr S 1993 Physiotherapy in the critically ill patient. Care of the Critically Ill 9: 128–131

Rapper S, Maynard N 1992 Feeding the critically ill patient. British Journal of Nursing 1: 273–280

Raymond S 1995 Normal saline instillation before suctioning: Helpful or harmful? A review of the literature. American Journal of Critical Care 4: 267–271

Rees J 1993 Guillain–Barré syndrome: the latest on treatment. British Journal of Hospital Medicine 50: 226–229

Rudy E B, Turner B S, Baun M, Stone K S, Brucia J 1991 Endotracheal suctioning in adults with head injury. Heart and Lung 20: 667–674

Scadding J W 1990 Neurological disease. In: Souhami R L, Moxham J (eds) Textbook of medicine. Churchill Livingstone, Edinburgh, ch 23

Sciaky A J 1994 Mobilising the intensive care unit patient. Physical Therapy Practice 3: 69–80

Singer M, Vermaat J, Hall G 1994 Haemodynamic effects of manual hyperinflation in critically ill mechanically ventilated patients. Chest 106: 1182–1187

Tharakan J, Ferner R E, Hughes R A C, Winer J, Barnett M, Brown E R, Smith G 1989 Plasma exchange for Guillain–Barré syndrome. Journal of the Royal Society of Medicine 82: 458–461

Thomas S 1991 The gift of life. Nursing Times 87: 28–31

van-der-Meche F G A, Schmitz P I M 1992 High dose intravenous immunoglobulin versus plasma exchange in Guillain–Barré syndrome. New England Journal of Medicine 326: 1123–1129

Watson G R, Wilson F M (1989) Guillain–Barré syndrome: an update. New Zealand Journal of Physiotherapy Dec: 17–24

West J B 1995 Respiratory physiology, 5th edn. Williams & Wilkins, Baltimore, p 35

Young C S 1984 A review of the adverse effects of airway suction. Physiotherapy 70: 104–106

FURTHER READING

American Association for Respiratory Care (AARC) Clinical Practice Guidelines 1993 Endotracheal suctioning of mechanically ventilated adults and children with artificial airways. Respiratory Care 38: 500–503

Edwards S 1996 Neurological physiotherapy, a problem-solving approach. Churchill Livingstone, Edinburgh

Ellis E, Alison J (eds) 1994 Key issues in cardiorespiratory physiotherapy. Butterworth-Heinemann, Oxford

Evans T W, Haslett C 1996 ARDS acute respiratory distress in adults. Chapman & Hall, London

Ganong W F 1995 Review of medical physiology, 17th edn. Appleton & Lange, Connecticut

Gower P 1991 Handbook of nephrology, 2nd edn. Blackwell Scientific Publications, Oxford

Hinds C J, Watson D 1996 Intensive care, 2nd edn. Saunders, London

Levick J R 1995 An introduction to cardiovascular physiology, 2nd edn. Butterworth-Heinemann, Oxford

Lindsay K W, Bone I, Callander R 1991 Neurology and neurosurgery illustrated, 2nd edn. Churchill Livingstone, Edinburgh

Marino P 1991 The ICU book. Lea & Febriger, Philadelphia

Moxham J, Goldstone J (eds) 1994 Assisted ventilation, 2nd edn. BMJ Publishing Group, London

Nunn J F 1993 Nunn's applied respiratory physiology, 4th edn. Butterworth-Heinemann, Oxford

Oh T E (ed) 1997 Intensive care manual, 4th edn. Butterworths, London

Singer M, Webb A 1997 Oxford handbook of critical care. Oxford University Press, Oxford

West J B 1992 Pulmonary pathophysiology, 4th edn. Williams & Wilkins, Baltimore

West J B 1995 Respiratory physiology, 5th edn. Williams & Wilkins, Baltimore

12

Surgery for adults

Sarah C. Ridley

INTRODUCTION

Advances in less invasive surgery and improved anaesthetic and pain management of the surgical patient have led to changes in physiotherapy practice. Treatment should never be routine but in response to individual patient assessment and the identification of a patient's particular problems. Communication with members of the multidisciplinary team is an essential element of good quality care.

To avoid repetition in this chapter, general physiotherapy management is discussed and for individual surgical procedures the physiotherapy key points are given additionally.

GENERAL ANAESTHESIA

The main objectives of a general anaesthetic (GA) are reversible loss of awareness and temporary blockade of gross response to stimulation. In other words, while the patient is anaesthetized, skeletal muscular contraction and autonomic responses such as increased heart rate, blood pressure and sweating are inhibited. A general anaesthetic may be divided into three main components: coma, muscular relaxation and analgesia (Forrest et al 1995). Current anaesthetic agents enable proportional adjustment of each component to suit the patient and the procedure. The actual course of a GA may be divided into different stages.

Premedication

The premedicant drugs provide reduction in anxiety, pain relief, sedation and encouragement of amnesia. Other desired effects may be prevention of bradycardia, excess salivation and antiemesis.

Induction

The aim at this point is to start the anaesthetic process rapidly and pleasantly. Usually this is by intravenous injection of a short-acting coma-inducing drug such as propofol. Occasionally anaesthetic vapours may be inhaled to the same effect. Anaphylaxis characterized by severe hypotension, hypoxia and bronchospasm can be a rare but life-threatening reaction.

Maintenance

This follows induction and is the stage when surgery commences. A combination of inhaled drugs (e.g. halothane/nitrous oxide) and intravenous analgesics (e.g. morphine/fentanyl) may be given with muscle relaxants to enable controlled ventilation of the lungs.

Reversal

The reversal of the effects of a GA is a short but potentially hazardous period. The concentration of the inhaled anaesthetic will be reduced and drugs such as neostigmine are given to reverse the effect of muscle relaxants. Occasionally when a spontaneous respiratory rate has been re-established but is less than 6–8 breaths per minute, a narcotic antagonist may be given to reverse the respiratory depressant effect of the narcotic. Unfortunately this will also abolish the analgesic effect. Extubation is carried out once the protective laryngeal reflexes have returned. The patient is normally positioned in side lying to reduce the risk of aspiration and given supplemental oxygen, while the upper airway is maintained by jaw thrust, head tilt or an oropharyngeal airway.

Effects of general anaesthesia on respiratory function

Under GA the functional residual capacity (FRC) may be lowered by up to 30% at 24 hours postoperatively and remain reduced for several days. This is related to diaphragmatic dysfunction which is thought to be associated with increased abdominal tone (reflex muscle spasm) and/or a reflex reduction in phrenic nerve activity (Craig 1981). This reduction in lung volume also reduces lung compliance, increases airway resistance and hastens atelectasis. Indeed, basal lung collapse occurs within minutes of IV or inhalational GA (Lunn 1991).

There is also a reduction in lung recoil pressure especially in overweight patients. Narcosis reduces the sensitivity of the respiratory centre and decreases the efficiency of the elimination of CO_2. A decrease in cardiac output potentially reduces pulmonary blood flow and alveolar perfusion thus increasing physiological dead space. Ventilation/perfusion ($\dot{V}/\dot{Q}$) mismatch is accentuated by the patient being supine on the operating table, respiratory depression and reduced cardiac output.

Inhalation of dry, cold gas which bypasses the warming/humidification effect of the upper airways will increase mucus viscosity and a high inspired FiO_2 over a period of hours will slow down mucus velocity. Mucociliary clearance ceases altogether after 90 minutes of a GA (Lunn 1991).

The cough reflex is dampened centrally by sedation/opiates and peripherally by any abdominal/thoracic wounds. The resultant reduction in inspiratory and expiratory volumes makes it more difficult to generate pressure to detach mucus from the airways.

If infection ensues, this is primarily caused by *Streptococcus pneumoniae* or *Haemophilus influenzae*.

SPINAL ANAESTHESIA

During spinal anaesthesia a needle is inserted between the spinous processes of the lumbar vertebrae, passing through the ligamentum flavum, the epidural space and the dura–

arachnoid and into the subarachnoid space (Fig. 12.1a). The correct position of the needle can be confirmed by the escape of cerebrospinal fluid. The third and fourth lumbar vertebrae are normally selected, as in adults the spinal cord has ended usually around the first lumbar vertebra (L1), thus reducing the risk of neurological complications. The spread of local anaesthetic solution, e.g. lignocaine or bupivicaine, is determined by the dose, volume, puncture site and position of the patient. It will result in sensory, motor and sympathetic blockade of the specific nerve roots as they pass from the cord through the intervertebral foramen. Disturbance of sympathetic outflow may result in hypotension and bradycardia (Lunn 1991). Generally spinal anaesthesia is carried out for operations performed below the level of the umbilicus. It is most suitable as an alternative to general anaesthesia for high-risk and elderly patients. Neurological complications are rare.

EPIDURAL ANAESTHESIA/ ANALGESIA

This procedure involves a needle being inserted, at the appropriate level of the spinal column, into the epidural space, i.e. passing through the ligamentum flavum but not the dura–arachnoid (Fig. 12.1b). A band of anaesthesia will form depending on which nerve roots have been selected. Commonly this is done in the lumbar region but the epidural space can be approached from any level. If anaesthesia/analgesia is required for a period of hours or days following the operative procedure, a fine catheter is inserted over the needle as it is withdrawn. This enables repeated injections or continuous infusion of

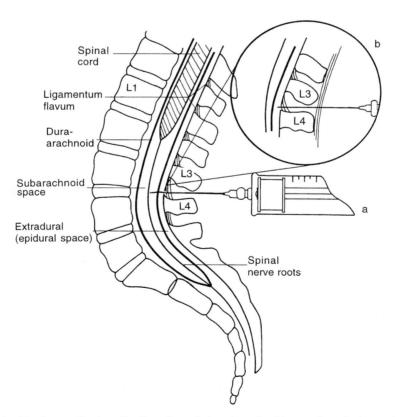

Fig. 12.1   Spinal and epidural anaesthesia. **a** Position of needle in subarachnoid space for spinal anaesthesia. **b** Position of needle in epidural space for epidural anaesthesia/analgesia.

local anaesthetic, with or without the addition of an opioid. Current epidural protocols recommend mixtures of potent local anaesthetics such as bupivicaine and very small doses of opioids to limit the opioid levels in the circulation (de Leon-Casasola et al 1994). It is suggested that epidural anaesthesia in abdominal surgery appears to decrease length of stay and pain experienced by patients postoperatively and results in a more rapid return of bowel function (Scott et al 1996).

Physiotherapy key points
• The patient may get up after a spinal anaesthetic once the effects have worn off. If, however, a post-dural puncture headache occurs secondary to leakage of cerebrospinal fluid, the patient is advised to lie flat until the symptoms have resolved. The dural hole can be sealed with a clot, by injecting some of the patient's own blood into the space, which is referred to as an epidural blood patch (Lunn 1991).
• In the recovery period after a spinal anaesthetic, patients will require care of their lower limbs owing to temporary sensory and motor loss as well as monitoring of potential postural hypotension. This is another reason why patients should not sit up until the spinal block has worn off.
• Respiratory depression can occur if opioids are being given via an epidural.
• A patient will experience pain if the epidural catheter becomes displaced or blocked or if a 'top-up' bolus of the anaesthetic/analgesic agent is required.

INTRAVENOUS REGIONAL ANAESTHESIA

This type of anaesthesia is used for simple limb surgery or manipulation of closed fractures. It involves the limb being injected with local anaesthetic while a tourniquet renders it ischaemic for the duration of the procedure.

Another procedure involves injection of a local anaesthetic into the main nerve supplying the area under operation and is termed a nerve block. Examples of this technique include brachial plexus, intercostal nerve and ilio-inguinal blocks.

TOPICAL ANAESTHESIA

Local anaesthetic agents in the form of solutions or creams may be applied to the skin or mucosa and are absorbed into the affected area. Lignocaine is commonly used and may also be administered as a spray/gargle/gel or soaked pieces of cotton wool. The effect is rapid and lasts approximately 30–60 minutes.

MANAGEMENT OF ACUTE POSTOPERATIVE PAIN*
Effects of pain

It is essential that pain relief is managed well, especially over the immediate postoperative period when the patient may be spending more time in a bed or chair than walking around the ward. This is when patients are at greater risk of developing atelectasis and subsequent pulmonary infection.

Acute pain is a complex process affected by the physiological reaction to injury or disease, as well as psychological and social factors. An individual's perception of pain may depend on his previous experience of pain as well as his current degree of control over his particular situation.

Pain following surgery may also indicate that a complication has occurred. The diagnosis of surgical complications should not be obscured by good pain control, providing the patient's overall condition is assessed regularly (Attard et al 1992). If postoperative pain is not managed appropriately the following effects may occur:

• Increased patient anxiety leading to fatigue and possible loss of confidence in the staff providing care

---

* I am grateful to Dr John McClure and the postoperative pain group of the Royal Infirmary of Edinburgh NHS Trust regarding this section on pain management which is based on their 1995 second edition of 'Guidelines for the Management of Postoperative Pain'.

- Increased heart rate and blood pressure resulting in increased myocardial oxygen consumption
- Decreased movement therefore increased risk of deep venous thrombosis (DVT), pulmonary embolus (PE), breakdown of pressure areas and increased dependency on staff
- Increased respiratory complications
- Disturbance of sleep pattern.

Assessment of pain

As pain is a subjective experience it should be assessed by recording the patient's current perception of the pain using either a visual analogue scale or a verbal descriptor scale.

Comparison of scores before and after administration of analgesics will provide essential information regarding the effectiveness of the pain relief. In some centres, as nausea and vomiting are common side-effects of analgesia and potentially more distressing than the actual pain, they will also be assessed on a scale and be dealt with appropriately. A minimum of 1–4-hourly assessment of pain is recommended but should be tailored to meet the individual's needs.

Non-pharmacological treatment

Emotions such as anxiety, fear and loss of autonomy are known to increase pain perception. Methods to reduce this include:

- Provision of accurate information preoperatively regarding expected methods of pain relief and where the pain is most likely to occur; advice on positioning, moving and wound support, etc. is also beneficial
- Explanation of pain scales and the importance of reporting pain as early as possible
- Awareness of side-effects such as nausea and vomiting
- Acupuncture and TENS are alternatives to medication
- Techniques which promote relaxation such as self-hypnosis.

Drug therapy

Oral analgesia

As major surgery is often associated with gastro-intestinal dysfunction resulting in variable drug absorption, oral analgesia is reserved for minor surgery or a few days after major surgery when the gut is working again and the pain is expected to be less acute.

Non-steroidal anti-inflammatory drugs (NSAIDs)

NSAIDs reduce inflammation at the site of injury as well as providing some central analgesic activity. They may be given orally, by IM injection or rectally via a suppository. Side-effects include gastric irritation, increased broncho-spasm, decreased renal function and platelet dysfunction.

Opioids

This category is used to manage moderate to severe pain especially of visceral origin. Side-effects include nausea, vomiting, constipation, drowsiness and the possibility of upper airway obstruction during sleep leading to hypoxaemia.

Despite these effects, opioids are the most commonly used postoperative analgesic particularly over the first 3 days. Dosages required to relieve pain are very unpredictable and not necessarily linked to age, gender or body weight. They may be delivered orally, by IM injection or IV infusion. The aim of an IV infusion is to maintain constant plasma concentration of the opioid, therefore avoiding the peaks and troughs of intermittent regimens. It should be noted that analgesia should initially be established by bolus IV injection allowing the infusion to then maintain that level of pain relief. Additional subsequent boluses may be required depending on the patient's condition but the risk of res-piratory depression is high and patients should be observed closely. Oxygen therapy is also advised during the period of infusion. It should be noted that the pump should always be placed at or below the level of the patient's heart and an antisiphon valve incorporated into the system to avoid an inadvertent large bolus of opioid being delivered.

Patient-controlled analgesia (PCA). The syringe containing the drug is put in a microprocessor-controlled pump and connected to an intravenous cannula or IV infusion with a non-return valve. The pump is programmed to deliver a bolus dose and set with a minimum period between doses ('lockout' interval). Every time the patient presses the button on the control lead the preset dose is given unless the button is pressed during the 'lockout' period.

Each patient can administer as much or as little analgesia as may be needed according to pain and activity levels. This should be a safe technique if the patient is in control of the button, i.e. not staff or family members, because as consumption increases, sleepiness should prevent self-administration continuing to the point of respiratory depression.

PCA may not be suitable for patients who are unable to comprehend the system or unable to operate the hand trigger, e.g. owing to arthritis.

Entonox

Entonox is a mixture of 50% oxygen and 50% nitrous oxide and provides good analgesia for severe pain of brief duration. Entonox cylinder headsets have a demand valve which is patient activated on inspiration and should be administered 1 or 2 minutes before the painful procedure is carried out. As the mask is self-administered it will fall away from the face if the patient becomes too drowsy. Entonox is contraindicated if:

- There is a low cardiac output because of peripheral vasodilatation
- A pneumothorax or subcutaneous emphysema is present, as rapid diffusion of nitrous oxide impedes the absorption of air
- A patient requires more than 50% oxygen
- A patient is relying on his hypoxic drive to breathe.

If it is used in high dosages or over a protracted period of time it is associated with bone marrow suppression. As with any drug, Entonox must be prescribed by a doctor prior to administration.

Entonox can be particularly helpful during intermittent, relatively short episodes of pain such as removal of tubes or drains, coughing with fractured ribs, repositioning a patient and contraction pains during labour. Occasionally it may be appropriate to deliver Entonox through the ventilator circuit during manual hyper-inflation or in conjunction with IPPB.

Side-effects include nausea, euphoria (hence the lay term 'laughing gas'), tingling, numbness, light-headedness and auditory disturbances. Cylinders are stored horizontally and it is good practice to turn the cylinder upside down approximately three times prior to use to ensure mixing of gases (BOC 1990).

INCISIONS AND SUTURES

Some common incisional sites are illustrated in Figure 12.2. These may vary according to the individual surgeon's preferences although are designed to provide optimal exposure to the surgical area of interest.

Ideally, incisions are made along the lines of least tissue tension to enable prompt healing and a fine scar line. Transverse abdominal incisions cause less strain on the wound compared to vertical incisions (Garcia-Valdecasas et al 1988). Accurate suturing of the deeper layers of the wound facilitates the superficial skin layers coming together without tension and this allows apposition by adhesive tape or superficial sutures (e.g. silk or nylon). Deeper wound spaces that are unable to be obliterated by suture should be drained to reduce the danger of exudate accumulation and possible consequent infection.

Absorbable sutures such as catgut or Dexon are preferable for stitching deeper layers while stronger sutures are appropriate around joints and over the abdominal wall. Areas with a good blood supply such as the face and neck tend to heal quickly possibly enabling suture removal at 3–5 days. In contrast, more peripheral areas such as the leg and foot may require sutures in situ for up to 14 days. The abdominal and

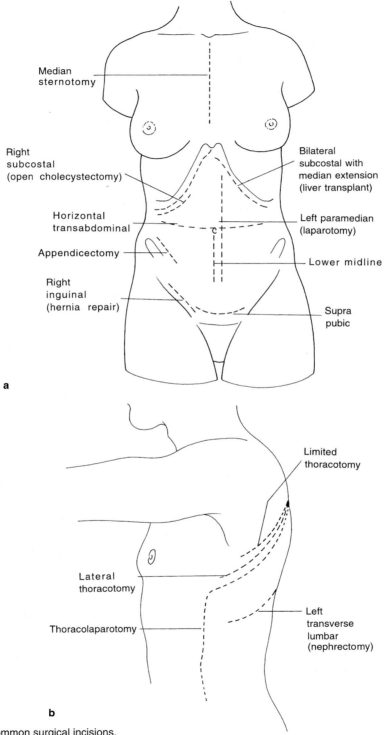

Fig. 12.2 a and **b** Common surgical incisions.

chest wound sutures generally need 7–10 days prior to removal (Forrest et al 1995).

A median sternotomy involves longitudinal division of the sternum and the aponeuroses of the pectoralis major muscle with all the thoracic muscles remaining intact. For this reason it is generally accepted that this incision is less painful than a thoracotomy or upper abdominal incision.

PREOPERATIVE PHYSIOTHERAPY MANAGEMENT

Appropriate patient selection

A number of factors should be taken into consideration when the physiotherapist is deciding which patients may be defined as 'high risk' and would benefit from input at this stage.

Incisional site

Several studies have shown that upper abdominal and thoracic incisions lead to a high incidence of respiratory complications (Craig 1981, Ford et al 1983). This may result from a decrease in FRC, change in the ventilatory pattern to rapid shallow breathing and impaired oxygenation. This is not the case with lower abdominal surgery (Dureuil et al 1987) but it may be appropriate to assess the patient who presents with other significant risk factors.

Pre-existing respiratory problems

Infection. Upper respiratory tract infection may result in excessive mucus secretion and reduction in mucociliary clearance. Lower respiratory tract infection may impair gas exchange leading to possibilities of hypoxia secondary to pneumonia and exacerbation of infection. The immunocompromised patient is more susceptible to infection.

Restrictive defects. Lung fibrosis and pulmonary oedema can cause restrictive defects. Patients with kyphoscoliosis and ankylosing spondylitis are especially at risk after upper abdominal surgery since almost all tidal volume may be dependent on diaphragmatic movement. A large pleural effusion may compress lung tissue thereby accentuating the reduced lung volume and leading to an increase in airways resistance and closure following anaesthetic induction.

Obstructive defects. A deeper anaesthesia may be required in asthmatic patients because of bronchial hyperreactivity. Patients with an FEV_1/FVC ratio of less than 35% are highly predictive of postoperative acute respiratory failure following thoracotomy (Brodsky 1995).

Obesity

Total lung compliance can be reduced to approximately one-third of the normal value owing to the additional weight of the chest wall (Selsby & Jones 1993) and this leads to an increased work of breathing and O_2 consumption. FRC decreases and closing capacity increases, thereby predisposing to atelectasis. A 60% reduction in FRC is often observed at anaesthetic induction and this leads to an increased risk of basal atelectasis (Damia et al 1988). Hypoxaemia can be found at rest in obese patients especially if they are supine and this further reduces the FRC.

Age

Increasing age is associated with increasing closing volume and loss of elastic recoil. At approximately 65 years of age, small airways close during resting tidal volume in seated subjects. Even from the age of 44 years and upwards airway closure is observed in the supine position (Leblanc et al 1970). With increasing age, the respiratory muscles weaken and the rib cage stiffens with a resultant decrease in excursion.

Smoking

Smoking results in small airways narrowing, increased mucus production, irritable airways, decreased mucus clearance and an elevated closing capacity. These factors predispose to a greater $\dot{V}/\dot{Q}$ shunt and impaired oxygenation during anaesthesia. Even a short period of abstinence from smoking (12–48 hours) is sufficient to decrease carboxyhaemoglobin (COHb) and nicotine levels and thus improve the work capacity of the myocardium (Anderson et al 1973). Six weeks' cessation of smoking is required to reduce the volume of sputum produced by the patient but it takes several months for mucociliary clearance to return to normal (Egan & Wong 1992, Morgan & Nel 1996).

Patient motivation

Patients affected by anxiety, depression, mental handicap or psychiatric disease may have a longer recovery period.

Nutritional status

Poor nutritional status has been shown to cause increased incidence of postoperative pneumonia. Impaired production of antibodies will also make these patients prone to infection. Protein and vitamin deficiencies can delay wound healing (Forrest et al 1995).

Reduced mobility and intercurrent disease

Diseases such as multiple sclerosis, parkinsonism and rheumatoid arthritis can increase the risk of complications through reduced mobility. Intercurrent disease, e.g. diabetes, leukaemia or haemophilia should also be taken into consideration.

Alcohol and drug dependency

Potential problems with withdrawal symptoms and the possible need for high levels of anaesthesia/analgesia should be anticipated.

Preoperative physiotherapy assessment

Once the appropriate patients have been identified, further questioning may be necessary concerning the patient's smoking and respiratory history including any relevant medications such as bronchodilators or steroids. It is important to establish the patient's exercise tolerance and to undertake a general examination of the musculoskeletal system. Examination of the chest (see Ch. 1) should also be carried out.

Teaching and information

Considering the amount of verbal information given to the patient at this stage, details should be brief and concise and ideally back-up written material should be provided. Preoperative explanation regarding the effects of surgery on respiratory function, the location of the wound, drips and drains may help to reduce pain, quicken recovery after the operation (Auerbach & Kilmann 1977). Nelson (1996) reported that 75% of patients who participated in a pre-admission education programme for patients undergoing cardiac surgery felt a resultant reduction in anxiety levels in response to the information that they received. The physiotherapist should also stress the importance of early mobilization (Mynster et al 1996), appropriate positioning while chair or bed bound, adequate pain control, regular thoracic expansion exercises and wound support during huffing or coughing if bronchial secretions are present. Close liaison with the nursing staff and provision of information leaflets will help to emphasize the importance of these activities to the patient.

Preoperative treatment

Occasionally a patient may need treatment to maximize pulmonary function in the preoperative stage because of, for example, a current chest infection or history of bronchiectasis. If major respiratory problems are anticipated postoperatively, a patient may benefit from instruction in the use of adjuncts such as periodic continuous positive airway pressure (PCPAP) or intermittent positive pressure breathing (IPPB). In elective cases, advice from the surgeon on cessation of smoking and weight reduction should ideally have been given weeks or months prior to admission.

POSTOPERATIVE PHYSIOTHERAPY MANAGEMENT

Generally the main aims in the postoperative phase are to promote the reinflation of areas of atelectasis and to maintain adequate ventilation, to assist in the removal of any excess bronchial secretions and to aid in the general positioning, bed mobility and early ambulation of the patient. Prevention of reduced joint movements or poor posture secondary to incisions or tubes, monitoring of adequate pain relief and appropriate oxygen therapy and humidification are also very important.

Physiotherapy techniques which help to achieve these aims include:

Early mobilization. With the development of laparoscopic surgery, improved anaesthetic and pain management many patients are often able to mobilize independently from a very early stage postoperatively. Some patients will require assistance because of the presence of the various drips and drains and it is sometimes safer to have two people assisting for the first stand or walk because of the patient's general fatigue and the risk of postural hypotension. A graduated walking programme adapted to suit each patient should be encouraged with the introduction of stair climbing at an appropriate stage.

Bed mobility/positioning. Advice on optimum and regular change of position while the patient is in bed is essential for patients in the early stages of recovery. Appropriate use of overhead 'monkey poles', rope ladders and cot sides can reduce the patient's reliance on staff to be 'mobile' if confined to bed. Suitable seating at a height appropriate to the individual can also improve patient independence, particularly for those patients after upper abdominal surgery (UAS) who find it difficult to move from sitting in a low chair to standing but are fully independent once up on their feet. Simple advice on how to get in and out of bed without putting undue strain on an abdominal wound can also be of great value to the patient.

Thoracic expansion exercises. See page 141.

Patients who are unable to be frequently mobile in the ward and are at risk of developing atelectasis, should be encouraged to carry out regular thoracic expansion exercises (e.g. three to four at least every hour) preferably with an end-inspiratory hold of a few seconds. Regular breathing exercises can also alert patients to the fact that their analgesia may be wearing off and

that they need to inform a member of staff or require to self-administer the patient-controlled analgesia (PCA) system.

Incentive spirometry/periodic continuous positive airway pressure/intermittent positive pressure breathing. See Chapter 8.

These techniques may be introduced for immobile patients who are unable or ineffective in carrying out thoracic expansion exercises and are showing signs of unresolved atelectasis.

Clearance of bronchial secretions. If sputum retention persists or difficulty in clearing secretions is still a problem, despite adequate analgesia and appropriate advice on thoracic expansion exercises, forced expiration technique (FET) and wound support, suction via the nasopharynx or oral airway may be an option. If it is anticipated that this may be required more than once or twice, minitracheotomy should be considered.

POSTOPERATIVE COMPLICATIONS

The following section highlights the general complications following surgery:

Atelectasis and infection. The main postoperative respiratory problems are decreased lung volume leading to atelectasis and infection. Any abdominal distension will tend to exacerbate these problems. See page 296 for effects of GA on the respiratory system.

Pulmonary oedema. Excessive administration of fluid in the early postoperative period may result in an increased workload for the heart and lungs and may lead to pulmonary oedema.

Myocardial infarction. Evidence suggests that a recent MI plays a major part in prediction of postoperative myocardial dysfunction and death (Mearns 1995).

Cardiovascular problems. Hypertension, ischaemic heart disease/angina, valvular heart disease, conduction defects and pacemakers may carry a risk to the patient.

Dysrhythmias and hypotension. Cardiac dysrhythmias may be associated with hypotension.

Deep venous thrombosis (DVT)/pulmonary embolus (PE). A number of surgeons use low-dose heparin in patients undergoing a GA and who are over the age of 40 years. If thrombosis develops and a clot is situated in the calf veins there is a low risk of embolism. In this situation, ambulant patients are given thromboembolic deterrent (TED) stockings and encouraged to continue mobilizing. Immobile patients would be considered for systemic heparinization. If the thrombus is affecting the ileofemoral segment of the deep veins, there is a high risk of embolism in this situation, so patients are anticoagulated and advised to rest in bed for 48 hours with slight elevation of the foot of the bed. All patients who suffer a PE will require warfarin therapy for approximately 3–6 months.

Haemorrhage. The amount of blood draining from bottles or bags should be monitored regularly as well as any signs of internal bleeding.

Acute renal failure. Impairment of renal function results from inadequate perfusion of the kidneys owing to hypovolaemia or sepsis.

Reduced gut motility. Paralytic ileus is characterized by reduced or absent bowel sounds and may result in considerable abdominal distension.

Nausea and vomiting. Gastrointestinal upset is experienced in about one-third of patients undergoing surgery.

Peripheral nerve injuries. Peripheral nerve injuries can be caused by stretching or compression of nerve trunks as a result of poor positioning of limbs on the operating table.

Pressure areas. Injury to the skin and subcutaneous tissues may occur over bony prominences. The back of the head should not be forgotten when assessing for pressure areas.

Loss or chipping of teeth. Tooth fragments may be aspirated inadvertently into the respiratory tract.

Myalgia. Neck, chest and abdominal muscle pain may last up to 1 week if the muscle relaxant drug suxamethonium is given during anaesthesia.

THORACIC SURGERY

Intercostal chest drainage

Many thoracic surgical procedures and traumatic conditions require intercostal drainage. The main aim of intercostal chest drainage is to remove air and/or fluid from the pleural space in order to restore subatmospheric intrapleural pressure, thus enabling re-expansion of the deflated or compressed lung.

Chest tube

The chest tube should be clear, of adequate diameter (6–11 mm internal diameter in adults) with a radio-opaque strip to outline the tube itself and the side holes should lie within the pleural space. Any connectors should also be clear to prevent blockage going undetected. Apical tubes are positioned to drain air while basal drains are intended to drain fluid (Fig. 12.3).

Underwater seal drainage

To ensure that the air removed from the pleural space during expiration is prevented from re-entering during inspiration, the drainage system must have an underwater seal. To achieve this the pleural drain is attached to a tight-fitting connector on the bottle neck (Fig. 12.4). This is

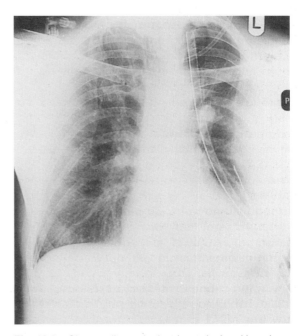

Fig. 12.3 Chest radiograph showing apical and basal drains.

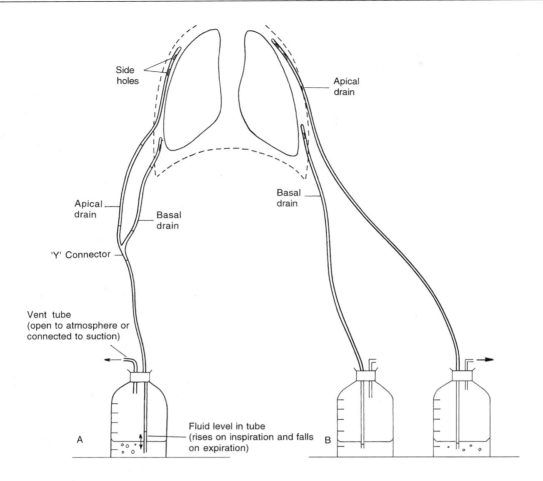

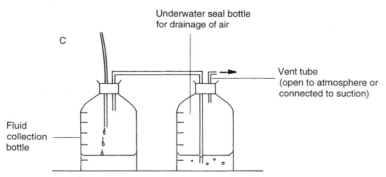

Fig. 12.4 Underwater seal chest drainage. **a** Single bottle system allowing use of one bottle via a 'Y'
connector to drain fluid and air. **b** Two separate bottles enabling drainage of air from the apical drain and
fluid from the basal drain. **c** Two-compartment drainage system where two bottles are connected in
series, the first collecting fluid and the second acting as the underwater seal drainage for air.

connected to a rigid tube which is submerged about 2 cm below the surface level of the water thus creating an underwater seal. The air is expelled against the hydrostatic resistance of the water and out into the atmosphere via the vent. The vent is essential to avoid build-up of pressure within the container. It is important that the distal end of the underwater seal tube is always submerged but that the length of the tube below the water level is as short as possible whilst maintaining the seal as this reflects the work required to expel air or fluid from the pleural space.

Fluids will drain by gravity and not spill back into the pleural space if, as recommended, the bottle is always kept below the level of the patient's chest.

Fluctuations in the level of the water column reflect the change in pleural pressure during breathing. In self-ventilating patients the intrapleural pressure becomes more negative during inspiration and the fluid column will rise. During expiration the intrapleural pressure is less negative causing the fluid level to fall. If air is seen to bubble through the water it indicates a hole in the visceral pleura. If the air leak stops suddenly, kinking or blockage of the tube should be suspected. A more gradual cessation of bubbling usually means that the lung has fully re-expanded.

The simplest form of underwater seal drainage system consists of one bottle serving as both collection container and underwater seal drain for evacuation of fluid and air. This system is adequate if minimal drainage of fluid is expected. If a 'Y' connector is incorporated into this system, two separate intercostal drains may be attached to a single bottle (Fig. 12.4a). Alternatively two separate bottles may be used, enabling drainage of air from the apical drain and fluid from the basal drain (Fig. 12.4b). In a two-compartment system fluid is collected in the first container via the chest tube and air is bubbled through to a second container via a connecting tube where it can be vented to the atmosphere (Fig. 12.4c). The advantage of this system is that both containers have underwater seals, but the separate container for drainage of

fluid only allows accurate monitoring of volume and expelled matter, e.g. pus, fibrin or blood clots. Three- and four-compartment systems are also available but are seldom seen in practice.

Suction

Free drainage depends on gravity to expel air and fluid from the pleural space. In the presence of excess volume of fluid to be drained or a large air leak, suction may be applied to the vent tube at recommended pressures of between 10 and 20 cmH$_2$O. Greater pressures may be necessary for the management of a persistent air leak. To maintain patency of the tube it is advisable that it be intermittently compressed and released by gentle hand squeezing to dislodge any clots. 'Milking' or stripping of drains with rollers is thought to create high negative pressures which could result in pulmonary trauma (Kam et al 1993).

Clamping

Clamping of tubes is generally avoided except:

- When the bottle needs to be temporarily lifted above the level of the patient's chest
- When the drainage container needs replacing
- When the drain has been inserted after a pneumonectomy
- When accidental disconnection of tubing or breakage of containers occurs
- When determining the absence of a pneumothorax on the chest radiograph prior to drain removal
- During chemical pleurodesis.

As there is a potential risk of a tension pneumothorax developing in the presence of a continuous air leak when the tubes are clamped, this procedure should be undertaken for very brief periods only.

It is essential that clamps are always readily available for any patient with an underwater seal drain in situ. In the situation where the intercostal drain is still within the patient's chest wall but has become disconnected or the bottle has broken, the tube should be clamped as close as possible to the patient's chest wall. The tubing should then be cleaned and reconnected or a new system applied as quickly as possible, if it is broken, and the tubing then unclamped. If, however, the intercostal drain has become completely detached from the patient, he is requested to breathe out while at the same time pressure is applied to the wound at the end of expiration. While maintaining the pressure on the wound, the patient is encouraged to breathe normally while medical help is obtained.

Drain removal

Tubes that have been used solely to drain fluid will be removed once they are producing 10–20 ml/hour or less. In the case of empyema where pus is being drained into a bag ('*open drainage*'), the length of the tube within the chest is gradually shortened, externally, by a few centimetres until the infection has resolved.

Air drainage tubes are removed once the lung has fully re-expanded and the air leak has stopped. To avoid unnecessary reinsertion of a chest drain, the tube may be clamped for a period of 12–24 hours and a radiograph taken to confirm that the lung has not deflated without the aid of the chest drain which may therefore be removed. If a pneumothorax has reoccurred, the tube is simply unclamped for a further period of drainage.

As the tube has normally been sewn into position with a 'purse-string' suture, the patient is asked to breathe in deeply and hold at full inspiration as the tube is taken out and the sutures pulled together to avoid air escaping back into the pleural space. Adequate analgesia should be ensured for this procedure.

Physiotherapy key points
- Advice should be given on postural correction and upper limb exercises. Occasionally inappropriate taping of the drains with sleek around the chest wall can limit the patient's range of movement and should be redressed.
- Care should be taken when handling patients so that the tubes are always visible, to avoid kinking, stretching or disconnection.
- Bottles should be at the side of a patient's bed and not hidden underneath, to avoid

crushing of the container if the bed is inadvertently lowered too far.
- Observation of changes in air leaks and drainage should be made before, during and after physiotherapy intervention.
- In the presence of an air leak, positive pressure techniques are usually avoided as they may perpetuate the problem.
- Patients requiring wall suction may compensate for lack of mobility by walking on the spot. Alternatively, having sought approval from the medical staff, the suction tubing may be disconnected from the vent tube, enabling the patient to mobilize. It must be stressed to the patient that the drains are held below the level of the chest and that clamps should be available at all times.

LUNG CARCINOMA

Lung carcinoma may be classified as:

- *Squamous (epidermoid) carcinoma.* This is the most common type of lung 'cancer' (45–55%) (Forrest et al 1995). It is rarely seen in non-smokers. Most tumours arise centrally in lobar and main stem bronchi. Secondary pneumonia and abscess formation occur frequently.
- *Small-cell (oat-cell) anaplastic carcinoma.* The majority of lesions arise proximally. It is highly malignant and at presentation more than 50% of patients will have widespread metastases. Subsequently radiotherapy and chemotherapy rather than surgery are the treatment options.
- *Adenocarcinoma.* This is most likely to present in peripheral lung regions. More common in women.
- *Large-cell carcinoma.* 90% of these patients are smokers. This form of cancer is highly malignant and does not respond to radiotherapy.
- *Bronchioalveolar carcinoma.* This is a rare type of tumour that spreads along the alveolar septal framework and can be easily confused with secondary tumours.

Staging and investigations

Clinical staging classifications define the tumour size, location and the presence or absence of metastases and facilitate the decision as to which patients should be referred for surgery. The assessment, management and prognosis of the disease depend largely on the cell type and whether there has been metastatic spread. The TNM staging system (T = description of the primary tumour, N = extent of regional lymph node involvement and M = the absence or presence of metastases) identifies those patients who, following resection, will have improved survival compared with the natural history of the disease (Tisi 1985).

Non-surgical treatment of lung carcinoma

If surgery is not appropriate, alternative treatments include radiotherapy and chemotherapy. Endobronchial treatment also offers a variety of options for advanced lung tumours such as thermal resection with high-powered lasers (neodymium–yttrium–aluminium–garnet (Nd-YAG) and carbon dioxide) for acute intrinsic obstruction of the airway, photodynamic therapy (PDT) where low-powered lasers are used to activate light-sensitive drugs which are preferentially retained by tumour cells, and fluorescence tumour detection which identifies tumour tissue through using certain drugs which will fluoresce if illuminated at the appropriate wavelength. Brachytherapy involves the implantation of radioactive isotopes (e.g. radioactive gold grains) into the tumour which is then allowed to naturally decay. The patient has to be isolated for several days to avoid staff and other patients being affected by the radiation. Insertion of expanding metal or Silastic stents may also relieve the pressure exerted on the airway by extrinsic tumours.

LUNG SURGERY

In addition to lung surgery for carcinoma, localized bronchiectasis, sequestrated lobe and benign tumours may also be suitable for surgical intervention.

Thoracic incision

Access to the lung may be obtained through a full posterolateral or anterolateral thoracotomy, limited thoracotomy (Fig. 12.2) or thoracoscopy.

The posterolateral approach involves muscular division of trapezius, latissimus dorsi, serratus anterior, the intercostals and erector spinae. A rib retractor will be used to spread the intercostal space. Whole or partial (2–4 cm) rib resection may be necessary to improve exposure of the lung. The anterolateral approach requires pectoralis major and minor, serratus anterior and the intercostal muscles to be cut.

Thoracoscopy

The main advantages of thoracoscopic techniques is that they offer minimal surgical trauma, and are associated with less pain and respiratory embarrassment, a stronger cough and reduced recovery time in comparison to open thoracotomy (Mack et al 1992, Smith et al 1993). It is an option for patients who are too severely compromised by their lung function to undergo open surgery.

Diagnostic thoracoscopy may be carried out with a single direct viewing thoracoscope but other techniques need video thoracoscopy and simultaneous use of more than one port of access through trocars to manipulate instruments.

The following are some of the procedures performed under thoracoscopy:

- Pericardial window/pericardectomy for recurrent pericardial effusions
- Pleurectomy for recurrent pleural effusions
- Lung and mediastinal resection
- Resection of bullous emphysema.

Lobectomy

This is the removal of an entire lobe. Generally two intercostal drains are placed in the pleural space at the time of operation to evacuate air and fluid/blood from the space (Fig. 12.4). The drains may be attached to low continuous suction (10–20 cmH$_2$O) to aid re-expansion of the remaining lung tissue. Normally the hemidiaphragm on the affected side will rise slightly owing to the subsequent loss of lung volume.

Sleeve resection

In this operation a section of the bronchus is removed, with or without a lobectomy, as a 'sleeve' and a primary bronchial re-anastomosis is carried out to preserve the remaining lung tissue. The procedure is commonly carried out for tumours affecting the right upper lobe with spread into the right main bronchus.

Segmentectomy

Segmentectomy is the excision of one or more of the ten bronchopulmonary segments. The subsequent loss of lung tissue is minimal. An air leak may persist for several days requiring an extended period of intercostal chest drainage.

Wedge resection

This entails the removal of a small, usually non-malignant, localized tumour or section of lung tissue for biopsy.

Physiotherapy key points
• Breathing exercises should be started on the day of surgery if possible.
• For many patients, the use of the active cycle of breathing techniques (ACBT) at frequent intervals in the sitting position and early mobilization (Fig. 12.5) may be all that is necessary to restore lung volume and clear secretions which will probably be bloodstained. Others who show signs of lung collapse may benefit from carrying out the ACBT while lying on the unaffected side (Fig. 12.6). Adjuncts such as IPPB or PCPAP may be considered with caution owing to the risk of perpetuating or increasing an air leak. Often lower pressures are therefore used to avoid this effect.
• Adequate wound support for huffing and coughing should be taught. The physiotherapist can offer assistance by placing one hand posteriorly below the thoracotomy incision and the other hand anteriorly to provide counter-pressure (Fig. 12.7).
• Damage to the recurrent laryngeal nerve can lead to reduced effectiveness of coughing and retention of secretions may be a problem

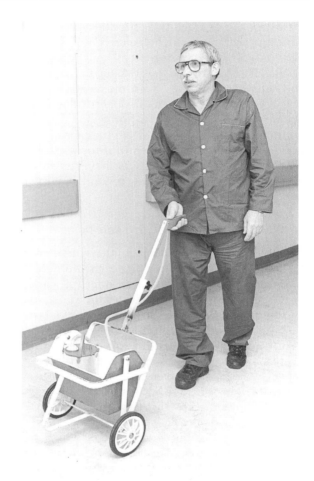

Fig 12.5   Walking with trolley for drainage bottles.

following surgery. Huffing rather than coughing is better tolerated. Nasopharyngeal suction or minitracheotomy may have to be considered.
• Early mobilization progressing to stair climbing, often as soon as the third day post-operatively, is encouraged. Exercise using a bicycle ergometer (Fig. 12.8) may be appropriate for some patients with persistent air leaks or those who cannot mobilize adequately if it is not appropriate to detach the drains from wall suction.
• Active / auto-assisted or resisted movements using proprioceptive neuromuscular facilitation techniques for the shoulder and shoulder girdle are encouraged from the day of surgery. Postural

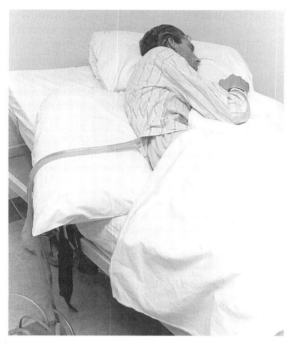

Fig 12.6 Use of positioning following thoracic surgery.

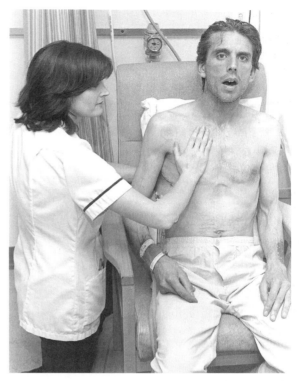

Fig 12.7 Wound support following thoracotomy.

correction is often needed as patients tend to side flex the trunk toward the thoracotomy incision.

- TENS for poorly controlled pain may be beneficial in the early postoperative stage.
- Thoracic mobilizations, TENS or acupuncture may be beneficial for patients with persistent chest wall pain.
- Segmental resections often result in a larger air leak and more pleural exudate compared with a lobectomy.
- Home advice should be tailored to suit each patient regarding postural, shoulder and general mobility exercises.

Pneumonectomy

This entails the removal of a whole lung. Bronchial closure may be achieved by using either mechanical staples or sutures. Bloody fluid collects within the pneumonectomy space and the remaining air is progressively absorbed. The rate at which the fluid rises and the air

is absorbed determines the position of the mediastinum. Some surgeons choose to insert a drain at the time of operation. The drain is usually in situ for 24 hours and is kept clamped except for 1–2 minutes every hour to allow a gradual build-up of fluid in the space, therefore maintaining an optimal mediastinal position. Usually after this 24-hour period, the air/fluid level in the space is at mid-hilar level. Monitoring of this position is aided by serial chest radiographs and palpation of the trachea to detect deviation. If the fluid accumulates too quickly the mediastinum will be pushed towards the unaffected lung resulting in tracheal deviation and possible compression of the remaining lung. If a chest drain is not in situ, the mediastinal position may be altered by aspiration of air from the space until the pressure is negative in both phases of respiration. Normally after 6 weeks the air will have been reabsorbed with subsequent loss of fluid level and complete

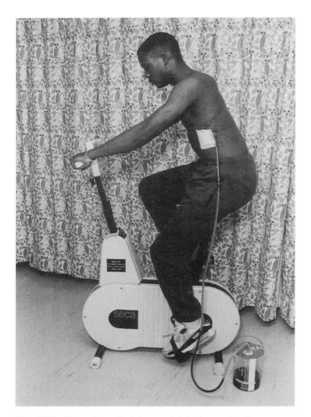

Fig 12.8 Exercise with intercostal drainage in situ.

opacification of the hemithorax on radiograph. Over the following months organization of the pleural fluid takes place which may result in complete fibrosis of the space. Consequently the pneumonectomy space contracts with progressive crowding of the intercostal spaces, elevation of the hemidiaphragm and possible mediastinal shift toward the side of surgery.

Physiotherapy key points
- The key points are similar to those under Lobectomy, Sleeve resection, etc. on page 310.
- If tracheal deviation occurs, especially in the early postoperative period, the effectiveness of the cough mechanism may be reduced.
- Huffing rather than coughing is encouraged to minimize the increase in intrathoracic pressures created during clearance of secretions.
- If suctioning, either via the nasopharynx or a minitracheotomy, is indicated to clear

sputum, great care must be taken to avoid trauma to the pneumonectomy stump, especially if the right lung has been removed.
- Avoidance of side lying in the first week postoperatively may be requested by some surgeons because if the patient lies on the non-thoracotomy side, the bronchial stump may become bathed in space fluid. Others believe that if the suture line is secure the patient is not at risk and may lie on whichever side is more comfortable. For patients who have had part of their pericardium removed at the time of operation, there may be a chance of cardiac herniation in the side lying position.
- Breathing control with stair climbing may increase exercise tolerance.

Lung volume reduction surgery

In patients with severe lung emphysema it is suggested that lung volume reduction surgery (LVRS) will restore the thoracic configuration to a more normal functional capacity (Teschler et al 1996, Thompson 1996).

Bullous emphysema is the presence of thin-walled air sacs under tension that impede surrounding lung tissue, causing compressive atelectasis. They may be single or multiple and can increase in size. The large bulla can impede lung function owing to its poor ventilation and perfusion. Only a few patients with this diagnosis benefit from corrective surgery. The main aim of surgery is to ligate or plicate the bulla using sutures or stapling devices preferably by removing the least possible amount of healthy lung tissue. The incision may be via a median sternotomy, thoracotomy or video thoracoscopy.

As an alternative method of treatment a tube may be inserted into the bulla followed by injection of a sclerosing agent causing it to gradually collapse. This allows the healthier lung tissue to re-expand to fill the space.

Following these procedures an air leak may persist for many days but as these patients are severely disabled by the disease, any subsequent improvement in lung function and exercise tolerance can lead to considerable patient benefit.

Physiotherapy key points
- Patients who require this form of surgery usually present with severe lung disease and are at risk of developing complications. Breathlessness is often one of the main symptoms which may be alleviated by instruction in breathing control at rest and on exercise.
- Pulmonary rehabilitation programmes are usually associated with lung volume reduction surgery.

PLEURAL SURGERY
Pleurectomy

Pleurectomy is an open procedure requiring thoracotomy where partial stripping of the parietal pleural layer enables the visceral pleura to stick to the subsequent raw surface of the chest wall. If at operation any blebs or bullae are identified these will be dealt with by oversewing, stapling, resection or ablation.

Pleurodesis

This entails the insufflation of a chemical irritant such as fibrin glue or iodized talc via a chest drain or thoracoscope. The latter technique has the advantage of being able to deal with any blebs or bullae identified at the time (see pleurectomy).

Decortication

This may be necessary for patients presenting with chronic empyema. Rib resection is often required, via a thoracotomy, and once the thickened pleurae are removed, the previously restricted lung may re-expand. Any remaining pus must be drained.

Physiotherapy key points
- As for Lobectomy, Sleeve resection, etc. (p. 310).

CHEST WALL SURGERY
Pectus excavatum

The primary defect results from the costal cartilages forming in a concave manner therefore depressing the sternum. Most patients have few symptoms despite several studies showing that cardiac and respiratory function tend to be marginally below normal.

On the whole, the primary indication for surgery is cosmesis because of psychological distress associated with altered body image (Sabiston 1990). Surgical correction involves a midline or transverse inframammary incision down to the periostium of the sternum. All cartilages are resected subperichondrially and the sternum repositioned. In adults internal fixation is carried out using retrosternal struts, plates or steel wires which can be removed during elective day surgery 18 months later. The cartilages regenerate rapidly within several months resulting in a firm anterior chest wall.

Physiotherapy key points
- Pulmonary atelectasis with fever may occur, therefore early mobilization is essential.
- On discharge patients are advised to avoid contact sports for several months or until the plate or wire, if in situ, has been removed.

Pectus carinatum

This is also commonly described as 'pigeon chest'. It is less common than pectus excavatum and is characterized by sternal protrusion caused by an upward curve of the 4th–5th costal cartilages. This usually results in reduced flexibility of the chest impeding inspiratory expansion. The operative procedure is similar to that for pectus excavatum except that the sternum is manipulated into a normal position without the insertion of a plate or wire. Postoperative complications are rare.

Thoracoplasty

Thoracoplasty is the removal of ribs in order to collapse the underlying diseased lung. Originally the operation was devised as primary treatment for pulmonary tuberculosis prior to the availability of antituberculous chemotherapy. Nowadays it may be undertaken for treatment of bronchopulmonary fistulas and empyemas in patients who are immunosuppressed. This often applies to patients suffering from acquired immune deficiency syndrome (AIDS) where tuberculosis and atypical mycobacterial infections do not respond well to chemotherapy and the patients are unable to withstand resectional surgery.

The procedure will result in irreversible loss of lung function to the affected area. In the past the operation was staged where only three to five ribs would be resected at a time. Today the two to three stages are often undertaken simultaneously.

Physiotherapy key points
• As for Lobectomy, Sleeve resection, etc. (p. 310).
• Postural re-education is extremely important due to the high risk of deformity following this procedure. If the first rib and distal attachments of the scalene muscles have been removed, the head and neck are pulled over to the non-affected side. As the rhomboids have been cut, the shoulder on the affected side is raised and medially rotated. To counteract the head displacement, the trunk leans towards the affected side. Postural correction should be achieved in standing and maintained when walking. Early correction with the aid of a mirror will minimize the deformity but the postural exercises may need to be continued by the patient for about 2 months.
• A firm pad should be applied if there is paradoxical movement of the chest wall.
• Shoulder girdle and arm movements should include depression of the shoulder girdle on the side of the thoracoplasty, retraction of the scapulae, bilateral full range movements and neck lateral lean towards the side of the operation.

SURGERY FOR THE DIAPHRAGM AND OESOPHAGUS

Diaphragm

Traumatic rupture of the diaphragm, more commonly the left hemidiaphragm, occurs because of injury to the chest or abdomen following a road traffic accident (RTA) or from a penetrating wound. Herniation of visceral/abdominal contents into the thoracic cavity may not occur instantly and is therefore often misdiagnosed. The affected lung may collapse as a result, with mediastinal shift away from the rupture site. Repair of the diaphragm will be carried out via a thoracotomy with or without an abdominal incision.

Physiotherapy key points
• There is a risk of empyema developing if stomach contents have ruptured into the pleural space.
• Preoperative chest radiograph may reveal a fluid level secondary to stomach or bowel contents in the thoracic cavity.

Nissen fundoplication for hiatus hernia

This procedure corrects herniation of the stomach through the oesophageal hiatus in the diaphragm. Symptoms of gastric reflux and oesophagitis increase with stooping, straining, coughing and pregnancy. It is corrected via a thoracic or abdominal incision.

Oesophagectomy

Surgical correction involves two main incisions via a laparotomy and a thoracotomy with two small neck incisions posterior to sternomastoid. The resected portion of affected oesophagus may be replaced by a tube of stomach or colon, anastomosed to the oesophageal stump or pharynx if a total resection has been carried out. Resection of oesophageal carcinoma carries a high mortality rate and a 5-year survival rate of less than 5% (Forrest et al 1995).

Physiotherapy key points
• The head-down position is avoided to prevent gastric reflux which could lead to pulmonary infection secondary to aspiration and/or breakdown of the anastomosis.
• If dysphagia has been a problem preoperatively, patients are often malnourished and weak which can lengthen the recovery period.

• Extreme care must be taken if naso-pharyngeal suction is indicated, as accidental entry of the catheter into the oesophagus may traumatize the anastomosis. Minitracheotomy may be a preferable option if secretion retention is a problem.

• Restriction of particular neck movements, usually extension, to avoid possible tension on the anastomosis is requested by some surgeons.

Complications of thoracic surgery

Pain. Extrapleural bupivicaine infusion is an increasingly popular method of pain control following a thoracotomy.

Bronchial secretions. The appropriate timing and selection of minitracheotomy can help reduce the incidence of sputum retention.

Pneumonia is a serious complication with a high mortality rate.

Atrial fibrillation is common with extensive resection in the elderly. Onset is usually 2–5 days postoperatively.

Wound infection is a problem in 10% of pulmonary resections. This percentage is reduced with the administration of prophylactic antibiotics at the time of anaesthetic induction.

Haemorrhage. Significant bleeding, usually involving the bronchial arteries, occurs in 1–2% of patients. It is more likely after a pneumonectomy.

Empyema. This occasionally presents a few weeks following surgery.

Bronchopleural fistula (BPF) is rare following a lobectomy. It is seen more commonly after a pneumonectomy and if it occurs in the early postoperative period is likely to be directly linked to the surgical closure of the stump. A classic sign on the chest radiograph is a drop in the fluid level in the pneumonectomy space and is usually associated with the patient coughing up loose brown liquid, i.e. space fluid, through the BPF. This fluid could potentially spill over into the healthy lung and therefore must be drained out through an intercostal drain. Surgical repair of a chronic bronchopleural fistula may be carried out by stump suturing with or without vascularized pedicle flaps of omentum (Sabanathan & Richardson 1994).

Surgical emphysema. The presence of air in the soft tissues is expected locally around wounds and will be absorbed over a few days. However, if surgical emphysema increases, review of intercostal chest drainage is necessary.

Recurrent laryngeal nerve damage. Palsy of the vocal cord may reduce the effectiveness of the cough mechanism and cause a weak or hoarse voice.

CHEST TRAUMA

There are many causes of chest trauma. The main areas of classification include stab/gunshot wounds, RTA or other accidents and blast injuries.

Simple rib fracture

Rib fractures are the most common thoracic injury and unless they are causing chest wall instability (flail) or associated with major intra-thoracic injury, the main aim is to relieve pain and thereby prevent pulmonary complications such as atelectasis and infection.

Pain control is paramount and should not be overlooked even with a single rib fracture as this can produce respiratory complications, especially in the elderly.

Physiotherapy key points
• A great deal of injuring force is required to fracture the first rib, therefore visceral injury is likely to be present. Brachial plexus deficit, absent radial pulse, pulsating supraclavicular mass or widening of the superior mediastinum on radiograph should always be reported to medical staff.

• Intercostal nerve blocks can be a very effective form of pain management in this group of patients.

• Patients will benefit greatly from early mobilization.

• Patients should be taught how to support the chest wall to facilitate an effective cough.

• Taping or restriction of the chest wall to

reduce pain is not advised as this may lead to further respiratory complications. Other methods of pain relief should be considered.

Flail chest

A flail chest may be caused by multiple continuous, comminuted or segmented rib fractures resulting in paradoxical movement of the chest wall, i.e. the flail segment is 'sucked in' during inspiration and 'blown out' during expiration. This can also occur because of disruption of cartilaginous or ligamentous rib attachments. Although paradoxical movement may be marked, the main concern is often pulmonary contusion resulting in reduced lung compliance and atelectasis. If pain and respiratory fatigue are not addressed promptly, respiratory decompensation may ensue a few hours or days later.

Physiotherapy key points
- Effective pain management is essential to maintain adequate ventilation and effective clearance of secretions.
- A cough pad may be supplied to ease the discomfort of coughing.
- Shakings and percussion are usually inappropriate as patients will tend to 'splint' their chest in response to any increase in discomfort.
- Early mobilization is of great benefit.

Pulmonary contusion

Pulmonary contusion is a major component of chest trauma. Parenchymal damage consists of interstitial oedema and haemorrhage which can result in obliteration of the alveolar space and large areas of consolidation. Hypoventilation and significant pulmonary shunting can occur. The contusion may present as unilateral or bilateral depending on the nature of the injury.

Chest radiographic findings of varying degrees of patchy consolidation may be very similar to that of adult respiratory distress syndrome (ARDS) and they often coexist. Close monitoring of fluid balance to avoid pulmonary oedema in lungs that may already have reduced compliance is essential. SaO_2 monitoring may be very useful in the early stages to detect any signs of respiratory decompensation.

Pneumothorax

A pneumothorax can be classed as open, tension or partial (Fig. 12.9).

Open pneumothorax

If an open chest wound is sufficiently large, intrapleural pressure will remain equal to atmospheric pressure and, with each breath, air will be sucked in and out of the chest wall, resulting in marked paroxysmal shifting of the mediastinum with each respiratory effort. The subsequent hypoventilation and decreased cardiac output can be life threatening. In the emergency situation closure of the wound by any means should be attempted, followed by surgical closure and insertion of an intercostal drain.

Tension pneumothorax

Injury to the lung results in a continuing air leak which acts as a one-way valve, allowing air to progressively accumulate in the pleural space. This creates positive intrathoracic pressure leading to mediastinal shift and compression of the remaining lung. These increasing pressures, if not corrected, can invert the diaphragm, cause subcutaneous emphysema and ultimately a cardiorespiratory arrest. Signs and symptoms include surgical emphysema, absent breath sounds on the affected side, mediastinal shift and tracheal deviation to the opposite side and acute respiratory distress. When an intercostal drain is inserted into the pleural space, the air is released under pressure.

Partial pneumothorax

This occurs with partial collapse of the lung away from the chest wall but is not 'under tension'. However, the pneumothorax may increase in size at any time and has the potential to develop into a tension pneumothorax.

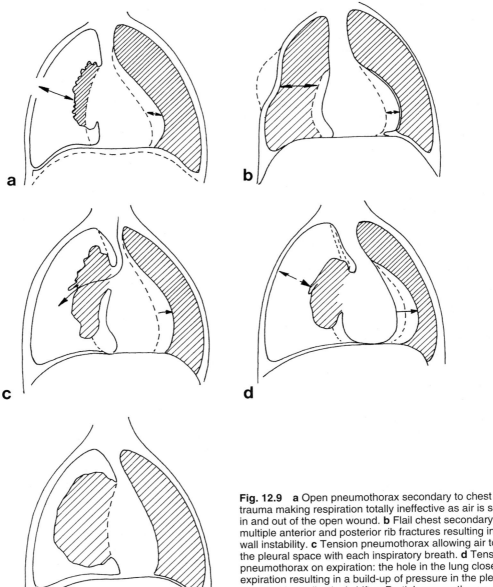

Fig. 12.9 **a** Open pneumothorax secondary to chest trauma making respiration totally ineffective as air is sucked in and out of the open wound. **b** Flail chest secondary to multiple anterior and posterior rib fractures resulting in chest wall instability. **c** Tension pneumothorax allowing air to enter the pleural space with each inspiratory breath. **d** Tension pneumothorax on expiration: the hole in the lung closes on expiration resulting in a build-up of pressure in the pleural space with mediastinal shift. **e** Partial pneumothorax: partial collapse of the lung away from the chest wall but not under tension.

Haemothorax

This involves accumulation of blood in the pleural space. Approximately 300–500 ml may be present before being evident on an erect chest radiograph. If a supine film is taken a haemothorax of up to 1000 ml may be missed. The source of bleeding may be attributed to the heart, aorta, intercostal arteries or internal mammary artery if a penetrating wound was the cause. It is often associated with a pneumothorax. Surgery to control bleeding will be considered if the immediate loss is greater than 1 litre or if the gradual loss is greater than 100 ml/hour for 4 hours or more (Hood 1990). If the blood has become clotted and unable to be cleared with an intercostal drain then thoracic evacuation of the pleural space will be necessary to avoid formation of a fibrothorax or empyema.

Tracheal injuries

These may take the form of a crushing injury to the larynx, a transverse tear or complete separation with retraction of the distal segment into the mediastinum.

Main causes are RTA and direct trauma to the neck. Resuturing will be carried out with some patients requiring tracheostomy postoperatively.

Major bronchial injuries

These are normally caused by blunt trauma to either main bronchus resulting in circumferential laceration with complete or partial separation. Lobar bronchi are less commonly affected. An incomplete laceration heals with stricture formation resulting in recurrent collapse/infection leading to parenchymal destruction. A sleeve resection may be necessary (p. 310). In the case of complete laceration both ends of the severed bronchus granulate and heal. The distal bronchial tree fills with mucus and the affected lung collapses. Early surgery is required to carry out re-anastomosis.

Cardiac and great vessel injury

This is usually secondary to RTA where the steering wheel compresses the heart between the sternum and the vertebrae. As a result, myocardial contusion with or without tamponade commonly occurs. There is usually associated trauma to the anterior chest wall. Emergency thoracotomy is required to drain the blood from the pericardium. Cardiac tamponade is suspected if there is profound shock and low cardiac output. This is manifested by hypotension, tachycardia, elevated jugular venous pressure, poor urinary output and low temperature due to impaired skin perfusion.

Thoracic aorta and branches

Injury occurs secondary to flexion or torsional forces. Aortic rupture results in immediate death unless a false aneurysm has formed in the periaortic tissue and pleura. In these cases immediate surgery is necessary but carries a high risk of fatal bleeding. For this reason patients are put onto partial bypass so that the aorta is cross-clamped enabling an end-to-end anastomosis or Dacron patch to be performed.

CARDIAC SURGERY

Owing to advancements, over the years, in anaesthetic, cardiopulmonary bypass and myocardial management many patients undergoing heart surgery can now expect shorter operating times with fewer complications.

The commonest indications for adults undergoing heart surgery are coronary artery and valve disease. Surgery for correction of rhythm disorders, ventricular aneurysms and aortic coarctation will also be encountered. See Chapter 13 for management of congenital heart defects.

Cardiopulmonary bypass

Open heart surgery requires exposure of the heart and great vessels most commonly via a median sternotomy in order to carry out cardiopulmonary bypass. This involves placing a cannula in the right atrium to drain blood away from the heart to a machine where it is oxygenated and filtered before pumping it back into the systemic circulation via another cannula into the ascending aorta. Administration of cold cardioplegic solution and topical cooling will result in a hypothermic diastolic arrest enabling the surgeon to operate on a non-beating, bloodless heart. The lungs are redundant during this procedure as oxygenation of the blood is being carried out by the bypass machine and therefore are partially or totally collapsed. At the end of the operation, systemic rewarming is commenced until the heart reverts spontaneously, or with the aid of direct current (D/C) conversion, to sinus rhythm. Cardiopulmonary bypass causes derangements of intrinsic coagulation and fibrolytic systems. In some centres there has been renewed interest in carrying out cardiac surgery without the aid of cardiopulmonary bypass (Westaby 1995).

If appropriate at the time of operation, temporary pacing wires will be attached to the ventricle or atrium and pericardial, mediastinal and pleural drains inserted as necessary. The sternum is closed with steel wires.

Coronary artery revascularization

Coronary artery bypass grafting

The principal indications for coronary artery bypass grafting (CABG) are angina pectoris and failed medical and/or previous surgical management. The preferred conduits for grafting are either reversed segments of the patient's own saphenous vein (SV), providing it is free from varicosities and DVT, or the internal mammary arteries (IMA) which have a much higher patency rate. At 10 years the patency rate for a SV graft is 40–60% compared to greater than 90% for an IMA graft (Lytle & Cosgrove 1992). The IMA graft appears especially suitable for grafting of the anterior descending coronary artery. However, owing to the delicate structure of the IMA, a longer operating time is required for mobilization of the vessel and a pleural drain is often required because the pleural space has been entered. Synthetic conduits such as Gore-Tex and biological grafts are usually unsatisfactory owing to their high risk of occlusion. Generally 95% of patients undergoing CABG are either completely free from symptoms or greatly improved at 1 year following surgery. Approximately 90% of patients are alive at 5 years, 75% at 10 years and 60% at 15 years (European Coronary Surgery Study Group 1980). Video-assisted endoscopic techniques are beginning to be used in surgical correction of coronary or cardiac lesions that do not need cardiopulmonary bypass (Lin et al 1996).

Myocardial revascularization with laser

Transmyocardial laser revascularization involves the creation of laser channels to increase the blood flow to an area of ischaemic myocardium (Frazier et al 1995).

Percutaneous transluminal coronary angioplasty (PTCA)

This technique is generally carried out on coronary arteries with proximal, localized lesions. A small balloon is inserted under radiological control until positioned across the stenosis, whereupon it is inflated thus compressing or displacing the plaque.

Coronary laser angioplasty

This technique has been developed whereby a laser rather than a balloon is used to vaporize and ablate atheromatous tissue (Topaz 1996).

Coronary stenting

This involves intravascular stents being used to support and maintain the calibre of diseased coronary arteries (de Cesare et al 1996).

Valvular heart disease

The commonest causes of diseased heart valves are childhood rheumatic fever, congenital abnormalities, endocarditis, collagen vascular disorders e.g. Marfan's syndrome, and ischaemic heart disease.

The valves may become incompetent leading to regurgitation or stenosis with or without calcification. Breathlessness, fatigue and cyanosis due to increased workload of the myocardium and lungs are the commonest symptoms. There is a high risk of sudden death associated with aortic stenosis even if the patient is free of symptoms.

Surgical management

Valvuloplasty. Balloon valvuloplasty entails a small balloon flotation catheter crossing the interatrial septum, enlarging the opening and then passing a larger balloon which is inflated through the orifice. This technique has virtually negated the need for closed valvotomy via a thoracotomy.

Annuloplasty. This is the refashioning of the annulus which is part of the valve apparatus which may become calcified or dilated.

Open valvotomy. Requires cardiopulmonary bypass and the valve is incised under direct vision.

Valve replacement. Replacement valves may be classed as mechanical prostheses or bio-prostheses (tissue valves). Mechanical valves are categorized into two major groups: the caged-ball, e.g. Starr–Edwards which has a durability of up to 35 years; and the tilting disc, e.g. St Jude. Lifelong anticoagulation is required following an insertion of a mechanical valve. Tissue valves were developed to overcome the risk of thrombo-embolism and may be divided into two groups, the first of those being porcine heterografts which are preserved in glutaraldehyde and mounted on a strut e.g. Carpentier–Edwards. Anticoagulant therapy is still necessary in some cases. The second group are classed as homo-grafts as they are harvested from human cadavers and placed in situ without the aid of a strut.

Coarctation of the aorta

This is a localized thickening and infolding of the media of the aortic wall which causes obstruction to aortic flow at the site where, postnatally, the ductus undergoes obliteration. Resection of the narrowed portion is advised to avoid systemic hypertension and its inherent risks. An end-to-end anastomosis is normally carried out with occasional insertion of a Dacron graft.

Ventricular aneurysms

The aneurysm usually occurs as a result of trans-mural myocardial infarction which leads to an area of ventricular scar tissue. Consequently the affected area is unable to contract effectively. Repair is carried out by resection or patching.

Surgical treatment of tachyarrhythmias

The aim of surgery is to excise, isolate or inter-rupt tissue in the heart responsible for triggering the tachycardia, while preserving or improving myocardial function. The appropriate layer of endocardium may be peeled off or cryoblation used to isolate areas of the ventricle that cannot be resected.

Postoperative management

Extubation within 3 hours of cardiac surgery is preferable in most non-complicated cases (Higgins 1992). Patients may remain in the recovery area for a few hours or on the intensive care unit (ICU) for up to 12–24 hours depending on their cardiovascular status before being transferred to the high-dependency area or post-operative ward. Continuous monitoring of the patient's cardiac status is necessary until the patient is stable.

See Chapter 5 for mechanical circulatory support devices.

Complications of cardiac surgery

Perioperative myocardial infarction can have major adverse effects on early and late prognosis.

Bleeding. 2–5% of CABG patients are reopened for control of bleeding (Shainoff et al 1994). Cardiac tamponade occurs owing to haemor-rhage into the pericardium causing pressure on the heart and preventing it from filling during diastole. Cardiac arrest may result if the heart is not reopened to remove clots and stop the bleeding.

Hypertension is a problem in up to one-third of patients. The actual mechanism for this rise in blood pressure is unknown (Colvin & Kenny 1989, Heuser et al 1989).

Low cardiac output occurs secondary to hypo-volaemia or failure.

Atrial fibrillation presents in approximately 40% of patients within 2–3 days of surgery (Frost et al 1992).

Lower lobe collapse, particularly of the left lung, is present in the majority of patients, owing to the compression of the lower lobe during surgery and/or damage to the phrenic nerve through trauma or cold injury secondary to cardioplegia (Markand et al 1985).

Reduced lung volumes are thought to be attributable to alterations in rib cage mechanics.

Pulmonary infection.

Pulmonary oedema/pleural effusions may occur secondary to excessive fluid replacement to correct low volume states.

Pneumothorax/haemothorax is often a consequence of opening the chest wall.

Impairment of renal perfusion due to low cardiac output or vasoconstriction secondary to inotropic support may require temporary renal replacement therapy.

Major wound complications such as mediastinitis and/or wound dehiscence affect 1% of patients (Loop et al 1990). After sternotomy the sternum may fail to unite requiring rewiring.

Intellectual dysfunction in the early postoperative period occurs in 75% of patients but major long-term problems are uncommon (Shaw et al 1986a). It is thought to be secondary to impaired cerebral perfusion during cardiopulmonary bypass.

Stroke occurs in 1–5% of patients and is age related (Shaw et al 1986b).

Physiotherapy key points

• For management of physiotherapy problems on the intensive care unit, see Chapter 11. The guidelines for pre- and postoperative physiotherapy management are similar to those discussed for the general surgical patient (pp. 302–305) but the following points should be noted.

• The physiotherapist may find Box 12.1 useful in assessment of the postoperative cardiac surgical patient.

• Patients who require intra-aortic balloon pump support (IABP) are normally nursed supine and are too unstable to tolerate change of position. Manual hyperinflation may further compromise the low cardiac output. If the IABP catheter has been inserted into the femoral artery, hip flexion of that limb could result in kinking of the tube. Any technique which disrupts the ECG signal, e.g. shakings/vibrations may interfere with the IABP trigger and function of the machine.

• Monitoring of blood pressure is essential

Box 12.1 Postoperative observations following cardiac surgery

• Respiration: spontaneous or mechanical
• Level of consciousness
• Colour
• Arterial blood gases (SaO_2)
• Pulse and temperature
• Blood pressure/central venous pressure
• Urinary output
• ECG
• Pacemaker/intra-aortic balloon pump
• Drugs including analgesia
• Incisions and drains
• Chest radiograph
• Bronchial secretions
• Auscultation

---

to avoid excessive pressure on newly grafted vessels. The head-down position increases atrial pressure and is usually not indicated or tolerated by patients after cardiac surgery. Periods of unexplained hypertension may occur in patients following resection of aortic coarctation.

• Reduced or bronchial breath sounds, especially in the left lower lobe, are a common finding and may persist even in an ambulant, apyrexial patient.

• In uncomplicated cases, advice and monitoring of early ambulation, regular thoracic expansion exercises and positioning during rest periods in bed or a chair may be all that is necessary. Stair climbing is introduced once the patient is cardiovascularly stable when walking for a reasonable distance on the flat. This generally occurs on the fourth or fifth day after surgery.

• The use of PCPAP, IPPB or IS may be indicated in persistent, problematic lung collapse where the patient is unable to mobilize adequately or participate in the ACBT.

• Support of the sternal wound may be carried out by the patient using a pillow, 'coughlok' or towel to assist huffing and coughing when clearing bronchial secretions. Particular attention should be paid to sternal support if a sternal click is heard or palpated. It should always be stressed that the 'cough-lok' should be tightened for coughing and any situations which may induce unwanted movement of the sternum such as straining or getting in/out of bed and loosened in between use.

• Postural correction and gentle shoulder girdle exercises are encouraged. If shoulder joint stiffness is a problem then gentle, bilateral shoulder exercises are taught. It should be noted that some surgeons who perform IMA grafting may request that shoulder movements be limited in the early postoperative period. For those patients with persistent chest wall pain of musculoskeletal origin, manual therapy techniques may help relieve symptoms (Ch. 8, p. 192).

• It is common for patients to feel depressed after the first couple of days following surgery. The patient is often reassured to know that this is a recognized feature of the recovery period.

• Prior to discharge the patient will be given advice regarding management of activities of daily living. A graduated, daily walking programme is generally advised but should be combined with rest periods of up to 1–2 hours each day. The distance walked should be increased at the patient's discretion but it is hoped that the majority of patients should be able to manage 3–4 miles after 6 weeks (barring any complications and/or past medical history which could inhibit their progress). Common sense should prevail for those living in hilly areas, e.g. if possible, being driven to a flatter area to carry out the exercise programme. Patients themselves should not drive for at least 6 weeks to allow sternal healing. It is for this reason also that heavy work or lifting should be avoided for approximately 3 months. Sexual activity may be resumed as soon as the patient feels able. Depending on the patient's occupation, the majority will return to work at around 3 months after surgery but where heavy physical tasks cannot be avoided, alternative employment may be advisable. Some centres offer cardiac rehabilitation but in the long term all patients who are able, would benefit from regular exercise such as swimming, walking and cycling. Advice/information on a general healthy lifestyle should also be made available to patients and their families.

ABDOMINAL SURGERY

Over the last 5 years, there has been a trend in general surgery towards minimally invasive surgical procedures. Laparoscopy has been applied in both the diagnostic and therapeutic fields. The technique is usually performed under general anaesthesia with a small incision being made to introduce a cannula to facilitate the insufflation of carbon dioxide or nitrous oxide into the peritoneal cavity. A pneumoperitoneum is created so that the peritoneal cavity may be visualized through a laparoscope and video camera and the picture is transmitted onto a monitor. Most procedures require additional punctures for passage of instruments including diathermy devices and retractors. The main advantages of this technique are the resultant reduction in postoperative pain, pulmonary complications and hospital length of stay, improved cosmesis and an earlier return to work compared with open procedures (Sawyers 1996). The disadvantages are the cost of training surgeons and the instrumentation, the duration of the operation and the possibility that the procedure may have to be converted to an open procedure if difficulties arise (Sawyers 1996).

The majority of patients undergoing laparoscopic surgery do not require physiotherapy input as they are normally fully mobile from a very early stage postoperatively. However, if a patient presents with other high-risk factors as discussed on page 302 or develops unexpected complications, physiotherapy may be appropriate.

ADULT LIVER TRANSPLANTATION

Liver transplantation is indicated in irreversible (acute or chronic) end-stage liver disease which is unable to be treated by conventional medical or surgical therapy and when life expectancy is judged to be less than 1 year. The patient's quality of life must also be taken into consideration since this may become unacceptable owing to a variety of associated symptoms. These include extreme disabling lethargy, progressive muscle wasting, intractable pruritus, recurrent oesophageal variceal bleeding, ascites and hepatic encephalopathy. Fulminant hepatic failure (FHF) is a less common but important indication and is defined as the development of hepatic encephalopathy within 8 weeks of the onset of symptoms in a patient without previous liver disease. In the UK, paracetamol overdose is the commonest cause of FHF (Mutimer 1994). Cumulative survival rate reported in transplant recipients since 1988 varies from 71% at 1 year to 63% at 3 years (European Liver Transplant Registry 1992) but has improved steadily over recent years.

Orthotopic liver transplantation (OLT)

This is the standard procedure where the whole diseased liver is removed and replaced by a cadaveric liver in the same position. This procedure represents one of the most major surgical insults which can be perpetrated on the ill patient. The incision is a bilateral subcostal incision with median extension to the xiphoid process. Many surgeons use venovenous bypass whereby blood is diverted from the liver via the inferior vena cava and returned to the circulation via the axillary vein thus ensuring portal and systemic decompression. The procedure is lengthy and may last up to 10 hours during complex transplants.

Patients are routinely sent to ICU postoperatively for ventilation but in uncomplicated cases, the patient may be extubated within 24 hours. For patients with FHF, signs of encephalopathy may be evident for several days following the procedure and there may often be a need for prolonged ventilation. British studies suggest that patients spend an average of 4 days in ICU and a median total hospital stay of 43 days (Burroughs et al 1992).

Physiotherapy key points

The majority of elective patients will be assessed during the preoperative work up period. Guidelines are similar to those for any patient undergoing major upper abdominal surgery but the following points should also be noted:

- Patients with chronic end-stage liver disease can present with very poor mobility and exercise tolerance secondary to long-term malnourishment, progressive muscle wasting and excessive fatigue. Muscle wasting may be 'masked' by generalized oedema.
- Some patients suffer from depression, often linked to their poor quality of life, and this should always be taken into consideration.
- Arterial hypoxaemia is relatively common in liver disease patients; therefore pulse oximetry may be advisable, in some cases, when assessing exercise tolerance.
- Some patients may be at high risk of oesophageal variceal bleeding. If nasopharyngeal suction is indicated, close liaison with medical staff and extreme caution is advised owing to the risk of the catheter entering the oesophagus and causing a massive, life-threatening bleed.
- Postoperative pulmonary complications are common secondary to the lengthy anaesthetic and prolonged supine position on the operating table.
- The right phrenic nerve can be damaged during the procedure, leading to a raised right hemidiaphragm and lower lobe collapse.
- If ascites is present, this can result in reduced chest wall compliance and static and dynamic lung volumes.
- There is always increased risk of infection secondary to immunosuppression.
- The majority of patients will develop a right pleural effusion but less than one-third are clinically significant.
- Pressure on the common peroneal nerve is a relatively common event during and after surgery in the iller patient and the temporary use of drop foot splints may be appropriate.
- Liver biopsies are carried out in the early postoperative period. Owing to the risk of bleeding, patients may need a period of bed rest for a few hours and ideally, physiotherapy should be avoided at this time.
- In uncomplicated cases patients are often independently mobilizing around the ward within a few days. However, certain patients need weeks or sometimes months of rehabilitation.

HEAD AND NECK SURGERY

Tumours of the head and neck may involve the oral cavity, oropharynx, larynx and hypopharynx.

Resection with primary closure may be adequate to clear some tumours. If, however, there has been metastatic spread to other tissues, a partial or radical neck dissection or the more extensive commando procedure may be indicated (Maran 1995).

When reconstructive surgery is necessary this may take the form of:

- Split skin grafting
- Pedicle or myocutaneous flaps using pectoralis major or less commonly trapezius and latissimus dorsi
- Free tissue transfer, e.g. a section of fibula may be used to reconstruct the jaw bone
- Organ transposition of the stomach or colon requiring major upper abdominal and/or thoracic incisions.

If the larynx has been removed this will result in loss of speech and a permanent tracheostomy. For patients undergoing surgery which does not entail a laryngectomy, a tracheostomy may still be required. This may only be on a temporary basis to protect the airway from aspiration and compression from swelling in the surrounding structures over the early postoperative period. Speech and language therapists will be involved with patients who have subsequent swallowing defects and those who require training in voice restoration. This can be achieved by oesophageal speech or by a laryngeal speech aid.

Physiotherapy key points
- See Chapter 11 for tracheostomy management.
- Until the patient's airways have become accustomed to the loss of upper airway humidification during the early postoperative period following laryngectomy, adequate fluid intake should be monitored. Provision of continuous, heated humidification via a tracheostomy mask should also be made available.
- Patients requiring a tracheostomy permanently or over an extended period will be taught general tracheostomy management including

how to carry out suction. Family and carers may also be involved in the teaching sessions.
- Consideration must always be given to the devastating effect of loss of speech and possible severe facial disfigurement following some types of surgery.
- If the patient has undergone extensive surgical resection, respiratory complications are expected, especially if upper abdominal or thoracic incisions have been necessary. If indicated, incentive spirometers can be adapted for use by patients with a tracheostomy and/or laryngectomy (Tan 1995).
- Close liaison with the surgeon is essential where muscles have been resected or grafted, as postural, neck and shoulder exercises may initially have to be avoided or modified to ensure that the graft is established and that the brachial plexus is not stretched. If the spinal accessory nerve has been affected following surgery, shoulder abduction may be reduced. Rehabilitation of upper and lower limbs affected by the use of free tissue transfer technique may be necessary.

VASCULAR SURGERY

Aortic aneurysm

An aneurysm occurs as a result of degeneration of the media and elastica lamina of the arterial wall of the aorta leading to local dilatation. The majority of aneurysms occur in the abdominal aorta but can also affect the thoracic aorta. Patients who present as emergency cases with aneurysm rupture will be in hypovolaemic shock due to leakage or rupture of the aneurysm and require immediate surgical repair.

During surgical repair of an abdominal aortic aneurysm (AAA) a horizontal transabdominal or vertical incision is made and the aorta is cross-clamped above and below the affected area. The aneurysm is then opened longitudinally removing all thrombi and a Dacron tube sewn into the aorta. Alternatively a 'trouser' bifurcation graft may be anastomosed distally to the iliac and femoral arteries. Techniques involving implantation of an endovascular aortic graft via the transfemoral route for repair of AAA are undertaken in some centres (Parodi et al 1991, Chuter et al 1993).

If a thoracic aortic aneurysm is being repaired an aortic valve replacement may also be necessary at the time of operation.

A dissecting aortic aneurysm occurs if there is bleeding into the wall of the aorta resulting in separation of the media from the intima and the adventitia.

Dissecting ascending thoracic aneurysms may result in upper limb ischaemia. Descending aneurysms can lead to lower limb ischaemia or paralysis, acute renal failure if the renal arteries are affected and possible bowel ischaemia where the mesenteric arteries are involved.

Physiotherapy key points
• The majority of patients presenting with AAA are over 70 years old with varying degrees of arteriosclerosis so that decreased mobility/ exercise tolerance may be a problem pre- and postoperatively.
• Early mobilization, within the patient's capabilities, is important to avoid respiratory complications.

SURGERY IN THE ELDERLY

It has been estimated that 50% of people currently aged 65 years and over will undergo some form of surgery in their remaining lifetime (Davenport 1986). For elderly patients who present with no medical problems, their postoperative morbidity and mortality rates are good.

See page 302 for effects of age on the respiratory system.

The elderly surgical patient has reduced autonomic responses, therefore perioperative blood loss or fluid overload are poorly tolerated. Acute confusional state is more common with advancing age and may be secondary to infection, hypoxia, drugs, major organ failure or alcohol withdrawal. Older patients are more sensitive to narcotic analgesia and temperature control mechanisms are less effective. With elective surgery in this patient group the mortality rate is between two and seven times lower than that in emergency procedures (Seymour et al 1992).

Orthopaedic surgery

Elderly women with osteoporosis are the commonest group of patients to suffer from fractured neck of femur. Surgical treatment should be immediate and involve internal fixation of the femur, allowing early mobilization and thus reducing the risk of postoperative respiratory complications. Sepsis and pulmonary embolus after major orthopaedic surgery are two of the main causes of death in the elderly population. Although early mobilization alone is insufficient to prevent postoperative thromboembolism, the advantages regarding bone density, neuromuscular and respiratory function, skin integrity, increased independence and sense of well-being are invaluable (Devas et al 1992).

Physiotherapy key points
• Following fixation of the femur, mobilization, initially possibly just from bed to chair, should be started from the first postoperative day in non-complicated cases. Patients are normally partially weight bearing with a frame or crutches and will need regular encouragement/ assistance to mobilize and carry out the ACBT to help prevent respiratory complications.

ACKNOWLEDGEMENTS

The author would like to thank Marion Kieran, Patricia McCoy, Barbara Webber and Jennifer Pryor for the sections taken from 'Surgical patients and patients requiring intensive care' in the 1st edition of *Physiotherapy for respiratory and cardiac problems.*

Also the author would like to thank the following people for all their support and advice: David Lindsay, Professor Garden, Dr Swan, Dr Sim, Dr McClure, Professor Ruckley, Mr Campanella, Mr Purves, Ian Lennox and all the staff of the Physiotherapy Department of the Royal Infirmary of Edinburgh NHS Trust.

REFERENCES

Anderson E W, Andleman R J, Strauch J M et al 1973 Effect of low carbon monoxide exposure on onset and duration of angina pectoris. Annals of Internal Medicine 79: 46–50

Attard A R, Corlett M J, Kidner N J et al 1992 Safety of early pain relief for acute abdominal pain. British Medical Journal 305: 554–556

Auerbach S M, Kilmann P R 1977 Crisis intervention: a review of outcome research. Psychological Bulletin 84: 1189–1217

British Oxygen Company 1990 Entonox fact sheet. Guildford, Surrey

Brodsky J B 1995 Anaesthesia for thoracic surgery. In: Healy T E J, Cohen P J (eds) Wylie and Churchill-Davidson's a practice of anaesthesia, 6th edn. Edward Arnold, London, ch 57, p 1148

Burroughs A K, Blake J, Thorne S et al 1992 Comparative hospital costs of liver transplantation and the treatment of complications of cirrhosis: a prospective study. European Journal of Gastroenterology and Hepatology 4: 123–128

Chuter T A M, Green R M, Ouriel K et al 1993 Transfemoral endovascular aortic graft replacement. Journal of Vascular Surgery 18: 185–197

Colvin J R, Kenny G N C 1989 Automatic control of arterial pressure after cardiac surgery. Anaesthesia 44: 37–41

Craig D B 1981 Post-operative recovery of pulmonary function. Anaesthesia and Analgesia 60: 46–52

Damia G, Mascheroni D, Croci M et al 1988 Peri-operative changes in functional residual capacity in morbidly obese patients. British Journal of Anaesthesia 60: 574–578

Davenport H T 1986 Anaesthesia in the elderly. Heinemann, London

de Cesare N B, Bartorelli A L, Galli S et al 1996 Treatment of ostial lesions of the left anterior descending coronary artery with palmal-slatz coronary stent. American Heart Journal 132: 716–720

de Leon-Casasola O A, Parker B, Lema M J et al 1994 Post-operative epidural bupivicaine–morphine therapy. Experience with 4227 surgical patients. Anesthesiology 81: 368–375

Devas M, Plumpton F S, Seymour D G 1992 Orthopaedics. In: Crosby D L, Rees G A D, Seymour D G (eds) The ageing surgical patient: anaesthetic, operative and medical management. John Wiley, Chichester, ch 11

Dureuil B, Cantineau J P, Desmonts J M 1987 Effects of upper and lower abdominal surgery on diaphragmatic function. British Journal of Anaesthesia 59: 1230–1235

Egan T D, Wong K C 1992 Perioperative smoking cessation and anesthesia: a review. Journal of Clinical Anesthesia 4: 63–72

European Coronary Surgery Study Group 1980 Prospective randomized study of coronary artery bypass surgery in stable angina pectoris. Lancet 2: 491–495

European Liver Transplant Registry 1992 (Update 30/6/1992). Hopital Paul Brousse, Villejuif, France

Ford G T, Whitelaw W A, Rosenal T W et al 1983 Diaphragm function after upper abdominal surgery in humans. American Review of Respiratory Disease 127: 431–436

Forrest A P M, Carter D C, Macleod I B 1995 Principles and practice of surgery, 3rd edn. Churchill Livingstone, Edinburgh

Frazier O H, Cooley D A, Kadipasaoglu K A et al 1995

Myocardial revascularisation with laser. Preliminary findings. Circulation 92: II58–65

Frost L, Molgaard H, Christiansen E H et al 1992 Atrial fibrillation and flutter after coronary artery bypass surgery: epidemiology, risk factors and preventative trials. International Journal of Cardiology 36: 253–261

Garcia-Valdecasas J C, Almenara R, Carbrer C et al 1988 Subcostal incision versus midline laparotomy in gallstone surgery: a prospective and randomized trial. British Journal of Surgery 75: 473–475

Heuser D, Guggenberger H, Fretschner R 1989 Acute blood pressure increase during the perioperative period. American Journal of Cardiology 63: 26C–31C

Higgins T L 1992 Pro: early endotracheal extubation is preferable to late extubation in patients following coronary artery surgery. Journal of Cardiothoracic and Vascular Anesthesia 6: 488–493

Hood R M 1990 Trauma to the chest. In: Sabiston D C, Spencer F C (eds) Surgery of the chest, 5th edn. W B Saunders, Philadelphia, ch 14

Kam A C, O'Brien M, Kam P C A 1993 Pleural drainage systems. Anaesthesia 48: 154–161

Leblanc P, Ruff F, Milic-Emili J 1970 Effects of age and body position on 'airway closure' in man. Journal of Applied Physiology 28: 448–451

Lin P J, Chang C H, Chu J J et al 1996 Video-assisted mitral valve operations. Annals of Thoracic Surgery 61: 1781–1787

Loop F D, Lytle B W, Cosgrove D M et al 1990 Sternal wound complications after isolated coronary bypass grafting: early and late mortality, morbidity and cost of care. Annals of Thoracic Surgery 49: 179–186

Lunn J N 1991 Lecture notes on anaesthetics. Blackwell Scientific Publications, Oxford

Lytle B W, Cosgrove D M 1992 Coronary artery bypass surgery. Current Problems in Surgery 29: 733–807

Mack M J, Aronoff R J, Acuff T E et al 1992 Present role of thoracoscopy in the diagnosis and treatment of diseases of the chest. Annals of Thoracic Surgery 54: 403–408

Maran A G D 1995 Head and neck surgery. In: Cuschieri A, Giles G R, Moossa A R (eds) Essential surgical practice, 3rd edn. Butterworth-Heinemann, Oxford, ch 42, p 1656

Markand O N, Moorthy S S, Mahomed Y et al 1985 Post operative phrenic nerve palsy in patients with open-heart surgery. Annals of Thoracic Surgery 39: 68–73

Mearns A J 1995 Tumours of the lung. In: Cushieri A, Giles G R, Moossa A R (eds) Essential surgical practice, 3rd edn. Butterworth-Heinemann, Oxford, ch 49, p 794

Morgan M, Nel M R 1996 Smoking and anaesthesia revisited. Anaesthesia 51: 309–311

Mutimer D 1994 Fulminant and subacute hepatic failure. In: Neuberger J, Lucey M (eds) Liver transplantation: practice and management. BMJ Publishing Group, London, ch 2, p 76

Mynster T, Jensen L M, Kehlet H et al 1996 The effect of posture on late post-operative oxygenation. Anaesthesia 51: 225–227

Nelson S 1996 Pre-admission education for patients undergoing cardiac surgery. British Medical Journal 5: 335–340

Parodi J C, Palmaz J C, Barone H D 1991 Transfemoral

intraluminal graft implantation for abdominal aortic aneurysms. Annals of Vascular Surgery 5: 491–499

Sabanathan S, Richardson J 1994 Management of post pneumonectomy bronchopleural fistulae. A review. Journal of Cardiovascular Surgery 35: 449–457

Sabiston D C 1990 Disorders of the sternum and the thoracic wall. In: Sabiston D C, Spencer F C (eds) Surgery of the chest, 5th edn. W B Saunders, Philadelphia, ch 15

Sawyers J L 1996 Current status of conventional (open) cholecystectomy versus laparoscopic cholecystectomy. Annals of Surgery 223: 1–3

Scott A M, Starling J R, Ruscher A E et al 1996 Thoracic versus lumbar epidural anesthesia's effect on pain control and ileus resolution after restorative proctocolectomy. Surgery 120: 688–697

Selsby D S, Jones J G 1993 Respiratory function and the safety of anaesthesia. In: Taylor T H, Major E (eds) Hazards and complications of anaesthesia, 2nd edn. Churchill Livingstone, Edinburgh, ch 4

Seymour D G, Rees G A D, Crosby D L 1992 Introduction and general principles. In: The ageing surgical patient: anaesthetic, operative and medical management. Wiley, Chichester, ch 1

Shainoff J R, Estafanous F G, Yared J P et al 1994 Low factor X111A levels are associated with increased blood loss after coronary artery bypass grafting. Journal of Thoracic and Cardiovascular Surgery 108: 437–445

Shaw P J, Bates D, Cartridge N E et al 1986a Early

intellectual dysfunction following coronary bypass surgery. Quarterly Journal of Medicine 58: 59–68

Shaw P J, Bates D, Cartridge N E et al 1986b Neurological complications of coronary artery bypass graft surgery. British Medical Journal 293: 165–167

Smith R S, Fry W R, Tsoi E K M et al 1993 Preliminary report on videothoracoscopy in the evaluation and treatment of thoracic injury. American Journal of Surgery 166: 690–693

Tan A K 1995 Incentive spirometry for tracheostomy and laryngectomy patients. Journal of Otolaryngology 24: 292–294

Teschler H, Stamatis G, El-Raouf A A et al 1996 Effect of surgical lung volume on respiratory muscle function in pulmonary emphysema. European Respiratory Journal 9: 1779–1784

Thompson A B 1996 Lung volume reduction surgery for emphysema: answers are beginning to accumulate. European Respiratory Journal 9: 1771–1772

Tisi G M 1985 Neoplastic diseases. In: Bordon R A, Moser K M (eds) Manual of clinical problems in pulmonary medicine, 2nd edn. Little Brown, Boston, ch 11, p 411

Topaz O 1996 Plaque removal and thrombus dissolution with photoacoustic energy of pulsed-wave lasers – biotissue interactions and their clinical manifestations. Cardiology 87: 384–391

Westaby S 1995 Coronary surgery without cardiopulmonary bypass. British Heart Journal 73: 203–205

13

Paediatrics

Annette Parker   Ammani Prasad

INTRODUCTION

Respiratory care in small children is very different from that in adults. There are anatomical and physiological differences which mean that additional criteria need to be used for assessment and treatment. The age of the child affects his ability to understand and cooperate with treatment. Fear of the unknown is even more acute in children than in adults.

At all times children should be handled with care and respect. They should be given information and explanation about their treatment appropriate to their age and understanding. It is always easier and more pleasant when a child is compliant with treatment. Cooperation can be obtained by persuasion, or by distraction, for example by games, television, cassette tapes, or reading books suited to the child's age and interest. Rewards can also be given for good behaviour or bravery, for example balloons or stickers. Occasionally children may refuse treatment (either because they simply do not want it or perhaps due to fear). However, if treatment is deemed essential it must be given, after thorough and careful explanation.

It is important to include parents, relatives, and carers as part of the care team. Parents should always have a full explanation of why treatment is required and how it is to be carried out. Parents are able to refuse physiotherapy treatment for their child but this rarely occurs in practice. Parents of sick children, particularly mothers who have recently delivered an ill baby, are extremely vulnerable to stress and should at all times be handled with tact and understanding. Parental stress may be manifested in different ways, for example hysteria, apparent lack of concern, or anger. Some parents are so distressed that they are unable to stay with or visit their sick child and may need special help to express their feelings of fear and panic.

Parents benefit from the physiotherapist's support when they are required to carry out physiotherapy treatment themselves at home. Fathers are frequently wary of participating in treatments and may need extra encouragement. When children and parents are intensively involved in treatment sessions, siblings may often feel left out. It is therefore important to include them in some way, perhaps even in helping with treatment.

A child's awareness of the implications of illness and treatment develops as he grows older. Explanations which are suitable for younger children will need to be expanded as the child grows older and begins to understand how his body works. Teenagers, particularly, have a more sophisticated understanding and may be beginning to think about the future and the impact of illness on school and social life, as well as body image. It is important for them to develop responsibility for their treatment, although they may often object to being told what to do or to being treated like a child.

The physiotherapist treating any child with acute or chronic respiratory problems must be aware of the psychological problems affecting the child and parents and adapt her approach accordingly.

DEVELOPMENT OF THE LUNGS

The development of the lung can be divided into four stages (Inselman & Mellins 1981):

- Embryonic period (weeks 3–5)
- Pseudoglandular period (weeks 6–16)
- Canalicular period (weeks 17–24)
- Alveolar sac period (week 24–term).

Embryonic period (weeks 3–5)

The lung bud starts as an endodermal outgrowth of fetal foregut. The single tube thus formed soon branches into two, forming the major bronchi. By cell division, the process of growth continues until, at the end of this period, the major lung branches are formed.

Pseudoglandular period (weeks 6–16)

During this period the airways grow by dichotomous branching so that by week 16 all generations of the airway from trachea to terminal bronchioles (i.e. the pre-acinus) are formed. During this period the pulmonary circulation also develops, cartilage and lymphatic formation occur, and cilia appear (week 10 onwards).

Canalicular period (weeks 17–24)

The respiratory bronchioles, alveolar ducts and alveoli (i.e. the acinus) start to develop during this time, simultaneously with the lung capillaries. The air-blood barrier first appears at week 19 and towards the end of this period surfactant synthesis begins.

Terminal sac period (week 24–term)

Development of the pulmonary circulation continues and the respiratory bronchioles subdivide to form air spaces. The air spaces are lined by two different types of cell (types I and II pneumocytes). Type-I pneumocytes flatten and elongate to cover the majority of the surface area of the saccular air spaces. Type-II cells only occupy approximately 2% of the surface and are responsible for surfactant synthesis and storage (Greenough 1996a). Surfactant is the phospholipid substance which stabilizes surface tension in the alveolus and prevents alveolar collapse on expiration. Small quantities of surfactant are present at weeks 23–24 of gestation and the amount present gradually increases until there is a surge at about week 30. Birth itself and the onset of respiration stimulate and mature surfactant production.

Towards the end of the terminal sac period, the air spaces have developed into primitive multilocular alveoli. After birth, alveoli increase in size and number. The average number of alveoli in the newborn is 150 million. By the age of 3–4 years, the adult number of 300–400 million alveoli has been reached, but alveolar growth continues until about 8 years of age.

ANATOMICAL AND PHYSIOLOGICAL DIFFERENCES BETWEEN CHILDREN AND ADULTS

There are several anatomical and physiological differences between children and adults that put children at an increased risk of respiratory problems.

Anatomical differences

• Differences in upper airway anatomy allow infants to feed and breathe simultaneously up to approximately 3–4 months of age. It has been thought that this effectively makes them 'obligatory nose breathers' so that any nasal blockage leads to apnoea. Though this concept has been questioned (Rodenstein et al 1987), during clinical observation infants with nasal passages occluded either by mucus or tubes have been noted to have an increased work of breathing and spells of apnoea.

• The lymphatic tissue (adenoids and tonsils) may be enlarged in the infant. The tongue is also relatively large. These factors may contribute to upper airway obstruction.

• The smaller diameter airways of infants, particularly those born preterm, offer very high resistance to airflow, and any mucosal oedema will significantly increase the work of breathing.

• Bronchial wall structure is different in infants. Cartilage is less firm and there are proportionately more mucous glands. Both these factors predispose to airway obstruction and collapse (Reid 1984).

• There are fewer alveoli in young children and, therefore, less surface area for gaseous exchange (Reid 1984).

• The collateral ventilatory channels between alveoli, respiratory bronchioles, and terminal bronchioles are poorly developed until 2–3 years of age, predisposing towards alveolar collapse.

• Infants' ribs are horizontally positioned (Fig. 13.1), therefore there is no 'bucket handle' movement of respiration. In addition weak intercostal muscles mean that the infant is

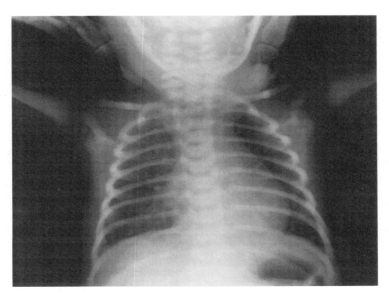

Fig. 13.1 Normal chest radiograph.

more reliant on the diaphragm for respiration. Adult rib configuration develops as the child adopts a more upright posture when gravity pulls the anterior ribs downwards.

• The horizontal angle of insertion of the diaphragm combined with the compliant cartilaginous rib cage of the infant means less efficient ventilation and distortion of chest wall shape on inspiration (Muller & Bryan 1979).

• The heart and other organs, e.g. thymus, are relatively large in infants and, therefore, there is relatively less space for lung tissue.

Physiological differences

• The lungs of infants are less compliant than those of older children and adults, particularly in preterm infants (< 37 weeks' gestation) where there may also be a lack of surfactant.

• Neonates, especially those born preterm, have irregular breathing patterns which may lead to apnoea. Although short spells of apnoea are considered normal, longer periods and those which require stimulation to restart breathing will need investigation.

• Anatomical differences in rib cage configuration do not allow the infant to increase lung volume to the same extent as an adult. Therefore when in respiratory difficulties, the infant must increase respiratory rate, rather than depth, to maintain minute volume.

• Neonates may sleep for up to 20 hours a day and 80% of this time may be in active (rapid eye movement, REM) sleep compared with 20% in adults. During active sleep there is a decrease in postural tone causing a drop in functional residual capacity, thereby increasing the work of breathing (Muller & Bryan 1979).

• The diaphragm in the adult is comprised of approximately 50% of fatigue-resistant type I muscle fibres whereas the neonate has only 25% and preterm infants may have as little as 10%. Therefore there is an increased susceptibility to fatigue of the diaphragm.

• Children have a higher resting metabolic rate with greater demand for oxygen. Any increase in demand can therefore cause hypoxia more rapidly than in adults. Hypoxia in infants causes bradycardia (less than 100 beats/min), rather than tachycardia as in adults.

• Infants and children preferentially ventilate uppermost lung regions, rather than dependent lung regions as in the adult (Davies et al 1985), although the pattern of perfusion is similar (Bhuyan et al 1989). This difference may persist as late as the second decade of life. In acutely ill children with unilateral lung disease, oxygenation may be optimized by placing the good lung uppermost.

• In the small infant the closing volume exceeds the functional residual capacity. In dependent regions airway closure may occur even during normal tidal breathing.

RESPIRATORY ASSESSMENT OF THE INFANT AND CHILD

Careful assessment is essential to identify a problem requiring physiotherapy intervention. Many aspects of assessment will be the same as in adults, but specific differences are listed below.

Medical notes

Information can be extracted from the medical notes relating to present condition and past medical history etc. When assessing a neonate, the following points are relevant:

1. History of pregnancy, labour, and delivery.
2. The Apgar score, which relates to heart rate, respiratory effort, muscle tone, reflex irritability, and colour, and gives an indication of the degree of asphyxiation suffered by the infant at birth.
3. Gestational age and weight.

Discussion with the relevant carers

Discussion with medical staff, nursing staff, and the parent/carer is essential to obtain correct information about recent changes. Questions may include:

1. How stable has the child's condition been over the last few hours?

2. How well is handling tolerated? Does the infant become rapidly hypoxic or bradycardic? How long does he take to recover from the handling episode?
3. Is the infant being fed? If so, is it via the oral, nasogastric, or intravenous route and when was the last feed?
4. Is the infant properly rested from the last handling episode?

Observation charts

Important information can be gained from nursing charts.

• Pyrexia may indicate a possible respiratory infection. In preterm infants, a temperature of less than 36.5°C indicates that non-essential handling should be delayed until the infant's temperature has risen. The core-to-peripheral temperature gradient should also be noted, particularly in the critically ill patient.

• Tachycardia may be due to sepsis or shock. It may also be caused by inadequate levels of sedation or analgesia. In preterm infants both self-limiting bradycardias and bradycardias requiring stimulation may be due to many causes, including retention of secretions.

• Apnoeic spells in the infant may indicate respiratory distress, sepsis, or presence of secretions in the upper or lower respiratory tract.

• The trend of arterial gases and their relationship to oxygen saturation and transcutaneous oxygen should be noted together with the degree and type of respiratory support.

Results of investigations and observations

Results of investigations and other relevant observations should be referred to as appropriate.

Examination

Examination of the older child is similar to that of the adult. The following specific considerations should be made:

Clinical signs. Clinical signs of respiratory distress are listed in Box 13.1.

Box 13.1 Clinical signs of respiratory distress

Respiratory
• Recession
  – intercostal
  – subcostal
  – sternal
• Nasal flaring
• Tachypnoea
• Expiratory grunting
• Stridor
• Cyanosis
• Abnormal breath sounds

Cardiac
• Tachycardia/bradycardia
• Hypertension/hypotension

Other/general
• Neck extension
• Head bobbing
• Pallor
• Reluctance to feed
• Irritability/restlessness
• Altered conscious level
• Headache

Recession occurs because of the high negative pressure generated on inspiration pulling on the soft, compliant chest wall and may be sternal, subcostal, or intercostal. Mild recession may be normal in preterm infants, but in older infants is a sign of increased respiratory effort.

Nasal flaring is a dilatation of the nostrils by the dilatores naris muscles and is a sign of respiratory distress in the infant. It may be a primitive response attempting to decrease airway resistance.

Tachypnoea (respiratory rate greater than 60 breaths/min) may indicate respiratory distress in infants. Normal values are listed in Table 13.1.

Grunting occurs when an infant expires against a partially closed glottis. It is an attempt to

Table 13.1 Normal values of heart rate, respiratory rate and blood pressure according to age

Age group	Heart rate (beats/min)	Respiratory rate (breaths/min)	Blood pressure (mmHg)
Preterm infants	120–140	40–60	70/40
Full-term infants	100–140	30–40	80/40
1–4 years	80–120	25–30	100/65
Adolescents	60–80	15–20	115/60

increase functional residual capacity and thereby improve ventilation.

Stridor is heard when there is partial obstruction of the upper trachea and/or larynx. Obstruction may be due to collapse of the floppy tracheal wall, inflammation, or an inhaled foreign body.

Cyanosis is an unreliable sign of respiratory distress in infants and young children as it depends on the relative amount and type of haemoglobin in the blood and the adequacy of the peripheral circulation. For the first 3–4 weeks of life, the newborn infant has an increased amount of fetal haemoglobin which has a higher affinity for oxygen than adult haemoglobin. The result is a shift of the oxygen saturation curve to the left in an infant.

Auscultation of the infant and young child may be difficult owing to the easy transmission of sounds. In the infant who is ventilated, referred sounds from the ventilator, including water in the expiratory tubing, make assessment difficult. It is often impossible to hear any breath sounds in the preterm infant who is breathing spontaneously. In the older child, secretions in the nose or throat may lead to referred sounds in both lung fields. Wheezing in the younger child or infant may be due to bronchospasm, but could also be due to retained secretions partially occluding smaller airways.

Cardiac manifestations of respiratory distress include an initial tachycardia and possible increase in systemic blood pressure. This changes with worsening hypoxia to bradycardia and hypotension.

Neck extension in an infant with respiratory distress may represent an attempt to reduce airway resistance.

Head bobbing occurs when infants attempt to use the sternocleidomastoid and the scalene muscles as accessory muscles of respiration. It is seen because the relatively weak neck extensors of infants are unable to stabilize the head.

Pallor is commonly seen in infants with respiratory distress and may be a sign of hypoxaemia or other problems including anaemia.

Reluctance to feed is often associated with respiratory distress, and infants may need to take frequent pauses from sucking when tachypnoeic.

Alterations in conscious level should be noted. A reduction in activity may be due to neurological deficit or following the use of opiate analgesia but can also be due to hypoxia and may be accompanied by an inability to feed or cry. Irritability and restlessness may also be indicative of a hypoxic state.

Other relevant observations. The behaviour and manner of a child can give important clues about his respiratory state. A child who is sitting up and playing happily is not usually distressed, whereas one who is agitated or irritable may be showing signs of hypoxia. The child in severe respiratory distress may be withdrawn and lie completely still as if saving all his energy for respiration.

It is important to note muscle tone and appearance in the infant or child with respiratory distress. A hypotonic child will have increased difficulty with breathing, coughing and expectorating. Children with hypertonia will also have difficulty with clearing secretions.

Abdominal distension can be a cause of respiratory distress in infants or can worsen an existing respiratory problem because the diaphragm, the main respiratory muscle in infants, is placed at a mechanical disadvantage.

PHYSIOTHERAPY TECHNIQUES IN INFANTS AND CHILDREN

Most physiotherapy techniques used in adults can be applied in children and the same contraindications apply. The possible deleterious effects of chest physiotherapy and suction mean that treatment should only be given when indicated and never as a 'routine'. Treatment should be performed prior to feeds or at least 1 hour following feeds to avoid the potential for aspiration of stomach contents.

Chest percussion

Chest percussion includes chest clapping using the hand or a face mask. It is generally well tolerated and can be extremely effective in the young child. Clapping should be one-handed in small children and infants. For preterm infants the first three or four fingers of one hand may be used, slightly elevating the middle finger (tenting) (Fig. 13.2a). Chest percussion can be applied using a cup-shaped object such as a face mask (Fig. 13.2b). This mask has a soft plastic cuff and so can be used over bare skin. The face mask has been shown to be a well-tolerated means of percussion (Tudehope & Bagley 1980) in the preterm infant.

Vibrations and shaking

The chest wall is very compliant in infants and young children, so vibrations can be very effective in removing secretions when the respiratory rate is normal or near normal (30–40 breaths/min).

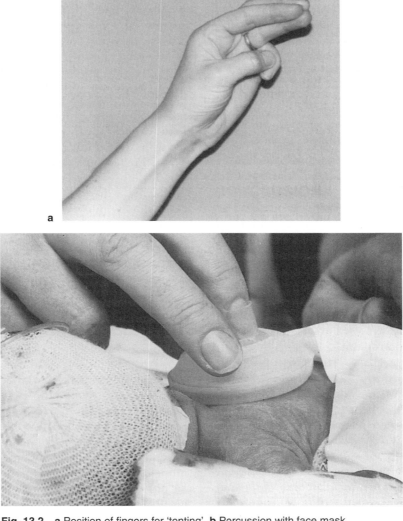

Fig. 13.2   **a** Position of fingers for 'tenting'. **b** Percussion with face mask.

If infants are breathing very rapidly, e.g. more than 60 breaths/min, the expiratory phase is so short that vibrations are neither easy to apply nor effective.

Precautions for chest percussion and vibratory techniques

- Children with dietary deficiencies, liver disease, or those who have been born preterm may develop rickets. Skeletal changes in rickets include general osteoporosis and softening of long bones and deformities of the thorax and pelvis; in these circumstances percussion and vibrations may be contraindicated.
- Very preterm infants have extremely thin skin which is easily bruised and damaged, thereby predisposing to infection. Chest percussion and vibrations may not be appropriate in these infants.
- Bronchospasm may be exacerbated by the use of chest percussion. Premedication with bronchodilator therapy is essential and it may be advisable to avoid percussion in some cases.

Gravity-assisted positioning (postural drainage)

Gravity-assisted positions can be used for children in the same way as for adults. The upper lobes, particularly the right side, are often more affected by respiratory problems in younger children, so gravity-assisted positions for these areas are important, particularly the posterior segments. A head-down tip should be avoided in children with raised intracranial pressure and in preterm infants who are at risk of periventricular haemorrhage. This position should also be avoided in infants and children with abdominal distension as this places the diaphragm at a mechanical disadvantage. Care should be taken in infants with a history of reflux. Whether the tipped head-down position should be used in infants with reflux remains unclear (Taylor & Threlfall 1997). Some evidence exists suggesting that its use may aggravate reflux and possible aspiration (Demont et al 1991, Button et al 1997) while other reports state that

this position has little effect on reflux (Phillips 1996). Reflux is particularly common in preterm infants, affecting approximately 80% (Newell et al 1989).

Positioning

Careful positioning is important to optimize lung function, and supine is the least beneficial position. Prone has been shown to be advantageous in terms of respiratory function (Dean 1985), gastro-oesophageal reflux (Blumenthal & Lealman 1982) and energy expenditure (Brackbill et al 1973), and should be used in infants with respiratory distress who are being closely monitored. However, parents should be advised against this position when babies are sleeping unattended because of its association with sudden infant death (Southall & Samuels 1992).

Owing to the differences in regional ventilation, care should be taken when positioning an affected lung segment/lobe uppermost as this may cause rapid deterioration of respiratory status in the acutely ill child.

Newborn infants are better oxygenated when tilted slightly head up (Thoresen et al 1988) and show a drop in PaO_2 if placed flat or tilted head down unless they are fully mechanically ventilated.

Manual hyperinflation

The same indications and contraindications apply for children as for adults when considering manual hyperinflation as a physiotherapy technique. 500 ml bags are used for infants and 1 litre bags are used for children. Bags may have valves or be open-ended for outlet of excess pressure, controlled by the operator's fingers. A manometer should be placed in the circuit whenever possible to monitor the inflation pressures being generated (Fig. 13.3). As a general guideline, the inspiratory pressure should be increased from the ventilator pressure by no more than 5 cmH$_2$O in an infant and 10 cmH$_2$O in an older child. In order to prevent airway collapse, some positive end-expiratory pressure (PEEP) should be maintained in the bag when-

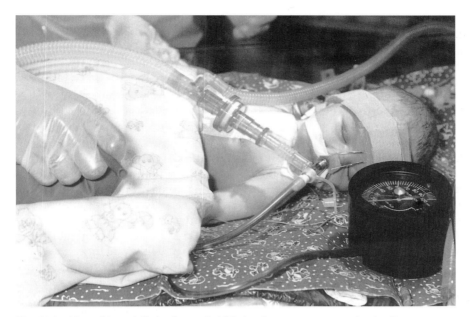

Fig. 13.3 Manual hyperinflation in small child showing pressure gauge in circuit.

ever possible. Self-inflating bags may be used in some units. The flow rate of gas is adjusted according to the size of the child: 4 l/min for infants increasing to 8 l/min for children. In situations where pulmonary blood flow is very high it is usually not advisable to use an FiO_2 of 1.0 during manual hyperinflation as this may further increase blood flow to the lungs.

Manual hyperinflation should only be carried out in children by staff experienced in its use.

Precautions of manual hyperinflation in children

• The lack of collateral ventilation means that air may not diffuse from inflated to collapsed alveoli, as air under positive pressure takes the path of least resistance. Manual hyperinflation may therefore over-distend areas already inflated but leave other areas collapsed. This increases the risk of pneumothorax and particular care should be taken in conditions causing hyperinflation, e.g. asthma and bronchiolitis.

• Manual hyperinflation should not be used as a physiotherapy technique in preterm infants whose delicate lung tissue is easily damaged by high inflation pressures.

Breathing exercises

Laughing and crying are very effective means of lung expansion in infants. It is possible to encourage children to deep breathe from about 2 years of age by using bubbles, paper windmills, etc., although whether these 'deep breaths' are effective is debatable. Incentive spirometers may be useful pre- and postoperatively (when early mobilization is not possible) or when teaching inhaler technique. Huffing can also be introduced at this age.

Older children can be taught the active cycle of breathing techniques. Since children use the diaphragm as the main inspiratory muscle, they find breathing control very easy. Encouraging them to 'fill up their tummy with air, like a balloon' works well, provided they are reminded not to use their abdominal muscles.

Coughing

Children from about 18 months of age can often mimic coughing if asked to do so, but it is often very difficult to persuade an acutely ill child to cough and expectorate.

Positioning or movement may cause mobilization of secretions which may stimulate a cough reflex. Secretions produced will be swallowed as the ability to expectorate does not often develop before 3–4 years of age. In children of less than 18 months of age, tracheal compression can be used to stimulate a cough. Gentle pressure with a sideways motion is briefly applied with a finger to the trachea below the thyroid cartilage. This causes apposition of the tracheal walls, which are soft and pliant in this age group, stimulating the cough reflex. This technique must be used with care and only in experienced hands as the infant can become bradycardic. If there is no effective cough and there are copious secretions, airway suction may be necessary.

Airway suction

This topic is also discussed in Chapters 8 and 11; however, particular points to note when performing airway suction in infants and young children are as follows:

- Preoxygenation is usually important to reduce hypoxia, but care should be taken in preterm infants to avoid hyperoxia. The inspired oxygen should therefore only be increased by about 10% in these infants. Hyperoxia, even for a short time, may lead to retinopathy of prematurity (Roberton 1996).
- Infants are at particular risk of infection, so great care must be taken with hand washing and wearing gloves, etc.
- The vacuum pressure should not be excessive but will need to be strong enough to draw secretions up very narrow bore catheters. Recommended values are 10–20 kPa (75–150 mmHg).
- Most commonly used catheters are 6 and 8 French gauge (FG). Size 5 FG and below are usually ineffective in removing thick secretions. Size 10 FG and above should be reserved for use with older children. When suctioning artificial airways the external diameter of the catheter should not exceed 50% of the internal diameter of the airway.

- Diluents and mucolytics, e.g. saline in aliquots of 0.5 ml (preterm infant) to 5 ml may be used to enhance secretion clearance. The efficacy of these is not conclusively proven (Ackerman 1985) and they should never be used routinely. Larger quantities of irrigants are sometimes used as part of bronchoalveolar lavage procedures but this should only be undertaken by experienced personnel and with great caution.
- Pneumothorax due to direct perforation of a segmental bronchus by a suction catheter has been reported in intubated preterm infants (Vaughan et al 1978). In this group of patients suction catheters should not be passed further than 1 cm below the tip of the endotracheal tube. Graduated catheters with centimetre markings are available or a measured catheter can be attached to the incubator so that staff can gauge how far to pass the catheter.
- The non-intubated child requiring nasopharyngeal suction should be wrapped in a blanket or held firmly by an assistant to avoid unnecessary struggling. The child should be positioned in side lying to avoid aspiration of gastric contents (Fig. 13.4). Constant reassurance should be given throughout the procedure. Supplemental oxygenation and resuscitation equipment should be available.
- Particular care should be taken with nasopharyngeal suction of neonates as reflex bradycardia and apnoea can occur.
- Nasopharyngeal suction should be avoided if the child has stridor or has recently been extubated as it may precipitate laryngospasm.

Passive movements

Passive movements and two-joint muscle stretches should be given regularly to older children in intensive care, although they are at less risk of developing joint stiffness than adults. Care should be taken when handling children and infants who are hypotonic in order to avoid soft tissue damage. Preterm infants are hypotonic and require minimal handling, so passive movements are not usually indicated.

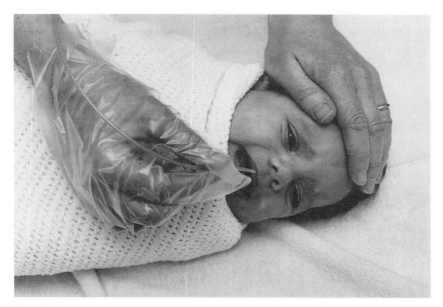

Fig. 13.4 Nasopharyngeal suction.

MANAGEMENT OF THE ACUTELY ILL INFANT OR CHILD

Respiratory failure in acutely ill infants and children may result from many different medical problems. In the neonate the most common causes are prematurity, respiratory distress syndrome, asphyxia and aspiration pneumonia. Under 2 years of age bronchopneumonia, bronchiolitis, status asthmaticus, croup, foreign body inhalation and congenital heart anomalies are more common aetiologies. In children over 2 years asthma, central nervous system infection (e.g. meningitis) and trauma are more frequent.

Equipment used in neonatal and paediatric intensive care

Physiotherapists working in an intensive care unit should be familiar with equipment used on that unit (Fig. 13.5). They should be able to respond when a problem is indicated by the equipment and be able to ascertain whether the problem is with the patient or the machine.

Incubators and radiant warmers

Infants may have difficulty maintaining their temperature, especially if they were born preterm. They are therefore nursed in incubators or under radiant warmers.

Incubators are enclosed units of transparent material with portholes in the sides for access. They can be warmed, and humidified air or oxygen can be delivered to the infant inside. The temperature inside an incubator is maintained in the thermoneutral range which is the environmental temperature at which oxygen consumption is minimal in the presence of a normal body temperature. This will vary according to the patient's gestation and weight.

A radiant warmer is an open-topped unit with a radiant heating device above it. It allows free access to the infant, but there is more convective heat loss and insensible fluid loss than with an incubator.

Phototherapy unit

These units consist of white or blue lamps which emit light of wavelength 400–500 nm. Light

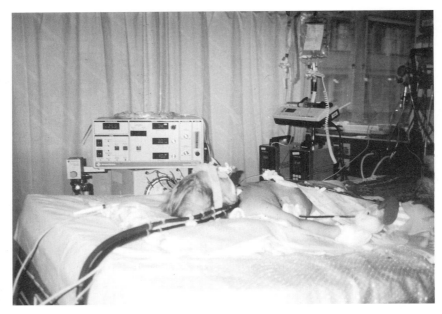

Fig. 13.5 Equipment used in a paediatric intensive care unit. Figure shows an infant undergoing extracorporeal membrane oxygenation and high-frequency oscillatory ventilation.

of these wavelengths oxidizes unconjugated bilirubin into harmless derivatives and so is very important in the treatment of jaundice in neonates. Infants receiving phototherapy have to be nursed naked, which can cause problems of temperature control. There is also increased insensible fluid loss and a theoretical risk of eye damage, so eye shields should be worn.

Electrocardiogram (ECG), respiratory and blood pressure monitors

These are similar to the monitors used on adults, although normal values vary according to age (Table 13.1).

Pulse oximetry

Pulse oximetry is a tool which non-invasively measures arterial oxyhaemoglobin (Ch. 4), giving a percentage value for oxygen saturation (SaO_2). The relative inaccuracy of these machines (i.e. their unreliability in reflecting arterial oxygena-

tion) means that they cannot be used as the only method of monitoring oxygen in the critically ill infant. They are, however, useful in terms of monitoring trends of change in arterial oxygenation in acutely ill infants and children.

Transcutaneous oxygen monitors

Most neonatal units use transcutaneous oxygen monitors to give an indication of oxygenation. These monitors provide a non-invasive means of measuring the partial pressure of oxygen (PaO_2) in arterialized capillaries through the skin. Transcutaneous oxygen (TcO_2) monitors have electrodes which are heated and placed on an area of thin skin, e.g. the abdomen. The heating produces a superficial erythema so that the PaO_2 in the dilated capillaries can be assessed by the machine and displayed on a visual monitor. Normal values are 8–12 kPa (60–90 mmHg). Accuracy is checked by regularly comparing with arterial blood gases. Electrodes need to be moved to a different position every 4 hours in order to prevent burning. In order to remain accurate the electrodes need careful positioning and calibration.

Carbon dioxide monitoring

When necessary it is possible to monitor CO_2 levels either transcutaneously or using end-tidal monitoring.

Respiratory support

Oxygen therapy

Supplemental oxygen therapy for the treatment of hypoxia may be administered by several means and is discussed in detail in Chapter 8. However, there are important points to consider when administering oxygen therapy to infants and children.

Oxygen can be delivered directly into an incubator via an inlet but it should be noted that such delivery can rarely exceed an FiO_2 of 0.4. Head box oxygen delivery via a clear plastic box placed over an infant's head (Fig. 13.6) is a very effective means of delivering supplemental oxygen, and FiO_2 levels of up to 0.95 can be effectively achieved. If used with small infants the humidification of inspired gas should be warmed. Other means include the use of a naso-pharyngeal catheter inserted 4–6 cm or paediatric nasal cannulae which can achieve an FiO_2 of 0.5 with a flow of 6 l/min. Older children are much more able to tolerate a face mask or nasal cannulae.

Humidification

Humidification of inspired gases is essential for infants and children as narrow bore endo-tracheal tubes (ETT) and small calibre airways can easily be blocked by thick secretions. Children requiring ventilation usually have a heated humidifier as part of the ventilator circuit. The amount of humidity received by the child is dependent upon the temperature of the humidifier, ambient room and/or incubator temperature, gas flow rate, level of water in the humidifier chamber, the length of ventilator tubing and the position of the temperature probe in the ventilator circuit (Tarnow-Mordi et al 1989). The optimum temperature of the inspired gas is unknown but temperatures greater than 36.5°C have been shown to reduce the incidence

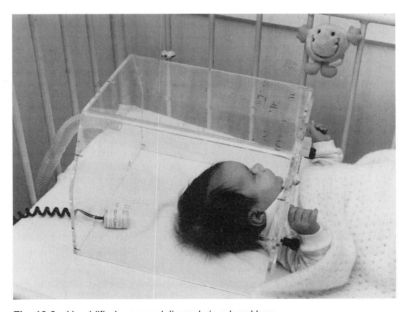

Fig. 13.6 Humidified oxygen delivered via a head box.

of chronic lung disease in infants weighing less than 1500 g (Tarnow-Mordi et al 1989).

Nitric oxide

Nitric oxide (NO) is a gas at room temperature which can be used to reduce pulmonary arterial pressures but has no effect on systemic pressure. It is delivered directly to the lungs during artificial ventilation and can be effectively used to treat pulmonary hypertension in infants and children (Zapol et al 1994).

Continuous positive airway pressure (CPAP)

CPAP (Chs 5 and 6) may be used as a first-line treatment in infants and children requiring respiratory support, or as part of the process of weaning from full ventilation. CPAP may be applied via an endotracheal tube, or in non-intubated infants, via a face mask or nasal prong.

Endotracheal intubation

Indications for endotracheal intubation are: (a) maintenance of a patient's airway; (b) protection of the airway in states of altered consciousness; (c) facilitation of pulmonary toilet; and (d) for mechanical ventilation due to inadequate spontaneous ventilation.

Tubes may be nasal (Fig. 13.7a) or oral (Fig. 13.7b) and in children below 8 years of age should be uncuffed to reduce the risk of damage to the tracheal mucosa and subsequent stenosis. It is important that a small air leak exists between the tracheal tissue and ETT to prevent mucosal damage; however, this does mean that the potential for aspiration is greater.

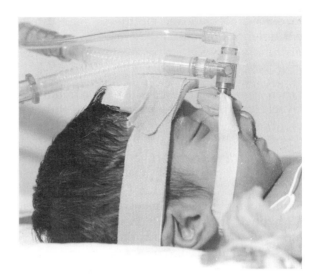
a

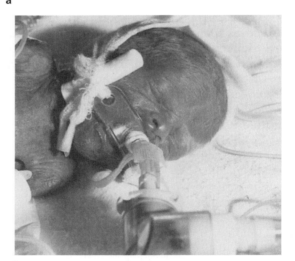
b

Fig. 13.7 **a** Nasal intubation. **b** Oral intubation of a preterm infant.

Conventional mechanical ventilation

A variety of mechanical ventilators are used in neonatal and paediatric practice. Pressure-limited ventilators avoid excessive inflating pressures and reduce the risk of barotrauma. There is a continuous flow of gas around the circuit which allows the infant to breathe spontaneously between ventilator breaths. However, if lung compliance decreases acutely (e.g. secretion accumulation), the tidal volume delivered will fall. This may go unnoticed as the ventilator continues to cycle at the preset pressure, and close monitoring is therefore essential. Time cycling allows the ratio of the inspiration to expiration to be controlled.

Volume-cycled (pressure-limited) ventilators deliver a preset tidal volume and are effective in situations where airway compliance is low and resistance is high. However, this can result in the delivery of excessively high inflation pressures which increase the risk of intrathoracic air leak and barotrauma.

The use of PEEP is standard when mechanically ventilating infants and children to prevent airway closure at end expiration as closing volume is much closer to FRC. Patient-triggered ventilation has been shown to be useful as an aid to weaning from conventional ventilation and in some mature infants during the acute stage of respiratory distress syndrome (RDS) (Greenough & Pool 1988). It is not as useful in the very preterm low birth weight infant whose respiratory efforts are often inadequate and inconsistent. Modified neonatal ventilators that respond quickly to small changes in airflow are needed in these infants.

In the newborn, ventilation is often started from birth in infants of birth weight less than 1000 g but otherwise the indications are:

- Deteriorating blood gases indicating respiratory failure, i.e. PaO_2 less than 8 kPa (60 mmHg) with an FiO_2 of 60% and/or $PaCO_2$ greater than 8 kPa (60 mmHg)
- Recurrent or major apnoea
- Major surgery pre- and/or postoperatively, e.g. cardiac lesions, diaphragmatic hernia.

Preterm low birth weight infants have been shown to be better oxygenated with fast rates of ventilation (60–150 breaths/min) using time-cycled, pressure-limited devices (Greenough et al 1987). This seems to allow the infant to synchronize with the ventilator and thus reduce the occurrence of pneumothoraces. If synchrony cannot be achieved it is necessary to use paralysing agents when ventilating these infants (Greenough et al 1984).

Weaning from ventilation in infants and small children is achieved by initial reduction of the inspiratory pressures and the inspired oxygen concentration. Intermittent mandatory ventilation (IMV) can then be used, followed by CPAP. Extubation is usually performed from CPAP via the ETT, but some infants require a period of support on CPAP via a nasopharyngeal airway (nasal prong) prior to unsupported spontaneous breathing. The weaning process in older children is similar to that in adults.

Negative extrathoracic pressure ventilation

Negative extrathoracic pressure ventilation (NEPV) was first used in the treatment of children with respiratory failure due to poliomyelitis. It has now been adapted for use in the management of respiratory failure due to a variety of causes (Samuels & Southall 1989), though its use is at present not widespread.

The equipment consists of a transparent Perspex box in which the infant's body is placed with the head remaining outside. An airtight seal around the neck is essential. There are portholes for access for nursing care and physiotherapy. A negative pressure is applied to the box so that the pressure inside becomes subatmospheric and assists with ventilation. It can also be applied via a rigid thoracic jacket (e.g. Hayek jacket or cuirass shell). The indications for the use of NEPV are:

- Respiratory failure due to myopathy or other neuromuscular disorder
- Congenital central hypoventilation (Ondine's curse)
- Bilateral phrenic nerve damage
- Weaning from positive pressure ventilation (e.g. in RDS or following cardiac surgery)
- Prevention of further lung damage due to positive pressure ventilation in infants with severe chronic lung disease.

High-frequency ventilation

High-frequency ventilation (using either jet, HFJV, or oscillatory ventilation, HFO) employs small tidal volumes (less than anatomical dead space) and high respiratory rates (60–3000/min) to achieve adequate ventilation. High-velocity ventilations result in increased mixing, gas diffusion and exchange. In theory ventilation is more evenly distributed while the airway pressures used are lower. High-frequency oscillation has been shown to be safe and effective in the treatment of respiratory failure in paediatric practice (Arnold et al 1993). The response to HFO in terms of improvement of oxygenation is also helpful in predicting outcome in children with potentially reversible lung disease and severe acute respiratory failure (Sarnaik et al 1996).

Extracorporeal membrane oxygenation

Extracorporeal membrane oxygenation (ECMO) is a technique which oxygenates blood outside the body and if necessary can also provide cardiovascular support (Ch. 5) for a limited period of time during which the underlying pulmonary disorder is expected to recover. It has been reported to be beneficial in some children with acute lung injury (Pearson et al 1993) and more recently a collaborative randomized trial of neonatal ECMO reported it to be clinically effective and a therapy which should be considered for neonates with severe but potentially reversible respiratory failure (UK Collaborative ECMO Trial Group 1996).

Liquid ventilation

It has been suggested that the use of liquid ventilation can improve ventilation–perfusion mismatch by promoting a more even distribution of pulmonary blood flow and improvement of compliance through the elimination of the gas–liquid interface. It may also be less damaging to the lungs when compared to gas ventilation. Ventilation using liquid perfluorocarbons has been reported as successful in infants and children with severe respiratory failure (Greenough 1996a).

Complications of ventilatory support

Pneumothorax

Pneumothoraces are a complication of positive pressure ventilation occurring mainly in preterm infants with immature lungs or in association with congenital bullae. A predisposing factor is the hyperinflation of alveoli occurring in conditions such as meconium aspiration and respiratory distress syndrome (RDS). They are also a complication seen in older children whose lung compliance is very poor and who require high inflation pressures.

Causative factors are high peak inspiratory pressures, positive end-expiratory pressure, long inflation times, and active expiration by the infant against the ventilator's inspiration (Greenough et al 1983). A tension pneumothorax will cause a sudden deterioration and should be drained as soon as possible with a chest drain and suction. Small pneumothoraces may not require drainage but the infant will need close monitoring.

Pulmonary interstitial emphysema

Pulmonary interstitial emphysema (PIE) occurs when gas leaks out of an alveolus, tracks along the cardiovascular bundle and remains trapped forming interstitial gas pockets. PIE is most common in preterm infants; the incidence is inversely proportional to gestational age.

Treatment is fast-rate, low-pressure ventilation with a longer expiratory than inspiratory time to prevent an increase in air trapping. In severe cases, where ventilation is becoming difficult, needle scarification of the lung surface may be helpful. Unresolved PIE may require surgical resection in severe cases.

Subglottic stenosis

Subglottic stenosis occurs in some infants following prolonged intubation and leads to upper airway obstruction. It should be avoidable by attention to tracheal tube placement and fixation, and care with suction (Albert 1995). Acquired neonatal tracheobronchial stenosis (particularly in preterm infants) has a poor outcome. Stridor is often present and may respond to adrenaline via a nebulizer. In more severe cases a tracheostomy may be necessary until the airway has increased sufficiently in size to allow adequate ventilation. Some patients will also require surgical laryngotracheoplasty before successful decannulation of the tracheostomy can be achieved. More recently, primary repair of subglottic stenosis with laryngotracheal reconstruction has been performed and can be effective.

Retinopathy of prematurity

This condition of preterm infants is seen when the delicate capillaries in the retina proliferate leading to haemorrhage, fibrosis and scarring. In the most severe form, this may result in permanent visual impairment. The cause is unknown but periods of hyperoxia (exact length of time unknown) with a PaO_2 of above 12 kPa are thought to be a major predisposing factor (Roberton 1996). Careful oxygen monitoring preferably using an arterial catheter is essential to attempt to prevent this condition. The damaged retina is treated with cryotherapy.

Chronic lung disease

Chronic lung disease (CLD) is defined as a requirement for ventilatory support at 1 month of age. Infants with the severest form who have specific radiographic changes are said to have bronchopulmonary dysplasia (BPD). The incidence of CLD varies between 4% and 40% according to the initial respiratory illness, birth weight and gestational age at delivery (Greenough 1996c). It is more common in preterm infants who have had acute RDS requiring oxygen and ventilatory support. High peak pressures in positive pressure ventilation cause barotrauma, and high inspired oxygen concentrations cause an acute inflammatory response leading to local tissue damage. Other precipitating factors are fluid overload, persistent ductus arteriosus (PDA), PIE and infection.

The infant with CLD shows an increased oxygen requirement and carbon dioxide retention and has decreased lung compliance with increased airway resistance. The infant is tachypnoeic with persistent sternal and costal recession. The condition may be progressive, requiring more ventilatory support and eventually leading to respiratory and cardiac failure.

Radiographic appearances can vary but include alternating areas of collapse and hyperinflation, widespread fibrosis, and scarring of the lung with compensatory emphysema.

Treatment consists of appropriate respiratory support which may be IMV, CPAP, HFO, NEPV or added oxygen via a head box or nasal cannulae. Good nutrition is essential and the infant may require fluid restriction and diuretics. Some infants respond to bronchodilators and steroids. Antibiotics may be required as these infants are prone to recurrent chest infections.

The prognosis is variable. Mortality may be as high as 40% in severe cases. Those who survive are often small and underweight, have recurrent upper and lower respiratory tract infections, wheezing and gastric reflux (Greenough 1996c). Some children may require oxygen for several years and are therefore managed at home if the family is able to cope with home oxygen therapy. The long-term prognosis for those who survive the first 2 years is good.

Physiotherapy. As infants with CLD are particularly prone to chest infections, physiotherapy may be indicated if excess secretions are a problem. These infants often have severe wheeze and airway collapse and physiotherapy techniques may not be appropriate. Careful assessment is important before any intervention. If wheezing is not too severe, careful treatment may be possible following bronchodilator therapy, providing the infant has a good response (O'Callaghan et al 1986, 1989). Modified gravity-assisted positions with chest percussion may be useful, and suction may be required. Infants having oxygen through nasal cannulae often have a problem with thick, dry nasal secretions. It is not possible to humidify oxygen effectively when using nasal cannulae as the water condenses in the small-bore tubing and cuts off the oxygen supply. Humidifiers which bubble oxygen through cold water counteract the absolute dryness of the oxygen to some extent but are not effective in loosening thick secretions. If necessary, the infant should have nasal cannulae while awake during the day to allow social interaction, but should have humidified oxygen via a head box for long periods of sleep. Normal saline via a nebulizer or saline nose drops can also be used but have a limited effect.

NEONATAL INTENSIVE CARE

Physiotherapists who may be called upon to treat

infants in a neonatal intensive care unit (NICU) should be fully aware of the problems these infants may have. Reasons for admission to a NICU include:

- Preterm delivery
- Low birth weight
- Perinatal problems
- Congenital abnormalities.

Preterm delivery

Preterm is defined as less than 37 completed weeks of gestation (full term is 38–42 weeks). In reality those preterm infants who may require admission to a NICU are likely to be less than 32 weeks of gestation and weigh less than 2500 g. Some infants are born after only 23 weeks of pregnancy and may weigh as little as 450 g. Causes of preterm birth may be antepartum haemorrhage, cervical incompetence, multiple pregnancies, or infection. There is also an association with deprived socioeconomic circumstances, and in some cases the cause of preterm delivery is unknown.

Low birth weight

Infants who are born preterm will have a low birth weight, but more mature infants may be of low birth weight due to intrauterine growth retardation. Causes include placental dysfunction, smoking, and intrauterine infection, e.g. rubella.

Perinatal problems

Problems occurring at or around the time of birth, e.g. birth asphyxia or meconium aspiration, may lead to an infant being admitted to the NICU.

Congenital abnormalities

Congenital abnormalities include congenital heart disease and diaphragmatic hernia and are discussed in the surgical section of this chapter (p. 350).

General problems of infants in the NICU

Parent–infant bonding

It is accepted modern practice for the newborn to remain with the mother and father, if present, after delivery. Infants who have been resuscitated and transferred to a NICU shortly after birth will not have had the chance for physical contact with their parents. Bonding is further hindered by the barrier of incubators and other equipment surrounding the infant.

Parents should be encouraged to give comfort to their infant by stroking etc., and to cuddle him when his condition is stable enough to do so. When parents are confident, they can be involved in their infant's care, e.g. nappy changing.

Handling

Handling of severely ill infants will cause their condition to deteriorate. For this reason, these infants should be left alone as much as possible. Physiotherapy and suction should only be carried out when there are definite indications, e.g. retention of secretions or lung collapse due to mucus plugging. Careful assessment is essential prior to intervention.

Problems of preterm and low birth weight infants

Respiratory distress

The main cause of respiratory distress in preterm infants is respiratory distress syndrome. The primary cause of this syndrome is lack of surfactant in the immature lung. The more preterm the infant, the higher the incidence of RDS. Steroids should be administered to women in preterm labour in order to enhance lung maturation (Crowley 1995).

RDS develops within 4 hours of delivery with sternal and costal recession, grunting, and tachypnoea. The chest radiograph shows a 'ground glass' appearance due to lung collapse (Fig. 13.8). Many preterm infants, however, are 'electively' intubated and ventilated at birth and thus never develop these classical signs.

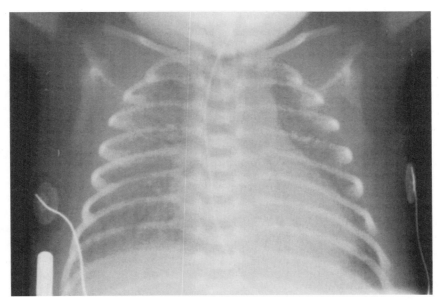

Fig. 13.8 Chest radiograph of respiratory distress syndrome.

Treatment includes giving supplemental oxygen to avoid hypoxia, which hinders surfactant production. These infants should be handled as little as possible. Mildly affected infants may only require humidified oxygen via a head box, but more severely affected infants will require ventilatory support of some kind such as positive pressure ventilation or continuous positive airway pressure.

The natural history of the syndrome is that surfactant will start to be produced in the lung 36–48 hours after birth, regardless of gestational age. The more mature infant will start to recover at this time. Very preterm infants who have other problems compounding their respiratory distress or infants who have developed complications of treatment may require ventilatory support for much longer.

During the last decade there have been many trials investigating the use of surfactant therapy to try to prevent or ameliorate RDS (Morley 1991). Natural or artificial surfactant in fluid form is introduced into the endotracheal tube prophylactically or after signs of RDS have appeared. Although these trials have shown a reduction in mortality in very preterm infants

given surfactant therapy, it is still unclear which is the best type of surfactant to use and how and when it should be given. Further trials are in progress.

As lung collapse in RDS is primarily caused by lack of surfactant, physiotherapy is not required for this condition. Secretions may become a problem after the infant has been intubated for more than 48 hours, owing to irritation of the tracheal mucosa by the endotracheal tube. These secretions may be cleared easily by suction alone. Physiotherapy should be given only when suction is not adequately clearing secretions.

Respiratory distress in the preterm infant can also be caused by pneumonia. Organisms causing pneumonia may be bacterial, viral, or fungal and may be acquired before, during or after birth. The most serious bacterial cause is group B *Streptococcus*. The presenting features of this pneumonia are similar to RDS with an indistinguishable chest radiograph. Group B streptococcal pneumonia can be rapidly fatal unless antibiotic therapy is started early. For this reason all infants presenting with respiratory distress are given antibiotics.

Periventricular haemorrhage and periventricular leukomalacia

Periventricular haemorrhage (PVH) is a major cause of mortality and morbidity in very pre-term and low birth weight infants. The incidence is inversely proportional to birth weight, occur-ring most frequently and severely in the smallest and least mature infant. It may occur sponta-neously, but particularly occurs in infants who have had episodes of hypoxia, hypotension, or apnoea causing surges in cerebral blood flow.

The haemorrhages arise from the fragile capillaries in the floor of the lateral ventricles. Fluctuations of cerebral blood flow are caused by marked changes in blood pressure, arterial oxygen, and carbon dioxide. These fluctuations cause the capillaries to burst and bleed into and around the ventricles.

There are four grades of severity:

- Grade I – bleeding into the floor of the ventricle
- Grade II – bleeding into the ventricle (intraventricular haemorrhage (IVH))
- Grade III – IVH with dilatation of the ventricle
- Grade IV – IVH and bleeding into the cerebral cortex causing areas of ischaemia.

Grades I and II may be asymptomatic and chances of recovery are good. Grades III and IV are likely to cause residual problems such as hydrocephalus or neurological deficit. Severe grade IV haemorrhage may result in the death of the infant.

Prevention of PVH is directed towards mini-mal handling of 'at-risk' infants and avoidance of hypoxic and hypotensive episodes.

Periventricular leukomalacia (PVL) may occur on its own or associated with PVH. Ischaemia of cerebral tissue adjacent to the ventricles causes formation of cystic lesions. There is an association with neurological problems particularly diplegia.

Regular cerebral ultrasound scanning shows the presence of PVH and PVL and their progression.

Temperature control

Preterm and low birth weight infants have difficulty in maintaining their body temperature because they have a large surface area relative to their body mass. They also have a smaller proportion of brown fat in comparison with full-term infants and easily lose heat through the skin by evaporation and radiation.

As hypothermia can cause acidosis, hypo-glycaemia, increased oxygen consumption, and decreased surfactant production, it is essential to maintain body temperature. Infants should therefore be kept in a thermoneutral environ-ment. To maintain a thermoneutral environ-ment, infants are nursed in incubators or under radiant warmers. Heat shields are used to reduce radiant heat loss and the ambient room tem-perature is kept high at 27–28°C. Draughts should be avoided and incubator doors should not be left open as the infant's temperature can drop dramatically. If the infant's temperature is less than 36.5°C physiotherapy should not be given unless essential.

Infection

The preterm infant is particularly vulnerable to infection. The skin is very thin and easily damaged. Cellular and humoral resistance to infection are also reduced.

The most important means of preventing and reducing cross-infection is by scrupulous hand washing by all staff and visitors. Regular use of a disinfectant solution is also necessary. Visitors should be kept to a minimum, for example parents, siblings, and grandparents. Anyone who has an infectious disease should not enter the unit.

Antibiotic therapy is frequently used to try to prevent infections becoming life threatening.

Jaundice

Physiological jaundice is common in the normal full-term infant owing to the breakdown of fetal haemoglobin causing a raised level of un-conjugated bilirubin in the blood. Physiological jaundice starts to appear 2 days after birth and has usually disappeared by days 7–10 of life.

If the level of unconjugated bilirubin is high

it may diffuse into the basal ganglia and lead to a condition called 'kernicterus'. Kernicterus is characterized by athetoid cerebral palsy, deafness, and mental retardation.

Preterm infants are particularly prone to developing jaundice and run an increased risk of subsequent kernicterus. To avoid this risk, daily serum bilirubin levels are taken by heel prick from jaundiced infants and treatment consists of phototherapy, or in severe cases exchange transfusion. In this procedure, blood is withdrawn from the infant in small amounts (5 or 10 ml) and replaced by donor blood until twice the infant's blood volume has been exchanged.

Nutrition

Adequate calorie intake and weight gain are important in preterm and low birth weight infants to avoid hypoglycaemia, persistent jaundice, and delayed recovery from RDS.

Feeding should be started as soon as possible, either enterally, in those who can tolerate it, or intravenously. Preterm infants have poor sucking, gag, and cough reflexes so will be fed nasogastrically until these reflexes develop. Continuous infusion of milk may be given rather than bolus feeds as bolus feeds can increase respiratory distress owing to abdominal distension. Pooling of milk in the stomach can also lead to regurgitation and aspiration. Feeds are often better tolerated when the infant is lying in the prone position. Orogastric tubes may be used rather than nasogastric ones in order to avoid blockage of the nostril in spontaneously breathing infants with respiratory distress.

Pulmonary haemorrhage

In this condition, fresh blood pours out of the lungs and the infant collapses. It is relatively uncommon but may occur after surfactant therapy.

Physiotherapy is contraindicated, although regular suctioning may be required to keep the airway clear. When fresh blood is no longer being aspirated, physiotherapy techniques may be required to aid removal of residual old blood. Prognosis is often poor.

Perinatal problems

Birth asphyxia

This occurs in about 10% of births. Infants who have been severely asphyxiated may require admission to the NICU. Careful monitoring will be required as these infants may develop cardiac failure, neurological damage, or renal failure. Some may have fits and will need to have anticonvulsant therapy. As these infants are often very irritable, handling should be kept to a minimum.

Meconium aspiration

This usually occurs in full-term infants who become hypoxic due to a prolonged and difficult labour. Hypoxia causes the infant to pass meconium into the amniotic fluid and to make gasping movements so that meconium may be drawn into the pharynx.

If the mother's liquor is meconium stained, a paediatrician should suction the infant's airway as soon as the head is delivered to prevent aspiration when the first breath is taken. Once delivered, the infant may require intubation for further suction. The irritant properties of meconium can cause a chemical pneumonitis and predispose to bacterial infection, especially *Escherichia coli*. A severely affected infant may require assisted ventilation, although ventilation is difficult because of the risk of pneumothorax due to gas trapping.

Physiotherapy. Physiotherapy is very important when meconium aspiration has occurred in order to remove the extremely thick and tenacious green secretions. Treatment consists of gravity-assisted positioning, as tolerated, with chest percussion and should be carried out as soon as possible after aspiration has occurred, preferably within 1 hour. Physiotherapy is often well tolerated in these cases as removal of meconium plugs allows the infant to be better ventilated.

SURGERY IN INFANTS AND CHILDREN

The effects of surgery, anaesthesia and immobility are the same in infants and children as in adults. Owing to the anatomical and physiological differences, however, the potential for respiratory complications is greater. Infants and children undergoing major surgery should, therefore, be regularly assessed by a physiotherapist.

Preoperative management

In some hospitals preoperative visits and handbooks are available which help to reduce some of the fear of being in hospital. Except in emergency situations, children and their parents should be seen by a physiotherapist preoperatively. Explanation of postoperative procedures should be given at a level appropriate to the child's understanding. Overloading the child with information which he does not understand only increases preoperative stress and anxiety. It is important that parents are fully aware of the need for postoperative physiotherapy intervention. Parents can play an important role in encouraging postoperative mobility.

Assessment by the physiotherapist should include respiratory function and motor development. Older children who are able to understand and cooperate may be taught the active cycle of breathing techniques. Incentive spirometry can be useful in children, especially those techniques specifically designed for their use, for example the 'Coach' incentive spirometer which has a spaceship which moves upwards on inspiration.

When a child has pre-existing pulmonary disease, for example cystic fibrosis, he may need to be admitted some time before surgery to clear his chest as effectively as possible. Some children may require physiotherapy and suction in the anaesthetic room following intubation and before entering the operating theatre.

Postoperative management

Children and infants should be regularly reviewed and intervention given as required. Effective pain relief is essential for children postoperatively prior to any intervention. It may be difficult to assess the severity of pain, as crying may be due to other causes, for example hunger. Lack of crying does not necessarily indicate lack of pain as children in pain are often totally withdrawn and immobile. Infants in pain may be tachycardic and tachypnoeic. Many children who have a fear of needles will deny pain in order to avoid injections.

Continuous opioid infusion, for example pethidine, is now used regularly in some hospitals following major surgery. It is an effective and continuous means of pain relief and fear of pain is not such a problem. This method of pain control means that the patient requires close monitoring owing to the risk of respiratory depression. The amount of drug delivered per hour to the child is gradually reduced as the pain lessens following surgery.

Treatment is directed towards regular position change; the 'slumped posture' position should be avoided at all times. When in bed, children should be comfortably positioned in alternate side lying or sitting upright. As soon as the condition allows, children should be sat out of bed, preferably on the first postoperative day. Walking should be started as soon as possible and drips, drains and catheters can all be carried to allow early ambulation. Attention to posture is important, particularly following thoracotomy when shoulder exercises to the affected side are also essential. Infants should have regular position changes and should be taken out of bed for a cuddle with parents as soon as the condition allows.

If sputum retention is a problem postoperatively, other techniques such as chest clapping may be required, but there should always be effective pain relief. A child often prefers not to have his wound supported or to support his wound himself. He may like to press a pillow or favourite soft toy to the area. At all times firm but sympathetic and gentle handling is important to avoid undue distress.

Congenital diaphragmatic hernia

In this condition intra-abdominal contents herniate through the diaphragm into the thoracic cavity, most commonly stomach or small bowel on the left side. The incidence is approximately 1 in 3000 births (Morin et al 1994). The abnormality may be diagnosed antenatally by ultrasound, or postnatally when the infant presents with respiratory distress (usually soon after birth). A chest radiograph will show abdominal viscera in the thoracic cavity. Unless the herniation has occurred late in pregnancy, which is very unusual, there will be associated pulmonary hypoplasia on the affected side as the abdominal viscera occupy the space normally available for the growing lung. The contralateral lung is also smaller than expected because of compression due to mediastinal shift during pregnancy.

The infant with diaphragmatic hernia is often very unwell, particularly as the bowel in the chest distends with air and further compresses the lungs, and requires immediate gastric decompression with simultaneous intubation and ventilation. Surgery is not carried out until the infant's condition is fully stabilized. Surgical correction is via a laparotomy. The abdominal viscera are carefully returned to the abdominal cavity and the defect in the diaphragm is closed.

Postoperatively, the infant may require ventilation for some time, depending on the amount of pulmonary hypoplasia. Prognosis is variable, and mortality for isolated hernias is about 45% (Wenstrom et al 1991).

Physiotherapy. Physiotherapy may be indicated postoperatively if retention of secretions is a problem. Manual hyperinflation is contraindicated because the lungs are hypoplastic and high inflation pressures should be avoided.

Other congenital anomalies of the lung

Congenital conditions of the lung such as lobar emphysema, lung cysts, and adenomata are very rare. They may be diagnosed by ultrasound antenatally, or by chest radiography postnatally. Treatment may involve surgical resection (lobectomy) if the condition is severe; however, in some cases the lesions appear to resolve spontaneously in infancy.

Acquired lobar emphysema and lung cysts are more common as complications of respiratory distress syndrome and its treatment. Most of these cases will resolve with medical therapy though some do require resection.

Physiotherapy. Physiotherapy may be indicated postoperatively if there is sputum retention, but manual hyperinflation is contraindicated if cysts are present.

Oesophageal atresia and tracheo-oesophageal fistula

There are five recognized types of this anomaly. In the most common variety the oesophagus ends in a blind proximal pouch and there is a fistula between the trachea and the lower section of the oesophagus. The incidence is approximately 1 in 3500 births (Depaepe et al 1993).

The infant presents soon after birth with respiratory distress due to an inability to swallow saliva with consequent overflow and aspiration. The first feed typically causes choking and coughing. The diagnosis is suspected by failure to successfully pass a nasogastric tube, which on chest radiograph appears curled in the upper oesophagus.

Surgical correction is usually attempted as soon as possible. Preoperatively the airway should be kept clear by continuous suction of the upper pouch, and the infant should be nursed head up to prevent reflux of gastric contents through the fistula.

In most cases surgical treatment consists of primary anastomosis of the oesophagus and closure of the tracheo-oesophageal fistula. Some anastomoses may have to be performed under tension and the infant has to be electively ventilated and paralysed with the neck kept in flexion postoperatively. In a few cases, where the gap between the two ends of the oesophagus is too large, primary anastomosis is not possible, and a feeding gastrostomy is performed. Oesophageal anastomosis or replacement by colonic, jejunal, or gastric interposition is delayed until a later date.

Physiotherapy. Preoperatively some patients may require physiotherapy if there are increased secretions or lung collapse due to reflux of gastric contents. Treatment must be carried out in the head-up position. Postoperatively the patient will be nursed in the head-up position for the first few days. Physiotherapy may be indicated but the head-down position should not be used because of the risk of reflux. Care must be taken not to extend the neck, especially in those patients whose anastomosis has been performed under tension. Naso- or oropharyngeal suction is usually limited to avoid passing the catheter into the oesophagus and damaging the anastomosis.

Gastroschisis and exomphalos (omphalocele)

These conditions are due to a defect in the abdominal wall and occur in approximately 1 in 4–6000 births (Lindham 1981, Baird & MacDonald 1982). The small and large bowel and sometimes the liver herniate through the anterior abdominal wall (gastroschisis). In exomphalos a membranous sac encloses the hernial contents. The defect is usually diagnosed antenatally by ultrasound.

Immediately after birth, the abdominal contents are covered to prevent heat and fluid loss until corrective surgery can be undertaken. In most cases primary repair is possible but where the defect is large a staged procedure is required.

Postoperatively the infant may require ventilation as the tightly packed, rigid abdomen causes respiratory embarrassment and compromises venous return. Where a staged procedure is necessary prolonged ventilation may be required.

Physiotherapy. These infants are particularly at risk from retention of secretions and lobar collapse due to the distended abdomen and lack of position changes. If treatment is required, techniques which increase intrathoracic pressure and consequently increase intra-abdominal pressure, such as vibrations, should be used cautiously, and manual hyperinflation is contra-indicated.

Congenital heart disease and cardiac surgery

Congenital heart disease is the most common congenital anomaly with an incidence of 8 per 1000 live births (Hoffman & Christianson 1978); however, only about one-third of these will require surgical intervention. The remaining cases will either resolve spontaneously or be haemodynamically insignificant and cause no problems. Major congenital cardiac defects can be detected antenatally by ultrasound examination in experienced hands. More minor defects may not be detected until the postnatal period. Diagnosis is usually confirmed by echocardiography. Postnatally these conditions are amenable to surgery and overall mortality has fallen to less than 5% in the best units (Elliott & Hussey 1995). Current preference is to perform an early complete repair whenever possible with the majority of operations being performed in the first year of life. The normal anatomy of the heart is shown in Figure 13.9.

On confirmation of the diagnosis it is vital that the family are well informed and a man-

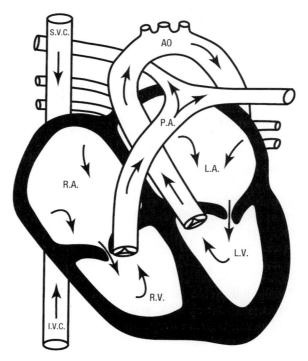

Fig. 13.9 Anatomy of the normal heart: AO, aorta; PA, pulmonary artery; SVC, superior vena cava; IVC, inferior vena cava; RA, right atrium; LA, left atrium; RV, right ventricle; LV, left ventricle.

agement plan made with the agreement of the cardiologist, surgeon and family. Each aspect of the child's care is an integrated process requiring the skills of a multidisciplinary team.

Palliative procedures

When a primary repair is not possible, palliative or staging procedures are indicated to deal with the problems of (a) excessive pulmonary blood flow, (b) inadequate pulmonary blood flow, or (c) inadequate mixing.

In circumstances where there is excessive pulmonary blood flow (such as large ventricular septal defects) the child may present with poor feeding, heart failure, tachypnoea and, if uncorrected, the defect results in pulmonary hypertension. If a corrective procedure is not possible pulmonary blood flow is restricted by banding the pulmonary artery (PA) via left thoracotomy. However, nowadays this procedure is rarely undertaken and is performed only in those at high risk or in preparation for right heart bypass surgery.

If pulmonary blood flow is inadequate the systemic circulation is insufficiently oxygenated, resulting in central cyanosis (e.g. tetralogy of Fallot, pulmonary or tricuspid atresia). If primary repair is not possible, the creation of a shunt between the systemic and pulmonary circulations results in an increase in blood flow and thereby significantly improves oxygen saturation. Most commonly a modified Blalock–Taussig shunt is performed which involves a thoracotomy and creation of a polytetra-fluoroethylene conduit between the subclavian and pulmonary arteries. The shunt is usually ligated at the time of definitive repair.

In defects such as transposition of the great arteries where there is inadequate mixing of oxygenated and deoxygenated blood within the heart, the foramen ovale may be enlarged using either a balloon atrial septostomy in neonates or surgically in older children via a Blalock–Hanlon septectomy.

Corrective surgery: closed procedures

Patent ductus arteriosus. The ductus arteriosus connects the main pulmonary trunk to the aorta, usually at a point distal to the origin of the left subclavian artery. It normally closes soon after birth but it may be artificially maintained by prostaglandin. If it persists pathologically the resulting left-to-right shunt can be associated with the development of pulmonary hypertension and pulmonary vascular disease. It may be possible to induce closure of the duct in preterm infants with indomethacin. Surgical correction involves left thoracotomy and ligation using silk ligature or a liga clip. In older infants closure may be achieved via cardiac catheterization using a double umbrella device.

Coarctation of the aorta. This is a congenital narrowing of the aorta. It usually occurs proximal to the junction of the ductus arteriosus and distal to the left subclavian artery origin. Neonatal presentation with symptoms of congestive heart failure requires early surgical repair. This is usually performed by resection of the stenosis and end-to-end anastomosis. If the aortic arch is hypoplastic a more extensive procedure, aortic arch angioplasty, is necessary. Repair of simple coarctation carries almost zero mortality; however, for severe forms of coarctation such as interrupted aortic arch (where upper and lower aortic arches are separated) the mortality rate is higher. Paraplegia is an extremely rare complication specific to correction of this defect (Brewer et al 1972) and may be associated with longer cross-clamping times.

Vascular ring. This defect is caused when abnormally routed mediastinal vessels (examples include double aortic arch, abnormally positioned innominate artery or abnormal course of the left pulmonary artery crossing behind the trachea) compress the trachea and oesophagus. Surgical treatment depends on the exact anatomy of the defect.

Corrective surgery: open procedures

Open procedures require cardiopulmonary bypass and use of this technique in children requires modification in terms of size, flow rate, perfusion, temperature and drugs (Elliott & Hussey 1995).

Atrial septal defect (ASD). This is one of the most common cardiac anomalies, characterized by a hole in the atrial septum. There are several types of ASD including those now known as partial ASD occurring within the ostium primum, ostium secundum defects due to failure of fusion of the two atrial septa, and patency of the foramen ovale. The defect is often detected at routine examination with discovery of a murmur. The natural course would be a slow development of symptoms as pulmonary artery pressure rises. Repair is undertaken via median sternotomy and is usually closed by direct suture. Recent developments have enabled repair of this defect to be undertaken via cardiac catheterization.

Ventricular septal defect (VSD). Ventricular septal defects (Fig. 13.10) are defined according to their position in either the perimembranous inlet, the trabecular portion or the muscular

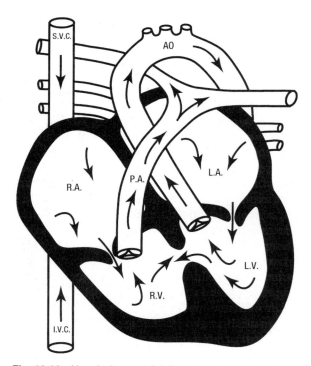

Fig. 13.10 Ventricular septal defect, showing mixing of blood between the left and right ventricle: AO, aorta; PA, pulmonary artery; SVC, superior vena cava; IVC, inferior vena cava; RA, right atrium; LA, left atrium; RV, right ventricle; LV, left ventricle.

outlet of the ventricular septum. This defect may be found in conjunction with other cardiac anomalies. Over 60% of VSDs close spontaneously (Elliott & Hussey 1995), but the larger ones require surgical intervention. The current preference is to perform a primary repair on presentation, though surgery can be undertaken at any age. All defects are repaired using Dacron, Gore-Tex or bovine pericardium patches via median sternotomy with care taken to avoid the Bundle of Hiss. Results for VSD repair are excellent, for isolated defects mortality approaches zero, but for multiple VSDs ('Swiss cheese defect') it is higher (8%) (de Leval 1994).

Atrioventricular septal defect (AVSD). Incomplete development of the inferior atrial septum, superior ventricular septum and atrioventricular valves result in a spectrum of anomalies termed atrioventricular septal defects. They may be associated with other cardiac defects (transposition of the great arteries, tetralogy of Fallot) and are also strongly associated with chromosomal abnormalities such as Down syndrome. High left-to-right shunting causes dyspnoea, recurrent chest infection and congestive cardiac failure. Partial AVSDs, where there is an intra-atrial communication, are managed by complete open repair using a patch method. Complete defects where there is a VSD in the inflow portion of the septum are managed using either a single or two patch technique where one patch is used to close the VSD and another for the atrial component. The recent trend is early complete repair and long-term survival is excellent for this anomaly.

Tetralogy of Fallot. In this anomaly four components are characteristic. These are a large VSD, right ventricular outflow obstruction, right ventricular hypertrophy and an overriding aorta (Fig. 13.11). The resulting inadequate flow to the pulmonary circulation and preferential flow of deoxygenated blood to the aorta leads to central cyanosis. Periodic spasm of the infundibulum leads to the rather alarming 'spelling' episodes; infants become irritable and continued crying leads to increasing cyanosis and eventual loss of consciousness. The spasm then relaxes and the child recovers slowly. In the older child adopting

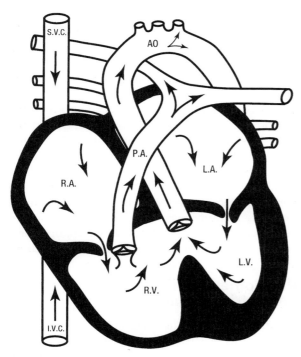

Fig. 13.11 Tetralogy of Fallot, showing VSD, right ventricular hypertrophy, aorta overriding both ventricles and stenosis of the pulmonary artery: AO, aorta; PA, pulmonary artery; SVC, superior vena cava; IVC, inferior vena cava; RA, right atrium; LA, left atrium; RV, right ventricle; LV, left ventricle.

the squatting position following exercise reduces blood flow to and from the lower extremities in an effort to compensate for the large oxygen debt accrued during physical activity.

Two approaches exist with regard to repair of Fallot's tetralogy. The more conservative approach involves an initial palliative shunt and complete repair at a later age, but many would advocate complete repair at any age. Long-term results are good with actuarial survival of 93% at 15 years and good quality of life (Castenda 1994).

Pulmonary atresia. This defect can occur with or without a VSD. In the presence of a VSD the anatomy differs little from that seen in tetralogy of Fallot except that the subpulmonary outflow tract is often hypoplastic or even absent and the pulmonary valve atretic. A staged approach to surgery is necessary to eventually link up all the lung segments with a vascular supply originating from the right ventricle. With an intact septum the right ventricle may be hypoplastic and repair is dependent on its salvability.

Transposition of the great arteries (TGA). The aorta originates from the right ventricle and the pulmonary artery from the left (Fig. 13.12). Babies therefore present soon after birth with severe cyanosis unless an additional defect (VSD, ASD or PDA) is present to allow adequate mixing of blood between the two circulations. The initial goal is to maintain this communication by using prostaglandin to keep the ductus arteriosus patent; this can be followed by a balloon atrial septostomy if necessary.

The arterial switch procedure is the management of choice for simple TGA or for TGA with VSD and is generally performed in the first 2–3 weeks of life, whilst the pulmonary vascular

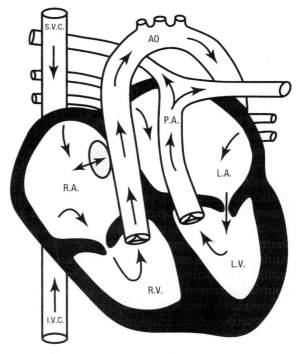

Fig. 13.12 Transposition of the great arteries. Shaded area shows position of either a patent foramen ovale or site of balloon septostomy allowing some mixing of oxygenated and deoxygenated blood between the systemic and pulmonary circulations: AO, aorta; PA, pulmonary artery; SVC, superior vena cava; IVC, inferior vena cava; RA, right atrium; LA, left atrium; RV, right ventricle; LV, left ventricle.

resistance is high and the left ventricle is 'trained' to receive the systemic workload. The aorta and pulmonary arteries (above the level of the coronary vessels) are transected and transferred and the coronary arteries themselves are also transferred to the appropriate position. Operative mortality is low (< 2%) and, though a relatively recently developed technique, the long-term results are very encouraging.

Prior to the switch procedure the defect was repaired by reversing the inflow to the ventricles using either a Mustard operation or a Senning procedure to redirect venous return via an intra-atrial tunnel (Jordan & Scott 1989). However, in the long term such procedures result in right ventricular failure amongst other complications.

Cardiac valve abnormalities

Aortic and pulmonary valve. Critical stenoses present neonatally with congestive cardiac failure and reduced peripheral pulses requiring immediate intervention. Less critical pulmonary stenosis may present later with breathlessness on exertion and fatigue. Aortic stenosis may not cause problems until adulthood though there may be left ventricular hypertrophy.

Critical aortic stenosis is managed by dilatation of the aortic valve or valvotomy. However, mortality is high (10%) (Elliott & Hussey 1995) and reoperation common. In older children the valve may be replaced with a homograft. Pulmonary stenosis is managed similarly to pulmonary atresia with an intact septum and homograft valve replacement may be required at a later stage.

Tricuspid valve. Tricuspid valve disease is rare in childhood but is seen in Epstein's anomaly. Patients present with severe cardiac failure, cyanosis and dysrhythmia. Neonatal surgery carries a high mortality and a palliative approach with a later Fontan procedure may be preferred. In the older child it is possible to perform a more complex repair of the anomaly.

Mitral valve. Mitral valve problems present either as stenosis or incompetence, usually associated with other cardiac anomalies. Repair is the preferred option though replacement may

be the only option. Early replacement is associated with a high mortality (20%) (Carpenter 1994).

Hypoplastic left heart syndrome. Aortic valve stenosis or atresia associated with severe left ventricular hypoplasia characterizes this defect. Until recently in the UK surgical intervention was not advised; however, some centres in the USA report survival rates of up to 95% following a first stage operation using a Norwood procedure and up to 70% for a second stage Fontan procedure (Norwood & Jacobs 1994). The corrective procedure aims to relieve the single ventricle of pulmonary flow (and allow passive venous return to the pulmonary circulation) and enable it to support only the systemic circulation.

Physiotherapy management of paediatric cardiac surgery

In addition to the altered pulmonary dynamics and resulting respiratory insufficiency seen after general anaesthesia, open heart surgery with cardiopulmonary bypass leads to further changes in respiratory function. Loss of perfusion and diminished surfactant production lead to poor compliance postoperatively. In addition the lungs may be compressed intraoperatively contributing to atelectasis. Pain due to the incision and presence of intercostal drains may cause splinting of the chest wall and reduced excursion.

Preoperative assessment

Preoperative assessment of both respiratory function and motor development is important. Any preoperative neurological problems or developmental delay should be documented and appropriate management plans formulated. The assessment of respiratory status may allow one to anticipate postoperative risks and occasionally it may be necessary to administer treatment preoperatively. The value of meeting the child and family preoperatively is to explain carefully the postoperative process and procedures, in order to prepare them and relieve some of the anxiety of the unknown.

Postoperative management

Thorough assessment prior to any physiotherapy intervention is essential in these patients who may be significantly haemodynamically compromised. Heart rate is an important component in determining cardiac output in infants whose ventricles are less responsive to filling pressure changes. Bradycardia can significantly compromise cardiac output and in infants is easily induced by hypoxia. Adequate pain relief must be ensured and in the immediate postoperative period continuous infusion is the method of choice. In the older child patient-controlled systems can be used.

Treatment should only be performed when the child is stable and never following any potentially destabilizing manoeuvres. Continuous observation of heart rate, blood pressure, pulmonary artery pressure and oxygen saturation should guide the progression of treatment. Treatment techniques have been discussed earlier but a few specific points should be noted:

- As soon as the child is relatively stable it is usually feasible to use the side lying position, with care not to kink or disrupt lines, wires or infusions, particularly neck lines, which may impede the delivery of inotropic agents. Hussey et al (1996) demonstrated a greater fall in oxygen saturation in children post-cardiac surgery who were turned as part of their physiotherapy treatment. More frequent but shorter episodes of treatment performed only in situ or allowing for sufficient time lapse between turning and continuing with treatment should be considered in the unstable child.

- Percussion and vibrations should be avoided if postoperative bleeding is persistent or excessive. Manual hyperinflation may be indicated to enhance secretion clearance and has been shown to have a negligible effect on oxygen saturation when used as part of a chest physiotherapy regimen for children post-cardiac surgery (Hussey et al 1996). However, care should be taken when cardiac output is low as the increase in intrathoracic pressure may decrease venous return, lowering the cardiac output further and leading to a fall in arterial oxygenation. Higher intrathoracic pressure may also decrease pulmonary blood flow and should be avoided in children with low pulmonary flow anomalies (e.g. tetralogy of Fallot, pulmonary atresia). In duct-dependent children manual hyperinflation with 100% oxygen should be avoided as the response of the specialized ductal tissue to oxygen is constriction and closure.

Specific considerations

Pulmonary hypertensive crises. This phenomenon is described as an acute elevation of the pulmonary artery (PA) pressure (owing to contraction of the arteriolar musculature) which restricts flow through the lungs. It is associated with a fall in left atrial pressure and a dramatic fall in cardiac output. PA pressure may approach or even exceed systemic pressure. It is seen in the presence of hypertrophic reactive arteriolar muscle in the lungs and is therefore common in those patients who have had significant left-to-right shunts (VSD, AVSD, truncus arteriosus). It is a critical, life-threatening event and prevention is the key to its management. Airway suction, and chest physiotherapy have the potential for precipitating a hypertensive crisis, perhaps due to a fall in oxygen saturation (as hypoxia is a known stimulant for pulmonary arteriolar vasoconstriction). Inspired oxygen should therefore be increased during chest physiotherapy (manual hyperinflation/hyperventilation) and treatment times kept to a minimum. Particular attention should be paid to oxygen saturation and the PA pressure in relation to systemic blood pressure.

Delayed sternal closure. Occasionally postoperative closure of the sternum is impeded by pulmonary, myocardial or chest wall oedema (due either to prolonged bypass times or particularly complicated intracardiac repairs). Sternal closure may constrict cardiopulmonary function. Closure may be delayed for up to 2 or more weeks. During this period children are paralysed, sedated and are preferentially nursed in supine. They are therefore at much greater risk of pulmonary complications. However, if stable and if the sternum is stented (to keep its edges separate) the child can with care be quarter turned into a side lying position. Manual hyperinflation is usually well tolerated and gentle posterior and posterolateral vibrations can be applied with care.

Phrenic nerve damage. Damage to the phrenic nerve is a well-documented complication of paediatric cardiac surgery (Main 1995). It occurs most commonly where dissection is required close to the mediastinal vessels and pericardium with which its course is closely associated. The result may be an inability to wean from mechanical ventilation or severe respiratory compromise once extubated. Upward paradoxical movement during inspiration may compress the ipsilateral lung and cause mediastinal shift to the contralateral side, causing a further loss in lung volume. Physiotherapy intervention will depend on clinical symptoms but it is important that the patient is positioned head up to relieve the pressure from the abdominal viscera and reduce the work of breathing. It is sometimes necessary to surgically plicate the affected diaphragm.

Transplantation surgery in children

The problems of transplant surgery in children are similar to those in adults, that is the availability of compatible donor organs and postoperative rejection (Ch. 16). An additional problem is finding a donor organ of a suitable size for the recipient.

The major concerns in paediatric transplantation are chronic rejection and the side-effects of long-term immunosuppression. Immunosuppressive therapies such as cyclosporin, corticosteroids, azathioprine and antithymocyte globulin are associated with renal and liver dysfunction, diabetes, tremors, hirsutism, osteoporosis and gastrointestinal ulceration. There is also an increased risk of malignancy associated with chronic immunosuppression.

Heart transplantation

Cardiac transplantation is undertaken when the heart is in terminal failure and no other treatment options are available (e.g. end-stage acquired or viral myopathy). Outcome is worst in patients who are transplanted at less than 1 year of age, with a 3-year survival of 60%. In children over 6 years of age, 3-year survival exceeds 70% (Hosenpud et al 1996). Coronary artery disease is not uncommon owing to chronic immunosuppression.

Lung and heart–lung transplantation

More children require lung or heart-lung transplantation than cardiac transplantation alone. However, fewer donors are available with lungs suitable for transplantation. Most children (two-thirds) requiring lung or heart–lung transplantation have cystic fibrosis (CF) (and usually the choice of procedure is limited by the availability of donor organs). Other indications include Eisenmenger's complex, fibrosing alveolitis, and interstitial pneumonitis. Early mortality is the same for all forms of transplantation (single/double lung or heart–lung) but bronchial anastomotic narrowing accounts for much of the late mortality in small children. In this group therefore 'en-bloc' heart–lung with a single tracheal anastomosis may be preferred. The 5-year survival for this group of patients is below 50% (Hosenpud et al 1996). Outcome post-transplantation for children with CF seems to be similar for both a younger and older age group, with survival at 3 years for children below 10 years of age recently reported as 41%, and 46% for older children (Balfour-Lynn et al 1997). The development of obliterative bronchiolitis seems to be the major obstacle to long-term success in this field.

Physiotherapy. Preoperative assessment and early postoperative management is again important and follows similar lines to that of any cardiac surgery. Additional advice on chest physiotherapy techniques and exercise where appropriate may also be offered pre-transplantation. As the timing of the actual surgery is unpredictable, preoperative physiotherapy assessment is undertaken during the initial admission for assessment for suitability for transplantation.

Early management aims to facilitate good thoracic expansion and clear any retained secretions. Careful attention should be paid to the increased risk of infection due to immunosuppression. In lung or heart–lung recipients the anastomosis may be distal to the end of the endotracheal tube and therefore suction should be performed with the greatest care. In the immediate postoperative period the anastomosis may not be 'air tight' and care should be taken when performing manual hyperinflation to ensure that excessive pressures are not delivered. Denervation below the anastomotic site may mean that the presence of secretions is not easily detected. Regular huffing and coughing to ensure the clearance of any secretions below the anastomotic site should be encouraged both following extubation and as a long-term measure.

Once extubated and off inotropic support an individually tailored graduated programme of rehabilitation can be instituted both to enable the child to regain confidence in his/her ability, and to achieve a good level of fitness. Bicycle ergometry is useful in the early stages and motivation may be enhanced by using charts to provide a measure of improvement in function. Chest physiotherapy is only required in the presence of infection and retained secretions.

Liver transplantation

Liver transplantation is used for chronic end-stage liver disease and fulminant hepatic failure. Shortage of paediatric donors means that more and more grafts are reductions of adult livers. In some situations one liver can be used for two patients.

Postoperative complications include bleeding and splinting of the right side of the diaphragm. Patients invariably develop a pleural effusion which is usually right sided but may be bilateral.

Acute rejection is common 5–7 days post-transplant. Some patients develop chronic rejection and require retransplantation (Salt et al 1992).

Physiotherapy. Physiotherapists may have the opportunity to assess these patients pre-operatively but often patients with fulminant hepatic failure are operated on as an emergency or are too ill to be seen preoperatively.

Postoperatively, the risk of bleeding in some patients means that handling is kept to a minimum. Patients are assessed regularly and treated as appropriate.

Following extubation, ambulation is encouraged as soon as possible. Large pleural effusions coupled with ascites mean patients are often very breathless and unable to mobilize.

TRAUMA

Accidents are the most common cause of child death after the first year of life; of these 50% are road traffic accidents. Children who have been severely injured may require intensive care and mechanical ventilation, particularly following a head injury.

Head injury

In the acutely head-injured child the primary injury refers to the damage sustained during trauma caused by bleeding, contusion or neuronal shearing. Secondary injury is due to the resultant complicating events. These may be either intracranial factors, such as bleeding, swelling, seizures and raised intracranial pressure (ICP), or systemic factors, such as hypoxia, hypercarbia, hyper- or hypotension, hyper- or hypoglycaemia and fever.

Raised ICP represents an increase in the volume of the intracranial contents due to a focal or diffuse cerebral process. In addition to trauma it can be caused by space-occupying lesions or encephalopathy. The normal value of ICP should be below 15 mmHg. Cerebral perfusion pressure (CPP) is the driving pressure for cerebral perfusion and is defined as the difference between mean arterial blood pressure and ICP. It is a crucial parameter which normally ranges between 50 and 70 mmHg.

Medical management aims to stabilize the child, avoid/minimize secondary brain injury, control ICP and maintain CPP. Immobility, impaired cough, depression of the respiratory centre and respiratory dysfunction due to anaesthetic and paralysing agents predispose these patients to pulmonary complications. The frequency of pneumonia in severely head-injured patients requiring prolonged mechanical ventilation may be as high as 70% (Demling & Riessen 1993).

Physiotherapy. Safe and effective treatment should be based on careful assessment and judicious use of appropriate physiotherapy techniques (Prasad & Tasker 1995). The use of bolus doses of analgesics and sedatives or, in more unstable cases, thiopentone prior to intervention can help reduce acute swings in ICP. Length of treatment time is an important factor, with longer treatment more likely to produce larger elevations of ICP. Sustained increases in ICP during cumulative interventions should be avoided by allowing a return to baseline values between procedures.

Careful monitoring of CPP during treatment is essential and treatment should be withheld or abandoned if levels fall below 50 mmHg.

A head-down position is generally considered to be contraindicated and any change in position should maintain the head midline in relation to body position. A 30 degree head-up tilt has been shown to significantly reduce ICP in the majority of patients (Feldman et al 1992). Chest clapping may be better tolerated than vibrations, and manual hyperinflation may be used with careful monitoring (Prasad & Tasker 1995). Endotracheal suctioning can have severe prolonged effects on ICP (Rudy et al 1986) and great care must be taken to avoid hypoxia. A protocol for physiotherapy management is shown in Figure 13.13.

RESPIRATORY DISEASE IN CHILDHOOD

Respiratory disease in childhood is very common. Most of the illnesses are mild; only a small proportion are more serious, involving the lower respiratory tract. The highest morbidity and mortality from lower respiratory tract disease occurs in the first year of life.

Respiratory disease is more common in children from a poor socioeconomic background, with a family history of respiratory disease, from an urban rather than country environment, with a school-age sibling, or with a mother who smokes.

Respiratory disease is more severe in infants with congenital heart or lung abnormalities, immunodeficiency, cystic fibrosis, or chronic lung disease.

Asthma

The incidence of asthma is increasing and the condition now affects about 20% of infants and children (Omran & Russell 1996). Air pollution may be identified as one of the causes of this increase.

Pathology

The main problem in asthma is bronchial hyperreactivity, where the smooth muscle in the bronchial wall overreacts to normal stimuli causing bronchoconstriction. This leads to hypertrophy of smooth muscle in the bronchial wall and an inflammatory response in the mucosa and submucosa. There is also hypertrophy of the mucus glands leading to mucus plugging. These changes cause airway obstruction which may become chronic and severe.

Aetiology

Children are more likely to develop asthma if parents or close relatives are asthmatic or atopic (allergic). There is an important link between atopy and bronchial hyperreactivity, as many children with asthma also have other atopic features such as eczema, food allergy, hay fever or urticaria. Exposure to specific allergens such as house dust mite, pollen and animal dander can precipitate bronchospasm and wheeze. Exercise, particularly running, can precipitate an acute attack (exercise-induced asthma, EIA) as can emotional upset or upper respiratory tract infections. There is also an increased incidence of asthma in children whose parents smoke.

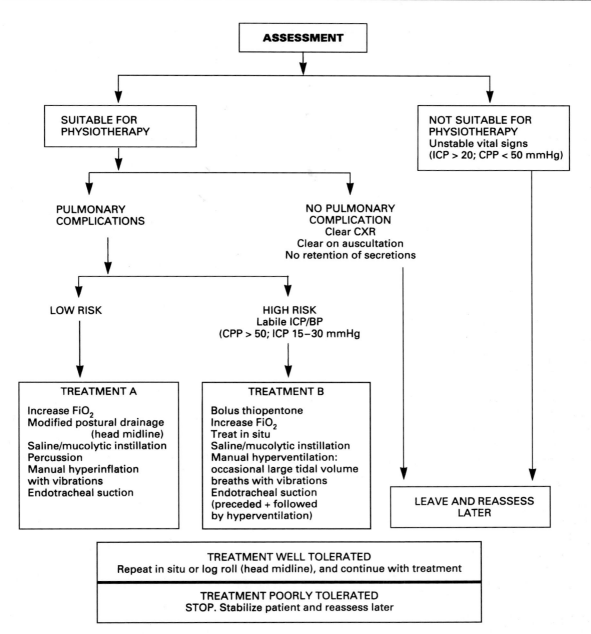

Fig. 13.13 Flow diagram of an approach to chest physiotherapy in children with raised intracranial pressure (reproduced with permission from Prasad & Tasker 1990 *Physiotherapy* 76: 250).

Management

The mainstay of asthma treatment is drug therapy and there are agreed guidelines on how asthma should be managed on a regular basis and during attacks (Rachelefsky & Warner 1993, British Thoracic Society et al 1997). Bronchodilator preparations are used to decrease bronchospasm and the most potent anti-inflammatory agents are corticosteroids. The use of continuous oral steroids for prophylaxis is unusual nowa-days, though more severely affected children may require them intermittently during exacer-bations. Administration of corticosteroids by the inhaled route is safer and results in fewer systemic effects. Their early use is indicated when there is insufficient response to initial treatment with bronchodilators and a trial of sodium cromoglycate. It is important when using inhaled corticosteroids in children that growth is carefully monitored.

Bronchodilators may be administered via the oral route in children under the age of 2 years and supplemented as necessary with nebulized bronchodilator and steroid preparations. In order that inhaled drug therapy can be effective, it is essential that the correct mode of delivery is chosen according to the age of the child. A metered-dose inhaler (MDI) with a spacer device (for example Nebuhaler or Volumatic and face mask) can be used to deliver bronchodilators or steroids to infants. The infant is placed in the supine position and the mask is held gently over the nose and mouth with the spacer held vertically. The drug can then drift down through the open valve to be inhaled. As infants can exhibit paradoxical bronchoconstriction following inhaled bronchodilators, the first dose should be given in controlled circumstances, for example in a hospital or clinic (O'Callaghan et al 1986, 1989).

From the age of 2–5 years, the spacer device can be used conventionally with the MDI (Fig. 13.14). Five tidal volume breaths are needed to inhale each dose of the drug (Gleeson & Price 1988). The click of the valve opening will be heard with each breath. It should be noted that different spacer devices have been shown to deliver varying drug doses (Barry & O'Callaghan 1996). From about 5 years of age, children's inspiratory flow rates will be fast enough to use powdered preparations in devices which are easy to use, such as a Rotahaler, Diskhaler or Turbohaler. The MDI without a spacer should not be used until the child is able to coordinate activation of the aerosol with inhalation.

In more severe cases or during exacerbations it may be necessary to deliver bronchodilators

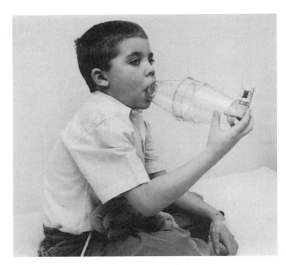

Fig. 13.14 Administration of bronchodilator by spacer device.

and steroids via a nebulizer, preferably with a mouthpiece (when the child is able to use one) to avoid drug deposition on the face.

Children with an acute severe attack may require admission to hospital. There are usually signs of respiratory distress, but wheezing may or may not be present as when there is severe airway obstruction with hyperinflation, airflow is so reduced that a wheeze may not be heard.

Physiotherapy. A crucial part of the manage-ment of asthma is education of the child and parents about the condition and its treatment. It is important that the physiotherapist is part of the team involved in that education. Physio-therapists are often involved in teaching children how to take their medication, although in some clinics this role is taken by a specialist asthma nurse.

Physiotherapists can also advise on exercise which is important in the asthmatic child to maintain general fitness. Where EIA is a prob-lem (Godfrey 1983), bronchodilators should be taken before beginning exercise. Swimming is the activity least likely to cause EIA. Some physio-therapists organize swimming and exercise classes specially designed for asthmatic children. These classes include instruction in drug therapy, progressive exercises to increase exercise tolerance, posture awareness, and breathing control to help cope with breathlessness during an acute attack. Peak flow is monitored regularly to judge effectiveness of treatment.

Apart from physical improvement, classes are also important psychologically, particularly for those with more severe asthma. These children are often afraid to exercise and lack confidence. Older children who do not have access to such classes should have the opportunity to consult a physiotherapist, if necessary, for education in breathing control and posture awareness.

The child with an acute attack may be severely ill. When bronchospasm is severe, tipping the child head down and encouraging coughing should not be attempted. Even in the ventilated patient it will not be possible to mobilize secretions until bronchodilatation has occurred. Younger children will not be able to cooperate with breathing control at this stage, but the physiotherapist may be able to advise on optimum positioning to reduce breathlessness.

When treatment is appropriate it should be given at least 15 minutes after inhaled bronchodilators and should proceed cautiously. If bronchospasm worsens treatment should be discontinued. Not all patients will require physiotherapy following an acute attack. Often effective bronchodilatation will allow the younger child to cough and clear secretions spontaneously.

Children with persistent areas of lung collapse following an acute attack will respond well to appropriate gravity-assisted positioning and chest clapping with the active cycle of breathing techniques. The pauses for relaxation and breathing control need to be emphasized to avoid any increase in bronchospasm. Parents may need to continue physiotherapy at home if excess mucus production is a chronic problem.

Bronchiolitis

Bronchiolitis is the most common severe lower respiratory tract disease affecting about 1% of infants less than 1 year of age (Dinwiddie 1997a). It occurs most frequently between October and March. The cause is viral with respiratory syncytial virus (RSV) being the main agent in more than 70% of cases. Other causes include parainfluenza, influenza and adenoviruses.

Pathology

Bronchiolar inflammation occurs with necrosis and destruction of cilia and epithelial cells leading to obstruction of the small airways. Ventilation and perfusion mismatch causes hypoxia and hypercapnia.

Clinical features

The initial presenting symptoms are coryzal, such as the common cold. The infant develops a dry irritating cough and has difficulty in feeding. As the disease progresses, the infant becomes tachypnoeic and wheezy with signs of respiratory distress. The chest radiograph shows hyperinflation and patchy areas of collapse or pneumonic consolidation. Widespread inspiratory crepitations and expiratory wheezes can be heard on auscultation.

Management

Management of this condition is mainly supportive. The infant is nursed in an upright position to assist respiration and is given humidified oxygen via a head box as required. Infants with severe respiratory distress will need blood gas monitoring and may require ventilatory support.

Most infants will have difficulty with feeding owing to respiratory distress. Milder cases may tolerate small, frequent nasogastric feeds, although the nasogastric tube causes obstruction of one nostril and may significantly increase the work of breathing. With enteral feeds there is always the risk of vomiting leading to aspiration. More severely affected infants will require intravenous nutrition.

Antibiotics are not required as the cause of the illness is viral, although they may be used if there is a secondary bacterial infection; many centres use intravenous antibiotics in these cases. If the infant is ventilated, there is an increased risk of secondary bacterial infection and many centres would use intravenous antibiotics for the ventilated patient.

Bronchodilators may be used in cases with severe wheeze, but effective response is variable and unreliable.

Ribavirin is an antiviral agent which has been shown to be effective in reducing severity and duration of the disease (Barry et al 1986). It is given in nebulized form for 18 hours per day for 3–5 days, and the drug is expensive. The complicated mode of delivery and cost of this drug means that its clinical use is limited to those infants with pre-existing cardiac or pulmonary problems, immunodeficiency or severe respiratory failure.

Physiotherapy. Physiotherapy is not indicated in the acute stage of bronchiolitis when the infant has signs of respiratory distress. A study comparing chest physiotherapy and no chest physiotherapy in infants with bronchiolitis showed no benefit in chest physiotherapy given routinely (Webb et al 1985).

The ventilated infant with bronchiolitis needs careful assessment, with physiotherapy techniques only being applied when sputum retention is a problem.

Pertussis

Pertussis, commonly called 'whooping cough', is caused by the organism *Bordetella pertussis*. It occurs in epidemics every 3–4 years and is largely preventable by immunization. Following adverse publicity about side-effects in the 1970s the uptake of immunization was greatly reduced, leading to an increased incidence of the disease.

Pertussis is particularly dangerous in infants less than 6 months of age and in children with other pulmonary problems, for example asthma and chronic lung disease.

Clinical features

The disease starts with coryza lasting 7–10 days during which the child is most infectious. The cough then becomes paroxysmal and can be provoked by crying, feeding or any other disturbance. It is particularly bad at night. The spasms of coughing may cause hypoxia and apnoea, especially in infants, and may lead to

further problems such as convulsions, intracranial bleeding, and encephalopathy.

At the end of the coughing spasm, the inspiratory whoop may occur, followed by vomiting. Some very thick, tenacious sputum may be expectorated. This phase of paroxysmal coughing may last for 6–8 weeks and is exhausting for the child and parents. The Chinese call pertussis the 'hundred day cough'.

Bronchopneumonia is the most common complication, particularly in infants and may be due to the disease itself or to secondary bacterial infection with *Staphylococcus*, *Haemophilus*, or *Pneumococcus*. The chest radiograph in severe cases shows hyperinflation and patchy areas of collapse and consolidation.

Management

Most children with pertussis will be managed at home. Infants and children with pneumonia may need admission to hospital. Treatment is supportive. Minimal handling in a quiet environment is essential for the infant with pertussis in order to reduce disturbance which may precipitate coughing. Nutritional and fluid support should be given throughout the stage of paroxysmal coughing. Antibiotics do not affect the course of the disease, but erythromycin may reduce infectivity and may also be given prophylactically to close contacts.

A small number of cases, particularly infants who have had frequent apnoeic attacks or hypoxic convulsions, will need intensive care and artificial ventilation.

Physiotherapy. Any physiotherapy manoeuvre during the acute phase precipitates the paroxysmal cough with its complications. Treatment is therefore contraindicated in infants during this stage and is of little use in older children.

If the child or infant requires ventilation, physiotherapy is very important to remove the extremely tenacious secretions which easily block large and small airways and endotracheal tubes. The paroxysmal cough is not a problem when the child is paralysed in order to be ventilated.

When the stage of paroxysmal coughing is

over, there may be persistent lobar collapse. This lung pathology responds to physiotherapy with appropriate gravity-assisted positions, and chest clapping with the active cycle of breathing techniques. Parents can be taught how to treat the child at home.

Pneumonia

The most common cause of pneumonia in the neonate is *Staphylococcus*, in the infant respiratory syncytial virus (RSV) or *Mycoplasma*, and in the child *Mycoplasma*, *Streptococcus*, or *Haemophilus influenzae*. Staphylococcal pneumonia can be an indication of underlying lung disease, for example cystic fibrosis. Children can become severely ill with pneumonia.

Clinical features

Presenting signs are pyrexia, dry cough, tachypnoea and sometimes recession of the ribs and sternum. The chest radiograph shows areas of consolidation. Chest signs are often minimal compared with the degree of illness. Children with underlying pulmonary disease are particularly at risk from pneumonia.

Management

Treatment is supportive with adequate fluid intake and humidified oxygen, if required. In younger children it is impossible to distinguish between viral and bacterial pneumonia and broad spectrum antibiotics are usually given.

Physiotherapy. In many cases of pneumonia there is consolidation of lung tissue with no excess secretions. Physiotherapy is therefore not indicated. Where sputum retention is a problem, appropriate gravity-assisted positions with clapping, and in the older child breathing techniques, can be used. Copious amounts of sputum may be cleared in one treatment following which the pyrexia may settle and the child will feel better. Reassessment of the child is often necessary as retention of secretions may become a problem as the pneumonia resolves.

Acute laryngotracheobronchitis (croup)

Croup is a common problem occurring between the ages of 6 months and 4 years. The illness is usually caused by viruses which produce acute inflammation and oedema of the airway.

Clinical features

The presenting symptoms are coryzal and later the symptoms include a harsh barking cough and hoarse voice. There may be fever. Stridor, initially inspiratory only, is much worse at night and may become inspiratory and expiratory. Signs of respiratory obstruction are seen and the severely affected child may develop respiratory failure. The acute stage of respiratory obstruction may only last 1–2 days, but the stridor and cough may continue for 7–10 days. Some children have recurrent bouts of croup.

Management

Mild cases can be managed at home. Extra humidity is often given, for example steam from a kettle, but there is no objective evidence of benefit from this treatment, and there are dangers of causing scalds from the steam.

More severely affected infants will be admitted to hospital and given humidified oxygen if hypoxic or distressed. Treatment is supportive, but with minimal handling as any disturbance which upsets the child will increase the laryngeal obstruction. Nebulized adrenaline may be given with careful observation. Antibiotics are not usually required unless there is some specific evidence of bacterial cause, for example purulent secretions. The use of oral or nebulized steroid therapy does have a beneficial effect on the course of the illness.

Very few children with croup who are admitted to hospital go on to require intubation to maintain the airway because of major respiratory obstruction. Some of these, particularly infants, may also require some additional form of respiratory support, e.g. IPPV or CPAP.

Physiotherapy. There is no place for physiotherapy in the non-intubated child with croup. Treatment may be required when the child is intubated if sputum cannot be cleared by suction alone.

Acute epiglottitis

Epiglottitis is an uncommon but very dangerous condition occurring between the ages of 1 and 7 years. The cause is usually *Haemophilus influenzae*, and the incidence is decreasing since the introduction of the Hib (*Haemophilus influenzae*) vaccine.

Clinical features

The onset is sudden. A severe sore throat develops with a high temperature. The child is systemically unwell and stridor and dysphagia develop rapidly. The child is unable to swallow saliva, and dribbles. The neck is held extended in an attempt to open the airway. Respiratory difficulty develops with hypoxia and hypercarbia. Acute and possibly fatal obstruction of the airway may develop at any time.

Management

The child with suspected epiglottitis must not be disturbed in any way. No attempt must be made to look down the throat as this may precipitate obstruction. Usual management is intubation with a nasotracheal tube, or tracheostomy if intubation is not possible. Ventilatory support may need to be given if the nasotracheal tube is very small. Intravenous antibiotics will be given.

The child may only require intubation for 3–4 days, following which there is usually complete recovery. Recurrence is rare.

Physiotherapy. Physiotherapy techniques may be required in the intubated child if secretions cannot be removed by suction alone.

Inhaled foreign body

Aspiration of a foreign body into the respiratory tract can occur at all ages, but is most common between the ages of 1 and 3 years. All types of foodstuffs may be aspirated, for example peanuts, pieces of fruit and vegetables, as well as small plastic or metal toys.

Objects are most commonly aspirated into the right main bronchus. The left main bronchus and trachea are the next most common, and smaller objects may be inhaled into right middle and lower lobe bronchi or occasionally into the left lower lobe bronchus.

When aspiration has been witnessed by parents or carers, the child should be taken immediately to hospital. On examination there may be wheeze and some signs of respiratory distress. Breath sounds may be reduced over the affected lung. The chest radiograph taken on expiration may show gas trapping in the area distal to the blockage.

In some cases the aspiration is not witnessed and the acute changes just described may be assumed to be the onset of a respiratory infection. Further changes then occur. The bronchial wall becomes oedematous, especially if the inhaled object is vegetable matter. Total obstruction of the bronchus gradually occurs and secondary pneumonic changes develop in the area distal to the blockage. After a few days the child becomes unwell with a persistent cough. The longer the obstruction remains the more permanent the lung damage, eventually leading to bronchiectasis (Dinwiddie 1997b). An inhaled foreign body should be suspected in a child with a pneumonia which does not respond to conventional treatment.

Management

All children who have aspirated a foreign body into the airway should have an urgent bronchoscopy for removal of the foreign body. If symptoms persist a repeat bronchoscopy may be necessary to ensure complete removal. Occasionally it may be impossible to remove the object by bronchoscopy and thoracotomy and bronchotomy may be required.

Physiotherapy. Physiotherapy is not indicated to attempt to remove the object before bronchoscopy. Usually physiotherapy is ineffective as the object is firmly wedged in the bronchus. More importantly, if the object is dislodged by physiotherapy manoeuvres it may travel up the bronchial tree and obstruct the trachea leading to respiratory arrest.

Following bronchoscopy, gravity-assisted positioning and chest clapping may be necessary to clear excess secretions, particularly if the object has been aspirated for some time and secondary bacterial infection has occurred.

Primary ciliary dyskinesia

Primary ciliary dyskinesia is a rare, inherited (autosomal recessive) condition in which cilial motility is severely reduced because of structural defects within the cilia.

Reduced cilial motility can lead to recurrent sinusitis and bronchiectasis due to decreased clearance of secretions. Males are usually infertile because of reduced cilial motility of the sperm tails. A classical triad of sinusitis, bronchiectasis, and infertility is known as 'Kartagener's syndrome', but only about 50% of patients with ciliary dyskinesia present with this picture. Cilia can be examined for motility using nasal epithelial brushings.

Infants with this condition may present in the neonatal period with pneumonia, but many children present later with chronic upper and lower respiratory tract infection. This condition is not curable, so treatment is directed towards preventing infection and chronic lung damage. Children will require daily physiotherapy (p. 468). Appropriate antibiotics will be required during periods of infection.

Cystic fibrosis

Cystic fibrosis is the most common inherited condition in Caucasians, occurring in about 1 in 2500 births. The major clinical and diagnostic features result from abnormalities of the exocrine glands, the most important areas affected being the respiratory and digestive tracts. 12% of children present at birth with meconium ileus, where thickened meconium causes blockage of the colon and ileum. The infant presents in the first day of life with abdominal distension, vomiting and failure to pass meconium. Nowadays the obstruction can often be conservatively managed but occasionally laparotomy may be required. Other modes of presentation include recurrent chest infections and/or failure to thrive.

Diagnosis of CF is confirmed with a sweat test and blood sampling for genotype.

Physiotherapy. Physiotherapy is essential from the time of diagnosis to try to prevent progressive lung damage caused by persistent airway inflammation and infection. Cystic fibrosis is fully described in Chapter 20.

CONCLUSION

Children are not just small adults. Their anatomical and physiological differences mean that their need for treatment and the response to it is variable compared with adults. The ability of children to understand and cooperate depends on their age and understanding. It is important for the physiotherapist to be aware of these differences and to adapt treatment so that it is appropriate and effective.

REFERENCES

Ackerman M H 1985 The use of bolus normal saline instillations in artificial airways – is it useful or necessary? Heart and Lung 14: 505–506

Albert D 1995 Management of suspected tracheobronchial stenosis in ventilated neonates. Archives of Disease in Childhood 72: 1–2

Arnold J A, Truog R D, Thompson J E, Fackler J C 1993 High frequency oscillatory ventilation in paediatric respiratory failure. Critical Care Medicine 21: 272–278

Baird P A, MacDonald E C 1982 An epidemiologic study of congenital malformations of the anterior abdominal wall in more than half a million consecutive live births. American Journal of Human Genetics 34: 517–521

Balfour-Lynn I M, Martin I, Whitehead B F, Rees P G, Elliot M J, de Leval M R 1997 Heart–lung transplantation for patients under 10 with cystic fibrosis. Archives of Disease in Childhood 76: 1–3

Barry P, O'Callaghan C 1996 Inhalational drug delivery from seven different spacer devices. Thorax 51: 835–840

Barry W, Cockburn F, Cornall R, Price J F, Sutherland G,

Vardag A 1986 Ribavirin aerosol for acute bronchiolitis. Archives of Disease in Childhood 61: 593–597

Bhuyan U, Peters A M, Gordon I, Helms P 1989 Effect of posture on the distribution of pulmonary ventilation and perfusion in children and adults. Thorax 44: 480–484

Blumenthal I, Lealman G T 1982 Effects of posture on gastro-oesophageal reflux in the newborn. Archives of Disease in Childhood 57: 555–556

Brackbill Y, Douthitt T C, West H 1973 Psychophysiological effects in the neonate of prone versus supine placement. Journal of Pediatrics 82: 82–83

Brewer L A, Fosburg R G, Mulder G A, Verska J J 1972 Spinal cord complications following surgery for coarctation of the aorta – a study of 66 cases. Journal of Thoracic and Cardiovascular Surgery 64: 368

British Thoracic Society, National Asthma Campaign, Royal College of Physicians of London, General Practitioner in Asthma Group, British Association of Accident and Emergency Medicine, British Paediatric Respiratory Society, Royal College of Paediatrics and Child Health 1997 The British guidelines on asthma management. Thorax 52(suppl 1): S1–S21

Button B M, Heine R G, Catto-Smith A G, Phelan P D, Olinsky A 1997 Postural drainage and gastro-oesophageal reflux in infants with cystic fibrosis. Archives of Disease in Childhood 76: 148–150

Carpenter A 1994 Congenital malformation of the mitral valve. In: Stark J, de Leval M (eds) Surgery for congenital heart defects, 2nd edn. W B Saunders, Philadelphia, ch 41, pp 599–614

Castenda A R 1994 Tetralogy of Fallot. In: Stark J, de Leval M (eds) Surgery for congenital heart defects, 2nd edn. W B Saunders, Philadelphia, ch 26, pp 405–416

Crowley P 1995 Update on the antenatal steroid meta-analysis. American Journal of Obstetrics and Gynecology 173: 322–335

Davies H, Kitchman R, Gordon G, Helms P 1985 Regional ventilation in infancy. Reversal of the adult pattern. New England Journal of Medicine 313: 1627–1628

Dean E 1985 Effect of body position on pulmonary function. Physical Therapy 65: 613–618

de Leval M 1994 Ventricular septal defects. In: Stark J, de Leval M (eds) Surgery for congenital heart defects, 2nd edn. W B Saunders, Philadelphia, ch 23, pp 355–371

Demling R H, Riessen R 1993 Respiratory failure after cerebral injury. Critical Care Medicine 1: 440–446

Demont B, Escarrou P, Vincon C, Cambas C H, Grisan A, Odievre M 1991 Effects of respiratory physical therapy and nasopharyngeal suction on gastrooesophageal reflux in infants less than one year of age with or without abnormal reflux. Archives Francaises de Pediatrie (Paris) 48: 621–625

Depaepe A, Dolk A, Lechat M F 1993 The epidemiology of tracheo-oesophageal fistula and oesophageal atresia in Europe. Archives of Disease in Childhood 68: 743–748

Dinwiddie R 1997a Respiratory tract infection. In: The diagnosis and management of paediatric respiratory disease, 2nd edn. Churchill Livingstone, New York, ch 6, pp 103–134

Dinwiddie R 1997b Aspiration syndromes. In: The diagnosis and management of paediatric respiratory disease, 2nd edn. Churchill Livingstone, New York, ch 10, pp 247–260

Elliott M, Hussey J 1995 Paediatric cardiac surgery. In: Prasad S A, Hussey J (eds) Paediatric respiratory care.

Chapman & Hall, London, ch 8, pp 122–141

Feldman Z, Kanter M J, Robertson C S et al 1992 Effect of head elevation on intracranial pressure and cerebral blood flow in head injured patients. Journal of Neurosurgery 59: 206–211

Gleeson J G, Price J F 1988 Nebuhaler technique. British Journal of Diseases of the Chest 82: 172–174

Godfrey S 1983 Exercise induced asthma. Archives of Disease in Childhood 52: 1–2

Greenough A 1996a Lung maturation. In: Greenough A, Roberton N R C, Milner A (eds) Neonatal respiratory disorders. Arnold, London, ch 2, pp 13–26

Greenough A 1996b Liquid ventilation. Care of the Critically Ill 12(4): 128–130

Greenough A 1996c Chronic lung disease. In: Greenough A, Roberton N R C, Milner A (eds) Neonatal respiratory disorders. Arnold, London, ch 26, pp 393–425

Greenough A, Pool J 1988 Neonatal patient triggered ventilation. Archives of Disease in Childhood 63: 394–397

Greenough A, Morley C J, Davis J A 1983 The interaction of the preterm infants spontaneous respiration with ventilation. Journal of Pediatrics 103: 769–773

Greenough A, Morley C J, Wood S, Davies J A 1984 Pancuronium prevents pneumothoraces in ventilated premature infants who actively expire against positive pressure inflation. Lancet i: 1–3

Greenough A, Pool J, Greenall F, Morley C J, Gamsu H 1987 Comparison of different rates of artificial ventilation in preterm neonates with respiratory distress syndrome. Acta Paediatrica Scandinavica 76: 706–712

Hoffman J I, Christianson R 1978 Congenital heart disease in a cohort of 19502 births with long term follow up. American Journal of Cardiology 42: 641–646

Hosenpud J D, Novick R J, Bennett L E, Keck B M, Fiol B, Daily O P 1996 The registry of the international society for heart and lung transplantation: thirteenth official report. Journal of Heart and Lung Transplantation 15: 655–674

Hussey J, Hayward L, Andrews M, Macrae D, Elliott M 1996 Chest physiotherapy following paediatric cardiac surgery: the influence of mode of treatment on oxygen saturation and haemodynamic stability. Physiotherapy Theory and Practice 12: 77–85

Inselman L S, Mellins R B 1981 Growth and development of the lung. Journal of Pediatrics 98: 1–15

Jordon S C, Scott O 1989 Cyanotic lesions with increased pulmonary blood flow. In: Jordon S C, Scott O (eds) Heart disease in paediatrics, 3rd edn. Butterworths, London, ch 10, pp 170–185

Lindham S 1981 Omphalocele and gastroschisis in Sweden 1965–1976. Acta Pediatrica Scandinavica 70: 55–60

Main E 1995 Phrenic nerve latency testing: assessing post operative diaphragmatic function in infants. MSc Thesis University of London

Morin L, Crombleholme T M, D'Alton M E 1994 Prenatal diagnosis and management of fetal thoracic lesions. Seminars in Perinatology 18: 228–253

Morley C J 1991 Surfactant treatment for premature babies: a review of clinical trials. Archives of Disease in Childhood 66: 445–450

Muller N L, Bryan A C 1979 Chest wall mechanics and respiratory muscles in infants. Pediatric Clinics of North America 26(3): 503–516

Newell S J, Booth W, Morgan M E, Durbin G M, McNeish A S 1989 Gastro oesophageal reflux in preterm infants.

Archives of Disease in Childhood 64: 780–786

Norwood W I, Jacobs M L 1994 Hypoplastic left heart syndrome. In: Stark J, de Leval M (eds) Surgery for congenital heart defects, 2nd edn. W B Saunders, Philadelphia, ch 40, pp 587–598

O'Callaghan C, Milner A, Swarbrick A 1986 Paradoxical deterioration in lung function after nebulized salbutamol in wheezy infants. Lancet ii: 1424–1425

O'Callaghan C, Milner A, Swarbrick A 1989 Paradoxical bronchospasm in wheezing infants after nebulized preservative-free iso-osmolar ipratropium bromide. British Medical Journal 299: 1433–1434

Omran M, Russell G 1996 Continuing increase in respiratory symptoms and atopy in Aberdeen school children. British Medical Journal 312: 34–35

Pearson G A, Grant J, Field D, Sosnowski A, Firmin R K 1993 Extracorporeal life support in paediatrics. Archives of Disease in Childhood 68: 94

Phillips G 1996 To tip or not to tip? Physiotherapy Research International 1(1): 1–6

Prasad S A, Tasker R C 1990 Guidelines for physiotherapy management of critically ill children with acutely raised intracranial pressure. Physiotherapy 76(4): 248–250

Prasad S A, Tasker R C 1995 Neurological intensive care. In: Prasad S A, Hussey J (eds) Paediatric respiratory care. Chapman & Hall, London, ch 9, pp 142–149

Rachelefsky G S, Warner J O 1993 International consensus on the management of pediatric asthma: a summary statement. Pediatric Pulmonology 15: 125–127

Reid L 1984 Lung growth in health and disease. British Journal of Diseases of the Chest 78: 113–132

Roberton N R C 1996 Intensive care. In: Greenough A, Roberton N R C, Milner A (eds) Neonatal respiratory disorders. Arnold, London, ch 13, pp 174–195

Rodenstein D O, Kahn A, Blum D, Stanescu D C 1987 Nasal occlusion during sleep in normal and near miss for sudden death syndrome in infants. Bulletin European Physiopathologie Respiratoire 23: 223–226

Rudy E B, Baun M, Stone K, Turner B 1986 The relationship between endotracheal suctioning and changes in intracranial pressure: a review of the literature. Heart-Lung 15: 488–494

Salt A, Noble-Jameson G, Barnes N D et al 1992 Liver transplantation in 100 children: Cambridge and King's College Hospital series. British Medical Journal 304: 416–421

Samuels M P, Southall D P 1989 Negative extrathoracic pressure in the treatment of respiratory failure in infants and children. British Medical Journal 299: 1253–1257

Sarnaik A P, Meert K L, Pappas M D, Simpson P M, Lieh-Lai M W, Heidemann S M 1996 Predicting outcome in children with severe acute respiratory failure treated with high-frequency ventilation. Critical Care Medicine 24(8): 1396–1402

Southall D P, Samuels M P 1992 Reducing risks in the sudden infant death syndrome. British Medical Journal 304: 260–265

Tarnow-Mordi W O, Reid E, Griffiths P, Wilkinson A R 1989 Low inspired gas temperature and respiratory complications in very low birthweight infants. Journal of Pediatrics 114: 438–442

Taylor C J, Threlfall D 1997 Postural drainage techniques and gastro-oesophageal reflux in cystic fibrosis. Lancet 349: 1567–1568

Thoresen M, Cavan F, Whitelaw A 1988 Effect of tilting on oxygenation in newborn infants. Archives of Disease in Childhood 63: 315–317

Tudehope D I, Bagley C 1980 Techniques of physiotherapy in intubated babies with RDS. Australian Medical Journal 16: 226–228

UK Collaborative ECMO Trial Group 1996 UK collaborative randomised trial of neonatal extracorporeal membrane oxygenation. Lancet 348: 75–81

Vaughan R S, Menke J A, Giacoia G P 1978 Pneumothorax a complication of endotracheal suctioning. Journal of Pediatrics 92: 633–634

Webb M S C, Martin J A, Cartlidge P H T, Ng Y K, Wright N A 1985 Chest physiotherapy in acute bronchiolitis. Archives of Disease in Childhood 6: 1078–1079

Wenstrom K D, Weiner C P, Hanson J W 1991 A five-year statewide experience with congenital diaphragmatic hernia. American Journal of Obstetrics and Gynecology 165: 838–842

Zapol W M, Rimar S, Gillis N, Marletta M, Bosken C H 1994 Nitric oxide and the lung. American Journal of Respiratory and Critical Care Medicine 149: 1375–1380

FURTHER READING

Dinwiddie R 1997 Diagnosis and management of paediatric respiratory disease, 2nd edn. Churchill Livingstone, New York

Grenough A, Roberton N R C, Milner A 1996 Neonatal respiratory disorders. Arnold, London

Prasad S A, Hussey J 1995 Paediatric respiratory care. Chapman & Hall, London

14

Pulmonary rehabilitation

Julia Bott   Sally J. Singh

DEFINITION AND AIMS OF PULMONARY REHABILITATION

Pulmonary rehabilitation is an holistic, complex, multidisciplinary therapy providing comprehensive treatment for the patient with chronic pulmonary disease. It is an integration of both physical and emotional therapy and support and usually consists of a combination of exercise and education. Programmes were originally developed for patients with chronic obstructive pulmonary disease (COPD), but the principles can be applied to those with other conditions (Petty 1993a).

Pulmonary rehabilitation has been redefined as 'a multidimensional continuum of services directed to persons with pulmonary disease and their families, usually by an interdisciplinary team of specialists with the goal of achieving and maintaining the individual's maximal level of independence and functioning in the community' (Fishman 1994).

The aims of pulmonary rehabilitation are:

- To maximize independent functioning in activities of daily living and minimize dependence on significant others and community agencies
- To evaluate and initiate, as appropriate, physical training to increase exercise tolerance and encourage efficient energy expenditure
- To provide educational sessions for patients, families and significant others regarding disease processes, medication and therapeutic techniques (Harris 1985).

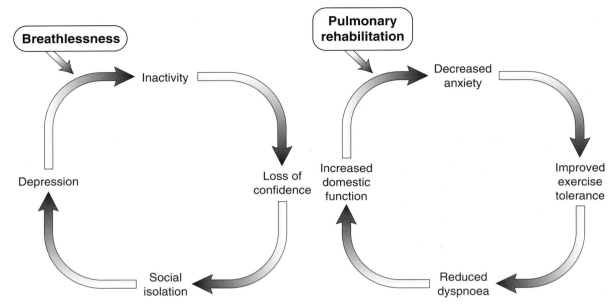

Fig. 14.1 Vicious circle of COPD and the circle of rehabilitation.

In essence, the patient with chronic lung disease enters the vicious circle of inactivity and the aim of pulmonary rehabilitation is to reverse that trend (Fig. 14.1).

The concept of exercise in pulmonary 'invalids' had been advocated as long ago as 1895, although pulmonary rehabilitation as a comprehensive therapy was not documented until the 1960s (Petty 1993b). However, difficulties in providing substantive data, owing to lack of control groups and the inability to separate the multidisciplinary components of programmes, caused interest to wane (Muir & Pierson 1993). Interest was revived during the following decade and Make (1986) maintained that 'after optimising medication, it is still possible to produce improvements in severe COPD with pulmonary rehabilitation'.

BENEFITS OF PULMONARY REHABILITATION

The results of early studies of rehabilitation were often viewed with scepticism because rehabilitation did not alter the pathophysiological state of the disease, traditionally measured using lung function tests. More recently a number of well-conducted randomized controlled trials have been published documenting the improvements achieved by graduating from a course of rehabilitation (Goldstein et al 1994, Reardon et al 1994, Wijkstra et al 1995). These studies and others report the benefits of rehabilitation to include:

- An improved quality of life
- A reduction of anxiety and depression
- Improved exercise tolerance
- Reduction in breathlessness and other associated symptoms
- An enhanced ability to perform activities of daily living.

Traditionally improvements in rehabilitation have been measured by changes in exercise capacity; however, more recently the measurement of quality of life has become increasingly important (Muir & Pierson 1993). The cost–benefit analysis is also being investigated. Experience from the United States of America (USA) would suggest that a typical outpatient rehabilitation programme costs in the region of $1000 (Petty 1993a). This may seem expensive but can be offset against the cost of one brief hospital admission, since evidence from the USA would suggest that rehabilitation reduces the number of hospital days compared with a control group (Hudson et al 1976). Even though the majority of patients referred for rehabilitation are retired, there is the potential for the younger participants to return to employment (Haas & Cardon 1969). While there is a large body of literature now available on the outcomes in COPD (Casaburi & Petty 1993, Lacasse et al 1996, Simonds et al 1996), there is very little on the outcomes in non-obstructive lung conditions (Foster & Thomas 1990, Novitch & Thomas 1993, Simonds 1996), but the reported findings indicate a similar level of improvement irrespective of the underlying condition (Foster & Thomas 1990).

SETTING UP PULMONARY REHABILITATION

Resources

Before embarking on any pulmonary rehabilitation programme it is essential that careful planning is done to ensure the success of the programme. The first step is providing adequate resources. Staffing is the most expensive resource and local factors will dictate who is involved, but the team is commonly drawn from the following professionals: physician (respiratory), physiotherapist, occupational therapist, pharmacist, dietitian, social worker, nurse, psychologist, medical laboratory scientific officer, and administrator/secretary. Precise roles will be determined by interest, availability and experience. Box 14.1 highlights the essential and desirable non-staffing resources required. Access to the venue including issues such as parking, public transport and ambulance or hospital car service are important considerations.

Selection of patients

The second step is identifying potential patient cohorts and defining suitable entry criteria (Box 14.2). Motivation of the individual to join a programme and to integrate into a group are key factors. Awareness of the extent of disability

---

Box 14.1 Resources for pulmonary rehabilitation

Desirable resources
- Access/transport/parking
- Floor space
  - non-slip
  - large enough for walking/exercising
- Equipment
  - supportive comfortable seating
  - quoits/sandbags/weights
  - step/low stool
  - wall space
  - writing materials
- Refreshments

Optional equipment
- Wall bars
- Bed/plinth
- Mini-trampoline
- Stationary bicycle
- Stairs
- Multi-gym
- Mats
- Treadmill
- Cassette player/music

Essential/emergency equipment
- Bronchodilator drugs
- Nebulizer and air compressor
- Pulse oximeter
- Oxygen/portable O_2
- Resuscitation equipment/trolley
- Emergency policy

Documentation
- Travel/location details
- Programme details
- Assessment forms
- Exercise sheets/booklets
- Progress report forms
- Patient information material

---

and possible denial need to be handled with sensitivity. Smoking is a contentious issue but is one which must be addressed particularly as the success of pulmonary rehabilitation depends largely on self-motivation and lifestyle change. If patients are not interested in attempting to stop smoking the question of whether they are prepared to embark on any form of self-help must be brought into question. Whether such patients are enrolled in any programme is up to the individual centre. In the case of a patient who is still smoking but is keen to stop and needs help, it is essential that this help is provided. This help can be provided in the form of counselling, either individual or group, smoking cessation programmes if available, or nicotine patches.

Box 14.2 Criteria for entry to a pulmonary rehabilitation programme

Psychological/practical
• Motivated to embark on self-help
• Motivated to make lifestyle changes
• Can hear or communicate adequately in a group setting
• Personality suitable for group work
• Able to attend for required period

Medical
• Shortness of breath and reduction of activity causing concern
• Stable and on optimum medication
• On O_2/non-invasive ventilation if indicated

Exclusions
• Patients with progressive diseases, e.g. cancer or neuromuscular disease
• Patients with conditions where exercise is contraindicated, e.g. certain cardiac disorders

---

Box 14.3 Preliminary assessment for pulmonary rehabilitation

• Past medical history
• Smoking history
• Medication
• Spirometry (FEV_1/FVC)
• Blood gas analysis/resting oxygen saturation/heart rate
• Perceived breathlessness
• Quality of life (general/disease specific)
• Exercise tolerance
• Previous hospital admissions
• Height/weight (to calculate BMI)

The issue of smoking can be addressed in the education sessions and reinforced by support from other patients who can help one another and often provide tips that they used to give up.

Issues such as age groups and disability levels will need to be considered by the team. It may be that patients with similar ages and those with similar levels of disability will bond better and feel less self-conscious. The emotional impact of being in prolonged contact with someone with the same condition and much worse than yourself should not be underestimated. The patient with a greater disability represents what may happen in the future and can be frightening. For the patient with the greater disability the issue is how it feels to be watching someone who can perform better. However, in real life, it is not often possible to separate patients into such discrete groups. It merely needs to be highlighted that the team members must be aware of this and the emotional impact on the individuals in the group. For a detailed discussion on selection and assessment the reader is referred to Singh (1997).

PATIENT ASSESSMENT FOR PULMONARY REHABILITATION

The type of information collected at the time of the initial assessment is summarized in Box 14.3. The assessment of the individual's past and current medical history requires little explanation and is discussed in Chapter 1. The patients should, on referral to the rehabilitation team, be clinically stable and their medical management optimal. This precludes any benefits of rehabilitation being assigned to manipulation of their medication. Smoking is a controversial issue, should smokers be included. This is often resolved locally. The measurement of resting heart rate, oxygen saturation and breathlessness score form the baseline upon which to judge any relative changes during exercise.

Exercise tolerance

The assessment of exercise tolerance is vital at the beginning of a rehabilitation programme. Indeed one of the aims of rehabilitation is to increase an individual's ability to perform physical activity. Domestic activity may not be reflected by the results of an exercise test but a test is important to:

• Assess the level of disability
• Identify the limitation to continued exercise
• Aid in the prescription of a training regimen
• Identify any benefits of rehabilitation.

There are many exercise tests to choose from, ranging from a laboratory-based test to a simple field test. The choice for a physiotherapist developing a rehabilitation service is most likely to be restricted by the availability of laboratory-based equipment. Maximal oxygen uptake is the 'gold' standard measure secured during laboratory-based testing. This point in healthy individuals is recognized by a 'plateauing' of oxygen consumption despite an increase in workload. For patients with COPD this point is rarely achieved and so the comparable point is defined as the peak oxygen consumption. It is frequently assumed that exercise is curtailed prematurely by deficits in the respiratory system; reasons can be defined in terms of abnormal gas exchange, altered respiratory mechanics and respiratory muscle dysfunction. Less frequently documented but equally important reasons are peripheral fatigue, poor motivation, poor co-ordination and chest pain (Killian et al 1992). Realistically, it is very unlikely that there will be access to sophisticated laboratory-based tests employed to assess the precise cardiorespiratory response to exercise. Therefore the physiotherapist must consider a test that can be performed in either the physiotherapy gymnasium or a hospital corridor.

As an outcome measure for rehabilitation a simple measure of performance is required that can be carried out easily and frequently; therefore field exercise tests are most commonly employed. The information collected during a field exercise test can be enhanced by the use of a portable pulse oximeter, heart rate monitor and subjective scores of dyspnoea. It is possible to measure ventilation and oxygen consumption. There is a spectrum of exercise tests that can be applied in the field. These can be broadly divided into maximal capacity and endurance tests. The 6- or 12-minute walking test (McGavin et al 1976, Butland et al 1982) is a simple self-paced corridor walking test. Owing to self-pacing, a patient's performance on this test may lie at any point of the range between maximal capacity and endurance and can be influenced by motivation and encouragement. Because of its lack of pacing, this type of test may define an individual's domestic function more accurately than a laboratory-based test. Reproducibility of this test is moderate, requiring up to three practice walks (Swinburn et al 1985). More recently, the shuttle walking test has been described and is both reproducible after one prac-

tice walk and correlates well with peak oxygen consumption (Singh et al 1992, 1994). This test requires the patient to walk around a 10 m course at speeds dictated by signals played from a cassette tape. Both the 6-minute walking test and the shuttle walking test appear to be sensitive enough to detect change as a consequence of rehabilitation (Goldstein et al 1994, Singh et al 1996) (see Ch. 3 for further details of exercise testing).

Assessment of dyspnoea

The experience of breathlessness is almost without exception a sensation experienced by the patient with COPD. It is the single most important symptom that provokes a medical consultation. One of the understated aims of rehabilitation is to assist the individual in controlling his breathlessness and to reduce the sensation. Studies have employed measures of dyspnoea as an outcome measure for rehabilitation (Reardon et al 1994). How an individual reacts to his dyspnoea is multifactorial, depending upon his emotional, physical and psychological state. Patients with COPD commonly avoid situations that will provoke this sensation. In the early stages of the disease individuals may even assign this sensation to one of 'old age'. Inevitably the precise measurement of dyspnoea is difficult; like the sensation of pain it is subjective and the magnitude of the discomfort is only apparent to the individual. Over the last 20 years a variety of instruments have been developed to assess dyspnoea. Perhaps the most simple is the visual analogue scale (VAS), consisting of a 10 cm line with descriptors 'not at all breathless' and 'extremely breathless' at either end. The individual is required to mark the line corresponding to his sensation of dyspnoea. The Borg breathlessness scale (Borg 1982) is another simple measure. This scoring system, originally designed as a 20 point scale for exertion and modified for breathlessness, comprises a 10 point scale (0–10) with descriptors at most of the values, for example 'moderate' (3),'severe' (5) and 'maximal' (10). This score is easy to employ and reproducible, and may be useful for exercise prescription. Both of these scales are useful because, not only can they be used at rest, but also meaningful data can be collected during or immediately after exercise. The Medical Research Council scale (Medical Research Council 1966) is a useful tool to identify the level of disability imposed by the sensation. Symptom severity is scored on a five point scale. It has recently been suggested that this scale may be a useful mechanism by which to select patients for rehabilitation (Bestall et al 1996).

Quality of life

Health-related quality of life (HRQL) can be assessed by several possible measurement tools. Most common are the questionnaire or interview, or a combination of the two. There are numerous general health questionnaires available (Bowling 1997) and a few disease-specific ones (Hyland et al 1994, Bowling 1995), usage varying with location, personal preference and desired information. Further discussion is beyond the scope of this chapter and the reader is referred to the referenced authors for details of these measures.

Musculoskeletal assessment

Many respiratory patients have problems of stiffness or abnormalities of the thoracic vertebrae, rib cage and sternal joints. This may be partly due to poor posture, decreased levels of activity and decreased respiratory muscle strength. In addition, given the likely advanced years of the majority of patients participating in pulmonary rehabilitation groups, there will be many patients who have musculoskeletal problems in addition to their respiratory one. It is imperative that the physiotherapist clearly understands which problem is producing the limiting factor to the patient's exercise tolerance and functional activities so that this can be taken into account during exercise prescription. Should a patient be suffering from musculoskeletal problems, or pain of any description, it is important that this is assessed and treated, preferably before entering the programme. There is increasing interest within the physiotherapy profession

in manual mobilization techniques for musculoskeletal problems (see p. 192) and alternative pain control methods such as acupuncture (see p. 202). Thoracic stiffness will lead to a reduction in functional capacity and therefore needs to be treated with gentle exercise including rotation and lateral flexion exercises.

STRUCTURE OF PULMONARY REHABILITATION

From the literature it would seem that small groups are optimal, four to eight being a good number to provide a group structure with bonding possibilities and small enough to allow individualization (Petty 1993a). Group size may, in reality, be dictated partly by space and economic considerations. Rehabilitation can be provided on an outpatient or inpatient basis. The outpatient format is most commonly provided and less costly. Given the length of time for physiological changes to take place and for lifestyle alterations to be made, the prolonged time of an outpatient programme allows the patient to see greater change during the course of the programme. In the USA, it is not uncommon for 4-week inpatient programmes to be offered. The inpatient programme increases cost, but has the advantage of being intensive and allowing contact with staff and group members to be prolonged with plenty of opportunity for discussion and sharing, and this may prove helpful.

If the programme is to be offered on an outpatient basis, consideration needs to be given to the most appropriate time of day, not just for the organization and its own timetable, but for those who attend. As patients with respiratory disease, and those who are elderly, are not uncommonly reluctant to venture out of their homes after dark, it is sensible to consider providing the programme during daylight hours. Many patients with severe respiratory disorders find getting up in the morning, getting washed, dressed, breakfasted and taking medication a slow and difficult process and this needs to be taken into account. In addition, it helps patients not to have to travel during peak hours. Should the programme be after lunch it is important to advise patients to have only a light meal so that exercising is not contraindicated.

The duration of such a programme is commonly 2–3 hours, with a mixture of exercise and education at the same session. This, however, can and does vary, with some centres providing education and exercise at separate sessions. Programmes can be offered any number of times a week with the most commonly reported in the literature being twice a week. In order to provide a comprehensive variety of education sessions and, owing to the time taken for exercise to have benefit, twice a week over 6–8 weeks is a very common time frame for a programme. The issue of the increased risk of an acute exacerbation occurring over a longer period needs to be taken into account when planning the length of a programme.

Pulmonary rehabilitation team

The rehabilitation team is drawn from the professionals listed earlier in this chapter. Precise roles and input will depend on expertise, interest and availability. However, three roles in particular will be discussed here.

Physician (respiratory)

A physician needs to be involved in any pulmonary rehabilitation programme, ideally a specialist chest physician with an interest in rehabilitation. Medical input could be to facilitate referral to the programme and to screen patients for suitability, to exclude or treat other disorders, to optimize medication, to ensure that long-term oxygen therapy (LTOT) or ventilatory support is provided if necessary and to provide general medical support for the programme. This physician or other nominated colleague may provide at least one or more of the educational sessions.

Physiotherapist

The physiotherapist should play a key role in any pulmonary rehabilitation programme and it may well fall upon the physiotherapist to be the coordinator or leader of such a programme. It is the physiotherapist who will be providing and supervising the exercise sessions and therefore needs to be present at every session, while it is unlikely to be the case for any other of the disciplines contributing to the programme. In addition to providing the exercise prescription and, if used, the respiratory muscle training, the physiotherapist is likely to be the person to provide training in breathing techniques, positions to adopt when breathless and some of the coping strategies. The physiotherapist will also assess and supply appropriate aids to assist with mobility. These may take the form of items such as walking sticks, walking frames, or any other suitably adaptable device to help with the patients' general functional mobility. For further discussion on the potential role of physiotherapy the reader is referred to Bott (1997).

Occupational therapist

Occupational therapy, when available, provides a very valuable dimension to the programme. Should an occupational therapist not be available to assist with the programme, it may be the physiotherapist who provides this input. The occupational therapist traditionally assesses patients for activities of daily living both in terms of self-caring and their domestic situation. The occupational therapist may provide the education on energy conservation techniques and include teaching of activities such as pacing, and organizing tasks, and may need to do a home assessment and organize the fitting of aids such as bath or shower rails or seats.

Exercise component

Effects of exercise

The rationale for rehabilitative exercise in patients with COPD is to improve exercise capacity and enhance the performance of activities of daily living. It is by offering a pulmonary rehabilitation programme that the vicious circle of breathlessness, inactivity, lack of fitness, social isolation and depression can be reversed (Fig. 14.1).

However, there has been some difficulty in identifying the precise physiological mechanism that can account for the improved exercise tolerance observed so often in rehabilitation programmes. Each bout of exercise stimulates beneficial short-term responses of the cardiovascular system as well as metabolic effects which, when repeated, can produce a desensitization to dyspnoea. Other potential mechanisms include greater neuromuscular coordination and increased confidence. Casaburi et al (1991) and Cox et al (1993) have produced some evidence to suggest that a physiological training response can be observed in certain groups of patients with COPD, but the groups studied tended to be younger than the average patient recruited to a rehabilitation programme. The authors observed a decrease in blood lactate concentrations and thus a decreased level of ventilation at a given work rate. One of the great difficulties in comparing outcomes of rehabilitation is that several outcome measures are employed. Some authors report incremental exercise test protocols (which measure peak performance) while others report constant intensity (endurance) tests. Inevitably the causes for the termination of exercise are not the same in all studies. Recently there was an attempt to combine the results of all the randomized controlled trials examining the benefits of rehabilitation (Lacasse et al 1996). The study assessed the effect of pulmonary rehabilitation on exercise tolerance and health-related quality of life. The ensuing meta-analysis attempted to identify the minimum clinically important difference, i.e. the smallest difference defined by the patient as being important. By pooling the results of 14 separate studies the authors concluded that rehabilitation relieves dyspnoea and improves the feeling of control over the disease, but failed to identify the value of the observed improvements in exercise capacity, particularly maximal capacity.

Exercise prescription

Celli (1995) summarized the physiological basis of exercise prescription for patients with COPD – specificity, intensity and reversal. Taken in order,

specificity relates to the measurable response to exercise training. The effect is 'training specific'; thus the benefit of an upper limb programme will not be apparent if a walking test is used to identify any changes in capacity. Secondly, the intensity of training has to be sufficient to produce a training effect. Finally, reversal of the training effect; once the regimen is discontinued the training effect will disappear. This has been extensively reported for a normal population. After knee surgery and subsequent immobilization for 4–6 weeks the cross-sectional area of skeletal muscle can reduce by 25% (Saltin & Gollnick 1983). In addition inactivity reduces the metabolic efficiency of the muscle and thus reduces endurance capacity (Henriksson & Reitman 1977).

There are several approaches adopted to improve the individual's exercise capacity, which range from whole body exercise to very specific muscle training. In addition to the different modes of training, different intensities can be applied, e.g. strength training (high intensity) or endurance training (low intensity). Perhaps most importantly the exercise prescription needs to be individualized. However, it appears that two schools of thought have developed for training patients with COPD; one adopts a fairly structured approach while the other is much more relaxed without specific training programmes identified.

Aerobic training. This type of training is widely recommended for a healthy population and is commonly associated with whole body exercise, i.e. the involvement of large muscle groups. In healthy individuals aerobic training provokes physiological and structural changes that will improve endurance performance. These changes centre around the trained muscles (an increased capillary network, mitochondrial density and concentration of oxidative enzymes) and the cardiovascular system (increased stroke volume). As outlined above, the changes that occur in patients with COPD remain unclear. Muscle biopsy studies have failed to identify an increase in the oxidative enzymes after a period of training (Belman & Kendregan 1981). The American College of Sports Medicine (ACSM) (1991) proposes that aerobic training should be performed for 20–30 minutes, three to four times a week at an intensity that corresponds to approximately 50% of the individual's maximal oxygen consumption, if these effects are to be observed. For patients with chronic respiratory disease it may be possible to prescribe aerobic exercise, most commonly walking or cycling (i.e. lower limb activity, Fig. 14.2). A measure of peak oxygen consumption can be secured either directly or indirectly (laboratory- or field-based respectively) and thus an estimate of workload (i.e. speed of walking, resistance on cycle ergometer) at a level of 50% predicted peak oxygen consumption. Punzal et al (1991) suggested that it may be possible to train patients successfully at a higher level of predicted peak oxygen consumption. Although this intensity of training may be maximally effective in enhancing functional capacity, it may carry an increased risk of poor compliance and injury. For the majority of patients, frequent bouts of moderate intensity exercise will produce worthwhile effects. However, the optimal exercise intensity, duration and frequency has yet to be determined.

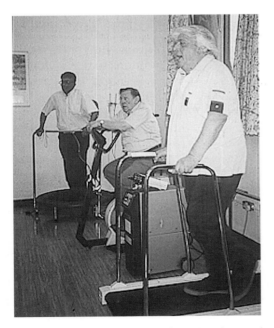

Fig. 14.2 Patients participating in an exercise session – aerobic exercise.

It is important that patients undertake exercise at home in between the hospital sessions. The duration, frequency and intensity of these home sessions must be identified and a record of the activity kept by the patient in an attempt to monitor progress and increase adherence. A typical programme for patients severely disabled by their disease may require them to walk for just 2–3 minutes at a steady pace twice daily, while for the more able patient, walking at the appropriate speed for 10 minutes daily may be indicated. Once the patient is able to achieve 20 minutes, the frequency can be reduced to five times weekly, as suggested by the ACSM (1991).

Prior to any bout of aerobic training a warm-up period is recommended (ACSM 1991). This brief 5- to 10-minute session is to increase the resting metabolic rate to an appropriate level for exercise training. The session can include gentle conditioning and stretching exercises; likewise a cool-down period is advisable, comprising activities that are less demanding than the training session and may even culminate in a period of relaxation.

Upper limb exercise. To perform activities of daily living a certain amount of upper limb strength and coordination is required. This is frequently lacking in patients with COPD, not least because of the dual action of many of the muscles around the shoulder girdle. In patients with COPD these muscles (accessory muscles) frequently assist the muscles of respiration. Therefore, by performing arm activities this support is lost and the load is forced back to the respiratory muscles and, of course, the diaphragm. Celli et al (1986) reported that upper limb activity hampers an already struggling diaphragm. Arm exercises appear to provoke a greater level of dyspnoea than leg exercises for a given energy expenditure. Not surprisingly, it is hypothesized that by training the upper limbs to be more efficient, the ventilatory requirements would be reduced for a similar level of work and the performance of the activities of daily living would improve. Lake et al (1990) randomized patients into one of three groups, upper limb activity, combined upper and lower limb training and a control group. Arm training improved upper limb endurance, but only the combined training regimen improved walking distance; i.e. the response is training specific. Results from the quality of life questionnaire revealed that an improvement in this parameter was observed again only in the combined training group. Interestingly a study by Ries et al (1988) reported that despite an improved cycle ergometer performance after upper limb training, the patients did not appear to improve their performance of the upper limb-based activities of daily living. All upper limb exercise needs to be combined with the regulation of respiration to produce exhalation on stretching or effort (Fig. 14.3).

Strength training. The vast majority of rehabilitation studies focus on endurance training regimens, but there may be a place for strength training (Fig. 14.4). Recently it has been suggested that fatigue of peripheral muscles could contribute to exercise limitation in patients with COPD. Gosselink et al (1996), following the work of Killian et al (1992), examined this relationship. The authors reported that in stepwise multiple regression, diffusing capacity, quadriceps force and the forced expiratory volume in one second (FEV_1) appeared to be significant determinants of maximal oxygen consumption. Simpson et al (1992) demonstrated the benefits of isolated muscle training (weight training) in patients with COPD. This study was able to report benefits measured as an increase in the strength of the muscle groups trained, an improved endurance capacity (cycle ergometer) and an improved quality of life. Clark et al (1996) have reported similar results for patients with mild COPD (FEV_1 64% predicted). An attractive feature of this study is that the exercise regimen can be replicated at home with ease, requiring no sophisticated equipment. The exercises incorporated into the programme were simple and included, for example, sitting to standing, walking on the spot, full arm circles and quadriceps exercises.

Ventilatory muscle training. The response of skeletal muscle training in pulmonary rehabilitation is well documented (Belman 1993). Respiratory muscles can be trained to improve strength and/or endurance in a similar way to skeletal muscle in other parts of the body

(Goldstein 1993). There is a suggestion that whole body exercise alone can improve respiratory muscle function. Martinez et al (1993) were able to demonstrate an improvement in inspiratory muscle strength and endurance after a rehabilitation programme incorporating unsupported arm exercises. It is believed that respiratory muscle training should result in

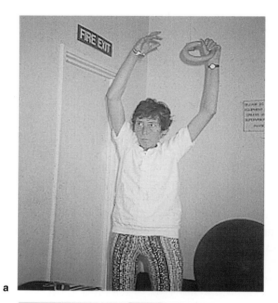

a

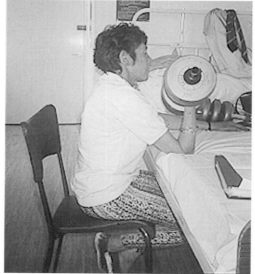

b

Fig. 14.3 Upper limb activity: **a** unsupported; **b** supported, resistive.

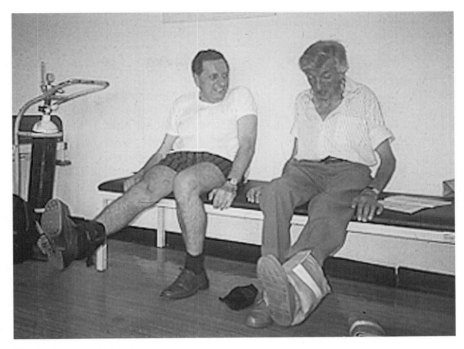

Fig. 14.4 Strength training.

improved function and thus decrease the effort of breathing, consequently reducing dyspnoea. In a similar way to conventional training, respiratory muscle training can be divided into strength and endurance training. Endurance training requires a low-intensity, high-frequency programme while a strength training programme requires a high-intensity load. This type of training has not gained acceptance in service-based rehabilitation programmes. This may in part be due to the lack of well-designed clinical trials and the vast repertoire of training methods. A report by Wanke et al (1994) suggested that respiratory muscle training may enhance the benefits acquired from an aerobic training programme. Considerably more research is necessary in this field before recommendations can be made about its inclusion into conventional pulmonary rehabilitation programmes.

Educational component

The education of patients with chronic disease is important regardless of the disease. Both the patients and their immediate carers and family need to understand about the disease itself and the management of it, the objectives of the programme, the methodologies to be used, and to jointly set and agree realistic goals that are achievable within the time frames set (Tiep 1993). The education in the programme needs to meet the health education aims of influencing beliefs, attitudes and behaviour (see Ch. 9) and a key feature of the health educators is to facilitate behaviour change (Kaplan et al 1993). Rehabilitation education may be individual but is more commonly offered in small groups (Petty 1993a). An example of the possible topics is given in Box 14.4. It is important that all the education provided to the patient is supplemented with handouts and pamphlets as patients need to be able to peruse the information at their leisure, to pick up things that they have missed in the session and to reinforce the information that they have gained. A few of these sessions are expanded below.

Box 14.4 Possible educational sessions within pulmonary rehabilitation

• Controlling breathlessness – breathing control/ positions
• Anatomy/physiology/pathophysiology
• Benefits of exercise
• Stress management/relaxation techniques
• Energy conservation/self-care/ADL/functional aids
• Airway clearance techniques
• Diet and nutrition – healthy eating/eating when unwell
• Medical management/when to seek help
• Medication
• Smoking
• Technological support:
  – O_2 (LTOT and portable)
  – nebulizers
  – ventilatory support
• Understanding physiological testing
• Social support network (benefits etc.)
• Psychological/emotional issues
• Self-help and support groups

Breathing retraining. Some form of breathing retraining, learning to control breathing and to pace activities are vital ingredients of any successful programme (Bott 1997). Teaching the patient to exhale on exertion and on bending and stretching activities will assist in the patient's ability to both exercise and perform functional tasks. Some physiotherapists may choose to teach pursed-lip breathing, commonly used in pulmonary rehabilitation programmes in the USA. Many patients with obstructive airways disease adopt this pattern of breathing quite naturally. However, Georgopoulos & Anthonisen (1991) reported that patients who do not naturally adopt pursed-lip breathing, but are taught it, do not find it helpful. It has been shown to have many beneficial effects, to decrease respiratory rate, increase tidal volume, increase oxygen saturation and decrease breathlessness during exercise (Thoman et al 1966, Mueller et al 1970, Tiep et al 1986). In addition, it has been shown to decrease ventilatory requirements. However, it has been postulated that pursed-lip breathing may produce a decrease in pulmonary blood flow and consequently cardiac output (Cameron & Bateman 1983). Should the client group require it, airway clearance techniques

can be included. Many of these patients will not suffer from excess secretions regularly, but only during an exacerbation. They may need to be taught independent techniques and given tips on other ways to assist with clearance such as using steam inhalations at home.

Energy conservation, activities of daily living and functional aids. It is commonly overlooked that patients with respiratory disorders may need devices such as 'helping hands', jar openers and other labour saving equipment to assist with difficult day-to-day activities which either require strength that they do not have, or involve reaching or bending activities that induce severe breathlessness. Many patients will require aids in the home to assist with bathing and general self-caring activities. Task organization and simplification are helpful for finding ways around common and difficult daily activities. Collecting all the items for a task in one place simplifies the task and reduces the energy cost. General advice on bathing, such as collecting all the clothes in advance, using a towelling robe instead of a towel to dry off, and thereby avoiding excess energy expenditure, running a shallow bath to avoid breathlessness or substituting a shower are all useful hints. Advice on dressing, such as dressing the lower half first, then sitting to dress the upper body, should also be included. Where possible, sitting down to perform tasks involving use of the upper limbs conserves valuable energy and a perching stool could prove useful in, for example, the kitchen. In particular, supporting the elbows for activities such as peeling potatoes, shaving and hair grooming assists enormously with these activities and needs to be taught.

Medication. It is essential that the drug therapy is optimized for the patient prior to entry into pulmonary rehabilitation. However, educational sessions on medication, the use of inhalers and nebulizers and general queries regarding the common drugs that patients may take are useful. Action of drugs, side-effects and types of devices that the patient uses can be discussed.

Diet and nutrition. Many patients with chronic respiratory disease have nutritional problems or eating difficulties, despite apparent normal body weight. Advice on healthy eating and how to keep well nourished during bouts of extreme breathlessness and infection are important. Specific problems, such as the need to reduce or increase weight can be addressed, individually if necessary. Patients who are over- or underweight have additional difficulties and every effort should be made to assist with the understanding and correction of these problems.

Technological support. It may be that some of the patients within a pulmonary rehabilitation programme require equipment to assist their daily life. Some patients entering a pulmonary rehabilitation programme will fit the criteria for long-term oxygen therapy (LTOT) and will already be using oxygen at home. Discussion and education about the use of oxygen are an essential part of the programme in this instance. There is an increased benefit shown when oxygen is given in the ambulatory form (Nocturnal Oxygen Therapy Trial Group 1980). This may be an increase in exercise capacity, participation in normal activities and social pursuits (Petty 1993a). In addition, the correct prescription and provision of compressors and nebulizers are equally important. For some patients the use of non-invasive positive pressure ventilation at night is an essential part of their care to prevent worsening respiratory failure (Muir 1993).

Travel. It is helpful for patients to be aware of special equipment that may be necessary to enable them to travel, in addition to advice and help in arranging travel plans. Issues such as contacting the airline in advance if the patient wishes to fly, and arranging oxygen either on board a flight, boat, coach, etc. or at a destination, need addressing. It is advisable to be well rested before travelling and to arrive at the airport or station well in advance of the travel time. Airlines will need information such as age, gender, diagnosis and clinical state of the patient and the oxygen flow rate required if oxygen is to be provided. In addition an airline will need information on the equipment the patient will carry as some devices may interfere with aircraft equipment. Hypoglycaemia can be minimized by eating small amounts regularly. If flying, a low salt diet may minimize oedema and should be requested in advance (Smeets 1994).

Emotional/psychosocial support. Depending on experience and training, the social worker, the occupational therapist, the physiotherapist, the psychologist, or a combination of these professionals may provide psychosocial help for the patients in the programme. The psychosocial impact of chronic disease on an individual should not be underestimated. Individuals will find that their chest disease can be debilitating, decrease their energy levels and ability for self-expression, increase self-consciousness and neediness and may create dependency on others. They may question the changes they have had to make and what they have had to give up, and need help with coming to terms with grief and loss, which may involve a lot of pain, anger and sadness. The bereavement process is one commonly attributed to death, but is a process that individuals with disease need to go through when giving up something, either tangible, such as a limb, or intangible, such as a way of life or certain activities. Chronic respiratory disease is extremely debilitating and in some part may take away the common gender roles for some individuals. For men, the inability, for example, to wash the car, carry the shopping, perform simple 'do-it-yourself' (DIY) tasks is quite an emasculating process. For women, being unable to provide a spick and span house, shop and cook effectively and generally care for their household members may be equally problematic. The individuals providing the psychosocial support, and preferably the whole team, need to be aware of all these issues for the patients, encourage them to vocalize the things that are hardest for them to come to terms with, and help them talk about and deal with the difficulties, stresses and strains of living with such a disease.

The psychosocial support provided within the programme should be non-judgemental, warm and confidential; it should provide support, with structure, in a safe environment. Allowing patients to own and accept their feelings is vital, as is facilitating the contact and discussion with others, both health care workers in their role and other patients who are facing similar situations.

Communication skills are vital to the physio-therapist in this situation and the additional skill of counselling would prove helpful (see Ch. 9). As well as practical support with finances or employment issues, discussions around relationships and changing relationships because of the disease are important, both with partner or spouse, dependants, and extended family and friends. Not to be forgotten is the issue of 'self' such as body image, self-image and sexuality. Patients may have had plans, dreams and ambitions that have come to nought as their disease has taken hold of their life, and rather than being able to enjoy retirement and carry on with the activities they had promised themselves in their youth, they find that they are confined to a far less active lifestyle than they had envisaged. The group setting of pulmonary rehabilitation, with sensitive facilitation, can provide hope and 'growth'. It may be for many of these individuals the first shared experience of some of their more negative feelings connected with their disease. For the first time since having the disease they may feel able to give to others and contribute to the group, and the group may provide gentle encouragement to move on to self-help and new ideas in dealing with their condition. The group setting helps reduce isolation, which for many people is a big issue when confined to the house with a debilitating disease, helps reduce self-consciousness and create links with others in a similar situation. Patients may learn self-value again in supporting others, feeling needed and assisting the other members of the team in any way that they can.

Maintenance and support. It is essential for the success of any programme that the patients have access to a support group or some form of maintenance therapy following cessation of the programme. These opportunities are present in the most successful groups in the USA and social or self-help support systems may include self-help groups, newsletters, activities such as meetings or get togethers, talks on appropriate issues, social outings and celebrations (Petty 1993a).

OUTCOME MEASURES

There is increasing pressure upon the providers of a pulmonary rehabilitation service to supply tangible evidence of its effectiveness to purchasers of the service. Consequently there is a need to collect reliable meaningful data. Traditionally for rehabilitation this has taken the form of exercise testing, although increasingly the measurements of dyspnoea and quality of life are gaining importance. Outcome measures are broadly those measurement tools employed at the time of the initial assessment and repeated at the time of graduation with additional follow-up assessment visits being a possibility. Information on the cost–benefit analysis, of obvious interest to the purchasers, is currently sparse but needs to be addressed by the collection of such data as hospital admissions and clinic and general practitioner visits.

CONCLUSION

It can be seen that pulmonary rehabilitation is a complex therapy providing a holistic approach to treatment with the vital ingredient of a multi-disciplinary input. The professionals need to impart to patients all the information and resources that they have available to them to assist the patients in maximizing their function and activities. It needs to be personally oriented and comprehensive and provide a form of integrated care beyond ordinary outpatient care (Petty 1993a), incorporating both physical and emotional support, and education.

REFERENCES

American College of Sports Medicine 1991 Guidelines for exercise testing and prescription, 4th edn. Lea & Febiger, Pennsylvania
Belman M J 1993 Pulmonary rehabilitation in chronic

respiratory insufficiency: 2 – exercise in patients with chronic obstructive pulmonary disease. Thorax 48: 936–946
Belman M J, Kendregan B A 1981 Exercise training fails to increase skeletal muscle enzymes in patients with chronic

obstructive pulmonary disease. American Review of Respiratory Disease 123: 256–261

Bestall J C, Garrod R, Garnham E A, Paul E A, Jones P W, Wedzicha J A 1996 The MRC breathlessness score as a means of stratification of COPD patients for pulmonary rehabilitation. European Respiratory Journal 9: 383s

Borg G A V 1982 Psychophysical basis of perceived exertion. Medicine Science Sport Exercise 14: 377–381

Bott J 1997 Physiotherapy. In: Morgan M D L, Singh S J (eds) Practical pulmonary rehabilitation. Chapman & Hall, London

Bowling A 1995 Measuring disease: a review of disease specific quality of life measurement scales. Open University Press, Buckingham

Bowling A 1997 Measuring health: a review of quality of life measurement scales, 2nd edn. Open University Press, Buckingham

Butland R J A, Pang J, Gross E R, Woodcock A A, Geddes D M 1982 Two-, six- and twelve-minute walking tests in respiratory disease. British Medical Journal 284: 1607–1608

Cameron I R, Bateman N T 1983 Respiratory disorders. Edward Arnold, London, p 75

Casaburi R, Petty T L (eds) 1993 Principles and practice of pulmonary rehabilitation. W B Saunders, Philadelphia

Casaburi R, Patessio A, Ioli F, Zanaboni S, Donner C F, Wasserman K 1991 Reduction in exercise lactic acidosis and ventilation as a result of exercise training in patients with chronic lung disease. American Review of Respiratory Disease 143: 9–18

Celli B R 1995 Pulmonary rehabilitation in patients with COPD. American Journal of Respiratory and Critical Care Medicine 152: 861–864

Celli B R, Rassulo J, Make B J 1986 Dyssynchronous breathing during arm exercises but not leg exercises in patients with chronic airflow obstruction. New England Journal of Medicine 314: 1485–1490

Clark C, Cochrane L, Mackay E 1996 Low intensity peripheral muscle conditioning improves exercise tolerance and breathlessness in COPD. European Respiratory Journal 9: 2590–2596

Cox N J M, Hendricks J C, Binkhorst R A, van Herwaarden C L A 1993 A pulmonary rehabilitation program for patients with asthma and mild chronic obstructive pulmonary diseases (COPD). Lung 171: 235–244

Fishman A P 1994 Pulmonary rehabilitation research. NIH workshop summary. American review of Respiratory Disease 49: 825–830

Foster S, Thomas H M 1990 Pulmonary rehabilitation in lung disease other than chronic obstructive pulmonary disease. American Review of Respiratory Disease 141: 601–604

Georgopoulos D, Anthonisen N R 1991 Symptoms and signs of COPD. In: Cherniack N S (ed) Chronic obstructive pulmonary disease. W B Saunders, Philadelphia, p 357

Goldstein R S 1993 Pulmonary rehabilitation in chronic respiratory insufficiency: 3 – ventilatory muscle training. Thorax 48: 1025–1033

Goldstein R S, Gort E H, Stubbing D, Avendano M A, Guyatt G H 1994 Randomised controlled trial of respiratory rehabilitation. Lancet 334: 1394–1397

Gosselink R, Troosters T, Decramer M 1996 Peripheral muscle weakness contributes to exercise limitation in COPD. American Journal of Respiratory and Critical Care Medicine 153: 976–980

Haas A, Cardon H 1969 Rehabilitation in chronic obstructive pulmonary disease; a five year study of 252 patients. Medical Clinics of North America 53: 593–607

Harris P L 1985 A guide to prescribing pulmonary rehabilitation. Primary Care 12(2): 253–266

Henriksson J, Reitman J S 1977 Time course of changes in skeletal muscle succinate dehydrogenase and cytochrome oxidase activities and maximal oxygen uptake with physical activity and inactivity. Acta Physiologica Scandinavica 99: 91–97

Hudson L D, Tyler M L, Petty T L 1976 Hospitalisation needs during out patient rehabilitation programme for severe COA. Chest 70: 606–610

Hyland M E, Bott J, Singh S, Kenyon C A P 1994 Domains, constructs and the development of the breathing problems questionnaire. Quality of Life Research 3: 245–256

Kaplan R M, Eakin E G, Ries A L 1993 Psychosocial issues in the rehabilitation of patients with chronic obstructive pulmonary disease. In: Casaburi R, Petty T L (eds) Principles and practice of pulmonary rehabilitation. W B Saunders, Philadelphia, pp 356–359

Killian J, LeBlanc P, Martin D H, Summers E, Jones N, Campbell E J M 1992 Exercise capacity and ventilatory, circulatory, and symptom limitation in patients with chronic airflow limitation. American Review of Respiratory Disease 146: 935–940

Lacasse Y, Wong E, Guyatt G H, King D, Cook D, Goldstein R 1996 Meta-analysis of respiratory rehabilitation in chronic obstructive pulmonary disease. Lancet 348: 1115–1119

Lake F R, Henderson K, Briffa T, Oppenshaw J, Musk A W 1990 Upper limb and lower limb exercise training in patients with chronic airflow obstruction. Chest 97: 1077–1082

McGavin C R, Gupta S P, McHardy G J R 1976 Twelve-minute walking test for assessing disability in chronic bronchitis. British Medical Journal 1: 822–823

Make B J 1986 Pulmonary rehabilitation. Clinics in Chest Medicine 7: 519–702

Martinez F J, Vogel P D, Dupont D N, Stanopoulos I, Gray A, Beamis J F 1993 Supported arm exercise vs unsupported arm exercise in the rehabilitation of patients with severe chronic airflow obstruction. Chest 103: 1397–1402

Medical Research Council 1966 Committee on research into chronic bronchitis: instructions for use on the questionnaire on respiratory symptoms. W J Holman, Devon

Mueller R E, Petty T L, Filley G F 1970 Ventilation and arterial blood gas changes induced by pursed lips breathing. Journal of Applied Physiology 28: 784–789

Muir J F 1993 Pulmonary rehabilitation in chronic respiratory insufficiency: 5 – home mechanical ventilation. Thorax 48: 1264–1273

Muir J F, Pierson D J 1993 Pulmonary rehabilitation in chronic respiratory insufficiency: introduction. Thorax 48: 854

Nocturnal Oxygen Therapy Trial Group 1980 Continuous or nocturnal oxygen therapy in hypoxemic chronic obstructive lung disease: a clinical trial. Annals of Internal Medicine 93: 391–398

Novitch R S, Thomas H M 1993 Rehabilitation of patients with chronic ventilatory limitation from non-obstructive lung diseases. In: Casaburi R, Petty T L (eds) Principles and practice of pulmonary rehabilitation. W B Saunders, Philadelphia, pp 416–423

Petty T L 1993a Pulmonary rehabilitation in chronic respiratory insufficiency: 1 – pulmonary rehabilitation in perspective: historical roots, present status, and future projections. Thorax 48: 855–862

Petty T L 1993b Pulmonary rehabilitation – a personal historical perspective. In: Casaburi R, Petty T L (eds) Principles and practice of pulmonary rehabilitation. W B Saunders, Philadelphia, pp 1–8

Punzal P A, Ries A L, Kaplan R M, Prewitt L M 1991 Maximum intensity exercise training in patients with chronic obstructive pulmonary disease. Chest 100: 618–623

Reardon J, Awad E, Normandin E, Vale F, Clark B, ZuWallack R L 1994 The effect of comprehensive outpatient pulmonary rehabilitation on dyspnea. Chest 105: 1046–1052

Ries A L, Ellis B, Hawkins R W 1988 Upper extremity exercise training in chronic obstructive pulmonary disease. Chest 93: 688–692

Saltin B, Gollnick P D 1983 Skeletal muscle adaptability: significance for metabolism and performance. In: Peachey L (ed) Handbook of physiology – skeletal muscle. American Physiological Society, Bethesda, Maryland, pp 555–631

Simonds A K 1996 Pulmonary rehabilitation in non-COPD disorders. In: Simonds A K, Muir J F, Pierson P J (eds) Pulmonary rehabilitation. BMJ Publishing Group, London, pp 212–235

Simonds A K, Muir J F, Pierson P J (eds) 1996 Pulmonary rehabilitation. BMJ Publishing Group, London

Simpson K, Killian K, McCartney N, Stubbing D G, Jones N L 1992 Randomised controlled trial of weight lifting in patients with chronic airflow limitation. Thorax 47: 70–75

Singh S J 1997 Patient selection and assessment. In: Morgan M D L, Singh S J (eds) Practical pulmonary rehabilitation. Chapman & Hall, London

Singh S J, Morgan M D L, Scott S C, Walters D, Hardman A E 1992 The development of the shuttle walking test of disability in patients with chronic airways obstruction. Thorax 47: 1019–1024

Singh S J, Morgan M D L, Hardman A E, Rowe C, Bardsley P A 1994 Comparison of oxygen uptake during a conventional treadmill test and the shuttle walking test in chronic airflow limitation. European Respiratory Journal 7: 2016–2020

Singh S J, Smith D L, Morgan M D L 1996 Out-patient pulmonary rehabilitation without maintenance in the UK: immediate and long term gains. European Respiratory Journal 9: 382s

Smeets F 1994 Pulmonary rehabilitation in chronic respiratory insufficiency: 6 – travel for technology-dependent patients with respiratory disease. Thorax 49: 77–81

Swinburn C R, Wakefield J M, Jones P W 1985 Performance, ventilation and oxygen consumption in three different types of exercise tests in patients with chronic obstructive lung disease. Thorax 40: 581–586

Thoman R L, Stoker G L, Ross J C 1966 The efficacy of pursed-lips breathing in patients with chronic obstructive pulmonary disease. American Review of Respiratory Disease 93: 100–106

Tiep B L 1993 Pulmonary rehabilitation program organization. In: Casaburi R, Petty T L (eds) Principles and practice of pulmonary rehabilitation. W B Saunders, Philadelphia, p 302

Tiep B L, Burns M, Kao D, Madison R, Herrera J 1986 Pursed lips breathing training using ear oximetry. Chest 90(2): 218–221

Wijkstra P J, Ten Vergert E M, Van Alten A R, Otten V, Kraan J, Postma D S, Koeter G H 1995 Long term benefits of rehabilitation at home on quality of life and exercise tolerance in patients with chronic obstructive pulmonary disease. Thorax 50: 824–828

Wanke T, Formanek D, Lahrmann H, Brath H, Wild M, Wagner C, Zwick H 1994 Effects of combined inspiratory muscle and cycle ergometer training on exercise performance in patient's with COPD. European Respiratory Journal 7: 2205–2211

15

Cardiac rehabilitation

Helen McBurney

INTRODUCTION

Since the realization in the 1940s and 1950s that long-term bed rest, the standard medical practice of the times for post-myocardial infarction (MI) patients, was in fact detrimental both physically and psychologically (Levine & Lown 1952, Newman et al 1952), efforts have been made to address these problems. Cardiac rehabilitation, including secondary prevention has become an important part of the management of patients both post-MI and post-coronary artery bypass graft surgery (CABGS).

Goals of cardiac rehabilitation

In 1993 the World Health Organization (WHO) defined cardiac rehabilitation as: 'the sum of activities required to influence favourably the underlying cause of the disease, as well as the best possible physical, mental and social conditions so that they may, by their own efforts preserve or resume when lost, as normal a place as possible in the community.'

Thus the major goal of a comprehensive cardiac rehabilitation programme is the achievement of an optimal health status for each patient, and the maintenance of this status, not only physically and psychologically but also in social, vocational and economic terms.

More specific goals of a cardiac rehabilitation or secondary prevention programme may include:

• The limitation of adverse effects of illness

- Efficient and effective symptom management
- Stratification of risk for a further cardiac event to assist in clinical decision making regarding further treatment
- Modification of cardiac risk factors to prevent progression of ischaemic heart disease as far as possible.

In order to achieve both a good functional capacity and a good quality of life, cardiac rehabilitation should not be equated with exercise alone but should also include education and counselling so that patients eventually become responsible for a large part of their own management. Ideally, rehabilitation should begin at the time of admission to hospital and continue after discharge (Hare 1990).

Cardiac rehabilitation team

A comprehensive cardiac rehabilitation programme will include a wide range of skilled health professional staff with a flexible approach to the provision of rehabilitation services. The patient's support people, family and / or close friends are an important part of any rehabilitation team and can greatly influence outcome.

The larger the team the greater the need for clear, concise communication between staff, patient and support persons to clarify problems, goals, treatment and outcomes.

In a smaller setting a wide range of professional staff may not be available. Overlap in the training of health professionals assists in the provision of quality care. Sometimes it will be necessary for staff to recognize their lack of expertise in a specific area and refer the patient on for specialist assistance. However, not every patient will require the help of every profession.

Role of the physiotherapist

The physiotherapist is primarily concerned with physical aspects of recovery, especially minimizing the deconditioning effects of bed rest and enhancing cardiovascular and musculoskeletal functioning. Initially this will involve assessment, perhaps breathing exercises and assisted or active exercises for some patients, supervised ambulation, stair climbing and other activities. Instruction in home exercise, self-monitoring and provision of activity guidelines are important functions.

The physiotherapist may encourage attendance at an outpatient programme and should report on the patient's physical progress to the team. Worcester (1986) found it appropriate that the physiotherapist should coordinate and conduct the exercise programme, liaising with other staff as required, because of the significant physiological and medical components of a physiotherapist's training. Other aspects of cardiac rehabilitation which may be carried out by the physiotherapist include: relaxation training, investigation of work potential and simulated work testing and, where specifically trained, exercise testing.

RATIONALE FOR CARDIAC REHABILITATION

Early ambulation

Early management of the post-MI patient is based on two conflicting needs: the need for restricted activity to avoid complications and the need for activity to avoid the undesirable effects of bed rest. Levine & Lown (1952) and Newman et al (1952) recognized this problem in their clinical settings and began supervised activity programmes for their post-MI patients, provided that they were not suffering any complications.

A randomized controlled trial of early mobilization after acute MI was conducted by Bloch et al (1974). Patients ($n = 154$) were assigned either to an early mobilization group which began supervised activity on day 2 or 3 post-MI, or to a usual hospital care group who underwent 3 weeks of strict bed rest. The authors found no differences in complication rates in the first 6 months, a significant decrease in the duration of hospitalization for the early ambulation group, and significantly greater disability in the control group on follow-up. The results of this study confirmed clinical observations of the benefits of early mobilization.

Many authors such as Haskell (1994) confirm that this approach is safe. Fears of exercise having adverse effects such as weakening of the healing myocardium, myocardial rupture or major arrhythmias should be allayed by the number of well-designed and positive trials.

Exercise training

In the post-MI and post-CABGS period the natural process of recovery and resumption of normal physical activity will result in some improvement in functional capacity. DeBusk et al (1979) found an increase of one third in exercise tolerance between weeks 3 and 11 post-MI. Training augmented improvement in exercise tolerance by a small amount (DeBusk et al 1979). Lipkin (1991) reported 15–25% increases in exercise tolerance associated with physical training in the short term. Increased maximal oxygen uptake can be achieved in the coronary heart disease patient via the same mechanisms of peripheral adaptation as in normal subjects. Astrand & Rodahl (1986) detail these changes. The principal advantage of training is an increased tolerance for usual activity, which requires a lower percentage of maximal oxygen uptake. In patients with angina pectoris, increases in activity before onset of symptoms are usually noted.

Habitual physical activity has been shown to lower the risk of coronary heart disease (Blair et al 1995). Risk factors favourably altered by exercise included blood pressure, weight and blood lipid profiles. Importantly these studies demonstrated that moderate intensity exercise is sufficient to provide significant risk reduction, so that high levels of physical fitness are not necessary for a favourable outcome. In contrast to previous belief it appears that the total weekly exercise energy consumption is more important than the duration and intensity of each individual exercise session.

Another reason often given for exercise training in cardiac rehabilitation is that of improved psychological well being. Newman et al (1952) and Levine & Lown (1952) certainly noted deleterious psychological effects of prolonged bed rest on their subjects and commented that these were lessened by activity programmes. Oldridge & Rogowski (1990) demonstrated an increase in self-efficacy scores associated with a ward ambulation programme for post-MI patients. Lavie & Milani (1995) showed improvement in quality of life measures in post-MI patients after a cardiac rehabilitation and exercise programme. At present there is no evidence in favour of rehabilitation programmes based purely on psychological therapy, counselling, relaxation training and stress management (Jones & West 1996).

Secondary prevention

There is evidence that regular exercise reduces the possibility of recurrence of MI, other clinical signs of ischaemic heart disease and associated mortality. Supporting data are provided by Leon et al (1987) who have demonstrated the necessity for long-term moderate exercise in the population at large in order to reduce the risk of coronary heart disease and have shown that current habitual activity level is the important factor. Participation in exercise even at an elite athletic level in the past has little bearing on current risk. Kallio et al (1979) and Hamalainen et al (1989) have used a multiple risk factor intervention approach in two Finnish populations. At follow-up the cumulative mortality rate was significantly smaller in the intervention group.

Education

The current emphasis in health care is on individuals making informed decisions regarding their management and taking responsibility for their own health and care (Doughty 1991).

Education, especially information regarding smoking, diet, weight, blood pressure and exercise is important for effective secondary prevention (Worcester 1986). To facilitate return to normal living, most patients post-MI or post-CABGS will require some information and guidelines to resume driving, work and other activities. Motivation to comply with advice has been linked to the understanding of illness and the need for risk factor modification (Worcester 1986).

The responsibility for patient education can be shared by all disciplines involved in cardiac rehabilitation (Davidson & Maloney 1985). It is important that advice is consistent and not confusing. Verbal, written and audiovisual material may be used. Worcester (1986) advocates the use of small discussion groups as active involvement achieves better understanding and opportunity for clarification than a lecture format.

The inclusion of partner, family or friend is recommended (Davidson & Maloney 1985, Worcester 1986) as this lessens misunderstandings during convalescence and the support of a partner can enhance motivation and adoption of a healthy lifestyle.

Caine et al (1991) found that attention to the quality of information given to CABGS patients, relatives and the community, especially employers, helped to improve outcome. Post-discharge depression, denial or anxiety may make this time especially difficult for the partner and participation in an outpatient programme can support both patient and spouse.

MANIFESTATIONS OF ISCHAEMIC HEART DISEASE

Ischaemic heart disease (IHD) is used synonymously with the term 'coronary heart disease' and refers to impairment of the cardiac muscle due to imbalance between coronary blood flow and myocardial needs caused by changes in the coronary circulation (Joint International Society 1979).

The various forms or manifestations of IHD are usually defined separately and include:

- Cardiac arrest
- Angina pectoris
- Myocardial infarction.

Cardiac arrest

This is a sudden event where there is no evidence for any other diagnosis. If resuscitation is not attempted or is unsuccessful then this is usually referred to as sudden death.

Angina pectoris

This is a symptom of myocardial ischaemia, episodic in nature and classically described as central chest or retrosternal pain. Angina can vary considerably from person to person, but usually remains constant in the individual patient (Gazes 1990). Angina may be described according to its location, quality, duration, intensity, and precipitating factors.

Location. Classical angina is retrosternal but it may radiate to or only be felt in the jaw, neck, back, shoulders and arms, more commonly on the left. Differential diagnosis is therefore extremely important in patients presenting with intermittent pain in these areas.

Quality. The sensation of angina is not always described by patients as 'pain'. Common alternatives are discomfort, burning, pressing or a squeezing sensation.

Duration. Angina is intermittent and onset is usually associated with a critical level of physical activity. The feeling may develop gradually and mount in intensity, but subsides quickly with rest or with sublingual nitroglycerin.

Intensity. Angina is often variously described as a 'mild ache', pressing or constricting but is rarely excruciating or intolerable.

Precipitating factors. Angina is usually brought on by an increase in myocardial work so that local oxygen consumption exceeds the supply capacity of the coronary vessels. Exercise is the most common precipitating factor. Some patients may have spontaneous or rest angina which occurs without apparent relation to increased myocardial work and may be due to factors such as coronary artery spasm.

Angina may be classified as 'stable' when the same factor induces the same sensation repeatedly, or 'unstable' when the sensation occurs spontaneously or is occurring with increasing frequency or severity or is caused by a lessening amount of effort.

Myocardial infarction

The clinical diagnosis of acute myocardial infarction (MI) is usually based on the patient history, electrocardiograph (ECG) changes and the elevation of serum enzymes.

History. The pain associated with myocardial infarction is usually similar in location to that of angina but is more severe and prolonged (more than 30 minutes). It is not relieved by nitroglycerin and may be accompanied by sweatiness, pallor, nausea and vomiting.

ECG. Unequivocal changes involve the development of persistent abnormally large Q waves. The evolution of ST/T wave changes with concomitant enzyme changes is also diagnostic.

Serum enzymes. These are released from irreversibly damaged myocardial cells into the circulation. The rise and fall of serum enzyme levels should be related to the time of cellular injury and is specific for each enzyme measured.

The Joint International Society (1979) states that diagnosis of definite acute MI requires unequivocal ECG changes and/or unequivocal enzyme changes with or without a typical history.

Physical complications. These are many and may include:

1. Rhythm and conduction disturbances – when the conduction system is involved in the MI or if a portion of the myocardium becomes less electrically stable.
2. Heart failure – the consequence of which may be minor or may include pulmonary oedema or shock.
3. Recurrent MI – occurs in 15–20% of MI patients during their initial hospitalization, especially in those who experience unstable angina early post-MI, who have a subendocardial (partial wall thickness) infarct and in those who experience angina and/or breathlessness on early mobilization (Jelinek 1988).
4. Pericarditis (p. 257).
5. Rupture of the myocardial wall – occurs in about 1% of patients and can cause tamponade or a ventricular septal defect. Rupture of papillary muscles may allow valvular regurgitation.
6. Systemic or pulmonary thromboembolism.

Other complications of MI may be anxiety and depression, and/or economic problems due to temporary or permanent loss of earnings.

Cardiac surgery

Many patients with some form of cardiac disorder may undergo cardiac surgery. This may be coronary artery bypass grafts, valvular repair or replacement, or repair of a congenital defect. The early postoperative management of these patients is discussed in Chapter 12.

Many of these patients require ongoing rehabilitation similar in principle to that of any medical cardiac patient in order to make long-term lifestyle adjustments. There are a few postoperative problems which will need consideration and have important implications for a postoperative programme.

Pain. Because consolidation of the sternum takes 2–3 months, many patients will experience pain in this area for this time. Muscular aches and pain in the chest, shoulders, neck and back, and rib pain are also common. Management should include the use of pain-relieving medication, especially prior to activity and continuation of range of movement exercises, until full active range of movement is achieved without pain. Soft tissue techniques such as massage may also be of use.

Fatigue. This is common in the early postoperative period. It is important that there is a balance between activity and rest and a conscious effort should be made to increase activity gradually.

Mood. After discharge from hospital mild depression is common. Most patients will recover spontaneously and find the stimulation of attending a cardiac rehabilitation programme helpful. A few will have a deep and persistent problem requiring professional help.

Visual changes. Blurring of vision may occur postoperatively but should resolve spontaneously over the first few months.

Concentration and memory. These are often poor in the early postoperative phase but should improve slowly.

Constipation. This is not unusual in patients taking some pain-relieving medications, but it may cause discomfort and require the use of a laxative.

Palpitations. Many patients are more aware of their heart beat postoperatively as it is often faster for the first few months. Frequent or persistent bouts of palpitations should be reported to the doctor for investigation and management.

Drugs to control the cardiovascular system

Medications involved in the control of the cardiovascular system are too numerous to mention individually, so only those categories of medication which affect exercise are mentioned here.

Beta-adrenergic blocking agents

Beta blockers are used to reduce myocardial oxygen demand by decreasing myocardial contractility, heart rate and systolic blood pressure.

Beta-blocking medication can be cardioselective and specifically act to inhibit β receptors which mediate cardiac stimulation, or it may be non-selective and act on both β_1 and β_2 receptors so that vascular and bronchial smooth muscle contraction is affected. The selectivity of all beta-blocking medications has been noted to be dose related, as the dose increases selectivity decreases. At high doses or with a non-selective beta blocker, bronchospasm and peripheral vasoconstriction may be undesired side-effects (Frishman & Teicher 1985).

Beta blockers have been shown to lower heart rate substantially both at rest and at any given exercise intensity. Exercise prescription for a patient on beta blockers should be made with this in mind. The lower heart rate and blood pressure will reduce myocardial oxygen demand and may allow the patient to achieve a higher workload before exertional angina is experienced. However, the peak workload achieved by a patient on beta blockers may be less than without the medication. Beta blockers reduce myocardial contractility and thus may precipitate or potentiate cardiac failure. As beta blockers vary in duration of action, exercise sessions performed hours after taking medication may result in a greater heart rate response than exercise performed close to the time of taking medication.

Some distressing side-effects may be experienced by patients taking beta blockers, including fatigue, bradycardia, impotence and vivid dreams. Sudden cessation of this type of medication can cause rebound phenomena such as reflex tachycardia, hypertension or angina.

Heart rate may not accurately reflect the exercise stress imposed by a given level of work in a patient taking beta blockers. Rating of perceived exertion (RPE) and/or respiratory rate are alternative forms of monitoring (Eston & Connolly 1996).

Nitrates

Nitrates cause dilatation of both the arterial and venous circulation by relaxation of smooth muscle in vessel walls and thereby reduce work of the heart by decreased peripheral resistance and decreased venous return. This may allow an improved exercise capacity by increasing the anginal threshold. Nitrates can be used prior to exercise to eliminate or reduce the likelihood of occurrence of angina. Hypotension may occur in patients on nitrates if they cease exercise abruptly, so an effective cool-down is important.

Vasodilators

Other vasodilating medications also have the potential to produce post-exercise hypotension if activity is abruptly ceased. Allowance for an adequate cool-down should effectively prevent this.

PHYSIOTHERAPY

Assessment

Cardiac rehabilitation may be commenced before a patient with angina experiences any further event, or more often commences during an inpatient stay after an acute MI, percutaneous transluminal coronary angioplasty (PTCA) or CABGS. In any situation some basic assessment is necessary prior to beginning a rehabilitation programme.

Demographic data. These can usually be

obtained from the patient's medical record and should include age, address and some social information, especially occupation, interests and the main support person or people who should be included in as much of the cardiac programme as is practicable.

In order to define the scope of cardiac dysfunction, information regarding the cardiac status of the individual should be sought.

Date of cardiac event. This should be considered. In a surgical patient rate of healing of the sternum may alter activities. The question of whether the surgical patient has had a previous, intra- or postoperative MI and the functional outcome after this should also be investigated. In a medical patient, some natural recovery of ventricular function will occur with time.

Site of MI. This may affect the outcome and may be roughly mapped out from a consideration of 12-lead ECG traces showing changes post-MI. More detailed mapping of the site of myocardial damage may be obtained from investigations such as radionuclide ventriculography or ^{99}Tn infarct imaging.

Size of MI. This may be estimated from the amount of serum cardiac enzyme elevation in a patient not given thrombolytic therapy.

Current management. At the start of the programme this will include therapy aimed at reduction of cardiac risk factors, such as medications, exercise, diet and smoking cessation. Some patients will experience considerable difficulty and stress in undertaking many major lifestyle changes at one time. These people may need additional support and assistance with many aspects of their management and may find it better to concentrate on one problem at a time.

Current signs and symptoms. The signs and symptoms presenting at the time of beginning a programme and the level of activity at which these occur can give a guide to the level at which exercise should be started. In particular, any anginal symptoms or symptoms of cardiac failure (undue breathlessness, pallor, dizziness, coldness and undue perspiration) associated with activity should be noted. It is helpful to have exercise test results to guide exercise prescription, but often these are not available. A record

of recent premorbid activity and any limitations to this may be helpful.

Medications. These are frequently prescribed for the management of the cardiovascular system and for any other medical condition of patients involved in a cardiac rehabilitation programme. Some of these medications will have an impact on the cardiovascular, respiratory and/or metabolic response to exercise.

Familiarity with medications enables the physiotherapist to provide a better service through comprehensive evaluation, increased awareness of potential problems or necessary treatment programme modifications related to medication, feedback to the physician regarding the efficacy or side-effects of medication changes, patient education to improve compliance and enhanced safety of a treatment programme (Ice 1985).

Occupational and recreational activities. These are important to the individual and should be considered in defining goals for outcome. Driving a car, sexual activity and occupation are major concerns of many patients. The demands of these activities may need assessment on an individual basis. Astrand & Rodahl (1986) have established that a work level of 30–40% of maximum aerobic capacity can be sustained for an 8-hour day without symptoms of fatigue.

Current functional level. This needs to be clearly defined at the start of any programme. Subjective and objective information may be used to establish this.

Functional physical capacity was defined by the New York Heart Association (NYHA) on a simple four-class scale assessing symptoms of fatigue, palpitations, breathlessness and angina (Hurst 1974). This is now referred to as the 'Old NYHA scale' (Hurst et al 1990). The criteria for classification of each class are outlined in Table 15.1. Although this classification system was superseded in 1973 by a broader approach, it is often still referred to clinically. The Canadian Cardiovascular Society used a similar four-point scale to describe the amount of effort needed to produce angina. This is outlined in Table 15.2. These scales are intended to classify patients by rating the severity of their symptoms.

Table 15.1 Old New York Heart Association criteria for classification of functional capacity

Class I	Patients with heart disease who have no symptoms of any kind with ordinary physical activity
Class II	Patients who are comfortable at rest but have symptoms with ordinary physical activity
Class III	Patients who are comfortable at rest but have symptoms with less than ordinary activity
Class IV	Patients who have symptoms at rest

Table 15.2 Canadian Cardiovascular Society Classification of angina pectoris

Class 1	Ordinary activity does not cause angina. (Angina may occur with strenuous or prolonged or rapid exertion)
Class 2	Slight limitations to ordinary activity. (Angina with walking or stair climbing rapidly, walking uphill, walking or stair climbing in cold or wind or after a meal)
Class 3	Marked limitation of ordinary activity. (Angina on walking one to two blocks on the level or climbing a flight of stairs at normal pace)
Class 4	Inability to carry out physical activity without discomfort. (Angina may be present at rest)

Exercise testing

Formal laboratory exercise testing is considered by many to be mandatory prior to any exercise programme. However, this is not universal and some authors such as Miller & Borer (1982) question the value of such tests. In a 1986 survey of Australian hospital practice Worcester found that only 11% of hospitals exercise tested most of their inpatients post-MI and that, in fact, 84% of hospitals tested less than half of their inpatient post-MI population.

The safety of exercise testing as early as 3 days post-MI has been clearly established (Miller & Borer 1982). Early exercise testing is advocated to provide both prognostic and therapeutic information. The American College of Sports Medicine (1995) recommends diagnostic exercise testing in the presence of a physician for patients with known cardiac disease in order to make decisions about the need for further evaluation or intervention. Functional exercise testing, with patients remaining on their usual medications,

should be used to determine the exercise capacity of patients requiring activity guidelines and exercise prescription.

The risks of testing are considered high in patients with post-MI complications. Absolute contraindications to testing include unstable angina and uncontrolled arrhythmias. In the North American literature a medical decision not to perform an exercise test is an independent factor denoting a high risk of a further cardiac event (DeBusk 1989).

The reliability of an exercise test as a diagnostic tool is compromised when ECG interpretation is difficult, for example in the presence of some dysrhythmias or after a large anterior MI. In this situation the test may provide some useful information regarding exercise capacity, and haemodynamic and respiratory function, but other forms of exercise investigation such as radionuclide ventriculography or echocardiography may be of greater use.

Protocol. In theory, any type of exercise can be used as long as a set reproducible protocol is followed. In practice, the majority of exercise tests are performed on a treadmill or bicycle, beginning at a low level of work and increasing in 2- or 3-minute stages. The Bruce protocol (Bruce et al 1973) is commonly used and is given as an example in Table 15.3. A variety of protocols have been developed and may be easily found in texts such as the American College of Sports Medicine (1995). Common criticisms of the Bruce protocol are that the first stage is too hard for many patients and that the jumps in workload are too great between stages. A modification of the Bruce protocol to answer the first criticism is to begin with a stage '1/2' with the treadmill at a speed of 1.7 mph and a slope of 5%, for 3 minutes.

Table 15.3 The Bruce Exercise Test protocol for a treadmill

Stage	Speed (mph)	Slope (%)	Time (min)
1	1.7	10	3
2	2.5	12	3
3	3.4	14	3
4	4.2	16	3
5	5.0	18	3
6	5.5	20	3

Table 15.4 Borg rating of perceived exertion scale

Category		Category-ratio	
6		0	Nothing at all
7	Very, very light	0.5	Very, very weak (just noticeable)
8		1	Very weak
9	Very light	2	Weak (light)
10		3	Moderate
11	Fairly light	4	Somewhat strong
12		5	Strong (heavy)
13	Somewhat hard	6	
14		7	Very strong
15	Hard	8	
16		9	
17	Very hard	10	Very, very strong (almost maximal)
18		•	Maximal
19	Very, very hard		
20			

Treadmill protocols commonly increase both the speed and slope of the machine; bicycle protocols increase workload by increasing resistance against which the subject is pedalling, whilst requiring that rhythm is maintained.

Monitoring of the subject is by continuous ECG, heart rate, blood pressure, symptoms, rating of perceived exertion (RPE) (Table 15.4) and appearance. Some laboratories will also include the direct measurement of oxygen uptake as a part of their protocol for exercise testing of cardiac patients.

Cessation of an exercise test may be at a predetermined arbitrarily selected end-point, for example a heart rate of 130 beats/min or a set workload, in which case the test is considered submaximal if the subject reaches this point without problems.

Maximal or symptom-limited tests require the subject to exercise until unable to continue due to fatigue, breathlessness or angina or the test is stopped by the physician at the expected maximal heart rate or because of ECG abnormalities.

Interpretation of exercise test results is critical to the value of the test as a diagnostic or therapeutic tool. Hare (1990) advocates the use of exercise testing for its effect on patient confidence, especially when implications of the test are discussed with patient and partner.

Reliability, sensitivity and specificity of the test are jeopardized when insufficient attention is paid to test details. False negative test results are associated with insufficient workload, insufficient number of ECG leads and failure to use all the available information in test interpretation. False positive results are associated with cardiac hypertrophy, an abnormal resting ECG and cardiomyopathy (American College of Sports Medicine 1995).

Information obtained from an exercise test can be compared with normal values for the population where these are available. Bruce (1956) used the concept of 'functional aerobic impairment' to describe the percentage that an individual's functional capacity falls below that expected for age and sex.

Walking tests such as a 6-minute walk (p. 66) may be useful for quantification of functional capacity in those patients not considered for a formal exercise test because of their level of functional impairment (Lipkin et al 1986a). The reliability of walking tests for cardiac patients is the subject of current investigations and is being advocated for the assessment of patients with cardiac failure (Shephard 1997).

Desired functional level. This should be discussed realistically with the individual patient, and should be related to premorbid activities and fitness as well as to current level of exercise tolerance. Attainable short-term goals as steps towards the desired outcome will help the patient feel a sense of achievement and progress with any programme. Unrealistic goals such as returning to cross-country skiing after a 40-year gap should be discouraged.

Other points. Other points to be included in assessment may relate to other cardiac risk factors such as smoking and obesity or may relate to other medical problems suffered by the patient. In particular, any disability which may affect the ability of the patient to exercise should be clearly documented.

DeBusk et al (1986) suggested that the clinical judgements of physicians regarding the capacity of their patients to safely resume their usual activities after MI are generally correct, but that this judgement can be refined by the use of exercise test results.

McBurney (1994) presented the results of a study to assess the ability of clinicians to judge physical work capacity of post-MI patients. 10 clinicians working in cardiac rehabilitation were asked to predict exercise test times for patients, using only data available from the medical record. All of the clinicians obtained high positive correlations with the actual exercise test time. Interviews with these clinicians revealed that all had slightly differing decision-making strategies but that the most common reference points were: age, date and site or size of infarct, premorbid activity levels, current activity levels and any current symptoms of IHD.

Recording

Database

The individual patient database will be compiled over time as information becomes available. Initial recording should include as much information relating to the preceding assessment points as possible. Analysis of the recorded findings allows an individual treatment plan to be formulated.

Ongoing information

Ongoing notes should include recording of the amount of activity performed in any exercise session, an objective measure of effect such as heart rate or respiratory rate and any other signs or symptoms associated with activity. A baseline or resting level of the parameter selected should be recorded before, during and 2–5 minutes after cessation of activity.

Home activity diary

The completion of a home exercise diary could assist some patients to continue their programme, and if kept conscientiously is often a good marker of progress.

Treatment

Type of activity

Activities which give the best cardiovascular protection involve regular and rhythmical use of large muscle groups. Such activities include walking, running, swimming, dancing, cycling and rowing. The most common and safest form of exercise is walking.

In order to meet needs associated with daily activities it may be necessary to ensure that some arm exercise is included as part of a whole body exercise programme. Arm exercise has been shown to impose a greater stress on the heart than the same amount of leg exercise (Astrand & Rodahl 1986), so a lesser intensity of arm exercise should be used to be safe and effective.

Large increases in blood pressure have been found in association with isometric activity such as heavy weightlifting and thus sustained and high-intensity isometric exercise has been discouraged for cardiac patients. Verrill et al (1992) cite a number of studies in which circuit weight training programmes using isotonic activities have been assessed in patients post-MI and post-CABGS. These programmes have been shown to be safe and to improve muscular strength and endurance. Further evidence for the inclusion of low- to moderate-intensity strength training in cardiac rehabilitation programmes is provided by studies such as Daub et al (1996).

Frequency, intensity, duration

The frequency, intensity and duration of exercise which should be recommended are factors which have been well investigated over a number of years. The threshold of exercise for cardiovascular protection has been reviewed by Haskell (1985), who concluded that an exercise threshold of about 630 kJ/day is required to decrease the risk of IHD. It appears that regular physical activity is beneficial, but that at high and vigorous levels there are no great gains and an increased risk of injury compared with moderate levels of activity. Leon et al (1987) found that a moderate level of leisure time physical activity was associated with fewer deaths than low levels of activity and with a similar rate of fatality as high levels of activity. Moderate-level activity involved the expenditure of an average 6300 kJ/week. This compared with an average of 2100 kJ in the low activity level group.

Common recommendations for exercise to improve and maintain fitness are for a target of exercising three to five times per week for a 5- to 10-minute warm-up, a 15- to 60-minute training session at 40–85% of functional capacity and a 5- to 10-minute cool-down. It now appears, however, that these guidelines can be modified. DeBusk et al (1990) found that men completing three 10-minute bouts of exercise each day showed the same improvements in fitness as men completing one 30-minute bout of exercise per day. Current recommendations are concentrating on total daily or weekly energy expenditure in exercise.

Goble et al (1991) reported the results of a study in which 308 men were randomly assigned to either an aerobic exercise group or a light exercise group for their 8-week cardiac reha- bilitation exercise programme after an anterior MI. The groups were well matched. Aerobic exercise was conducted at a gymnasium three times per week according to the guidelines of the American Heart Association. Light exercise was conducted two times per week in the physio- therapy department and involved flexibility exercises, stationary cycling, stairs, light hand weights and rowing machine activity interspersed with rest periods. Both groups were advised to walk at a comfortable pace for 30 minutes each day. The effects of the programmes were measured by treadmill exercise test times prior to the start of exercise, at the completion of the 8-week programme and at a 1-year follow-up. The only statistically significant difference in exercise capacity was a small and temporary advantage in the aerobic exercise group at the end of the training period. Physical benefits at 1 year were equally well achieved in the light exercise group.

Recommendations for exercise now also include an initial phase involving multiple short bouts of low-intensity exercise, distributed throughout the day (American College of Sports Medicine 1995), until the participant is used to the activity and the supervisor is accustomed

to his response. It is often necessary to point out to cardiac patients that, although some exercise is good, more is not necessarily better. This may relate to intensity, frequency and/or duration of activity.

Environmental factors may also be important in determining the amount of exercise to be undertaken at any one time, as variables such as wind, terrain, humidity, altitude and tem- perature extremes are known to affect the body response to exercise.

Intensity of exercise should be monitored and it is appropriate that the patient learns at least one way to do this. Recommended methods are by heart rate, rating of perceived exertion (RPE) or by the use of metabolic equivalents (METs). Heart rate is usually determined by direct measurement from ECG monitoring, radiotelemetry or palpation. In a group situation, palpation of the radial artery and counting the pulse for 15 seconds and then multiplying by four is the simplest method. The formula often used clinically (220 – age in years) is not recommended by the American College of Sports Medicine. Several alternative procedures to determine suitable exercise training heart rates are outlined by the American College of Sports Medicine (1995). The use of heart rate to monitor exercise intensity is simple and has the advantage that as exercise tolerance increases patients will be able to do more before reaching their training heart rate, so that frequent revision of exercise prescription is not necessary.

Monitoring of exercise intensity by RPE has similar advantages and has been found to be a reliable indicator of intensity of effort. Most patients would exercise at the lower end of the 12–16 RPE range.

METs are sometimes used to monitor exercise intensity and rely on the use of tables which give MET values for common activities. Examples are given by the American College of Sports Medicine (1995) and Greenland & Chu (1988). One MET is equal to the resting level of oxygen uptake which is approximately 3.5 ml/kg·min^{-1}. The use of METs to monitor exercise intensity does not make any allowance for environmental factors and does not allow for body adaptations to exercise so that there is a frequent need to review the level of exercise prescribed in this way.

Phases of recovery

Cardiac rehabilitation is often divided into three periods which are not defined by time. They are defined in American and Australian literature as: phase I – the time of inpatient management; phase II – outpatient recovery; and phase III – long-term maintenance. However, the British Association of Cardiac Rehabilitation continues to classify four phases of rehabilitation as: phase I – hospital inpatient period; phase II – immediate post-discharge; phase III – intermediate post-discharge; and phase IV – long-term maintenance (Stokes et al 1995).

In hospital. Inpatient physiotherapy is usually directed at preventing or treating the sequelae of bed rest. This may include techniques to prevent lung collapse, especially in patients with pericarditis, and simple assisted or free range of movement activities. This phase may last from a few hours to days or weeks.

Activity should be slowly increased and include a graduated exercise and mobilization programme, so that by discharge the patient is able to attend to his own activities of daily living, is ambulant and able to negotiate stairs.

Exercise in this phase can often be directed at negating old wives' tales or myths such as 'reaching your arms above your head will cause death'. A potential outline of inpatient activities is shown in Figure 15.1. Advice for home activity and exercise must be given pre-discharge, and preferably some formal arrangement made for follow-up as an outpatient.

After hospital discharge. Continuation of cardiac rehabilitation may be by attendance at an organized education and exercise session one or more times per week for 1–2 months, supplemented by home exercise, or it may be feasible to use a home-based exercise training programme such as that studied by Miller et al (1984). Suitable activities include stretches, flexibility and coordination exercises for warm-up and cool-down and an aerobic component which may utilize one or a combination of activities such

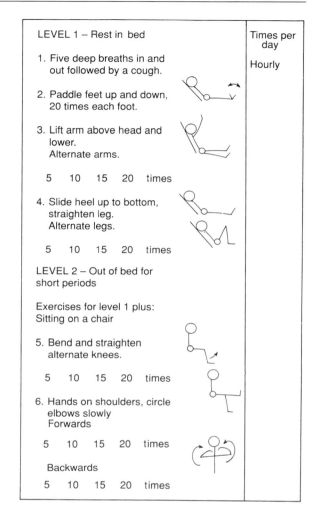

Fig. 15.1 Sample inpatient activity sheet (prior to ambulation).

as walking, minitrampoline, exercise cycle, and rowing machine (Figs 15.2 and 15.3). Miller et al (1984) found that patients training at home or in a group programme had significant improvements in functional capacity over patients not training or in a control group. Home training patients were monitored twice weekly by telephone.

Long-term continuation of exercise is desirable for stable post-MI and post-CABGS patients as well as for the community in general. Many phase III long-term exercise programmes specific to cardiac patients are now available. Many peo-

Exercise at a comfortable pace.

Repeat each exercise for:

    30 seconds

    1 minute

    2 minutes

STANDING

1. Legs apart, hand on hips. Bend left knee, straighten. Bend right knee, straighten. Keep trunk upright and facing forward.

2. Hands on shoulders. Turn upper body side to side easy and relaxed to warm up.

3. Quarter squat. Head up, back straight.

4. March on the spot. Lift knees, swing arms.

5. Arm circles forwards backwards

FLOOR

6. Bridging. Knees bent, lift bottom. Return to floor.

7. Modified push up - sitting back on to heels then return to floor.

Continue as appropriate.

The floor exercises (6&7) are not suitable for every patient.

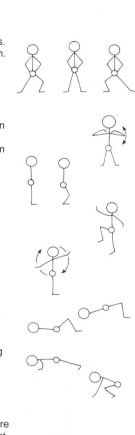

Fig. 15.2 Sample outpatient exercise (in addition to a walk).

ple find the stimulus of company assists in long-term motivation to exercise and benefit from an appropriate community exercise programme.

Supervision

There are many aspects of patient monitoring useful for cardiac patients. Direct visual super-

vision is difficult in a large group situation, so it is recommended that exercise classes be kept small and be organized so that all participants can be seen.

Telemetry is a useful facility for allowing direct ECG recordings to be made at a central monitor whilst the patient exercises at a distance. This is recommended for patients with poor left ventricular function, resting or exercise-induced ventricular arrhythmias, decreased systolic blood pressure during exercise, and survivors of cardiac arrest (American College of Cardiology 1986).

Individual supervision may be necessary for patients with special needs or problems, especially those whose functional level is extremely low.

Home exercise has been found to be an acceptable alternative for those unable to attend group activities. Regular telephone contact allows the patient to keep in touch with staff.

Monitoring

The level of exercise achieved in any session is an important part of monitoring and should always be recorded. This might be the distance covered in a given time for walking or the number of repetitions of an exercise.

Signs and symptoms. Signs and symptoms occurring with any level of activity should also be recorded. Angina in particular should be noted, together with the level of activity at which it occurs and, if possible, some objective measure such as heart rate at the time.

Heart rate. Heart rate is known to correlate with activity level (Astrand & Rodahl 1986) and is a useful measure of the stress imposed on the body by exercise. Resting, peak exercise and recovery heart rates associated with activity are useful measures (Fig. 15.4).

Many heart rate monitors are commercially available. Leger & Thivierge (1988) studied the validity and stability of measures from a wide range of monitors and found excellent correlations between ECG and monitors using chest electrodes. Monitors using finger or ear probes were found to be unsatisfactory during exercise.

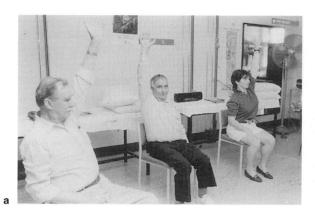

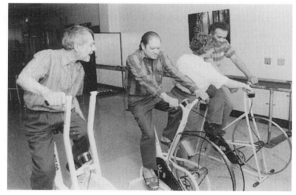

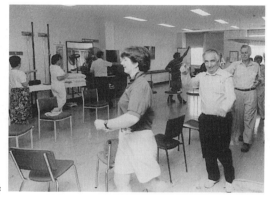

Fig. 15.3 Group outpatient exercise programme: **a** warm-up; **b** major aerobic activity; **c** cool-down.

Should the patient be taught to take his pulse? Some authors argue that this is mandatory and others suggest that it increases anxiety. Patients who have silent ischaemia certainly need to be able to regulate their exercise level reliably so that their activity is below the ischaemic threshold. Heart rate measurement is one way of doing this. It is quick and easy, reliable and requires only a watch with a second hand.

Rating of perceived exertion (RPE) could be an alternative to this. In patients on beta-blocking medications, heart rate response to exercise will be attenuated and other objective measures such as respiratory rate or RPE may be more reliable and sensitive.

Rating of perceived exertion. RPE scales were developed by Borg to rate intensity of exercise. The RPE Category Scale (Borg 1982) uses 15 grades ranging from 6 to 20 to describe intensity of effort, whilst the Category-Ratio Scale uses grades ranging from 0 to 10. These scales are shown in Table 15.4 (p. 395). The RPE scales are simple and practical for clinical use. Gutmann et al (1981) investigated the relationship between RPE and heart rate during exercise testing and training in a group of post-CABGS patients. They found that patients perceived exercise similarly at given heart rates, but that with recovery, time and further training the same RPE was given for higher heart rate levels. This finding is consistent with improvement in fitness. Studies cited in Williams & Eston (1989) have found that RPE can be used to control intensity of exercise. A rating of 12–13 (3–4) is equal to 60–80% of maximal oxygen uptake in most individuals, while 16–17 (7–8) has been found to correlate to 90%. A general conclusion reached by Williams & Eston (1989) is that the Borg RPE

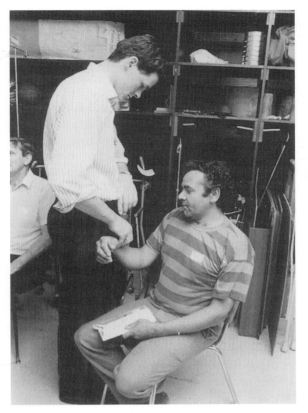

Fig. 15.4 Heart rate monitoring by radial pulse palpation pre- or post-exercise.

scale is a valid measure of exercise intensity for both indicating and regulating intensity of effort. It is worth noting that it may take several training sessions for an individual to become reliable at regulating his exercise effort by using this scale.

Breathlessness. Breathlessness is normally associated with exercise, especially when the activity is vigorous or prolonged. Respiratory rate is another measure which can be used to assess exercise effort. If the cardiac patient is exercising at a moderate level he should not be so breathless that he is unable to talk. In fact, the ability to answer a simple question verbally whilst exercising is a simple clinical method for assessment of breathlessness.

Blood pressure. Blood pressure usually rises gradually with 'aerobic style' exercise and should not drop dramatically during activity. Monitoring of blood pressure is a part of comprehensive patient monitoring, but is usually only performed at initial inpatient exercise sessions unless there is a problem with stability. If the patient complains of lightheadedness or dizziness his blood pressure should be checked.

Other signs. Pallor, fatigue and excessive perspiration are all signs associated with inability of the heart to maintain adequate cardiac output and should be treated as indicators of poor exercise tolerance.

Crackles. Crackles associated with cardiac failure are also an important sign which should be checked in patients who are extremely breathless with activity but have no respiratory disorder.

Angina. Angina is a major sign of myocardial insufficiency and if it occurs with activity the patient should stop and rest. If rest is not sufficient to relieve angina then sublingual nitroglycerin should be available for use. Angina occurring with exercise should be documented and discussed with the relevant medical personnel.

Outcome evaluation

The impact of a cardiac rehabilitation programme may be measured in a number of ways, on the basis of outcome for an individual or for the programme as a whole. In general these may be categorized as: health, clinical or behavioural. Examples of each may be: quality of life (health), change in fitness (clinical) and change in exercise activity (behavioural). It is important that target outcomes are identified to attain baseline measures in the desired variable(s) before any intervention occurs.

Quality of life is not easy to define, but some authors have studied this in relation to cardiac rehabilitation. Measures used by Oldridge et al (1991) included a specifically developed quality of life questionnaire which had 97 items of possible concern to patients. Mortality and work status were monitored and exercise tolerance was measured for a rehabilitation and a control group. The rehabilitation programme was found to accelerate recovery at 8 weeks post-MI but by 12 months all measures had improved significantly in both groups. The Short Form-36, a generic measure of health status has been used as an indicator of overall function in cardiac patients before and after cardiac rehabilitation. Spertus et al (1994) have found that it is not as sensitive to change in cardiac patients as a more specific assessment tool.

Return to work is often used as a marker of cardiac rehabilitation success. There is certainly a question as to whether this is valid as specific interventions to facilitate employment are often not a part of a programme. Hedback & Perk (1987) reported a 5-year follow-up of a cardiac rehabilitation programme and found that in patients aged less than 55, more patients in the rehabilitation group returned to work than in the control group. In patients over this age, a large number of other factors were important in the decision to return to work.

The use of medical services by rehabilitation and non-rehabilitation groups has not been studied by many workers. Levin et al (1991) reported a cost analysis of their cardiac rehabilitation programme and found that the rehabilitation programme did not increase the costs of post-MI care as these costs were balanced by a decrease in readmissions for cardiovascular diseases. Ades et al (1992) found that the participants in a comprehensive cardiac rehabilitation programme had significantly lower cardiac rehospitalization costs in the years after a coronary event than non-participants.

Beneficial physiological alterations associated with exercise training have been well documented over many years (Astrand & Rodahl 1986). Objective measures such as exercise heart rate and respiratory rate for a given level of activity decrease with training. Subjective decreases in perceived effort are also reported.

Many of the benefits of cardiac rehabilitation have only been reported in studies with long-term follow-up (Hedback & Perk 1987, Levin et al 1991). It appears that long-term follow-up is necessary to maintain benefits of a programme and that analysis of effect and costs are best demonstrated in this way.

Effectiveness of education is again an area in which there has been little formal evaluation. Studies on the effects of outcomes from education and studies on the effects of education programmes on both knowledge and behaviour are lacking.

Morbidity and mortality are also frequently used as markers of success in assessment of cardiac rehabilitation programmes. Hedback & Perk (1987) found no difference in mortality between their rehabilitation and their reference groups but the recurrence rate of non-fatal MI and the total cardiac event rate was lower in their intervention group.

Complications of exercise

Adverse effects of exercise are noted within both the normal and cardiac populations. In particular, orthopaedic breakdown is more common in middle-aged or older patients and is more likely with frequent or prolonged activity. Adequate warm-up and cool-down can reduce the incidence of orthopaedic problems.

Cardiovascular complications are less common but serious. Sudden death is defined as unexpected and atraumatic death within 6 hours of a normal state of health (Amsterdam 1990). This includes fatality during or within 30 minutes of concluding exercise.

Haskell (1994) reported the incidence of death during exercise of cardiac patients as 1 per 787 305 patient-hours. More recent reports cite lower event rates than studies prior to 1980. Sudden death during exercise is usually associated with structural heart disease and the usual mechanism is ventricular fibrillation; however, malignant arrhythmias may occur throughout the spectrum of cardiac disease. Many exercise-related deaths in cardiac patients occurred with activity in excess of normal exercise and with failure to heed symptoms induced by exercise.

OTHER CONSIDERATIONS
The older patient

There are no specific age-related contraindications to joining a cardiac rehabilitation programme.

Lavie et al (1993) have demonstrated that the older cardiac population can benefit from an outpatient cardiac exercise programme to the same extent as younger patients.

There are some general considerations which may apply to any population, but are more prevalent in the elderly. Older people may have more than one chronic condition which limits their exercise ability, for example osteoarthritis, peripheral vascular disease or pulmonary disease. Modification of an exercise programme on an individual basis may be necessary.

Landin et al (1985) cite evidence that the older population will have lost work capacity and suggest that 50% of the diminished function in muscle strength and mass, cardiac output and heart rate, respiratory capacity, bone mass and joint flexibility may be attributed to disuse. Stretches, flexibility exercises and range of movement activities should be incorporated as a part of an exercise programme.

Older patients will usually start their cardiac exercise programme at a lower level than their younger counterparts. This will often necessitate both a lower workload and an interval programme of shorter duration and with longer rest periods. At a lower exercise intensity patients can be encouraged to exercise daily (Williams et al 1984b) in order to encourage improvement without untoward effects.

Older patients can gain significant improvement in functional status with a lower intensity, longer-term exercise programme. This may contribute to the patient's ability to maintain an independent lifestyle.

Cardiac failure

Heart failure is a complex and increasingly prevalent clinical syndrome. The basic cause of the inability of the heart to pump blood at a rate sufficient for the needs of the body may be cardiac or extracardiac in origin. Cardiac disturbances may be related to muscle contractile failure due to ischaemic heart disease, myocarditis or cardiomyopathy, or to disorders causing impaired filling or emptying of the cardiac chambers such as valvular stenosis or regurgitation. Extracardiac disorders which may cause failure include hypertension, anaemia and thyrotoxicosis. This discussion will focus only on failure due to reduced ability of the myocardium to pump blood. An increased survival rate after myocardial infarction of patients with ventricular dysfunction and the ageing of the population are two major factors contributing to the increased incidence of cardiac failure.

Reduction in symptoms and improvement in functional capacity are the goals of treatment most appreciated by patients. Without these outcomes the prolongation of survival is considered less desirable.

Until the past decade patients with cardiac failure were excluded from cardiac exercise programmes because of concern regarding the risks of exercise-related arrhythmias and death and the possibility of further damage to the myocardium. Current medical practice as outlined by Shabetai (1988) involves bed rest during an acute unstable phase, with no subsequent limitations on usual physical activity.

The exercise capacity of patients with chronic heart failure is usually limited by breathlessness and/or fatigue, although the mechanisms which cause these limitations are still not clearly understood.

Exercise ability in patients with cardiac failure is widely variable. Franciosa et al (1981) have demonstrated that indices of left ventricular performance such as resting left ventricular ejection fraction do not correlate with exercise capacity in patients with heart failure. In clinical practice some patients with cardiac enlargement and a poor resting left ventricular ejection fraction will be able to perform near normal levels of exercise. In other patients, activities of daily living are a substantial physiological stress causing breathlessness and fatigue.

The physiological exercise responses of patients with coronary artery disease including left ventricular dysfunction have been shown to be identical to those of age-matched normals and patients with coronary artery disease without left ventricular dysfunction (Kellerman et al 1988).

Many studies have now demonstrated that exercise training is a safe and effective method of improving functional capacity in patients with impaired ventricular function (Shephard 1997). Sullivan et al (1988) found that exercise training induced adaptations in peripheral musculature which contributed to the improvement in exercise ability.

In prescribing exercise for a patient with ventricular dysfunction Mathes (1988) suggested that special consideration must be given to factors such as usual activity level and body weight. General debility may necessitate the initial use of very low level interval training, with the use of exercise such as stationary cycling where carriage of body weight is almost eliminated. In general, the principles of exercise prescription will be the same as those for other cardiac patients. The rate of exercise may determine the limiting symptoms in patients with heart failure. Lipkin et al (1986b) found that fast exercise was usually limited by breathlessness and slower or endurance exercise by fatigue. Fatigue that continues for hours or days after a particular bout of exercise is considered by Dubach & Froelicher (1989), an indicator that the amount of work was excessive either in workload, time or both.

Exercise training at an appropriate level in patients with stable compensated heart failure may have a major impact on quality of life with only a small increase in functional capacity. Patients who require a low level, long-term, small and slow increment exercise programme may be major beneficiaries of cardiac rehabilitation (Dubach & Froelicher 1989), especially if exercise training is combined with other measures to improve symptoms and quality of life such as dietary and vocational advice and instruction in energy conservation techniques.

Valvular heart disease

Some patients with valvular disorders have concomitant coronary artery disease and may benefit from the full range of services offered in cardiac rehabilitation. Other patients with valvular disorders may also benefit from an exercise programme for general fitness, dietary advice or work simplification. Valvular heart disease has not been studied as extensively as coronary artery disease, especially with respect to exercise ability; however, some useful information is available.

Mitral stenosis and regurgitation

A decrease in exercise performance has been noted in association with progressively severe mitral stenosis, with good correlation between symptoms of fatigue, weakness and exertional breathlessness, severity of valvular obstruction and decline in exercise tolerance or degree of valvular regurgitation and exercise tolerance (Lutz & Wenger 1985). Carstens et al (1983) performed pre- and postoperative exercise studies on 46 patients undergoing mitral valve replacement, 19 undergoing aortic and mitral valve replacement and 17 undergoing mitral valve reconstruction. Their postoperative evaluation generally found marked improvement in symptoms and some improvement in exercise performance. Disturbed haemodynamics persisted 6 months after surgery with elevated pulmonary artery pressures at rest which rose further during exercise and a low cardiac output at rest which failed to increase normally with exertion. The ability to exercise was generally significantly less than that of age-matched sedentary control subjects. The extent to which this reflects decreased fitness prior to surgery is unknown.

Aortic stenosis and regurgitation

Patients with severe aortic stenosis are rarely assessed with exercise because of the possibility that exercise-induced syncope and/or sudden cardiac death may occur secondary to an inability to increase stroke volume and an actual or relative decrease in cardiac output with exercise. Results of postoperative evaluation in 49 patients studied by Carstens et al (1983) showed a generally good exercise performance after surgery, although haemodynamics remained abnormal.

Impairment of exercise tolerance often occurs late in the natural history of aortic regurgitation. Krayenbuehl et al (1979) found significant improvement in left ventricular function after aortic valve replacement, with residual impairment being greater in aortic regurgitation than in stenosis or a combination of regurgitation and stenosis. The need for early operative intervention was not demonstrated by Henry et al (1980) in their prospective study of 42 patients.

Sire (1978) reported on 44 patients randomly assigned to either an exercise training or a control group after aortic valve replacement. At 12 months postoperatively the exercise training group had a significantly higher physical work capacity and were much more likely to be in paid employment than their control counterparts.

Double valve surgery

Carstens et al (1983) found that their 19 patients undergoing double valve surgery had an outcome similar to those undergoing mitral valve surgery. A significant improvement in symptoms was accompanied by a small improvement in exercise ability.

Exercise recommendations. A longer-term slow increment exercise programme is indicated for patients following valvular surgery because of their reduced functional ability preoperatively and the continued abnormal haemodynamics, particularly their inability to increase cardiac output with exertion. Goforth & James (1985) have found that a workload of 50% of the patient's maximum is one that nearly all patients with non-coronary heart disease can comfortably perform at the start of exercise training. This is usually achieved by brisk walking. As with patients post-MI, ejection fraction does not correlate with exercise tolerance (Lutz & Wenger 1985).

Congenital heart disease

A large number of cardiac surgical procedures are undertaken to repair congenital heart lesions. These patients may not require the full range of cardiac rehabilitation services, as they do not have coronary artery disease and many are infants at the time of surgery. However, many can benefit from general health advice and may have specific questions and problems.

In the paediatric population it has been noted that delayed motor development occurs in children with congenital heart defects (Box & Burns 1990). This may be related to the level of hypoxaemia associated with the defect, type of malformation, length of time prior to surgery or congestive heart failure.

Motor developmental delay was noted to persist for 2 or more years by Box & Burns (1990) after corrective surgery in children of below school age. The older the child at time of surgery, the greater the delay. These authors suggested physiotherapists should be involved in the long-term follow-up of children after congenital heart defect repair to minimize motor developmental delays.

Many patients with surgically corrected or repaired congenital heart defects are now adults or approaching adulthood and seek advice on safe and appropriate activity. They may be limited in their ability to perform work by residual deficits, but exercise should be encouraged in this population as part of a healthy lifestyle, and with the knowledge that training will assist in performance improvement.

Perrault & Drblik (1989) have reviewed much of the literature on this topic and found that maximum exercise tolerance after repair of congenital heart disorders is related in particular to three factors: age at time of definitive surgical repair (the younger the better); the severity of any lesions remaining after surgery; and the age of the patient at the time of investigation. While a normal maximal exercise capacity may be attained by some patients after surgical repair, they noted some important exercise-related differences in function: firstly that near normal exercise capacity does not imply normal exercise haemodynamic responses and secondly that in general there is some variance in exercise capacity when a comparison is made between people with corrected congenital lesions and age-matched normals.

Atrial septal defect

Lutz & Wenger (1985) note that even after closure of a large atrial septal defect (ASD) some patients will have a very low functional capacity. No limitations are usually placed on participation in physical activity and sport once the post-operative recovery phase is over. However, a good result is usually achieved with no significant difference in work capacity between patients and age-matched controls, especially if surgical correction occurred before 10 years of age.

Pulmonary stenosis

Little information is available on performance after repair of pulmonary stenosis. Early repair is now favoured as this seems to limit the long-term effects of obstruction to right ventricular ejection and thus minimizes right ventricular hypertrophy, hyperplasia and failure (Perrault & Drblik 1989). It appears that patients can safely participate in exercise and sport provided that right ventricular function is adequate.

Ventricular septal defect

The haemodynamic consequences of a ventricular septal defect (VSD) are largely determined by its size. Early correction lessens damage to the pulmonary vascular bed. Almost all patients have some ventricular conduction abnormality. Exercise tolerance after VSD repair is very variable and depends on the extent of any residual deficit, arrhythmias and pulmonary vascular resistance (Perrault & Drblik 1989). When pulmonary hypertension is present preoperatively this rarely alters after VSD repair.

Reports on postoperative function cited by Perrault & Drblik (1989) suggest that, while many patients will have a good outcome, in general their exercise tolerance is less than that of age-matched controls. Unless residual shunt or arrhythmias are present participation in sport and exercise is encouraged. An exercise test may be useful to identify activity-induced arrhythmias. Moller et al (1991) published the results of more than 30-years follow-up of 296 patients surviving closure of a VSD. The defect had completely closed in 80% of cases; 59 patients had died. Mortality was associated with high pulmonary vascular resistance (> 7 mmHg/1/min/m^2), complete heart block and being older than 5 years at the time of operation. Of the patients, 208 rated themselves in NYHA class I for function.

Tetralogy of Fallot

In patients exercising after a repair of Fallot's tetralogy the ability to perform is affected by the amount of residual circulatory deficit and by the severity of changes in left and/or right ventricular function in the preoperative period. In many patients excellent surgical results are obtained, allowing them to live a normal life, symptom and medication free (James et al 1976); however, cardiac output is lower in patients than in age-matched normals. A comparable aerobic performance may be found between patients with corrected Fallot's tetralogy and age-matched controls, but patients are unable to reach elite standards of performance because of the limitation of exercise cardiac output. Exercise participation should be encouraged at a level allowed by the success of the repair. James et al (1976) recommend a prior exercise test to identify patients who have developed arrhythmias following intraventricular surgery.

Exercise recommendations. In patients with congenital cardiac disorders undergoing exercise training either before or after surgery, special consideration must be given to the existing pathophysiology, keeping in mind that surgical intervention will not restore normal function to the heart. Goforth & James (1985) recommend submaximal activities with long, slow warm-up and cool-down periods. Training patients to be aware of symptoms and their level of perceived exertion may assist in keeping exercise at a submaximal level.

Compliance

When planning an exercise programme which requires long-term adherence, strategies to maximize compliance must be considered.

In a short-term study of patients after CABGS Shankar et al (1990) found that at one month following hospital discharge, self-reports of behaviour with respect to smoking, exercise and diet were consistent with physiological measurements in approximately 50% of subjects.

Oldridge et al (1991) reported a 46.5% drop-out rate of post-MI patients from an exercise programme at a 3-year follow-up. Investigation of their subject sample showed that those most likely to drop out were smokers and 'blue collar' workers. There was no difference in drop-out rate between the high-intensity and low-intensity exercise programmes.

An earlier study by the same group (Andrew et al 1981) had found that the three main reasons given for lack of compliance were:

- Inconvenience (of exercise centre, times, parking)
- Poor perception of the exercise programme (fatigue, lack of staff attention and enthusiasm, poor belief in need for exercise for health)
- Family and lifestyle factors (interfered with work, spouse negative or indifferent).

From these complaints some potential strategies to improve compliance might include: flexibility in timing of exercise programmes, staffing to meet the needs and interests of the participants, spouse involvement, feedback of improvement to maintain motivation, and the possibility of a home exercise programme.

Cost-effectiveness

In a time of economic restraint and burgeoning health care expenditure the costs and effectiveness of any programme should be considered. Does a programme have benefits worth the costs involved? In assessing the worth of any programme it is necessary to have well-defined and agreed outcome measures.

The assessment of effectiveness of cardiac rehabilitation has involved the use of a number of quite different outcome measures, for example: a decrease in morbidity and/or mortality (Marra et al 1985, Hamalainen et al 1989), improvement in functional capacity (Greenland & Chu 1988), return to work (Marra et al 1985, Oldridge et al 1991), reduction in risk factors (Hedback et al 1990), change in quality of life (Greenland & Chu 1988, Oldridge et al 1991) and the long-term utilization of health care services, especially hospital readmissions (Blodgett & Pekarik 1987, Huang et al 1990), outpatient and local doctor attendances.

The costs of each of these outcomes are difficult to assess in monetary terms as many health care choices are influenced by factors not easily quantified or given a monetary value. The importance and desirability of each of these outcomes also varies from individual to individual, across health care settings and between nations. Equally the patient's perception of costs and benefit should be considered. Is increased survival time worth the necessary effort to the individual?

Some of the beneficial evidence in favour of cardiac rehabilitation has already been presented in this chapter. Counting cost and benefit to the community is a much larger and more difficult issue. The costs associated with a cardiac rehabilitation programme include as a minimum those of the venue, equipment and personnel and to the patients those of their own time and effort.

Many studies of cardiac rehabilitation programmes like Marra et al (1985) have not demonstrated benefits in terms of morbidity and mortality like the studies of Hamalainen et al (1989) and Kallio et al (1979), but they have shown short-term improvement in functional capacity and psychosocial status. Oldridge et al (1988) believe that this is because trials have been too small and have used heterogeneous patient populations. The results of their meta-analysis suggest that comprehensive cardiac rehabilitation has a beneficial effect on mortality.

In considering the costs of cardiac rehabilitation, Worcester (1986) suggests that the reduction in indirect costs of cardiac illness (loss of income and social security payments) vastly outweigh the costs of a cardiac rehabilitation programme to the extent that $A100 of indirect cost could be saved for every dollar expended on the direct costs of effective cardiac rehabilitation. Huang et al (1990) found a 38% reduction in rehospitalization costs in his group of post-MI rehabilitation participants compared with a no-rehabilitation group. After adjustment for other factors, participation in an exercise programme was a favourable influence in longer-term cost reduction.

The strongest evidence of the cost-effectiveness of cardiac rehabilitation comes from the studies of Hedback & Perk (1987), Hedback et al (1990), and Levin et al (1991).

Legal aspects

Cardiac rehabilitation is a recently developed health care service and a diversity of programmes are offered across differing health care settings. Personnel, policies, procedures and methods of operation may differ from programme to programme, and certainly the law differs from country to country and state to state. There are a number of legal issues and concerns which should be addressed by cardiac rehabilitation providers.

Standards of care. Acceptable standards of conduct or of care in cardiac rehabilitation may be established by reference to respected authorities. Professional associations with expressed positions regarding protocols for cardiac rehabilitation programmes include the American Heart Association (1994), the American College of Cardiology (1986), the American Association of Cardiovascular and Pulmonary Rehabilitation (1990), the American College of Sports Medicine (1995) and the British Association for Cardiac Rehabilitation (Coats et al 1995). Unfortunately, the standards of these bodies are not uniformly consistent; however, they do provide some guidance for the development of local programme policies and procedures and point to areas of concern.

Policies and procedures. In developing policies and procedures, safe and appropriate patient care should be of paramount concern. Policies and procedures should be documented in writing with reference to the appropriate professional standards of care. The potential for serious adverse reactions to occur during exercise should alert all concerned to the necessity for and use of protocols.

Staffing. Programme personnel may come from a variety of professional backgrounds. In some countries statutes and laws may define the scope of a profession. Failure to comply with such laws may expose staff to legal action. Exercise prescription is considered in some countries to be a part of medical practice and in this situation exercise can only be prescribed by the physician. In any programme only properly authorized professionals should prescribe exercise. Appropriate monitoring while exercising patients is part of any reasonable standard of care.

Informed consent. Consent to treatment is another area of concern. Many patients enter cardiac rehabilitation with only a vague idea of what is involved and usually give written consent only for procedures such as exercise testing. The American College of Sports Medicine (1995) now suggest informed consent be obtained for a cardiac rehabilitation programme, and have developed forms for this purpose.

Shephard (1981) lists the common bases for legal claims against cardiac rehabilitation providers as: failure to detect pre-existing medical abnormalities contraindicating the proposed programme, failure to monitor the patient adequately before, during and after exercise, lack of skill or delay in handling an emergency, lack of equipment, drugs and trained personnel necessary for resuscitation, lack of informed consent and inadequate documentation of procedures.

Legal concerns for cardiac rehabilitation programmes can be minimized by good management practices within the programme.

CONCLUSION

Cardiac rehabilitation is only now being demonstrated to be a cost-effective form of management for the cardiac patient. The training of a physiotherapist gives an excellent background for integral involvement in multidisciplinary cardiac rehabilitation. Exercise is an effective and important way of altering cardiac risk factors and of optimizing function for cardiac patients, but should be applied judiciously.

REFERENCES

Ades P, Huang D, Weaver S 1992 Cardiac rehabilitation participation predicts lower rehospitalisation costs. American Heart Journal 123: 916–921

American Association of Cardiovascular and Pulmonary Rehabilitation 1990 Scientific evidence of the value of cardiac rehabilitation services with emphasis on patients following myocardial infarction – section 1: exercise conditioning component. Journal of Cardiopulmonary Rehabilitation 10: 79–87

American College of Cardiology 1986 Recommendations of the American College of Cardiology on cardiovascular rehabilitation. Journal of the American College of Cardiology 7: 451–453

American College of Sports Medicine 1995 Guidelines for exercise testing and prescription, 5th edn. Lea & Febiger, Philadelphia

American Heart Association 1994 Cardiac rehabilitation programs: a statement for health professionals from the American Heart Association. Circulation 90: 1602–1610

Amsterdam E A 1990 Sudden death during exercise. Cardiology 77: 411–417

Andrew G M, Oldridge N B, Parker J O et al 1981 Reasons for dropout from exercise programs in post coronary patients. Medicine and Science in Sports and Exercise 13: 164–168

Astrand P-O, Rodahl K 1986 Textbook of work physiology, 3rd edn. McGraw-Hill, New York

Blair S N, Kohl H W, Paffenbarger R S et al 1989 Physical fitness and all cause mortality a prospective study of healthy men and women. Journal of the American Medical Association 262: 2395–2401

Blair S, Kohl H, Barlow C et al 1995 Changes in physical fitness and all cause mortality. JAMA 273: 1093–1098

Blair S, Booth M, Gyarfas I et al 1996 Development of public policy and physical activity initiatives internationally. Sports Medicine 21: 157–163

Bloch A, Maeder J P, Haissly J C et al 1974 Early mobilisation after myocardial infarction. A controlled study. American Journal of Cardiology 34: 152–157

Blodgett C, Pekarik G 1987 Program evaluation in cardiac rehabilitation IV: efficiency evaluation. Journal of Cardiopulmonary Rehabilitation 7: 466–474

Borg G V 1982 Psychophysical bases of perceived exertion. Medicine and Science in Sports and Exercise 14: 377–381

Box R C, Burns Y R 1990 The motor performance of preschool aged children after surgery for congenital heart disease. Australian Journal of Physiotherapy 36: 235–242

Bruce R A 1956 Evaluation of functional capacity and exercise tolerance of cardiac patients. Modern Concepts of Cardiovascular Disease 25: 321–326

Bruce R A, Kusumi F, Hosmer D 1973 Maximal oxygen intake and nomographic assessment of functional aerobic impairment in cardiovascular disease. American Heart Journal 85: 546–562

Caine N, Harrison S C W, Sharples L D, Wallwork J 1991 Prospective study of quality of life before and after coronary artery bypass grafting. British Medical Journal 302: 511–516

Carstens V, Behrenbeck D W, Hilger H H 1983 Exercise capacity before and after cardiac valve surgery. Cardiology 70: 41–49

Coats A, McGee H, Stokes H, Thompson D (eds) 1995 BACR guidelines for cardiac rehabilitation. Blackwell Science, Oxford

Davidson D M, Maloney C A 1985 Recovery after cardiac events. Physical Therapy 65: 1820–1827

Daub W, Knapik G, Black W 1996 Strength training early after myocardial infarction. Journal of Cardiopulmonary Rehabilitation 16: 100–108

DeBusk R F 1989 Specialised testing after recent acute myocardial infarction. Annals of Internal Medicine 110: 470–481

DeBusk R F, Houston N, Haskell W et al 1979 Exercise training soon after myocardial infarction. American Journal of Cardiology 44: 1223–1229

DeBusk R F, Blomqvist C G, Kouchoukos N T et al 1986 Identification and treatment of low risk patients after acute myocardial infarction and coronary artery bypass graft surgery. New England Journal of Medicine 314: 161–166

DeBusk R F, Stenestrand U, Sheehan M, Haskell W L 1990 Training effects of long versus short bouts of exercise in healthy subjects. American Journal of Cardiology 65: 1010–1013

Doughty C 1991 A multidisciplinary approach to cardiac rehabilitation. Nursing Standard 5: 13–15

Dubach P, Froelicher V F 1989 Cardiac rehabilitation for heart failure patients. Cardiology 76: 368–373

Eston R, Connolly D 1996 The use of ratings of perceived exertion for exercise prescription in patients receiving β blocker therapy. Sports Medicine 21: 176–190

Franciosa J A, Park M, Levine T B 1981 Lack of correlation between exercise capacity and indexes of resting left ventricular performance in heart failure. American Journal of Cardiology 47: 33–39

Frishman W H, Teicher M 1985 Beta adrenergic blockade; an update. Cardiology 72: 280–296

Gazes P C 1990 Clinical cardiology, 3rd edn. Lea & Febiger, Philadelphia

Goble A, Hare D L, Macdonald P S et al 1991 Effect of early programmes of high and low intensity exercise on physical performance after transmural acute myocardial infarction. British Heart Journal 65: 126–131

Goforth D, James F W 1985 Exercise training in noncoronary heart disease. In: Wenger N K (ed) Exercise and the heart, 2nd edn. F A Davis, Philadelphia

Greenland P, Chu J 1988 Efficacy of cardiac rehabilitation services with emphasis on patients after myocardial infarction. Annals of Internal Medicine 109: 650–663

Gutmann M C, Squires R W, Pollock M L et al 1981 Perceived exertion–heart rate relationship during exercise testing and training in cardiac patients. Journal of Cardiac Rehabilitation 1: 52–59

Hamalainen H, Luurila O J, Kallio V et al 1989 Long term reduction in sudden deaths after a multifactorial intervention programme in patients with myocardial infarction: 10 year results of a controlled investigation. European Heart Journal 10: 55–62

Hare D L 1990 Cardiac rehabilitation. Australian Family Physician 19: 1043–1052

Haskell W L 1985 Physical activity and health: need to define the required stimulus. American Journal of Cardiology 5: 4D–9D

Haskell W L 1994 The efficacy and safety of exercise programs in cardiac rehabilitation. Medicine and Science in Sports and Exercise 26: 815–823

Hedback B E, Perk J 1987 5 year results of a comprehensive rehabilitation programme after myocardial infarction. European Heart Journal 8: 234–242

Hedback B E, Perk J, Engvall J, Areskog N-H 1990 Cardiac rehabilitation after coronary artery bypass grafting: effects on exercise performance and risk factors. Archives of Physical Medicine and Rehabilitation 71: 1069–1073

Henry W L, Bonow R O, Borer J S et al 1980 Evaluation of aortic valve replacement in patients with valvular aortic stenosis. Circulation 61: 814–825

Huang D, Ades P A, Weaver S 1990 Cardiac rehospitalisations and costs are reduced following cardiac rehabilitation. Journal of Cardiopulmonary Rehabilitation 10: 108

Hurst J W (ed) 1974 The heart, 3rd edn. McGraw-Hill, New York

Hurst J W, Schlant R C, Rackley C E (eds) 1990 The heart, 7th edn. McGraw-Hill, New York

Ice D 1985 Cardiovascular medications. Physical Therapy 65: 1845–1851

James F W, Kaplan S, Schwarz D C et al 1976 Response to exercise in patients after total surgical correction of tetralogy of Fallot. Circulation 54: 671–679

Jelinek V M 1988 Exercise after myocardial infarction: a practical guide to prescription. Patient Management Jan: 69–80

Joint International Society and Federation of Cardiology/World Health Organization Task Force on Standardisation of Clinical Nomenclature 1979 Nomenclature and criteria for ischaemic heart disease. Circulation 59: 607–609

Jones D, West R 1996 Psychological rehabilitation after myocardial infarction: multicentre randomised controlled trial. British Medical Journal 313: 1517–1521

Kallio V, Hamalainen H, Hakkila J, Luurila O J 1979 Reduction of sudden deaths by a multifactorial intervention programme after acute myocardial infarction. Lancet ii: 1091–1094

Kellerman J J, Shemesh J, Ben Ari E 1988 Contraindications to physical training in patients with impaired ventricular function. European Heart Journal 9(suppl F): 70–73

Krayenbuehl H P, Turina M, Hess O M et al 1979 Pre- and postoperative left ventricular contractile function in patients with aortic valve disease. British Heart Journal 41: 204–213

Landin R J, Linnemeier T J, Rothbaum D A et al 1985 Exercise testing and training of the elderly patient. In: Wenger N K (ed) Exercise and the heart, 2nd edn. F A Davis, Philadelphia

Lavie C, Milani R 1995 effects of cardiac rehabilitation and exercise training on exercise capacity, coronary risk factors, behavioural characteristics and quality of life in women. American Journal of Cardiology 75: 340–343

Lavie C, Milani R, Littman A 1993 Benefits of cardiac rehabilitation and exercise training in secondary coronary prevention in the elderly. Journal of the American College of Cardiology 22: 678–683

Leger I, Thivierge M 1988 Heart rate monitors: validity stability and functionality. The Physician and Sports Medicine 16(5): 143–151

Leon A S, Connett J, Jacobs D R, Rauramaa R 1987 Leisure time physical activity levels and risk of coronary heart disease and death. Journal of the American Medical Association 258: 2388–2395

Levin L-A, Perk J, Hedback B 1991 Cardiac rehabilitation – a cost analysis. Journal of Internal Medicine 230: 427–434

Levine S A, Lown B 1952 Armchair treatment of acute coronary thrombosis. Journal of the American Medical Association 148: 1365–1369

Lipkin D P 1991 Is cardiac rehabilitation necessary? British Heart Journal 65: 237–238

Lipkin D P, Scriven A J, Crake T, Poole-Wilson P A 1986a Six minute walking test for assessing exercise capacity in chronic heart failure. British Medical Journal 292: 653–655

Lipkin D P, Canepa-Anson R, Stephens M R, Poole-Wilson P A 1986b Factors determining symptoms in heart failure: comparison of fast and slow exercise tests. British Heart Journal 55: 439–445

Lutz J F, Wenger N K 1985 Use of exercise testing in noncoronary heart disease. In: Wenger N K (ed) Exercise and heart disease, 2nd edn. F A Davis, Philadelphia

McBurney H 1994 Clinical and statistical assessment of outcome in the post myocardial infarct population. PhD Thesis, La Trobe University

Marra S, Paolillo V, Spadccini F, Angelino P F 1985 Long term follow up after controlled randomised post MI rehabilitation programme: effects on morbidity and mortality. European Heart Journal 6: 656–663

Mathes P 1988 Physical training in patients with ventricular dysfunction: choice and dosage of physical exercise in patients with pump dysfunction. European Heart Journal 9(suppl F): 67–69

Miller D H, Borer J S 1982 Exercise testing early after myocardial infarction: risks and benefits. American Journal of Medicine 72: 427–438

Miller N H, Haskell W L, Berra K, De Busk R 1984 Home versus group exercise training for increasing functional capacity after myocardial infarction. Circulation 70: 645–649

Moller J H, Patton C, Varco R L, Lillehei C W 1991 Late results (30 to 35 years) after operative closure of isolated ventricular septal defect from 1954 to 1960. American Journal of Cardiology 68: 1491–1497

Newman B, Andrews M F, Koblish M S, Baker L A 1952 Physical medicine and rehabilitation in acute myocardial infarction. Archives of Internal Medicine 85: 552–561

Oldridge N B, Rogowski B L 1990 Self efficacy and inpatient cardiac rehabilitation. American Journal of Cardiology 66: 362–365

Oldridge N B, Guyatt G H, Fischer M E, Rimm A A 1988 Cardiac rehabilitation after myocardial infarction:

combined experience of randomised clinical trials. Journal of the American Medical Association 260: 945–950

Oldridge N B, Guyatt G, Jones N et al 1991 Effects on quality of life with comprehensive rehabilitation after acute myocardial infarction. American Journal of Cardiology 67: 1084–1089

Perrault H, Drblik S P 1989 Exercise after surgical repair of congenital cardiac lesions. Sports Medicine 7: 18–31

Shabetai R 1988 Beneficial effects of exercise training in compensated heart failure. Circulation 77: 775–776

Shankar K, Mihalko-Ward R, Rodell E et al 1990 Methodologic and compliance issues in post coronary bypass surgery subjects. Archives of Physical Medicine and Rehabilitation 71: 1074–1077

Shephard R 1981 Ischaemic heart disease and exercise. Croom Helm, London

Shephard R 1997 Exercise for patients with congestive heart failure. Sports Medicine 23: 75–92

Sire S 1987 Physical training and occupational rehabilitation after aortic valve replacement. European Heart Journal 8: 1215–1220

Spertus J, Winder J, Dewhurst T et al 1994 Monitoring the quality of life in patients with coronary artery disease. American Journal of Cardiology 74: 1240–1244

Stokes H, Turner S, Farr A 1995 Cardiac rehabilitation: programme structure, content, management and administration. In: Coats A, McGee H, Stokes H, Thompson D (eds) BACR guidelines for cardiac rehabilitation. Blackwell Science, Oxford

Sullivan M J, Higginbotham M B, Cobb F R 1988 Exercise training in patients with severe left ventricular dysfunction: hemodynamic and metabolic effects. Circulation 77: 506–515

Verrill D, Shoup E, McElveen G et al 1992 Resistive exercise training in cardiac patients. Sports Medicine 13: 171–193

Wenger N K 1989 Quality of life: can it and should it be assessed in patients with heart failure. Cardiology 76: 391–398

Williams J G, Eston R G 1989 Determination of the intensity dimension in vigorous exercise programmes with particular reference to the use of the rating of perceived exertion. Sports Medicine 8: 177–189

Williams M A, Maresh C M, Aronow W S et al 1984a The value of early outpatient cardiac exercise programmes for the elderly in comparison with other selected age groups. European Heart Journal 5(suppl E): 113–115

Williams M A, Esterbrooks D J, Sketch M H 1984b Guidelines for exercise therapy of the elderly after myocardial infarction. European Heart Journal 5(suppl E): 121–123

Worcester M 1986 Cardiac rehabilitation programmes in Australian hospitals. National Heart Foundation of Australia, Woden, Australia

World Health Organization 1993 Needs and action priorities in cardiac rehabilitation and secondary prevention in patients with coronary heart disease. WHO Technical Report Service 831, WHO Regional Office for Europe, Geneva

16

Cardiopulmonary transplantation

Catherine E. Bray

INTRODUCTION

The first human cardiac transplant was performed by Dr Christiaan Barnard and his team at Groote Schuur Hospital, South Africa, in 1967 (Barnard 1968). Despite initial enthusiasm, the problems of acute rejection and infection soon slowed the practice of the procedure. Several units continued with their programmes, gaining valuable clinical experience. However, it was the introduction of cyclosporin A, in the late 1970s, which significantly advanced immunosuppressive therapy and encouraged many centres world-wide to establish and continue heart transplantation programmes. This new age of transplantation also saw the first long-term survivors of heart–lung (Reitz 1982), single lung (Cooper et al 1987) and double lung (Patterson et al 1988) transplantation.

The transplantation of the thoracic organs is now an accepted practice in over 200 centres world-wide. In 1990, a total of 3054 heart, 194 heart–lung, 214 single lung and 60 double lung transplant procedures were registered as being performed on recipients, aged from newborn to 70 years (Kriett & Kaye 1991).

The primary indication for cardiac transplantation today, is for the relief of severe symptoms in individuals with end-stage dilated cardiomyopathy (Keogh et al 1991). Cardiopulmonary and pulmonary transplantation is increasingly utilized for patients with end-stage pulmonary disease which may or may not be associated with cor pulmonale. The indications for the various

Table 16.1 Indications for cardiopulmonary transplantation

Heart transplantation	Heart–lung transplantation	Single lung transplantation	Double/bilateral sequential single lung transplantation

End-stage heart failure as a result of:
  Post-viral cardiomyopathy
  Ischaemic cardiomyopathy
  Idiopathic cardiomyopathy
Disabling angina with inoperable coronary artery disease
	Pulmonary vascular disease, e.g. primary pulmonary hypertension Eisenmenger's syndrome Pulmonary parenchymal disease (with non-reversible cardiac dysfunction), e.g. bronchiectasis, cystic fibrosis, sarcoidosis, fibrosing alveolitis, chronic airflow limitation	End-stage fibrotic lung disease, e.g. pulmonary fibrosis, occupational lung disease, sarcoidosis, chronic airflow limitation	An alternative to heart–lung transplantation for patients with satisfactory right ventricular function and bilateral pulmonary sepsis, e.g. bronchiectasis, cystic fibrosis, chronic airflow limitation

forms of cardiopulmonary transplantation are outlined in Table 16.1.

ASSESSMENT

The assessment of potential recipients (which may be done on an outpatient basis) involves a review of the patient's past medical history and the results of previous investigations and interventions. Further investigations are carried out to define the following:

- Severity of cardiac and/or pulmonary dysfunction

- Identification of contraindications (Table 16.2)
- Immunological status (ABO group, human leucocyte antigen (HLA) tissue typing)
- Previous exposure to potentially complicating infections (cytomegalovirus (CMV), toxoplasmosis, hepatitis B, hepatitis C and methicillin-resistant *Staphylococcus aureus* (MRSA), and Epstein-Barr virus (EBV))
- Nutritional status
- Psychological status (Keogh et al 1991).

Once accepted for the active waiting list, potential recipients are reviewed every 1–3 months.

Table 16.2 Contraindications to transplantation (procedure-specific exclusion criteria)

General	Heart	Heart–lung	Single/double/bilateral sequential single lung
Absolute exclusion			
Irreversible renal dysfunction (except in combined heart–kidney transplantation) Irreversible hepatic dysfunction Active malignancy Immunodeficiency Alcohol/drug abuse Morbid obesity	Raised transpulmonary gradient (> 15 mmHg) and/or pulmonary vascular resistance (> 4 mmHg) (Patients who are excluded may be reconsidered for heterotopic heart or heart–lung transplantation)	Systemic corticosteroids (retard healing, especially tracheal or bronchial anastomosis)	Right ventricular ejection fraction < 25% (Patients who are excluded may be reconsidered for heart–lung transplantation) Systemic corticosteroids
Relative exclusion			
Active systemic infection Recent pulmonary infarction Insulin-dependent diabetes mellitus Peripheral or cerebrovascular disorders Psychological instability		Previous extensive pleural surgery Malnutrition Immobility Cachexia	Previous extensive pleural surgery Malnutrition Immobility Cachexia

THE TRANSPLANTATION PROCESS

Donors

Potential donors have been declared brain dead and have usually been the victims of a head injury or cerebrovascular accident. Table 16.3 outlines the transplant specific donor requirements. Another source of donor hearts is from heart–lung transplantation. In the 'domino' technique the heart from a patient undergoing heart–lung transplantation is utilized in a heart transplant.

When a potential donor becomes available, the donor hospital notifies a central organ transplant coordinator and provides information on the donor's age, weight, cardiopulmonary status and ABO blood grouping. The coordinator in turn contacts the transplant unit(s) that may utilize the organ(s) which are available.

All donor matching involves ABO blood group compatibility. Cardiac donor–recipient matching is done such that the donor weight is no more than 5 kg below that of the recipient. A positive donor weight advantage is necessary when the recipient's transpulmonary gradient is increased (Keogh et al 1991). Pulmonary donors are matched with the recipient's weight and dimensions of the thoracic cavity.

In the early days of transplantation it was necessary for the donor to be transported to the transplant centre. Today, hearts, heart–lung blocks, lungs and other transplantable organs/tissues are utilized via distant procurement procedures.

Operative procedures

Heart transplantation (HTx)

Orthotopic transplantation. Preparation of the heart (and heart–lung) transplant recipient is similar to that for any patient undergoing cardiac surgery (anaesthesia, median sternotomy and cardiopulmonary bypass). When the donor heart is present in the recipient theatre and has passed a final inspection, the recipient heart is removed, by incising the atria, pulmonary artery and aorta (leaving the posterior walls of both atria, including the sinoatrial (SA) node). The donor heart is sutured in place: the anastomoses joining recipient and donor atria, the pulmonary arteries and finally the aortas (Keogh et al 1986) (Fig. 16.1).

Heterotopic transplantation. Heterotopic transplantation is a less commonly used procedure than orthotopic transplantation. In this 'piggyback' procedure the recipient heart is left in place and the donor heart (connected to the recipient's in parallel by anastomoses made between the two hearts at the atria, pulmonary arteries and aortas) is positioned in the right chest. Both hearts contribute to the cardiac output (Weber 1990).

Heart–lung transplantation (HLTx)

The heart and lungs are excised separately, allowing identification and protection of the phrenic, recurrent laryngeal and vagus nerves,

Table 16.3 Donor selection criteria

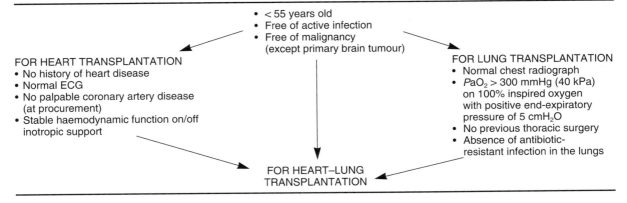

- < 55 years old
- Free of active infection
- Free of malignancy
  (except primary brain tumour)

FOR HEART TRANSPLANTATION
- No history of heart disease
- Normal ECG
- No palpable coronary artery disease
  (at procurement)
- Stable haemodynamic function on/off
  inotropic support

FOR LUNG TRANSPLANTATION
- Normal chest radiograph
- $PaO_2 > 300$ mmHg (40 kPa)
  on 100% inspired oxygen
  with positive end-expiratory
  pressure of 5 cmH$_2$O
- No previous thoracic surgery
- Absence of antibiotic-
  resistant infection in the lungs

FOR HEART–LUNG
TRANSPLANTATION

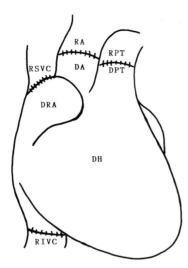

Fig. 16.1 Orthotopic technique: the donor heart following implantation: DH, donor heart; RPT, recipient pulmonary trunk; DPT, donor pulmonary trunk; RA, recipient aorta; DA, donor aorta; RSVC, recipient superior vena cava; DRA, donor right atrium; RIVC, recipient inferior vena cava.

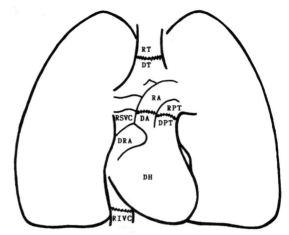

Fig. 16.2 The donor heart–lung block following implantation: DH, donor heart; RPT, recipient pulmonary trunk; DPT, donor pulmonary trunk; RA, recipient aorta; DA, donor aorta; RSVC, recipient superior vena cava; DRA, donor right atrium; RIVC, recipient inferior vena cava; RT, recipient trachea; DT, donor trachea.

a most critical part of the procedure. The heart is removed leaving the posterior wall of the right atrium. The left, then right lung is removed (following stapling of the bronchi, to minimize the risk of contaminating the area) and the trachea is divided above the bifurcation. The donor heart–lung block is implanted starting with the tracheal, then the atrial and aortic anastomoses. Ventilation is established (ensuring the patency of the airway anastomosis) and the heart resuscitated (Jamieson et al 1984) (Fig. 16.2).

Lung transplantation

Single lung transplantation (SLTx). The procedure commences as a lateral thoracotomy. The recipient's lung is removed and the donor lung positioned in the chest. Cuffs on the left atrium of the donor and recipient heart are joined. The pulmonary artery anastomosis is completed and circulation is restored to the lung, allowing for inspection of the arterial and atrial anastomoses. The bronchial anastomosis is performed and ventilation is resumed (Cooper et al 1987). Cardiopulmonary bypass is made available for the procedure but is rarely needed. Bronchial

healing may be promoted by the 'telescoping' of the donor and recipient bronchial anastomosis.

Double lung transplantation (DLTx) / bilateral sequential single lung transplantation (BSSLTx). The early experiences of DLTx involved the implantation 'en bloc' of both lungs via a median sternotomy utilizing an omental wrap to secure the tracheal anastomosis (Patterson et al 1988). In an effort to avoid the high incidence of airway complications associated with the original procedure, the technique of BSSLTx via anterolateral, bilateral thoracotomies with transverse sternotomy is now preferred. The procedure of direct revascularization of the bronchial arteries with the internal mammary artery is sometimes used to promote healing (Madden et al 1992). The donor procedure for double lung transplantation allows for the separate excision of the heart, facilitating the utilization of donor organs (Kaiser et al 1991).

Postoperative care

The intensive care area and ward management of the cardiopulmonary transplant patient is similar to that for any patient having undergone cardiac or thoracic surgery. The major differences include drug therapy and the intensive and comprehensive monitoring necessary because of the potential for rejection and infection. The degree and duration of protective isolation of recipients varies considerably between centres. Some units protectively isolate recipients in laminar airflow rooms, while others only require thorough hand washing before contact with the patient.

Rejection of the transplanted organs

The same immune response that protects the body against foreign chemicals and organisms, is also responsible for graft (transplanted organ) rejection. The presence of the transplanted organs triggers the immune system to respond, that is, to reject them. Both humoral (B lymphocyte mediated) and cellular (T lymphocyte mediated) immune responses may be involved in graft rejection. Rejection may occur at any time following transplantation, but the risk is greatest in the first 10–18 days post-transplantation (Weber 1990).

Acute rejection

Acute rejection occurs within the first 3 months after transplantation. Most recipients can anticipate two or more episodes of this cell-mediated immune response. The patient may be asymptomatic despite a definitive biopsy diagnosis.

In heart recipients it may be associated with malaise, shortness of breath, peripheral oedema, low-grade fever, nausea, vomiting, a voltage drop on ECG and/or an atrial arrhythmia (Keogh et al 1986). Endomyocardial biopsy (using a bioptome, passed down the right internal jugular vein and sampling tissue from the right ventricle) is currently the only way to objectively diagnose rejection. Biopsies are performed routinely on a regular basis for the first year following transplantation, and then only if indicated symptomatically.

A clinical diagnosis of acute lung rejection is usually made from a combination of findings

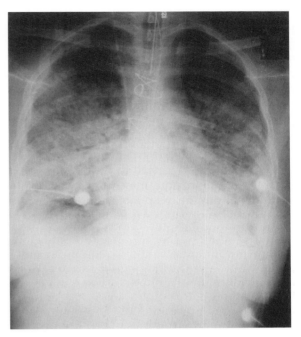

Fig. 16.3 A chest radiograph showing acute pulmonary rejection in a heart–lung recipient.

such as fever, shortness of breath, increasing infiltrates on chest radiograph, deteriorating gas exchange and lung function, the exclusion of infection and rapid symptomatic improvement with increased immunosuppression (Lawrence 1990) (Fig. 16.3).

To establish a diagnosis of lung rejection (and to identify infection) transbronchial lung biopsy may be utilized. There are, however, intrinsic difficulties in obtaining adequate tissue samples and in performing the procedure on critically ill patients. Transbronchial lung biopsies are carried out on a regular basis and when symptoms necessitate.

Chronic graft dysfunction

Chronic graft dysfunction occurs over months to years. In the transplanted heart it is characterized by diffuse and rapidly progressing coronary artery disease (CAD) manifesting in myocardial infarction, congestive heart failure or sudden cardiac death. CAD is postulated to be the result of chronic undetected rejection. It is a major factor limiting long-term survival and is seen in approximately 40% of patients 5 years following transplant (Squires 1990). Periodic coronary angiography is utilized for the diagnosis and monitoring of this process.

Obliterative bronchiolitis (OB), associated with lung transplantation, involves an inflammatory process in the small airways which leads to the obstruction and destruction of pulmonary bronchioles. It is suggested that OB is the result of 'late' rejection and may be advanced (or even triggered) by respiratory infection. It is one of the major factors influencing long-term survival of heart–lung and lung recipients.

Its successful management requires the close monitoring of pulmonary function and aggressive, early immunosuppression augmentation (Theodore et al 1990) as well as aggressive surveillance and treatment of infection (Fig. 16.4).

Immunosuppression

Immunosuppressive therapy is necessary for the rest of the recipient's life. Most maintenance immunosuppressive regimens utilize a combination of two or three drugs. By combining a number of drugs the doses of each can be adjusted to reduce associated side-effects (Table 16.4).

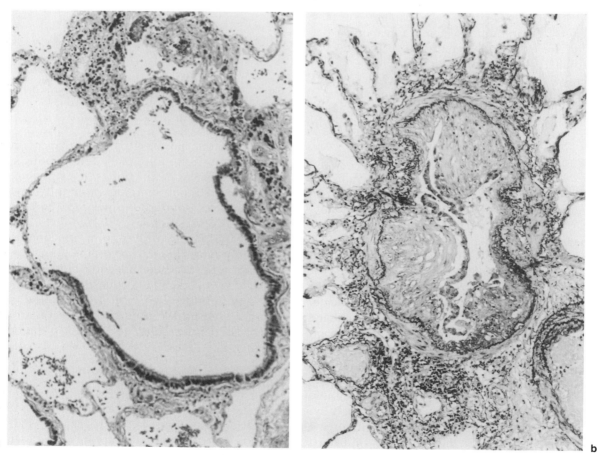

a   b

Fig. 16.4 **a** A normal bronchiole lined by ciliated, columnar epithelium deep to which there is a thin layer of smooth muscle. **b** Obliterative bronchiolitis: nodules of submucosal fibrous tissue have developed elevating the lining mucosa and substantially occluding the lumen.

Table 16.4 Immunosuppression

Drug	Effect	Side-effects
Maintenance immunosuppression		
Cyclosporin	T cell suppressor, lesser B cell effect	Nephrotoxicity, hepatic dysfunction, hirsutism, tremor, hypertension, susceptibility to malignant neoplasms
Azathioprine	Decreases the body's ability to generate T cells	Bone marrow suppression, hepatic dysfunction, nausea, anorexia
Corticosteroid (prednisolone)	Decreases antibody production and depresses the maturation of T cells	Water retention, hypertension, gastrointestinal ulceration, altered glucose metabolism, mood changes, osteoporosis
Anti-rejection therapy		
Corticosteroid (methyl prednisolone)	Reverses acute rejection as above	As above
Antithymocyte globulin (ATG)	T cell cytolytic (can be used in prevention)	Fever, rigors, neutropenia, 'serum' sickness
OKT3	For the management of cardiac rejection T cell cytolytic Blocks generation and function of T cells	Acute pulmonary oedema, fever, rigors, headache, tremor
FK506 (tacrolimus)	Blocks proliferation of T cells by inhibiting IL-2 secretion	Hypertension, diabetes, nephrotoxicity, increased malignancy risk, neurotoxicity
Mycophenolate mofetil	Inhibits T and B cell proliferation by blocking DNA replication	Diarrhoea, bone marrow suppression, opportunistic infection (especially tissue invasive CMV)
Methotrexate/cyclophosphamide	Cytotoxic to T and B lymphocytes	Bone marrow suppression, hepatic and renal toxicity

Infections

Infection continues to be a complicating and life-threatening feature of transplantation, especially in the first 3 months following the surgery. High-dose immunosuppressive therapy allows for the growth of opportunistic organisms (Table 16.5).

Patients can be discharged from the hospital to home (if within a 60-minute drive from the unit) or to the hospital accommodation as early as 5 days postoperatively. Patients continue to be closely monitored on an outpatient basis, usually for the first 3 months postoperatively. Regular follow-up continues until most patients can be reviewed on a 6- to 12-monthly basis. All patients are well informed of the signs or symptoms with which they must contact their carer centre.

SPECIAL CONSIDERATIONS FOR THE PHYSIOTHERAPIST

The key to a successful cardiopulmonary transplant programme is a well-informed, communicative, multidisciplinary team. With medical and nursing staff, social worker, pharmacist and dietitian the physiotherapist is vitally involved in the monitoring and education of the recipients, throughout each phase of the transplantation process. To do so effectively, the physiotherapist needs a strong knowledge base, particularly focused on the features of transplantation which will strongly influence the recipient's ability to participate in rehabilitation activities and later to resume employment and leisure activities. Physiotherapy specialization in this field, with continuity of care from assessment to postoperative rehabilitation, offers significant

Table 16.5 Common infections seen post-cardiopulmonary transplant

Infection	Common manifestation	Management
Bacterial (especially postoperative days 0–7)	Respiratory involvement; bronchial and/or lobar pneumonias	Specific antibiotic therapy
Viral Cytomegalovirus (primary or reactivation infection), especially subacute phase	Systemic, gastrointestinal inclusion/ulceration, pneumonitis (especially lung and heart–lung recipients)	Gancyclovir (intravenous twice daily, 10–14 days; prophylaxis, intravenous, 3 times weekly for donor–recipient cytomegalovirus mismatch)
Herpes (simplex and zoster)	Usual manifestations	Acyclovir
Epstein–Barr virus (primary or reactivation infection)	Lymphoma	Acyclovir
Fungal Candida	Oral, oesophageal	Nystatin, fluconazole, amphotericin B
Aspergillus	Respiratory, cerebral	Amphotericin B, itraconazole
Protozoal *Pneumocystis carinii*	Respiratory	Bactrim (treatment and prophylaxis)
Toxoplasma gondii	Systemic	As above

advantages in patient confidence, education and compliance.

Denervation of the heart/lungs

At rest. Most heart and heart–lung block recipients will have a higher than normal resting heart rate: they lack the inhibitory vagal influence. The lungs of heart–lung and lung recipients are denervated distal to the tracheal/bronchial anastomosis. As a result, the recipient's ability to cough spontaneously in response to secretions accumulating distal to the anastomosis is impaired.

Exercise. Denervation of the heart, in particular, has significant implications for the exercising of heart and heart–lung recipients. In the normally innervated heart it is changes in heart rate, not stroke volume, which account for the increase in cardiac output in response to dynamic exercise. There is substantial evidence that the denervated heart also increases its cardiac output in response to exercise. It does so early in the activity by increasing its stroke volume (based on the Frank-Starling mechanism). The heart rate of the recipient rises more gra-

dually than that of a normal individual following the commencement of exercise, does not reach a similar peak and slows more gradually once exercise is stopped. This pattern of heart rate response is primarily the result of changing levels of circulating catecholamines, which play an increasingly important role in increasing cardiac output at high workloads.

It is important to note that, although the transplanted heart does demonstrate compensatory exercise responses, the peak intensity of exercise and the duration of activity may be lower than that of normal individuals. If these limitations are present, it has been suggested that it may be the result of the donor heart having undergone an ischaemic period and reperfusion, myocyte necrosis as a result of acute rejection episodes, undetected or chronic rejection and/or diffuse CAD (Horak 1990, Squires 1990).

Denervation also prevents the transmission of pain from any ischaemic area of myocardium (Weber 1990). As a result patients should be advised against unsupervised exercise at high intensities for long periods. This is especially important if angiography indicates the presence of CAD.

Immunosuppression

It is important that physiotherapists working with transplant recipients are mindful of the effects of immunosuppressive drug therapy, particularly corticosteroids, on the musculo-skeletal system. The overall exercise capability of many transplant recipients is limited by peripheral musculoskeletal factors (Kavanagh et al 1988). Drug-related myopathy and prolonged periods of inactivity, pre- and postoperatively may be responsible for these limitations.

The contribution of corticosteroids to the process of osteoporosis must also be acknowledged particularly for those patients whose preoperative management (at any stage) has involved the prolonged use of steroid therapy. Special care when exercising and immediate and thorough investigation of reports of pain (especially back and hip pain) are essential for these patients.

When prescribing exercise and advising patients on resuming sporting activities, both physiotherapist and patient must be mindful of the inhibiting influence of steroid therapy on healing.

Infection/rejection

When a recipient is diagnosed as being in severe rejection (and provided that his cardiac rhythm and oxygen saturation are stable) his activity should be limited to walking at a slow, comfortable pace within the limits of the ward area. The rehabilitation programme is recommenced when the anti-rejection therapy is being reduced and the patient is asymptomatic.

In instances of minimal and moderate rejection or infection, exercise is continued according to the patient's presentation and symptoms. For lung and heart–lung recipients it is of paramount importance to monitor oxygen saturation regularly at rest, and throughout any exercise activities, even when they report no symptoms, but a biopsy has indicated an acute rejection episode. Again, monitoring of the patient's heart rate, rhythm and blood pressure is of importance.

PHYSIOTHERAPY MANAGEMENT

Physiotherapy has always played an important part in cardiopulmonary transplantation. The number of centres carrying out these procedures has expanded over recent years and so has the role of the physiotherapist within these units. Physiotherapy is now an integral part of all stages of the patient's management at assessment, preoperatively and at both the acute and rehabilitation phases of postoperative care.

Assessment

All patients referred for formal assessment are seen by the physiotherapist. The assessment of potential heart transplant recipients focuses on previous and current activity levels, muscle bulk and strength, and respiratory history and function. At this interview/assessment the physiotherapist may provide advice on dividing fatiguing activities of daily living (ADL) into more easily managed subtasks and outline a programme of stretches and exercises to maintain mobility, strength and muscle bulk.

All potential heart–lung and lung transplant recipients accepted for formal assessment are seen by the physiotherapist who assesses the patient's:

- Breathing pattern (at rest and while exercising)
- Cervical and thoracic spine posture and mobility
- Chest wall mobility
- Muscle range and strength (upper limb, trunk, quadriceps, etc.)
- Activity/exercise tolerance (including oximetry during a 'self-care' activity and a 6-minute walking test or shuttle walking test).

The findings are then reviewed with those of other team members in considering if the patient is an appropriate candidate for transplantation. The issue of patient compliance with both medical management and activity is an important issue with all team members.

Preoperative care

The goals in the preoperative period are to:

- Establish a good rapport between patient and physiotherapist
- Provide each potential recipient with a thorough understanding of his role in transplantation
- Improve and maintain the potential recipient's physical condition
- Assist the patient to use his time constructively
- Improve the potential recipient's (and support person/s') quality of life, while awaiting transplant.

All patients awaiting heart and lung transplants are included in a conditioning-rehabilitation programme (CRP). Patients living within ready access to the hospital (30% of patients on the active list) attend the gymnasium one to four times weekly and continue elements of the programme in a home routine. Patients who regularly attend other hospitals for ongoing outpatient treatment are supervised by their own physiotherapist in a modified form of the conditioning programme. Patients who live beyond the reach of regular hospital attendances are worked through a home conditioning programme and are managed and reviewed at clinic visits.

The CRP involves five treatment/training components: patient education, 'endurance' training, specific muscle training, thoracic mobility techniques and relaxation and stress management techniques. Each of the five components specifically addresses one or more previously identified problems and involves a number of techniques (Table 16.6). The patient's heart rate and rhythm,

Table 16.6 A conditioning–rehabilitation programme for potential heart–lung and lung recipients

Problem(s) addressed	Management/techniques
Component 1: Patient education	
Poor quality of life while awaiting transplantation	ADL advice Alternative strategies for recreational time Instruct family in massage and relaxation techniques
Fear of intubation/ventilation	Explanation of surgical and intensive care procedures Visit to intensive care unit Talk with (selected) recipients
Poor awareness of patterns of breathing	Review of chest anatomy, muscles of breathing, normal and abnormal breathing patterns Practice in 'isolating'/focusing on specific muscles and patterns of breathing
Component 2: Endurance training	
Poor endurance	Treadmill and bicycle ergometer programmes (intermittent work/rest periods) Home walking programme
Component 3: Specific muscle training	
Muscle weakness	Upper limb/trunk programme Abdominal programme Quadriceps programme Home weight programme
Component 4: Thoracic mobility techniques	
Preoperative musculoskeletal discomfort and postoperative pain	Soft tissue techniques Joint mobilization for cervical, thoracic, costal and sternal articulations
Component 5: Relaxation and stress management	
Preoperative respiratory crisis management and postoperative pain management	Relaxation techniques

blood pressure, oxygen saturation and rating of perceived exertion are checked before and during the gymnasium activities. Supplementary oxygen is used as appropriate.

The ongoing monitoring of all potential heart–lung and lung recipients is the responsibility of each team member who regularly reviews the patient. If significant deterioration in the potential recipient's functional status and/or physical condition is noted, an intervention strategy involving one or a number of intensive therapies may be devised in an effort to optimize the patient's condition. In particular cases of increasing hypercapnic respiratory failure the application of continuous positive airway pressure (CPAP or BIPAP) or intermittent positive pressure ventilation via a nasal mask during rest and sleep periods may provide ventilatory support, reducing respiratory muscle energy expenditure and allowing effective participation in preoperative rehabilitation (Carrey et al 1990). Nasogastric or gastrostomy feeding may be of benefit in these instances.

Increasingly, ventricular assist devices are being utilized to sustain patients awaiting heart transplant. These devices vary considerably with respect to the degree of mobility they afford the patient. Some require the patient to be maintained on complete bed rest whilst other devices allow the patient to ambulate. The obvious benefit of these ambulatory devices is that they allow the physical condition of the patient to be preserved during the waiting period.

Postoperative care

Acute care

The goals for the immediate postoperative period are to:

- Assist in weaning patients from mechanical ventilation and in establishing energy cost-efficient patterns of breathing
- Encourage and optimize secretion clearance
- Establish and progress pre-rehabilitation activities as soon as is appropriate
- Promote the patient's independence/self-reliance

- Consolidate and extend the information/education component of the preoperative programme.

For the majority of patients, postoperative physiotherapy is started immediately (30 minutes to 1 hour) post-extubation, which is usually 6–12 hours following transfer to the intensive care unit from theatre. There are occasions, however, when it may be necessary for the physiotherapist to be involved before extubation. This may be to facilitate the removal of secretions. More often, the treatment involves techniques of breathing control when a patient, weaning from ventilatory support, is showing signs of distress without obvious fatigue. Well-supported positioning, utilization of the stimulation and reassurance of hands-on instruction alternated with shoulder and cervical soft tissue techniques can bring about a change in respiratory pattern and rate, and positively affect arterial blood gases and the haemodynamic status. These techniques are especially effective when the physiotherapist–patient relationship has been well established in the preoperative period. In some instances it is also appropriate to encourage the patient to utilize the relaxation method he chose and practised in the preoperative conditioning programme.

Initial treatments involve:

- the active cycle of breathing techniques:
  - breathing control
  - thoracic expansion exercises
  - the forced expiration technique
  - gravity-assisted positions as appropriate
- active anti-gravity limb work as appropriate.

The frequency and duration of treatments in the early postoperative days are dependent upon the patient's presentation, needs and progress. Experience suggests that frequent, brief treatments are most beneficial. Thorough and comprehensive monitoring and reassessment of the patient by every health professional involved in the acute care are of paramount importance both to the individual patient and the auditing of the programme as a whole.

It is essential that the physiotherapist assesses and reassesses the patient at each treatment, remembering the vulnerability of the immuno-suppressed patient, both to infection and rejection. Subjective and objective assessment findings must be reviewed along with the latest microbiology results, arterial blood gases, chest radiograph, lung function measurements and oxygen saturation at rest and while mobilizing. Any changes, no matter how subtle should be noted and reassessed regularly. Effective communication between staff, particularly surgeon, physician, nursing staff and physiotherapist is essential for optimal patient care.

As a result of denervation of the lungs following transplantation (that is the absence of the recipient's ability to cough spontaneously in response to secretions accumulating distal to the anastomosis) it is essential that the physiotherapist evaluates (and educates the patient to do likewise) that their effective huff is dry sounding. If the huff is moist sounding, appropriate techniques should be employed to clear the bronchial secretions. Education regarding gravity-assisted positions and their utilization is usually of benefit at this stage.

Patients may be sat out of bed (depending on their cardiovascular stability) as early as 12 hours postoperatively. Patients usually start mobilizing from bed to chair on day 1. Recipients (especially the very debilitated patients) may commence a light upper limb weight programme as early as day 3, depending on their wound pain and stability (using weights of 1–1.5 kg).

Patients may be transferred to the ward as early as day 2 postoperatively. At this stage, patients are usually seen three or four times daily. Once free to mobilize from the bed area, patients are commenced on stair walking and gentle bicycle ergometer work. Usually on day 4 or 5, soft tissue (Chaitow 1988) and/or joint mobilization techniques (Maitland 1986) are commenced as indicated. These have proven particularly valuable with the SLTx and BSSLTx recipients whose primary pain following removal of the now routine epidural infusion appears to be associated with the articulations and muscle groups which have been stressed during surgery.

Should a patient require prolonged ventilatory support or reintubation, stretching, strengthening and mobilization work is started/continued as appropriate. Non-invasive ventilatory support (e.g. CPAP, BIPAP) is increasingly utilized at this stage and complements the emphasis of most programmes on promoting mobility.

Rehabilitation

The primary goals in the rehabilitation phase after transplantation are to:

- Improve the patient's physical condition (posture, strength and endurance)
- Improve the patient's (and support person/s') confidence in becoming involved in a full range of activities of daily living and appropriate exercise activities
- Nurture realistic expectations for employment, sport and leisure activities
- Promote independence in maintaining and monitoring the physical condition.

When the patients are allowed to mobilize from the ward area, they are commenced on a gymnasium-based rehabilitation programme. This may begin as early as day 3 postoperatively. Each patient's programme is tailored to suit his current physical status and is oriented toward his specific goals for employment and recreational pursuits. Even the most debilitated patient is included in the gymnasium programme and his support person/s are also encouraged to attend and become involved in supervising and encouraging exercise activities and in extending the patient's off-ward activities to include walking out-of-doors and eating 'out'.

Inpatients attend the gymnasium one or two times daily. Outpatients are encouraged to attend the gymnasium three to five times weekly, depending upon their condition and distance from the hospital, for a period of 8–12 weeks.

Each patient's gymnasium programme is based on varying times and intensities of work in a number of activities. The activities are introduced gradually according to the patient's physical condition, wound/musculoskeletal dis-

Table 16.7 Gymnasium activities utilized in the post-transplant rehabilitation programme

Activity	Purpose	Time/repetitions
Treadmill/bicycle ergometer	Warm up	12 minutes
Bicycle ergometer/treadmill	Endurance/aerobic fitness	5–40 minutes
Weights	Quadriceps strengthening Upper limb and shoulder girdle strengthening Glutei and lower limb strengthening	1–10 kg, 10–30 repetitions

comfort and level of confidence. Table 16.7 outlines the activities/equipment used, their primary purpose(s) and the varying duration of activities through which patients are progressed.

In our experience, the most effective way to determine the appropriate intensity of an activity has been to exercise according to a scale of perceived exertion such as the Borg scale (Borg 1970, Pandolf 1983). Activities are introduced at an intensity such that the patient's subjective description of his level of exertion is 'very light' or 'light'. The intensity is subsequently progressed to levels of exertion described as 'somewhat hard' and 'hard'. The same scale of exertion that is used in this rehabilitation phase is also used in the preoperative conditioning programme and the patient's home-based, maintenance work so that by the time a patient is ready for discharge from the immediate supervision of the gymnasium environment, he is well practised in judging and progressing activity intensity and is encouraged to apply this scaling to his recreational activities and workplace tasks.

Thorough supervision/monitoring of recipients before and while participating in gymnasium activities is of the utmost importance, especially in the early weeks of rehabilitation, while patients are unfamiliar with 'reading' the symptoms often associated with infection/rejection episodes. Prior to commencing their gym activities, patients are asked to comment on their ability to cope with activities of daily living and walking and how it compares with their performance in the previous days. Patients are checked for any change in weight, lung function tests (for heart–lung and lung recipients this includes twice daily self-monitoring of FEV_1 and FVC), blood pressure, heart rate and rhythm and resting oxygen saturation. Heart rate and blood pressure (and oxygen saturation for heart–lung and lung recipients) are monitored throughout the gymnasium session. Any uncharacteristic changes in the above parameters are noted as is any decline in a patient's ability to cope comfortably with an activity that previously has been well within his ability. Medical staff in the outpatients' clinic are notified and the patient is reviewed and investigated accordingly.

Patient participation in and progression through a rehabilitation programme needs to be flexible and readily modified and 'back tracked' to accommodate the sometimes unpredictable nature of the recipient's postoperative course. There will be occasions when patients are unable to exercise:

- immediately following cardiac or transbronchial biopsy (or other 'minor' procedures/investigations)
- when symptoms and/or a biopsy are indicative of a significant rejection or infection episode.

When exercise can be resumed, it will need to be at a lesser intensity than when the patient last participated in the activities and, as always, progressed considering the recipient's presenting condition. This is particularly important if the patient has just completed a course of intravenous steroid therapy and has noted symptoms of peripheral myopathy.

At 3–4 weeks postoperatively, abdominal and lower back strengthening exercises are added to the work-out. These exercises and upper limb weight work are outlined in each patient's maintenance programme, which is based on a once a day aerobic activity of the patient's choice, whether it be walking, cycling, swimming or running or a combination of these. Specific stretching/strengthening programmes are also outlined for patients returning to physically demanding employment and sporting activities.

CONCLUSION

Physiotherapy is an integral part of the management of the cardiopulmonary transplant recipient. The role of the physiotherapist has expanded considerably in the last 5 years and the future looks equally exciting. Nasal ventilation systems are being utilized in the pre- and postoperative phases to address sleep/ventilation problems which are prevalent amongst both pre- and postoperative patients. Physiotherapists

are in an ideal situation to involve themselves in these therapies. There are also numerous research opportunities available to physiotherapists working with transplant programmes.

The greatest challenge facing cardiopulmonary transplant programmes is the limited number of donor organs available for the ever expanding potential recipient waiting list. An essential part of addressing this dilemma is for units to ensure that maximal effort is made to optimize the physical condition of potential and actual recipients, providing the best possible situation for a successful transplant outcome. Physiotherapy has much to offer these patients and it is essential that the physiotherapist be actively involved in the cardiopulmonary transplant team.

ACKNOWLEDGEMENTS

I would like to acknowledge the assistance of Ms Jodie Partridge and Ms Megan Smith (physiotherapists), and Drs Peter Macdonald, Julie Mundy and Stephen Rainer in the preparation of this chapter.

It is also necessary to thank the entire Cardiopulmonary Transplant Team, St Vincent's Hospital, Sydney, Australia for their continued encouragement to develop physiotherapy in this challenging area.

REFERENCES

Barnard C 1968 Human cardiac transplantation. American Journal of Cardiology 22: 584–596

Borg G 1970 Perceived exertion as an indicator of somatic stress. Scandinavian Journal of Rehabilitation Medicine 2(3): 92–98

Carrey Z, Gottfried S, Levy R 1990 Ventilatory muscle support in respiratory failure with nasal positive pressure ventilation. Chest 97: 150–158

Chaitow L 1988 Soft-tissue manipulation: a practitioner's guide to the diagnosis and treatment of soft tissue dysfunction and reflex activity. Healing Arts Press, New York

Cooper J, Pearson F, Patterson G, Todd T, Glinsberg R, Goldberg M, DeMajo W 1987 Technique of successful lung transplantation in humans. Journal of Thoracic and Cardiovascular Surgery 93: 173–181

Horak A 1990 Physiology and pharmacology of the transplanted heart. In: Cooper D, Novitzky D (eds) The transplantation and replacement of thoracic organs. Kluwer, Lancaster

Jamieson S, Stinson E, Oyer P, Baldwin J, Shumway N 1984 Operative technique for heart–lung transplantation. Journal of Thoracic and Cardiovascular Surgery 87: 930–935

Kaiser L, Pasque M, Trulock E, Low D, Dresler C, Cooper J 1991 Bilateral sequential lung transplantation: the procedure of choice for double-lung replacement. Annals

of Thoracic Surgery 52: 438–446

Kavanagh T, Yacoub M, Mertens D, Kennedy J, Campbell R, Sawyer P 1988 Cardiorespiratory responses to exercise training after orthotopic cardiac transplantation. Circulation 77(1): 162–171

Keogh A, Baron D, Spratt P, Esmore D, Chang V 1986 Cardiac transplantation in Australia. Australian Family Physician 15(11): 1474–1481

Keogh A, Macdonald P, Chang V, Farnsworth A, Harvison A, Connell J, Jones B, Johnston R, Spratt P 1991 Seven years of heart transplantation in Australia – the St Vincent's Hospital experience. On the Pulse III(2): 2–7

Kriett J, Kaye M 1991 The registry of the International Society for Heart and Lung Transplantation: eighth official report, 1991. Journal of Heart and Lung Transplantation 10(4): 491–498

Lawrence E 1990 Diagnosis and management of lung allograft rejection In: Grossman R, Maurer J (eds) Clinics in chest medicine. W B Saunders, Philadelphia, vol II(2), pp 269–278

Madden B, Hodson M, Tsang V, Radley-Smith R, Khaghani A, Yacoub M 1992 Intermediate-term results of heart–lung transplantation for cystic fibrosis. Lancet 339: 1583–1587

Maitland G 1986 Vertebral manipulation. Butterworths, London

Noakes T, Kempeneers G 1990 Exercise rehabilitation. In: Cooper D, Novitzky D (eds) The transplantation and replacement of thoracic organs. Kluwer Academic Publishers, Lancaster

Pandolf K 1983 Advances in the study and application of perceived exertion. Exercise, Sports Science Review 11: 118–158

Patterson G, Cooper J, Goldman B, Weisel R, Pearson F, Water P, Todd T, Scully H, Goldberg M, Ginsberg R 1988 Technique of successful clinical double-lung transplantation. Annals of Thoracic Surgery 43: 626–633

Reitz B 1982 Heart and lung transplantation. Heart Transplantation 1(1): 80–81

Squires R 1990 Cardiac rehabilitation issues for heart transplantation patients. Journal of Cardiopulmonary Rehabilitation 10: 159–168

Theodore J, Starnes V, Lewiston N 1990 Obliterative bronchiolitis. In: Grossman R, Maurer J (eds) Clinics in chest medicine. W B Saunders, Philadelphia, vol II(2), pp 309–321

Weber B 1990 Cardiac surgery and heart transplantation. In: Hudak C, Gallo B, Benz J (eds) Critical care nursing: a holistic approach, 5th edn. J B Lippincott, Philadelphia

FURTHER READING

Cooper D, Novitzky D (eds) 1990 The transplantation and replacement of thoracic organs. Kluwer, Lancaster

Grossman R, Maurer J (eds) 1990 Clinics in chest medicine: pulmonary considerations in transplantation. W B Saunders, Philadelphia, vol II(2)

Kavanagh T, Yacoub M, Mertens D, Campbell R, Sawyer P 1989 Exercise rehabilitation after heterotopic cardiac transplantation. Journal of Cardiopulmonary Rehabilitation 9: 303–310

Keteyian S, Ehrman J, Fedel F, Rhoads K 1990. Heart rate-perceived exertion relationship during exercise in orthotopic heart transplant patients. Journal of Cardiopulmonary Rehabilitation 10: 287–293

Paul L, Solez K (eds) 1996 Organ transplantation long-term results. Marcel Dekker Inc, New York

Solez K, Racusen L, Billingham M (eds) 1996 Solid organ transplant rejection mechanisms, pathology and diagnosis. Marcel Dekker Inc, New York

Squires R, Allison T, Miller, Gau G 1991 Cardiopulmonary exercise testing after unilateral lung transplantation: a case report. Journal of Cardiopulmonary Rehabilitation 11: 192–196

Vibekk P 1991 Chest mobilisation and respiratory function. In: Pryor J (ed) Respiratory care. Churchill Livingstone, Edinburgh

17

Spinal injuries

Trudy Ward

INTRODUCTION

The prognosis for the patient sustaining spinal cord injury has until this century remained poor. An unknown Egyptian physician of 2500 BC describing spinal cord injury in the Edwin Smith Papyrus wrote: 'An ailment not to be treated' (Grundy & Swain 1993). This view continued until the work of Guttman and others encouraged development of special centres throughout the world and saw the problems associated with spinal cord injury at last being addressed, although the mortality from tetraplegia until the 1960s remained at 35% (Grundy & Swain 1993). Improvements in management at the time of the accident, technological advances in diagnosis and management approaches have contributed to the continuing fall over recent years in mortality and morbidity rates (Hornstein & Ledsome 1986).

The respiratory care of patients with spinal cord injury is examined in this chapter; however, the total management of patients requires a holistic, multidisciplinary approach to ensure effective rehabilitation.

MECHANICS OF RESPIRATION

In order to appreciate the effect of spinal cord injury on respiratory function it is necessary first to understand the mechanics of normal respiration. Table 17.1 illustrates the main muscles of respiration and their level of innervation.

Inspiration in the normal subject occurs as a

Table 17.1 The muscles of respiration

Respiratory muscle	Level of innervation	Respiratory action
Sternocleidomastoid	C1–3	Inspiration
Trapezius	C1–4	Inspiration
Diaphragm	C3–5	Inspiration
Scaleni	C4–8	Inspiration
Intercostals	T1–11	Expiration/inspiration
Abdominals	T2–L1	Expiration

result of the creation of negative intrapleural pressure. This may be achieved by contraction of the diaphragm causing it to descend, or by action of the intercostal muscles at lower lung volumes causing an increase in the lateral and anteroposterior diameter of the thorax (Morgan et al 1986). The intercostal muscles also work to stabilize the rib cage against the tendency for paradoxical inward movement caused by contraction of the diaphragm. Further stability is provided by the sternocleidomastoid, scaleni and trapezius muscles which assist the elevation and fixation of the ribs during forced or maximal inspiration, and will probably also act with other muscles in normal quiet respiration to ensure efficient movement of the chest wall (De Troyer & Heilporn 1980).

Expiration is normally a passive process, active muscle contraction being used during more forceful activities such as coughing or sneezing. The abdominals form the major muscles of expiration and also have an important role in maintaining the position of the diaphragm, so improving its efficiency. The intercostal muscles also have an expiratory function at higher lung volumes. Coughing and sneezing primarily rely for their powerful and explosive natures on the ability of respiratory muscles to generate sufficient inspiratory volumes, followed by the production of powerful expiration against controlled closure of the glottis (Braun et al 1984). The effectiveness of the cough depends on the linear velocity of the air in the airways. At high lung volumes, clearance will occur principally from the larger airways. At low volumes the effect is more marked in the smaller airways (Brownlee & Williams 1987).

EFFECTS OF SPINAL CORD INJURY

Following spinal cord injury, the muscles innervated below the level of injury will become weakened or paralysed (Loveridge et al 1992). The higher the level of injury, the greater the functional consequence on respiration. In addition, injury above T6 can cause disruption of the autonomic nervous system with loss of normal parasympathetic and sympathetic interaction, owing to sympathetic paralysis (Braddon & Rocco 1991).

Respiratory complications remain a major cause of death and morbidity for the patient with spinal cord injury, especially in the early and intermediate stages (Alvarez et al 1981, VanBuren et al 1994). Those particularly at risk are:

- Tetraplegic patients
- Patients with thoracic or lumbar lesions and rib or sternal injuries
- Patients with pre-existing lung disease.

For the tetraplegic patient, the ability to produce effective inspiration and cough will be severely impaired. This will be most marked during the phase of spinal shock when muscles below the level of injury are flaccid and the rib cage at its most mobile. Contraction of the diaphragm will therefore result in a marked paradoxical breathing pattern with limited apical expansion. Some improvement may occur as spinal shock resolves and the muscles become hyperreflexive or spastic (Mansel & Norman 1990). With time the tendons, ligaments and joints of the rib cage stiffen owing to decreased active movement. This, together with spasticity, will provide some compensation for loss of intercostal activity in stabilizing the rib cage (De Troyer & Heilporn 1980, Estenne et al 1983).

Transection of the cord above C4 will cause paralysis of the diaphragm, intercostal and abdominal muscles leaving the patient with sternocleidomastoid and trapezius for respiration. Unaided these are usually incapable of sustaining long-term ventilation, and for survival these patients will require mechanical assistance.

Patients with cervical lesions below C4 will have partial or total diaphragmatic action plus accessory muscles and can be ultimately independent of mechanical ventilation. Paralysis of the intercostal muscles will result in marked changes in the mechanical properties of the lungs as resultant paradoxical breathing (Fig. 17.1) will have a tendency to cause microatelectasis, and chest wall instability will add to the work of breathing (Fishburn et al 1990). A relatively minor insult to the respiratory system could therefore lead to major respiratory problems (De Troyer & Heilporn 1980). Effective cough for these patients requires the addition of external compression to produce the necessary large positive intrathoracic pressures (Braun et al 1984, De Troyer & Estenne 1991) and this is discussed later.

Patients with thoracic lesions will have some preservation of intercostal function but paralysis of the abdominal muscles. The lower the level of lesion the more inspiratory ability will approach normal values, although paralysis of the abdominal muscles will result in a decrease in potential expiratory effort. Damage below L1 has little effect on respiratory function.

THE EFFECT OF POSTURE

In the normal subject, mechanisms exist to ensure that adequate ventilation is maintained in all positions. In the supine position, contraction of the diaphragm displaces the abdominal contents without significantly expanding the rib cage, there being greater compliance of the abdomen than the rib cage. In standing, abdominal tone increases to support the abdominal contents, thereby decreasing abdominal wall compliance. Contraction of the diaphragm, intercostal and accessory muscles now cause greater rib cage expansion, resulting in an increase in vital capacity of about 5% (Chen et al 1990).

Positional changes will, however, affect the respiratory function of the tetraplegic patient. In supine, the weight of the abdominal contents forces the diaphragm to a higher resting level so that contraction produces greater excursion of the diaphragm. In sitting or standing, the weight of the unsupported abdominal contents increases the demand on the diaphragm which now rests in a lower and flatter position (Alvarez et al 1981, Chen et al 1990), decreasing effectiveness and restricting available excursion for creating negative intrapleural pressure. Chen et al (1990) recorded a 14% drop in predicted vital capacity in the tetraplegic patient on changing position from supine to sitting or standing. It is therefore important with these patients not to assume that ventilation will be sufficient in all positions.

RESPIRATORY ASSESSMENT

Accurate assessment and regular review of the respiratory status of a patient is vital. Initial assessment must be carried out as soon as possible to establish a baseline against which future deterioration or improvement can be monitored. Assessment procedure is discussed in Chapter 1.

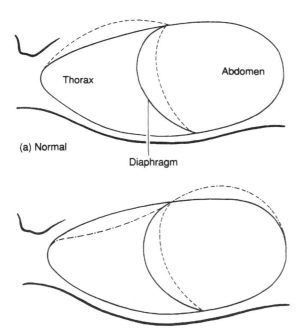

(a) Normal

Thorax

Abdomen

Diaphragm

(b) Paralysis below C5 showing paradoxical movement of the chest wall and abdomen

----- Active movement
—·— Passive movement

Fig. 17.1 Movement of the diaphragm, chest wall and abdomen: **a** normal; **b** paralysis below C5.

For complete assessment of the patient with spinal cord injury, the following details should be considered:

1. Motor and sensory neurological levels.

2. Associated injuries – rib fractures and flail segments are particularly likely in the patient with thoracic spinal injury and these may require modification of treatment techniques. Patients involved in diving accidents may present with the additional respiratory complications of water aspiration. The presence of intra-abdominal trauma or complications such as paralytic ileus, acute gastric dilatation or gastrointestinal bleeding will require modification to the techniques used by the physiotherapist, especially in assisted coughing.

3. Associated lung trauma – common injuries include pneumothorax, haemothorax and pulmonary contusion.

4. Pre-existing lung disease – problems such as asthma or chronic airflow limitation may exist and will be treated as indicated.

5. Presence of ventilatory support.

6. Psychological state – major psychological adjustment is required by the patient with spinal cord injury, not only to the injury itself, but also to the necessary treatment procedures. Sensory deprivation may cause loss of orientation, made worse by enforced immobilization and restricted visual input. Anxiety and interrupted sleep patterns caused by frequent turns and other procedures can result in increased patient confusion and fatigue. These factors will all affect respiratory function and must be considered by the physiotherapist to enable the most effective and appropriate planning of respiratory treatment.

7. Results of the chest radiograph and arterial blood gases, if available.

8. Altered levels of consciousness.

9. Respiratory rate at rest – with normal diaphragm activity the rate remains regular at 12–16 breaths/min. In the presence of a weak or fatiguing diaphragm the rate will increase (Alvarez et al 1981).

10. Assessment of breathing pattern to establish the degree of paradoxical movement or presence of unequal movement of the chest wall.

11. Assessment of diaphragm function, by inspection or palpation of the upper abdomen.

12. Assessment of cough to ascertain effectiveness.

13. Measurement of vital capacity – repeated measurement of vital capacity provides an indication of trends developing in respiratory function, and should be recorded in all the positions in which the patient may be nursed to detect postural variations (Morgan et al 1986). This will be especially pronounced in the presence of unilateral phrenic nerve damage. Values will vary depending on the level of injury. Ledsome & Sharp (1981) observed initial vital capacities of 30% of predicted normal value in C5/C6 patients, rising to 58% at 5 months. The high thoracic patient may be expected to have a vital capacity of around 80% of predicted normal (Bromley 1991). Vital capacity may fall over the first few days post-injury owing to factors such as muscle or patient fatigue, respiratory complications, or cord oedema which result in a rise in neurological level. Improvement is usually seen as oedema resolves and respiratory function stabilizes (Ledsome & Sharp 1981, Axen et al 1985). Vital capacity values of 500 ml or less may, in conjunction with clinical assessment, indicate the need for ventilation (Gardner et al 1986).

14. Auscultation of the chest to detect areas of lung collapse, pleural effusion or secretions.

PHYSIOTHERAPY TECHNIQUES

Respiratory management of the patient with spinal cord injury requires the application of the same principles as other respiratory problems; the skills used are discussed in Chapters 7 and 8. The goals of treatment include:

- Clearance of secretions from the lungs
- Improvement in breath sounds
- Increase in lung volumes
- Strengthening of the available muscles of respiration
- Improvement of pulmonary and rib cage compliance
- Education of the patient and his carer.

Treatment may be prophylactic or directed to treat specific problems.

Prophylactic treatment

This will include breathing exercises, modified postural drainage by regular turning and assisted coughing.

Breathing exercises to encourage maximal inspiration must be established at an early stage, although the absence of sensations below the level of injury may necessitate the use of overbed mirrors to supplement verbal and tactile feedback. Exercises are directed to improve lateral basal and apical chest wall expansion and diaphragmatic excursion, but care must be taken to avoid tiring the diaphragm. Patients with intercostal paralysis, however, are usually unable to perform localized breathing exercises.

Respiratory muscle training. Many articles have been written on the reduction of respiratory fatigue and increase in endurance achieved by respiratory muscle training (Cheshire & Flack 1978, Gross et al 1980, Hornstein & Ledsome 1986) (see also p. 168).

Gross et al (1980) used inspiratory muscle training in the form of variable resistance over a 16-week period and reported respiratory improvement in symptoms, endurance and inspiratory muscle strength. It was acknowledged, however, that continuous training would be necessary to maintain improvement, a statement supported by Ledsome & Sharp (1981).

Incentive spirometry enables respiratory training with immediate visual feedback to reinforce success. This can be particularly beneficial for the high tetraplegic patient for whom physical achievement is limited (Cheshire & Flack 1978). The use of incentive spirometry can be useful in involving relatives in respiratory rehabilitation at an early stage.

Intermittent positive pressure breathing (IPPB) can be used in conjunction with other methods of training, although work by Rose et al (1987) concluded that solely increasing lung volumes had no major effect on lung function in stable tetraplegics. IPPB may be useful in increasing inspiratory volume to aid the clearance of secretions in patients with sputum retention and lung collapse (p. 169), or in enhancing the administration of nebulized drugs in cases of ineffective inspiratory ability.

Glossopharyngeal breathing is another technique that can be used to increase lung volumes and assist secretion clearance (p. 159) in the high tetraplegic. Vital capacity may be increased by as much as 1000 ml (Alvarez et al 1981).

Assisted coughing

Assisted coughing is a vital inclusion in any respiratory programme. Patients may be able to clear sputum from small to large airways, but will need assistance to produce an effective cough for expectoration. Assistance is provided by the application of a compressive force directed in an inwards and upwards direction against the thorax to create a push against the diaphragm, thus replacing the work of the abdominal muscles. Pressure on the abdominal wall alone must be avoided. The sound of the resultant cough is the best indicator of the force required, but care must be taken to avoid movement of any fracture. Pressure directed down through the abdomen must be avoided, especially in the acute patient, due to the possibility of associated abdominal injury, or paralytic ileus.

Various methods of achieving assisted cough are described in the literature (Braun et al 1984, Brownlee & Williams 1987, Bromley 1991), Braun et al (1984) recording a 15% increase in peak expiratory flow using lower thoracic compression. The methods which may be used in the supine patient are illustrated in Figure 17.2.

If one person is assisting the cough, hands should be placed so that one rests on the near side of the thorax and the other on the opposite side of the thorax, with the forearm resting across the lower ribs (Fig. 17.2a). As the patient attempts to cough the physiotherapist pushes inwards and upwards with her forearm and stabilizes the thorax with her hands.

Alternatively, the hands are positioned bilaterally over the lower thorax (Fig. 17.2b) and with elbows extended the physiotherapist pushes inwards and upwards evenly through both arms.

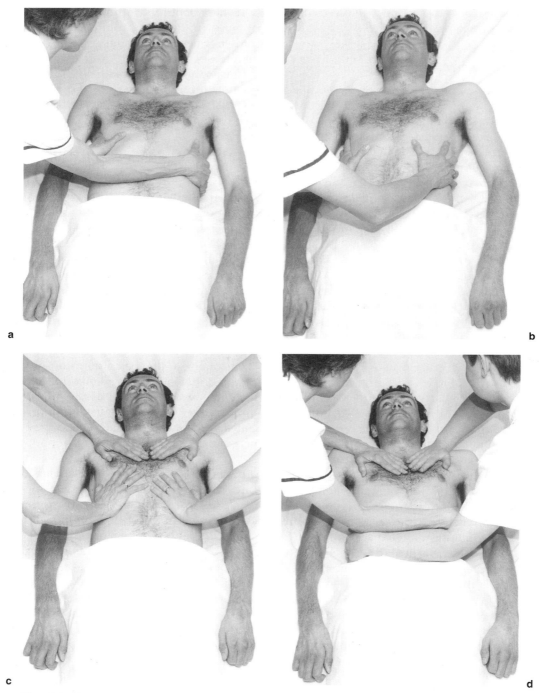

Fig. 17.2 Assisted coughing (see text).

In the case of the patient with a large thorax or having particularly tenacious sputum, two people may be required to produce an effective cough (Fig. 17.2c and d).

Care must be taken to avoid movement at the fracture site, and to synchronize the applied compressive force with the expiratory effort of the patient. Once the cough is completed, pressure must be lifted momentarily from the lower ribs, thus enabling the patient to use his diaphragm to initiate the next breath. If there is concern over fracture site stability or the amount of force needed for effectiveness, another person should be used to stabilize the patient by supporting his shoulders on the bed. In the presence of paralytic ileus or internal injury, extreme care must be taken during assisted coughing to avoid the application of pressure over the abdomen. Patients should be encouraged to cough three to four times per day, with nursing staff involvement in this process. If possible, patients should be taught self-assisted coughing when in a wheelchair, and relatives should learn how to assist the patient to cough in both lying and sitting.

Abdominal binders have been used on patients with high spinal cord injury for many years, both to minimize the effect of postural hypotension and aid respiration (Goldman et al 1986, Scott et al 1993). Their effect is achieved by providing support to the abdominal contents, decreasing the compliance of the abdominal wall and thereby allowing the diaphragm to assume a more normal resting position in the upright posture (Alvarez et al 1981). Goldman et al (1986) investigated the effect of abdominal binders on breathing in tetraplegic patients, and concluded that in the supine position there was no change, but when sitting there was a trend for improvement in lung volumes. This may help the patient considerably during the early stages of mobilization.

Treatment of the non-ventilated patient with respiratory problems

In the presence of respiratory problems such as retained secretions or lung collapse, sputum clearance is of paramount importance and vigorous, aggressive treatment is often needed. Physiotherapy treatment plans will be determined by ongoing assessment. Unless contraindicated by other complications, postural drainage either with an electric turning bed or manual turn into supported side lying should be used as appropriate. Great care must be taken to maintain spinal alignment and cervical traction throughout treatment. The effect of positioning on lung ventilation and perfusion must be considered (Ch. 7). Patients should never be left unsupervised during postural drainage in case of sudden sputum mobilization which could cause the patient to choke unless cleared by assisted coughing. Treatment may consist of vibration, shaking and chest clapping as necessary, followed by assisted coughing. 'Little and often' is the general rule as patients will tire quickly, but treatment must be effective, using two physiotherapists if necessary. Where possible, treatment should link in with planned turn times to allow some rest between various procedures.

Nasopharyngeal suction may be used if clearance by assisted cough alone is insufficient, but great care must be taken as pharyngeal suction can cause stimulation of the parasympathetic nervous system via the vagus nerve, resulting in bradycardia and even cardiac arrest. Hyperoxygenation of the patient with 100% oxygen prior to treatment will help minimize this possibility (Wicks & Menter 1986), but atropine or an equivalent drug should be available for administration intravenously should profound bradycardia occur.

Occasionally, bronchoscopy using a fibreoptic bronchoscope may be necessary to treat cases of unresolving lung or lobar collapse.

Care of the ventilator-dependent patient

Mechanical ventilation of the patient with spinal cord injury may be necessary in the following circumstances:

1. Injury to the upper cervical spine C1–C3, resulting in paralysis of the diaphragm.

2. Deterioration in respiratory function as a result of oedema or bleeding within the spinal canal causing the neurological level to rise so affecting the diaphragm. Patients are most at risk during the first 72 hours.

3. Respiratory muscle fatigue. The use of non-invasive positive pressure ventilation, e.g. a bilevel positive pressure device, may be helpful in providing ventilatory assistance without the need for full ventilation (Ch. 6). Tracheostomy may be beneficial in reducing the dead space by up to 50% (Bromley 1991).

4. Associated chest or head injuries which require management by elective ventilation.

Insertion of a minitracheostomy may be considered for patients with problems purely of retained secretions (Gupta et al 1989).

Physiotherapy goals for treatment for the ventilated patient are the same as those for the non-ventilated patient (p. 435). Treatment will include modified postural drainage, vibration and shaking with manual hyperinflation followed by suction to remove secretions. Frequency of treatment will be determined by assessment of the respiratory condition, but should not exceed 15–20 minutes. Patients requiring ventilation due to complications from spinal cord injury are often not sedated and a system of communication must be established before physiotherapy is started.

Ventilatory weaning considerations

A significant number of patients can be weaned from mechanical ventilation. In a study by Wicks & Menter (1986) factors which affected the predicted outcome of weaning included:

- Level of neurological injury
- Age less than 50 years
- Vital capacity improvement to 1000 ml.

There are other associated injuries and complications which may affect the results.

Weaning from the ventilator should start as soon as the patient's condition permits and is best performed with the patient supine, allowing the most effective diaphragm function (Mansel & Norman 1990). Weaning must take into account the possibility that the patient's respiratory muscles will have atrophied if ventilation has been prolonged. The goal must therefore be to achieve spontaneous breathing for short periods several times a day to avoid fatigue. Gardner et al (1986) suggested that spontaneous respiratory effort until the patient is tired may result in diaphragmatic fatigue, which may take about 24 hours to recover.

Additional mechanical assistance such as bilevel positive pressure, e.g. BiPAP, or continuous positive airway pressure (CPAP) will aid the patient during the weaning period, with emphasis being placed on psychological support and encouragement during this phase.

For the patient on long-term ventilation, a battery-driven ventilator may be attached to the wheelchair to enable mobility (Fig. 17.3). Home ventilation may also be a considered option,

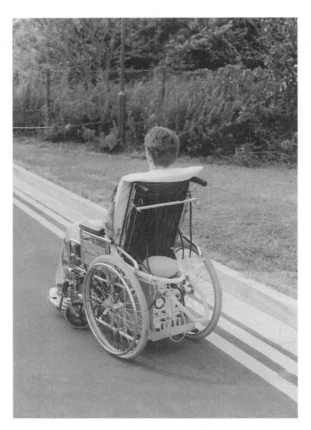

Fig. 17.3 Ventilated patient in a wheelchair.

although planning, education and support must be provided for all involved to achieve successful integration of the patient and his family back into the community.

The ethical dilemmas surrounding the ventilation of the high tetraplegic patient have challenged, and will continue to challenge, medical practice (Gardner et al 1985, Purtilo 1986, Maynard & Muth 1987, Gupta et al 1989). Only the ventilated tetraplegic knows what it is like to be a ventilated tetraplegic, and only his carer knows what it is like to care for him. In one review (Gupta et al 1989) of 21 patients who had required artificial ventilation, 18 stated that they would prefer a further period of continuous ventilation to being allowed to die. Sixteen of the 21 nearest caring relatives indicated that they were glad that their relative had been kept alive by ventilation. The study concluded that patients with spinal cord injury should be ventilated, provided that total emotional, educational and physical support could be given and maintained to all involved. This would seem to be most important.

In a case study, Maynard & Muth (1987) reveal how one individual's request to cease life-supporting ventilation was met. They suggest that 'if rehabilitation is defined as achieving optimal quality of life for people with severe disability then quality must be defined by the disabled individual'. An individual's perception of what constitutes acceptable quality of life will change over time (Purtilo 1986) and this poses the question of the feasibility of the involvement of the newly injured patient and relatives in the decision regarding ventilation, unable as they are to appreciate the global implications of tetraplegia. However, the patient and his family must be kept fully informed and their views taken into account before any decisions are made (Gardner et al 1985).

The ethical issues surrounding the high tetraplegic will continue to be debated but, ultimately, whatever is decided to be appropriate for an individual patient, psychological and physical support must be given to all involved (Gardner et al 1985).

Diaphragmatic pacing. Phrenic nerve pacing may sometimes be used on selected patients to free them from ventilatory dependence (Miller et al 1990). A paralysed diaphragm can be electronically stimulated if the phrenic nerve is intact and the cell bodies of C3, C4, C5 at the spinal cord viable. Electrodes may be placed to stimulate the phrenic nerve either in the neck or thorax, and are connected to a receiver embedded in the skin of the anterior chest wall. Stimulation is achieved by means of a radio transmitter placed over the receiver. Extensive postoperative training is necessary to increase diaphragmatic endurance, and teach the patient, his family and carers the necessary skills and understanding of the device.

For some patients, phrenic nerve pacing will provide an alternative to the ventilator, although this will remain as an emergency back-up. For others, pacing provides selective periods of freedom from mechanical ventilation enabling easier wheelchair mobility and improved psychological status.

CONCLUSION

Greater understanding of the problems of the spinal cord injured patient has led to continuing improvements in morbidity and mortality rates. Respiratory complications can now be managed more effectively as understanding of the problems facing these patients improves. Physiotherapists have, and will continue to have, much to offer in the respiratory care of the patient with spinal cord injury.

REFERENCES

Alvarez S, Peterson M, Lunsford B 1981 Respiratory treatment of the adult patient with spinal cord injury. Physical Therapy 61(12): 1737–1745
Axen K, Pineda H, Shunfenthal I, Haas F 1985

Diaphragmatic function following cervical cord injury: neurally mediated improvement. Archives of Physical Medicine and Rehabilitation 66(April): 219–222
Braun S, Giovannoni R, O'Connor M 1984 Improving the

cough in patients with spinal cord injury. American Journal of Physical Medicine 63(1): 1–10

Braddon R L, Rocco J F 1991 Autonomic dysreflexia: a survey of current treatment. American Journal of Physical Medicine and Rehabilitation 70: 234–241

Bromley I 1991 Tetraplegia and paraplegia. A guide for physiotherapists, 4th edn. Churchill Livingstone, Edinburgh

Brownlee S, Williams S 1987 Physiotherapy in the respiratory care of patients with high spinal injury. Physiotherapy 73(3): 148–152

Chen C, Lien I, Wu M 1990 Respiratory function in patients with spinal cord injuries: effects of posture. Paraplegia 28: 81–86

Cheshire D, Flack W 1978 The use of operant conditioning techniques in the respiratory rehabilitation of the tetraplegic. Paraplegia 16: 162–174

De Troyer A, Heilporn A 1980 Respiratory mechanics in quadriplegia. The respiratory function of the intercostal muscles. American Review of Respiratory Disease 122: 591–600

De Troyer A, Estenne M 1991 Review article: the expiratory muscles in tetraplegia. Paraplegia 29: 359–363

Estenne M, Heilporn A, Delhez L, Yernault J-C, De Troyer A 1983 Chest wall stiffness in patients with chronic respiratory muscle weakness. American Review of Respiratory Disease 128: 1002–1007

Fishburn M J, Marino R J, Ditunno J F 1990 Atelectasis and pneumonia in acute spinal cord injury. Archives of Physical Medicine and Rehabilitation 71: 197–200

Gardner B, Theocleous F, Watt J, Krishnan K 1985 Ventilation or dignified death for patients with high tetraplegia. British Medical Journal 291: 1620–1622

Gardner B, Watt J, Krishnan K 1986 The artificial ventilation of acute spinal cord damaged patients: a retrospective study of forty-four patients. Paraplegia 24: 208–220

Goldman J, Rose L, Williams S, Silver J, Denison D 1986 Effect of abdominal binders on breathing in tetraplegic patients. Thorax 41: 940–945

Gross D, Ladd H, Riley E, Macklem P, Grassino A 1980 The effect of training on strength and endurance of the diaphragm in quadriplegia. American Journal of Medicine 68: 27–35

Grundy D, Swain A 1993 ABC of spinal cord injury, 2nd edn. British Medical Journal, London

Gupta A, McClelland M, Evans A, El Masri W 1989 Minitracheostomy in the early respiratory management of patients with spinal cord injury. Paraplegia 27: 269–277

Hornstein S, Ledsome J 1986 Ventilatory muscle training in acute quadriplegia. Physiotherapy Canada 38(3): 145–149

Ledsome J, Sharp J 1981 Pulmonary function in acute cervical cord injury. American Review of Respiratory Disease 124: 41–44

Loveridge B, Sanii R, Dubo H I 1992 Breathing pattern adjustments during the first year following cervical spinal cord injury. Paraplegia 30: 479–488

Mansel J, Norman J 1990 Respiratory complications and management of spinal cord injuries. Chest 97(6): 1446–1452

Maynard F, Muth A 1987 The choice to end life as a ventilator dependent quadriplegia. Archives of Physical and Medical Rehabilitation 68: 862–864

Miller J, Farmer J, Stuart W, Apple D 1990 Phrenic nerve pacing of the quadriplegic patient. Journal of Thoracic and Cardiovascular Surgery 99: 35

Morgan M, Silver J, Williams S 1986 The respiratory system of the spinal cord patient. In: Bloch R, Bashaum M (eds) Management of spinal cord injuries. Williams & Wilkins, Baltimore

Purtilo R 1986 Ethical issues in the treatment of chronic ventilator dependent patients. Archives of Physical and Medical Rehabilitation 67: 718–721

Rose L, Geary M, Jackson J, Morgan M 1987 The effect of lung volume expansion in tetraplegia. Physiotherapy Practice 3: 163–167

Scott M D, Frost F, Supinski G, Gonzalez M 1993 The effect of body position and abdominal binders in chronic tetraplegic subjects more than 15 years post injury. Journal of American Paraplegia Society. (Abstract) 16(2): 117

VanBuren R, Lemons M D, Franklin C, Wagner M D Jr 1994 Respiratory complications after cervical spinal cord injury. Spine 19(20): 2315–2320

Wicks A, Menter R 1986 Long-term outlook in quadriplegic patients with initial ventilator dependency. Chest 3: 406–410

18

Care of the dying patient

Wendy Burford   Stephen J. Barton

INTRODUCTION

Palliative care is the essence of care for many people with respiratory conditions because so many of these diseases are disabling and incurable.

'The palliative care approach aims to promote both physical and psychosocial well being. It is a vital and integral part of all clinical practice, whatever the illness or its stage, informed by a knowledge and practice of palliative care principles. The key principles underpinning palliative care which should be practised by all health care professionals in primary care, hospital and other settings comprise:

• focus on quality of life which includes good symptom control
• whole-person approach taking into account the person's past life experience and current situation
• care which encompasses both the dying person and those who matter to that person
• respect for patient autonomy and choice (e.g. over place of death, treatment options)
• emphasis on open and sensitive communication, which extends to patients, informal carers and professional colleagues' (National Council for Hospice and Specialist Palliative Care Services 1995).

It is to be emphasized that it is the disease itself which is terminal and not the patient; because the disease is in the terminal phase this does not mean the withdrawal of appropriate treatment.

In 1992 the Standing Medical Advisory Committee and Standard Nursing and Midwifery Advisory Committee recommended that all patients requiring palliative care services should have access to them and that they should be developed as for patients with terminal cancer. To maintain contact with the patient, by a short visit, when it is no longer appropriate to continue active interventions is important to the patient, carer and physiotherapist.

Throughout the disease process it is important to maintain a holistic approach; the physical symptoms are often glaringly obvious but other components are often forgotten by the professionals. Good symptom control takes into account the physical, social, psychological and spiritual aspects affecting both the patient and those caring for him (Fig. 18.1).

PSYCHOLOGICAL FACTORS

The psychological factors of the disease process reverberate around the patient, relatives and the staff involved. For both the patient and the carer the grieving process begins with the diagnosis of a life-threatening condition. The patient anticipates lack of function and the thought of leaving the family, 'How will they cope without me?'. The family tree (Fig. 18.2) can be used to show who is important to the patient and if they have faced a significant loss before.

It is important to recognize that an understanding of the psychological aspects of dying is as important as the understanding of the physiological changes that are occurring within the dying patient.

When a patient and the family have been given the diagnosis of a terminal illness, and learn that the emphasis of treatment will now be aimed at palliative care and the effective control of symptoms, to allow for quality of life instead of a cure, the grieving process begins.

Effective care of the dying patient lies in the approach of the different members of the health care team's ability to understand the problems faced by each individual patient and family, and then to initiate the appropriate actions.

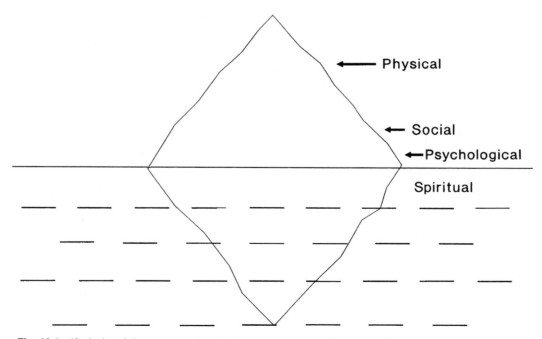

Fig. 18.1 'An iceberg' demonstrates how health care professionals perceive the physical, social, psychological and spiritual needs of patients.

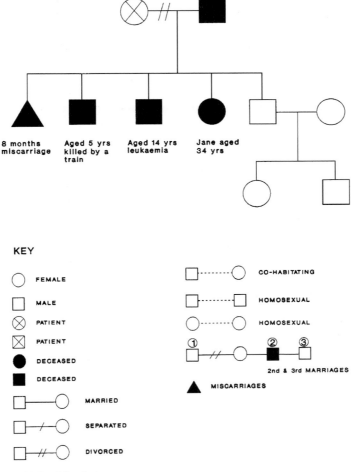

Fig. 18.2 A family tree.

The stages of the grieving process described below can occur at any time and in any order (Fig. 18.3).

Denial

After the initial shock that the patient has a terminal illness, the denial phase begins. 'There must be some mistake', 'They don't really mean me', or 'They must have someone else's results'. This behaviour continues in the hope that if it is denied long enough it will eventually go away, or the result will change.

It is a coping mechanism used to protect the individual from something unpleasant. It is hard to accept the news of a terminal disease if one has a sense of well-being and one's physical condition is not yet compromised by symptoms. For example, some newly diagnosed lung cancer patients present to their general practitioners with a cough that is not resolving or responding to conventional antibiotic therapy. The chest radiograph shows a mass, and subsequent fibreoptic bronchoscopy confirms that there is a tumour present. Cytology confirms small-cell (oat-cell) lung cancer. It is even harder for patients to accept that without treatment their life expectancy is approximately 3 months and with treatment probably between 12 and 18 months, especially if they are still able to lead a near normal lifestyle.

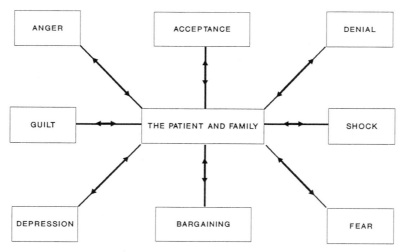

Fig. 18.3 The psychological components of terminal care.

Shock

No matter how much preparation is given before confirmation of bad news, it can still surprise and shock when given. The two most common reactions seen in hospital are the hysterical and inconsolable, or the numbing and emotionless response. Of these two responses the hysterical reaction is often the easier to deal with, once the patient and family are through the initial stage. Working with them it is possible to build up a relationship of mutual trust and respect and to help them come to terms with the future and what it may hold.

With the latter of the two responses, it may be impossible to help patients until they have let down the barriers that they are using to protect themselves. It will inevitably be a long process trying to win the patients' and relatives' confidence and so helping them face up to the future.

Anger

Anger may be felt by many people during the terminal phases of a person's life, varying from the patient to the immediate members of the family. Their reactions will be as diverse as their reasons for trying to understand what is happening.

The patient or relatives may initially become angry with the doctor or nurse when informed of the diagnosis, and although this anger is directed at them it should not be taken personally. It is usually an automatic response when given information that one cannot cope with. It may also be an aspect of some people's coping ability that they have to retaliate when faced with a situation that is alien to them. Often patients become angry and frustrated as the illness progresses, owing to a loss of their physical ability and independence, becoming more dependent on the carer either in the home or in hospital. It is therefore very important that both the patient and carer should be involved in all decisions made with regard to medical and nursing management and so help to retain autonomy of care.

The family may become angry and highly critical of the treatment and care being offered to their loved one. This anger may be as a result of their own feelings of guilt and inadequacy and inability to cope with the fact that their partner is actually going to die and leave them alone, and it is this fear that is presenting itself as anger.

Many parents when faced with the death of one of their children will initially respond with anger – anger at God for allowing this to happen, anger at the medical profession for not doing enough to help, and anger at each other for allowing this to happen by not caring enough.

Guilt

Guilt is an emotion common to all involved in the life of a terminally ill patient. The patients themselves may feel a sense of guilt for becoming a burden on their family. The burden may be physical because they are no longer able to look after themselves, or it may be financial, especially if they are the main breadwinner of the family. They may have feelings of guilt that they will eventually be leaving their partner to cope alone after they have gone.

The carers will often feel guilty if they are unable to cope with the patient in the community, and hospital admission is required. They often see this as letting their loved one down. There may also be feelings of guilt on the part of the family that they are being left behind and will have to cope.

Depression

Depression is the emotion that everyone expects to see at some time in someone faced with the prospect of dying. Depression can present in different forms and has many components that need to be considered. These vary from feelings of melancholia and somatic complaints to feelings of deep despair and suicidal tendencies.

The more common symptoms are changes in behaviour, with the person becoming withdrawn, having reduced concentration, loss of interest and increased irritability, for example laughter and the noise of children are no longer welcomed with a tolerant smile but arouse irritation and frustration. There may be changes in the sleep pattern which consist of early morning waking rather than difficulty in getting off to sleep. This can lead to insomnia which is highly resistant to hypnotics and, although the answer is in treatment of the underlying depression, the patient and the family cannot see this and often demand more powerful drugs.

Changes in appetite are commonly associated with depression and in mild cases compulsive eating may be witnessed with the patient helping himself to 'tit-bits from the biscuit tin'. Generally appetite is diminished and weight loss is more common, and in severe cases it can be dramatic.

Somatic complaints are multiple and range from the common tension symptoms, such as pain in the head, back and neck. The tension can manifest itself locally or can be very generalized.

Fear

Fear is a natural component of terminal care, and the uncertainty that people face. It may only be a temporary feeling or it can remain with the patient and family until the end. Usually this feeling can be overcome by a little thought on the part of the doctor and the nurse. Quite often a simple explanation of any procedures that are about to be performed will suffice to help and reassure the patient and carer. Honest and realistic answers to any of their questions will help reassure the patient and reinforce what is happening and what to expect.

Bargaining

Bargaining is a mental process that many people will experience when faced with a terminal disease. For example, the patient with lung cancer who promises to give up smoking if it will buy more time, or the frequent saying 'If only the doctor had done something earlier'. This process is often associated with feelings of guilt and will be faced by both the patient and the family.

Acceptance

Acceptance is the final stage of the grieving or bereavement process; it is the coming to terms with, the resolution of one's emotions or the resolving of conflicts. It is only when this phase is reached that patients can be at peace with themselves, accepting and preparing for death, a death with dignity. To allow for this to happen, all components have to be equal and when this equilibrium between physical symptoms and psychological state is balanced, then a peaceful death can follow.

PHYSICAL FACTORS

Respiratory conditions which physiotherapists

may see in the terminal care stage include lung cancer, cystic fibrosis, emphysema and crypto-genic fibrosing alveolitis. The period between the time of diagnosis of a terminal condition and the stage of terminal care varies from years to several weeks. Most patients with cystic fibrosis will have lived with the knowledge that their life expectancy is limited, but for patients with lung cancer the diagnosis will probably be a shock to them and to their families.

There are different types of lung cancer and these include squamous cell carcinoma, adeno-carcinoma, large-cell and small-cell carcinoma. Half of the lung cancers arise peripherally, but the others are situated more centrally, proximal to a segmental bronchus and are less often resectable. The cell type will be identified by histological or cytological investigation and will influence the treatment the patient will receive. Of all cases presenting, only about 25% are suitable for surgery. The majority of patients who develop lung cancer have a relatively poor prognosis (Mountain 1986).

Psychologically, patients who are found to have an inoperable tumour may find it difficult to accept that no 'active' treatment is offered whilst they remain asymptomatic. Radiotherapy in the treatment of lung cancer is primarily palliative but is reserved for the control of symptoms, that is haemoptysis, bone pain or nerve pain, superior vena caval obstruction, breath-lessness (intraluminal radiotherapy), dysphagia, cough, spinal cord compression, lymphangitis and cerebral metastases.

With small-cell (oat-cell) carcinoma there is usually evidence of disease elsewhere in the body at the time of diagnosis which therefore excludes surgery. The overall prognosis is very poor but the tumour does respond for a time to chemotherapy and/or radiotherapy.

Symptom control in lung cancer

Pain

Pain is the symptom most feared both by the patient and carer and once a diagnosis of cancer is made physical pain is the symptom which

they all anticipate, although one-third of patients with cancer do not experience any physical pain (Twycross & Lack 1990).

Pain is influenced by physical, social, psycho-logical and spiritual attitudes. Pain is whatever the patient says it is. It is individual and is affected by the patient's previous experience of pain, and there are racial and cultural differ-ences. Patients often fear the process of dying rather than death itself and it is important to emphasize that measures can be taken to control physical pain in the majority of patients.

Analgesics should be given on a regular basis, there is no place for 'as required' analgesia in the situation of chronic pain. The aim is to ensure that the patient is pain free and this can only be achieved by the regular administration of drugs, often in combination. Pain should be assessed regularly and adjustments made to the analgesia.

It is important to gain the patients' trust and confidence and to restore their sense of worth, well-being and self-esteem, thereby enabling them to feel more relaxed. Some patients find this by utilizing complementary therapies, for example aromatherapy, reflexology, gentle mas-sage and relaxation techniques (possibly includ-ing a relaxation tape). Time spent with patients allaying their fears will often enable a reduction in the amount of analgesia required.

Bone pain. This is usually the result of metastatic deposits (which may present as a pathological fracture and may require surgery). Radiotherapy as a single treatment is often very beneficial for bone pain. A non-steroidal anti-inflammatory agent combined with an opiate drug may control the pain. Bone pain related to hypercalcaemia may respond when a *bisphos-phonate* is administered (Bower & Coombes 1993).

Nerve pain. This is caused by the invasion or destruction of nerve fibres, for example supe-rior sulcus tumours (Pancoast tumour). These tumours grow in the apex of the lung and invade the brachial plexus. Mesotheliomas are tumours usually occurring in patients who have had exposure to asbestos. They grow in the pleura and cause intractable chest wall nerve pain.

Nerve pain can be difficult to control and is often opiate resistant. Drugs which may be helpful are tricyclic agents, anticonvulsants, corticosteroids and local anaesthetic congener drugs such as flecainide. Nerve blocks may be attempted and transcutaneous electrical nerve stimulation may bring some relief to this type of pain.

Liver pain. This is caused by metastases invading the liver capsule. This pain responds to corticosteroids.

Headaches. These may be caused by raised intracranial pressure from cerebral metastases. Corticosteroids and cranial irradiation will relieve this symptom.

Muscle spasm. This may be experienced following convulsions if the patient has cerebral metastases. Muscle relaxants (benzodiazepines) may be administered.

Drugs for the control of chronic pain must be given regularly (Fig. 18.4):

- mild analgesics – non-opioid – aspirin, paracetamol
- moderate analgesics – weak opioid – codeine phosphate, dihydrocodeine (DF 118), co-proxamol
- strong analgesics – strong opioid – morphine, diamorphine, methadone.

At all levels co-analgesics may be used for specific symptoms. There is no minimum or maximum amount of opiate which can be given. The advent of the syringe driver, which delivers a controlled regular amount of drug, has made it possible for many patients with terminal illness to be nursed at home until their death.

Nausea

Nausea may be a side-effect of chemotherapy or a result of the administration of opiates. It may also be caused by severe constipation,

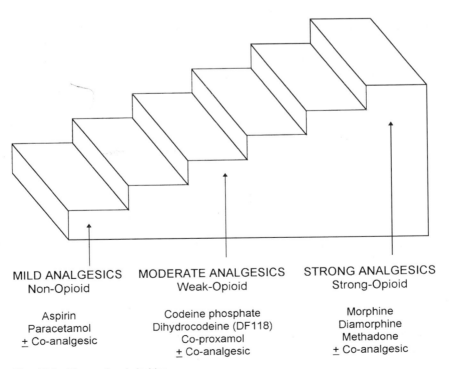

MILD ANALGESICS
Non-Opioid

MODERATE ANALGESICS
Weak-Opioid

STRONG ANALGESICS
Strong-Opioid

Aspirin
Paracetamol
± Co-analgesic

Codeine phosphate
Dihydrocodeine (DF 118)
Co-proxamol
± Co-analgesic

Morphine
Diamorphine
Methadone
± Co-analgesic

Fig. 18.4 The analgesic ladder.

electrolyte imbalance, or a raised intracranial pressure. Some patients obtain relief of nausea from antiemetic drugs and steroids. Dexamethasone may help to reduce a raised intracranial pressure. (Cold fizzy drinks, e.g. ginger ale, may be tolerated by the nauseated patient.)

Breathlessness

Positioning the patient plays a very important part and the high side lying position can be of great assistance to the breathless patient (Fig. 8.2, p. 139). Many patients prefer sitting upright in an armchair and may wish to sleep in the armchair at night. Some find resting on a pillow across a small table helpful (Fig. 8.6, p. 142).

Oxygen therapy may be necessary for patients with co-existing respiratory or cardiac conditions and patients with lymphangitis carcinomatosis, stridor or if they are continuously dyspnoeic. However, for many patients with lung cancer oxygen therapy is usually of no value except psychologically for the patient with terminal malignant disease and sets up yet another physical barrier between patients and their family/carer.

Occasionally when a tumour is causing tracheal obstruction heliox, a mixture of helium (79%) and oxygen (21%), is used to relieve respiratory distress (p. 188).

Opiate drugs can be helpful in the relief of breathlessness and may be administered either orally or by subcutaneous infusion. An anxiolytic may be of use, for example Valium. Nebulized morphine has been shown to relieve breathlessness in some patients with severe chronic lung disease (Young et al 1989).

Superior vena caval obstruction

Superior vena caval obstruction is caused by the spread of a tumour into the mediastinum or by enlarged lymph nodes. Pressure on the superior vena cava leads to oedema in the face, neck and arms. The patient may complain of difficulty breathing, headaches and feeling faint when he bends down. Stridor may be present.

Urgent treatment is necessary and radiotherapy is probably the most effective except for patients with small-cell carcinoma who usually respond to chemotherapy. Opiate and corticosteroid drugs may alleviate breathlessness. The head of the bed may be raised in an attempt to reduce the facial oedema during the night.

Death rattle

This noise is produced by the movement of secretions in the hypopharynx in association with the inspiratory and expiratory phases of respiration. This is heard in patients who are too weak to expectorate. Repositioning the patient is often effective in reducing the sound for both patient and family. Oropharyngeal suction is unpleasant for the patient, particularly if conscious, and is usually ineffective. Hyoscine may be given by subcutaneous injection. If the patient is unconscious and the syringe driver is being used, the administration of hyoscine subcutaneously is the treatment of choice and can be combined with diamorphine.

Physiotherapy

The physiotherapist may have been involved with the patient throughout his illness and there will be a stage when most physical treatment techniques are inappropriate, but it is important that the physiotherapist maintains contact with both the patient and the family during the terminal stages. Positioning the patient for comfort and relief of breathlessness, and assisting the patient to clear a plug of sputum may be beneficial. Even if the physiotherapist feels she is achieving very little, the patient would feel abandoned if her visits stopped.

SOCIAL FACTORS

Social factors affect the total well-being of the patient. The patient may be concerned about his inability to work and the financial implications which may affect the whole family. This can cause depression and it is important that the patient is aware of the social benefits to which he is entitled. Industrial claims can be instigated if it is an industry-related disease, for example mesothelioma. A social worker should be available and good communication among the multiprofessional team will lead to more effective treatment.

The patient may fear rejection by family, friends and colleagues and this may lead to social isolation. As the disease progresses the patient experiences a loss of libido and those who have received cytotoxic chemotherapy become sterile. This has implications for family life.

The control of symptoms enables a more socially acceptable lifestyle. Family and friends should be included in the decision making and care of the patient both at home and during hospitalization. This helps the carers to cope when death occurs.

SPIRITUAL CARE

To help a patient attain or maintain peace of mind it is important to be aware that the patient's personal value system may have been shaken as a result of the illness. 'It may be that the person's concept of God or his understanding of the spiritual dimensions of his life are stunted; that religious ceremonies are neither meaningful, nor supportive, nor a source of strength to him' (Kitson 1985).

Sensitive listening may enable the patient to express his fears, hopes and conflicts. The lack of a firm commitment to a religion does not mean that the patient does not have spiritual requirements. Religious practices should be observed and patients and families are usually happy to explain practices which are unfamiliar to members of the multiprofessional team of carers. Ministers and religious leaders should be available.

RESPONDING TO THE DYING PATIENT AND HIS RELATIVES

It is important to be natural and to spend time with the dying patient. You do not have to talk all the time, but give the patient an opportunity to express his fears and anxieties. Patients often ask questions which are uncomfortable to answer.

Am I going to die? The patient will put this question to the person he trusts, and an honest reply is being sought. The response 'Do you think you are?' gives the patient the chance to vocalize his fears and opens up an opportunity for you to say, 'Yes, but I don't know when' and to ask him if he is afraid. Many patients say that they are not afraid of death but of the process of dying.

When am I going to die? This is always difficult because we cannot predict the answer. We can say, 'Yes, you are very sick but we do not know when you are going to die'.

All questions should be handled very sensitively. Sit with the patient and do not rush away. It is not appropriate to tell patients not to worry, but listen to their fears and anxieties. You cannot say that you know how they are feeling because we all have individual ways of coping.

Tell the nurse who is looking after the patient about the type of questions you have been asked. Return to the patient later in the day as this will allow him to ask you more questions if he wishes and shows that you are offering him support at a difficult time.

How am I going to die? This is a question frequently asked by dying patients. Always be honest. Ask the patient how he feels he might die. This allows him to express his fears.

Many breathless patients lie awake at night, afraid to go to sleep in case they do not wake up. It is often the fear of dying alone, without anyone noticing, that keeps them awake. During the day there are people around. Breathless patients need reassurance that they are not going to suffocate and that drugs can be given to relieve symptoms.

If good symptom control is maintained the patient should die quite peacefully.

How to approach relatives before and after a death

The relatives should be kept informed of the patient's deteriorating condition and should be encouraged to participate in the care of the patient as much as they wish. In stressful situations we all behave differently and it is important to allow relatives to express their worries and fears. Many adults have never seen anyone die except on films or television where death is often portrayed as being frightening.

The staff should explain to the relatives how they think a patient will die, that the breathing will get slower and eventually stop. Following the patient's death the relatives should have the opportunity to stay with the patient until they feel ready to leave.

It is important to acknowledge what has happened. This may be verbally by saying how sorry you are to hear of the patient's death. Non-verbal communication can be very comforting. A gentle touch on the arm can convey more than a list of platitudes.

Support for staff

Staff need the opportunity to talk through the problems they are experiencing when working with the dying patient. This helps the individual to cope with their feelings and physiotherapists should be sensitive to these needs. It is particularly difficult when patients are young or in the same age group as the professional.

Many dilemmas have arisen for staff working with patients who are terminally ill but awaiting transplantation. When the patient's physical condition is deteriorating, what would normally be considered appropriate management may be withheld in anticipation of donor organs becoming available.

It is important that the patient is able to live until he dies. 'We cannot judge a biography by its length, by the number of pages in it; we must judge by the richness of the contents ... Sometimes the 'unfinisheds' are among the most beautiful symphonies' (Frankl 1964).

REFERENCES

Bower M, Coombes R C 1993 Endocrine and metabolic complications of advanced cancer. In: Doyle D, Hanks G W C, MacDonald N (eds) Oxford textbook of palliative medicine. Oxford University Press, England, ch 4: 11, p 449

Frankl V 1964 Man's search for meaning. Hodder & Stoughton, Bury St Edmunds, Suffolk

Kitson A 1985 Spiritual care in chronic illness. In: McGilloway O, Myco F (eds) Nursing and spiritual care. Harper & Row, London, ch 11, p 145

Mountain C F 1986 A new international staging system for lung cancer. Chest 89: 225S–233S

National Council for Hospice and Specialist Palliative Care Services 1995 Specialist palliative care, a statement of definitions. Occasional Paper 8, section 4.3, p 6

Standing Medical Advisory Committee and Standing Nursing and Midwifery Advisory Committee Joint Report 1992 The principles and provision of palliative care. HMSO, London, p 27

Twycross R, Lack S 1990 Therapeutics in terminal cancer, 2nd edn. Churchill Livingstone, Edinburgh, p 11

Young I, Daviskas E, Keena V A 1989 Effect of low dose nebulised morphine on exercise endurance in patients with chronic lung disease. Thorax 44: 387–390

FURTHER READING

Buckman R 1988 I don't know what to say. Papermac (Macmillan), London

Doyle D, Hanks G W C, MacDonald N (eds) 1993 Oxford textbook of palliative medicine. Oxford University Press, England

Hoogstraten B, Addis B J, Hansen H et al (eds) 1988 Lung tumours. Springer-Verlag, Berlin

Kübler Ross E 1970 On death and dying. Macmillan, New York

Lugton J 1987 Communicating with dying people and their relatives. Austen Cornish / Lisa Sainsbury Foundation, Great Britain

McGilloway O, Myco F (eds) 1985 Nursing and spiritual care. Harper & Row, London

Murray Parkes C 1986 Bereavement studies of grief in adult life, 2nd edn. Penguin, Harmondsworth

Souhami R, Tobias J 1986 Cancer and its management. Blackwell Scientific, Oxford

19

Hyperventilation

Diana M. Innocenti

INTRODUCTION

Hyperventilation is a 'physiological response to abnormally increased respiratory "drive" which can be caused by a wide range of organic, psychiatric and physiological disorders, or a combination of these' (Gardner & Bass 1989). It is a state of breathing in excess of metabolic requirements resulting in a lowering of the alveolar partial pressure of carbon dioxide ($PACO_2$) and arterial partial pressure of carbon dioxide ($PaCO_2$). 'Hyperventilation' is synonymous with 'hypocapnia'.

Acute hyperventilation is a normal physiological response to stress and may result in self-regulating paraesthesia, dizziness and palpitations. The disorder of chronic hyperventilation, or the spontaneous occurrence of prolonged hyperventilation with multiple and alarming symptoms, was described as the hyperventilation syndrome in 1937 (Kerr et al 1937). A syndrome is, by definition, identified by its combination of symptoms. It is not possible to contain it within a single diagnostic measurement and so it continues to be recognized clinically as a constellation of continuous or intermittent symptoms and physiological changes with or without recognizable provocative stresses (Magarian 1982) or known etiology.

The diagnosis was not uncommon in the past (Baker 1934, Wood 1941) but in the present technological era, hyperventilation in its chronic recurrent forms generally tends to go unrecognized and the diverse symptoms are labelled as functional; even though it has been shown that severe chronic hyperventilation with profound hypocapnia can be present in the absence of psychiatric, respiratory or other organic abnormalities (Bass & Gardner 1985).

Hyperventilation is more likely to be recognized in association with panic disorders or phobic states because of its causal, consequential or perpetuating relationships (Cowley & Roy-Byrne 1987) but still patients attend a succession of clinics, presenting with increasingly disturbing symptoms which appear to have no organic foundation and the patient receives no help. The anxiety aroused by the situation increases the hyperventilation and a hyperventilation–anxiety spiral is set up.

The spiral may be perpetuated by physiological and/or psychological causes, setting up conditioned reflexes of new and incorrect habitual patterns of breathing and a re-setting, or loss of fine tuning, of the respiratory centre's trigger mechanisms. (Fig. 19.1).

Signs and symptoms (Table 19.1)

Some patients present with a constant level of hypocapnia which drops further as a result of trigger mechanisms. Others present with resting levels of carbon dioxide within the normal range but with episodic lowering of the $PaCO_2$ to a level that precipitates symptoms.

Hypocapnia induces vascular constriction resulting in decreased blood flow and as a response to the Bohr effect there is inhibition of transfer of oxygen from haemoglobin in the circulating blood to the tissue cells. Most of the cerebral, peripheral and cardiac symptoms occur as a consequence. Fluctuations in $PaCO_2$ can have

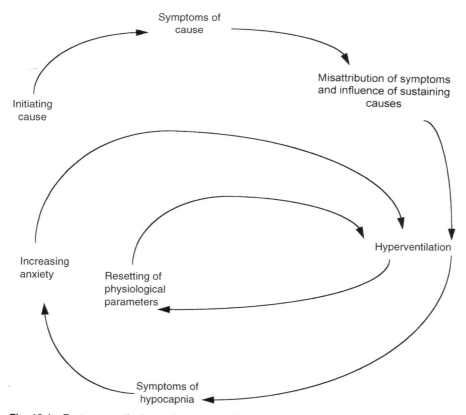

Fig. 19.1 Factors contributing to the hyperventilation–anxiety spiral.

Table 19.1 Commonly reported signs and symptoms can be loosely grouped into systems

System	Signs and symptoms
Cardiovascular	Palpitation
	Chest pain (pseudoangina)
	Peripheral vasoconstriction
Gastrointestinal	Dysphagia
	Dyspepsia
	Epigastric pain
	Diarrhoea
General	Exhaustion
	Lethargy
	Weakness
	Headache
	Sleep disturbance
	Excessive sweating
	Disturbance of concentration and memory
Musculoskeletal	Muscle pains
	Tremors
	Involuntary contractions
	Cramps
	Tetany (rarely)
Neurological	Paraesthesiae
	Lack of coordination
	Dizziness
	Disturbance of vision and hearing
	Syncope (rarely)
Respiratory	Breathlessness
	Difficulty in taking a satisfying breath
	Excessive sighing
	Chest pain
	Bronchospasm
Psychological	Anxiety
	Panic attacks
	Phobic states
	'Depersonalization'

a destabilizing effect on the autonomic system resulting in a sympathetic dominance (Freeman & Nixon 1985). The patients are often in a state of arousal. It has been shown (Folgering et al 1983) that the mean urinary excretion of adrenaline in a group of hyperventilators was three times as high as in a group of normals. The respiratory alkalosis associated with hyperventilation causes a lowering of calcium ions in the plasma which precipitates hyperirritability of motor and sensory axons (Macefield & Burke 1991). Altered patterns of breathing can cause musculoskeletal dysfunction with subsequent chest pain, which may be due to intercostal muscle tension, spasm or fatigue, costochondritis, costosternal, or costo-

vertebral joint pain. It has been suggested that hyperventilation increases circulating histamine, which may be causative in the high incidence of allergies reported and that as the cerebral symptoms of hypoglycaemia are similar to those of hypocarbia, the cerebral effects of hyperventilation are highlighted at times of low blood sugar (Lum 1994).

Causes of hyperventilation

It is necessary to recognize any specific organic, physiological or psychological causes (Table 19.2) and before embarking on a treatment programme to ensure that the patient has been suitably investigated to eliminate any underlying treatable disease or disorder. Other than hyperventilation being the main cause of the patient's symptoms it is not uncommon for hyperventilation to be a sustaining factor within a complex interaction of a number of physiological, organic and psychological disorders (Gardner 1994).

Personality

Why are some people more prone to respond to these and environmental stimuli with altered

Table 19.2 Some causes of hypocapnia

Drugs	Drug ingestion (causing acidosis or respiratory dyskinesia)
	Alcohol
	Caffeine
	Nicotine
Organic disorder	Anaemia
	Asthma
	Chronic severe pain
	Central nervous system disorders
	Diabetes mellitus
	Pneumonia
	Pulmonary embolus
	Pulmonary oedema (LVF)
Physiological	Altitude
	Pyrexia
	Pregnancy
	Luteal phase of the menstrual cycle
Psychiatric	Depression
	Anxiety
Psychological	Panic disorders
	Anxiety
	Phobic states

breathing patterns? Breathing is controlled by chemoreceptors in the medulla, mechano-receptors in the muscles, joints and lung tissue which modulate the rhythm generator in the medulla by reflex action; by behavioural and voluntary stimuli coming from the cerebral cortex and by temperature influences from the hypothalamus. Adaptation of any of the components of the neuro-pathways of respiration can influence or perpetuate disordered responses, breathing patterns and carbon dioxide levels, resulting in what appears to be a re-setting of the respiratory centre's triggering mechanisms.

One hypothesis is that the sensitivity of the respiratory centres may be greater than normal and be personality linked (Clark & Cochrane 1970). The type of person who presents with a chronic hyperventilation syndrome tends towards the perfectionist personality, one who functions at a high level of arousal to achieve self-set high expectations and unrealistic time frames. Another, and related hypothesis, is that there is an underlying biological and often inherited vulnerability, leading to a hypersensitive central nervous 'alarm system'. This system is triggered inappropriately causing the 'fight and flight' response (Cowley & Roy-Byrne 1987).

Diagnostic tests

There are no generally accepted measurable diagnostic criteria and it is probably not possible to devise satisfactory or conclusive diagnostic tests for the hyperventilation syndromes because of the multifactorial effects and complex systemic interactions.

The voluntary hyperventilation provocation test (HVPT)

The HVPT (Hardonk & Beumer 1979) records end-tidal $PaCO_2$ and all symptoms provoked during the test. Using end-tidal $PaCO_2$ recordings the patient is requested to hyperventilate for 3 minutes. If the $PaCO_2$ falls by at least 1.33 kPa (10 mmHg) and the rate of recovery is less than two-thirds of the former resting level after 3 minutes, the result is recorded as a positive diagnosis of a hyperventilation syndrome. However, as about a quarter of 'normals' also show this phenomenon, the test in this form is losing favour as an instrument for diagnosis.

Immediately after the voluntary hyperventilation the patient is asked to compare any symptoms provoked during the test with recognized complaints. When two major symptoms are reproduced the HVPT is considered positive. Generally, tingling of fingers and dizziness are not included because these symptoms occur in 'normal' subjects. Sometimes provoked symptoms are new experiences and not related to the patient's complaints. Caution should be exercised on using this test if the patient complains of cardiac symptoms or pseudoangina.

The Nijmegen questionnaire

This was first drawn up as a list of 16 complaints (Box 19.1), chosen by a team of specialists from different disciplines, from 45 clinically relevant symptoms related to hyperventilation syndromes (van Doorn et al 1982). The complaints fall into three categories or dimensions, corresponding with the classical triad of breathing disruption, paraesthesiae and central nervous system effects. The list does not include fatigue or behavioural disturbances. Patients score on a five-point scale from 0–4 (0 = never, 1 = rare, 2 = sometimes,

---

Box 19.1 Nijmegen questionnaire: the list of 16 symptoms

- Chest pain
- Feeling tense
- Blurred vision
- Dizzy spells
- Feeling confused
- Faster or deeper breathing
- Short of breath
- Tight feelings in the chest
- Bloated feeling in the stomach
- Tingling fingers
- Unable to breathe deeply
- Stiff fingers or arms
- Tight feelings round the mouth
- Cold hands or feet
- Heart racing (palpitations)
- Feelings of anxiety

3 = often, 4 = very often) against each of the 16 listed symptoms and a score over 23 is recognized as positive.

The questionnaire can be useful for physiotherapists to record symptoms and, if used at regular intervals, it could record the changing status in relation to treatment and a final score at discharge could be used as a semi-objective outcome measure. The efficacy of the questionnaire was investigated by comparing patients who hyperventilate with persons who do not. It showed a high ability to differentiate between the two groups (van Dixhoorn & Duivenvoorden 1985) and, although not conclusive, it was recognized that the questionnaire was suitable to be used as a screening instrument in diagnosing the syndrome when used with additional information. A correlation has been shown between positively rated Nijmegen questionnaire results (score of 24 or more) and positive HVPT results (recognition of at least two major symptoms) (Vansteenkiste et al 1991).

The 'Think test' (Nixon & Freeman 1988)

This provides a patient-specific stimulation which can have an advantage over unspecific challenges in testing for episodic hypocapnia. Approximately 3 minutes after a period of forced voluntary hyperventilation the patient is invited to close the eyes and to think about the circumstances, feelings and sensations surrounding or initiating the experience of symptoms. A fall in $PaCO_2$ greater than 1.33 kPa (10 mmHg) is considered to be significant.

Ambulatory monitoring of transcutaneous $PaCO_2$ $P_{Tc}CO_2$ (Pilsbury & Hibbert 1987)

The patient is attached to the apparatus and instructed on how to press the 'event button' and in the use of a diary. The 'event button' marks the recording tape and the diary entry records the type of symptoms, severity of symptoms (on a visual analogue scale 0–8), type of activity or non-activity and the extent of the physical exertion (visual analogue scale 0–8).

Breath-holding time

This is a semi-objective measure which generally shows a direct relationship between the maximum breath-holding time and the resting $PaCO_2$ (short breath-holding time is usually associated with a low or unstable resting $PaCO_2$).

Breathing patterns

Normal breathing patterns at rest involve an active inspiratory phase and a passive expiratory phase at approximately 8–14 breaths per minute. The body movement is predominantly a gentle swelling of the abdomen on inspiration which reflects the descent of the diaphragm, and it returns to rest on expiration. Thoracic movement is minimal at rest and increases on exercise. Rate, size and place of movement change with varying stimuli, disease or dysfunction.

The breathing patterns related to the chronic hyperventilation syndromes vary widely from gross upper thoracic movement with sternomastoid action at a rate of 50 breaths/min, to a near-normal rate and volume and minimal upper thoracic movement. The degree of lower thoracic movement and abdominal movement also varies from almost nil to normal.

The respiratory rate and volume may be extremely irregular and the pattern interspersed with sighs (Fig. 19.2). At the other extreme, once hypocapnia has been established, it may only require an occasional deep sigh to maintain the low levels of carbon dioxide and the general breathing pattern may appear normal.

The patterns vary with each patient and within the daily time span of each patient. The only constant feature in hypocapnia is that the patient moves more air than that which is required by the metabolic rate. There does not seem to be

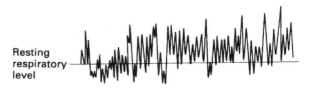

Fig. 19.2 Diagrammatic representation of an irregular pattern taken from a spirometry trace.

a strict correlation between the abnormality of the breathing pattern, the depression of $PaCO_2$ and the severity and type of symptoms.

TREATMENT

We have seen that there appear to be various groups of patients with symptoms related to hyperventilation. The disorder may be symptomatic hyperventilation without any underlying abnormalities or the hyperventilating component may be a part of emotional, psychiatric or behavioural disorders in causal, consequential or perpetuating relationship. The sooner a hyperventilating component is recognized and treated the less likely the situation will escalate. If there is related disorder then an interdisciplinary approach is helpful at most times (psychiatric, counselling, behavioural or speech therapy).

Whether the hyperventilation be the primary or secondary factor an improvement of subjective symptoms, exercise tolerance, general fitness and quality of life can be gained by re-educating the breathing pattern with the subsequent re-ordering of the patient's responses to the internal and external environment.

Re-education of the breathing pattern involves a conscious control of rate, volume and regularity of the breathing cycle devised to raise $PaCO_2$ by a small measure. A predominantly re-laxed, passive abdominal movement (reflecting the movement of the diaphragm) is preferred and movement directed away from the upper thorax. This abdominal pattern of movement may in turn help to induce physical and mental relaxation. Relaxation is often aided by a regular, slow pattern of breathing. It may be necessary with some patients to practise a relevant relaxation technique before, during or after the breathing control. The long-term goal is to decrease ventilation sufficiently to raise the resting $PaCO_2$ and re-establish a more normal pattern of movement.

In the short term, until the new pattern of breathing becomes the natural, constant, unconscious, spontaneous method of breathing, the patient will continue to experience episodes of symptoms. These symptoms may be related to certain recognizable situations, stresses or exercise. It is necessary to learn to control the breathing pattern at these times and/or take 'first aid' measures of breath holding or rebreathing expired carbon dioxide. In time, with reassurance and perseverance, it should be possible to control intermittent dropping of $PaCO_2$ by identifying the provoking situations and practising precautionary measures.

Assessment

The assessment should include:

- History
- Signs and symptoms
- Personality
- Physical examination.

History

It is helpful to ask open-ended questions to elicit when the patient was first aware of symptoms and the response to them. The first awareness may have been an acute 'attack', for instance driving home on the motorway on a Friday night after a stressful week and experiencing dizziness, tingling in the limbs and central chest pain. The response to this could be that of believing it to be a heart attack. This would be very understandable, especially if a member of the family had recently died of coronary disease. The anxiety would stimulate the respiratory rate further and the symptoms would increase, possibly to the point of admission to the nearest accident and emergency department.

Misrepresentation of the symptoms of an acute short-term episode of stress may cause a natural response to be transformed into a pattern of inappropriate responses in daily life.

Signs and symptoms may not present so dramatically. Commonly there is a history of glandular fever or a prolonged viral illness or fever. The patient never fully recovers and many of the listed signs and symptoms supervene. Symptoms may be traced back to a bereavement, change of lifestyle, job or house, family breakdown, frightening experience or prolonged emotional pressure. A definitive triggerpoint may not be found and the first experience of the disorder be related to an array of stimuli which happened together or in close succession. History of chronic pain should be noted as this may be the underlying cause (Glyn et al 1981). Hypermobility syndrome may have an effect on the ventilation because of abnormally compliant lungs and hypermobility of the thoracovertebral joints.

Family history. Have parents, siblings or more distant relatives experienced similar symptoms, allergy, cardiac or respiratory disease? Not uncommonly the habit of overbreathing can be traced back to family relationships.

Childhood history. General health, including illness patterns (especially respiratory problems), physical ability and exercise tolerance, should be recorded. History of premature birth, oxygen therapy or artificial ventilation immediately after birth are incidents which are increasingly reported.

Signs and symptoms

There may be difficulty in describing the symptoms, as many of them are not usually within our experience. The symptoms generally occur when the brain is trying to function in a hypoxic condition, causing difficulty in perception, retention and recall of phenomena. The symptoms should be recorded, listed and numbered in relation to severity, occurrence and concern. The degree that a symptom is incapacitating could rate 0–10 on a *disability scale* and the degree that a symptom is fear-provoking could rate 0–10 on a *distress scale*, while occurrence of the symptom could also be rated 0–10.

These records will give a guide to progress and ultimately give a semi-objective outcome measure.

Assessment of personality

A detailed analysis of the personality is neither possible nor necessary in this setting. However, a simple assessment may be made by noticing the posture, facial expression, demeanour of the hands, manner in which the history is given and the patient's emotional responses and reactions to the situations related in the history. One patient may be overtly obsessive and perfectionist and obviously reacting against the uncertainties of life, whilst another may be superficially tranquil, masking the underlying burden of troubles and emotions which are being carried. These may come spilling out at any time during the sessions.

Physical examination

It may not be appropriate to make a physical examination if pertinent information is given in the referral. When examination is deemed necessary and with the chest unclothed, note is made of:

1. The shape of the chest (including any physical deformity)
2. The findings from auscultation.

The pattern of breathing can be assessed with the patient dressed. The place of movement, size, regularity and rate of breathing should be recorded. The physiotherapist should have a watch with a second hand available to record the breathing rate per minute. The patient must not be informed at this stage of the rate per minute, as the re-education will take place at the level of the individual breath or phase of breath and a knowledge of the greater time scale can be damaging.

Treatment plan

The treatment plan will be agreed after discussion of symptoms and findings. The patient needs to highlight the greatest problem areas, related if possible to lifestyle and expectations. Treatment in the short term (to control symptoms) and in the long term (spontaneously to maintain a corrected pattern of breathing) will be described and agreed. Agreement will also be sought to look constructively at the activities of the day and to try to identify possible factors influencing the onset of symptoms. It is usually not difficult to obtain a firm commitment to take responsibility for the home treatment programme, as the patients are only too delighted to find a rationale for their symptoms and the recognition that it is possible to help themselves to gain a semblance of mastery over the symptoms and the environment. A fitness programme may be discussed at this stage, but it will not be introduced until later in the plan.

Breathing education

The most comfortable position for learning breathing awareness is lying with suitable support. Most people with chronic hyperventilation do not have respiratory disease and therefore can lie flat without distress. The suggested position is supported with one or two pillows under the head and a pillow under the knees. The knee pillow helps to prevent tension in the abdominal muscles and thus enables a natural passive abdominal movement during the respiratory cycle. For patients who find that this position is uncomfortable or if it precipitates breathlessness or a feeling of vulnerability another position should be found. Usually sitting with adequate support is acceptable.

Recognition of the relationship of body movements to the flow of air in breathing is the first step of awareness. Sensory input and body awareness is increased if the patient rests both hands on the abdomen. The physiotherapist lightly covers them with her hands. This light contact helps to bond the physiotherapist–patient relationship and allows the physiotherapist to feel, as well as observe, the movements related to the breathing cycle.

A simple description of respiration is given, relating the flow of air in and out, to the chest, diaphragmatic and abdominal movements. The transfer of oxygen and carbon dioxide should be described in lay terms so that the patient can relate this knowledge to the symptoms, which are secondary to the falling carbon dioxide levels.

Tuition and discussion will continue in this position until the physiotherapist is satisfied that the patient has grasped the basic information. Generally the patient has relaxed more

as the interaction has been a distraction from excess self-awareness.

Having had the breathing described the patient is asked to close the eyes and try to feel and sense what is happening with regard to the breathing. It may be necessary for the physiotherapist to relate what is happening. Care must be taken not to direct the pattern but merely to describe it:

> 'You are now breathing in and now you are breathing out'
> 'Your abdomen is swelling and now your abdomen is falling back to rest'.

At this early stage it is helpful for the patient to relate air movement with the associated body movement and to recognize that as the air moves 'in' the body moves 'out', and vice versa.

As soon as one becomes conscious of one's breathing there is a natural feeling of discomfort. Breathing is naturally reflex and subconscious but has a voluntary pathway. When it is brought into the consciousness, as it has to be for re-education, there is a discomfort which has to be recognized and at the same time accepted and yet disregarded. Re-education has to take place within this forum.

The patient is then asked to focus on the 'in breath' and notice when and how it starts and finishes. This 'quiet attentiveness' is then transferred to the 'out breath' and note taken of the beginning and end of this phase. Particular attention should be given to the end of the phase to recognize when the breath gently stops. The spontaneous rest point is identified as the natural rest point in the breathing cycle and the patient is helped to feel it as a relaxation place and not a place of tension. It may be helpful to practise general relaxation into this place of 'no movement'. Most patients can accept this experience and begin to recognize it as a welcome rest.

In order to recognize the full breathing capacity it is helpful to stop the breath at the upper point of the tidal volume and then to request a continuation of inspiration until full inflation is achieved. In this way it is possible to experience the inspiratory capacity. Similarly, the expiratory reserve can be experienced by breath holding at the bottom of the tidal volume and then exhaling entirely by using all the expiratory muscles.

Having practised these two manoeuvres the patient will also realize that the relaxed tidal volume is relatively easy compared with the muscle work needed above and below the tidal flows. Patients may be able to use this information to perceive a change in pattern before symptoms occur.

Breathing pattern re-education

The initial education and breathing awareness training is followed by re-education of the components that have been identified as being disordered. These components are:

- Flow rate
- Tidal volume
- Regularity
- Place of movement.

The new breathing cycle may be of two or three phases, depending on the patient's body preference. The two-phase cycle would consist of a gentle inspiration followed by a slow expiration. In a three-phase cycle the natural rest point at the end of expiration is used and extended. A gentle inspiration is followed by an easy (passive) expiration which naturally changes into the rest period which is extended until the next inspiration is gently initiated. Care has to be taken not to extend this rest to the point of stimulating a gasping inspiration.

Method

By this stage the patient and physiotherapist will be aware of the size, speed and rhythm of the breathing pattern. The physiotherapist will describe these components and clarify with the patient what changes need to be made. A change of volume, speed of flow, regularity and place of movement may be required. One component, a combination, or all of these may be involved. The new pattern will be re-made with the least possible interference.

As many patients who hyperventilate have a predominantly thoracic movement, this needs to be changed to a gentle passive movement of the abdominal wall. Some patients find it extremely difficult to obtain any abdominal movement and it may be necessary to spend several treatment sessions using different word combinations and images until a more relaxed abdominal movement is achieved. Large or forced movements must be discouraged. Any increase in ventilation will increase or precipitate symptoms. In general, most patients manage to recognize what is needed to change from a thoracic 'in and up' pattern to an abdominal 'in and down' pattern. A new pattern is introduced by gradual and patient work. It will be very individual. Guidance will be given breath by breath and phase by phase, relating which movement is good and which incorrect, thus reinforcing correct patterns of volume, movement and rest, which will of course be smaller and slower and more regular.

This decrease in ventilation will raise the $PaCO_2$. The higher level is uncomfortable at first. The patient is helped to accept the sensation of unease or discomfort as the sensation is described, discussed and understood.

It is necessary to experience this sensation at a minimal level while practising the corrected pattern. The decrease of ventilation should not create an unacceptably strong sensation as this would increase anxiety. It should be barely perceptible and acceptable. By maintaining the controlled pattern for as long as possible the respiratory centre can be reprogrammed to trigger inspiration at a higher level of carbon dioxide. The reprogramming is similar to that which occurs in patients with ventilatory insufficiency in chronic obstructive disease. An imperceptible increase in $PaCO_2$ over a period of time appears to condition the respiratory centre to accept higher levels before triggering inspiration.

If the desire to breathe becomes too great to contain, simple swallowing may ease the discomfort. If this is not sufficient, a slow, controlled deep breath may be taken. To compensate for moving this large volume of air a longer period of time must be used. It is helpful to hold the breath after expiration for a count of five or six

(2–3 seconds). In a normal subject the $PaCO_2$ drops as the result of a deep breath and takes 3–4 minutes to return to normal if no compensatory measures are taken. Patients need to learn of this phenomenon and to use the knowledge positively by compensating for deep breathing or sighing by breath holding (preferably at the point of expiration) for a count of five or six.

The stretch reflexes in the joints and muscles of the chest wall probably also play a part in the sensation of unease as the patterns of movement are altered.

Once a pattern has been found that fulfils the change criteria and suits the patient, it needs to be reinforced in the patient's mind. Some are able to recognize the pattern without external help; others find it difficult to recognize the time scale required. The correction in time may be helped by the physiotherapist guiding, by counting monotonously, the time span of the phases of each breath. The possibilities are many and individual. They may vary from *in out in out in …* to a slower more natural pattern of *in and out two three and rest and in and out two three* … (Fig. 19.3). The use of a tape recorder, to capture the timing of the pattern during a treatment session, may help the patient to practise more effectively at home.

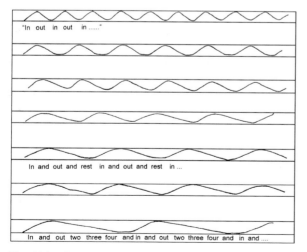

Fig. 19.3 Some suggested breathing patterns demonstrating a regular small tidal volume with various flow rates and rest periods.

The patient needs to learn to control the breathing pattern in sitting, standing, walking, during and after exercise and at times of stress and risk. It may be necessary to practise these activities during treatment sessions. Natural breathlessness will occur on exercise and should be recognized and accepted as normal. Some patients may feel better on exercise, as the body's metabolic needs rise to equilibrate with the respiratory physiology. Others may overbreathe on exercise which will be recognized by an increase in, or occurrence of, symptoms. Appropriate control measures will need to be introduced and practised. If the natural breathlessness does not subside within an acceptable time span, help may be given with control by changing one component at a time. First slow the rate, then decrease the volume, then slow the rate, etc., until control is achieved.

Treatment sessions will take approximately 1 hour. Outpatients will need to attend weekly at first. As the patient progresses the sessions will become less frequent. Some patients need only two or three sessions; others 12 or 14 spaced out over 12 or 18 months. At the time of discharge it is important for the patient to know where to telephone in an emergency for advice and review if necessary. Inpatients will probably be treated daily at first, with the time between sessions being increased as soon as possible to allow the patient responsibility for practice.

Compensatory procedures in the short term

If the patient falls back into the old habit (irregularity, deep breaths or frequent sighs) it may precipitate symptoms. One first-aid measure is a conscious compensation for the movement of a large volume of air by gentle breath holding. This is so planned that a natural size of breath is subsequently possible. Intermittent breath holding is a useful manoeuvre to practise throughout the day. It is not anticipated by a deep breath, rather the breathing cycle is stopped anywhere in the cycle for a count of two or three or such time that does not provoke a large following inspiration. It can be practised and linked to simple everyday activities until it becomes a conditioned reflex. The hypothesis of this manoeuvre is to raise the $PaCO_2$ minimally and regularly to help to lessen the falling of carbon dioxide to symptomatic levels as a result of overventilation and slow recovery times.

Planned rebreathing

It has been recorded that paper bag rebreathing may carry the hazard of hypoxia (Callaham 1989). However, poorly programmed rebreathing in acute hyperventilators who may have undiagnosed cardiac or respiratory conditions should not rule out the careful, controlled use of rebreathing therapy for chronic hyperventilators. There is a small group of people who cannot control the breathing pattern when it is most needed. There may be many reasons for this. One possibility is that the low $PaCO_2$ has an effect on memory programming and recall. If the $PaCO_2$ can be raised by rebreathing, the patient becomes more clear headed and can then remember the breathing control programme.

At times of acute distress or inability to control the disordered breathing, a bag of 25 cm × 30 cm minimum may be used as a rebreathing apparatus. The bag must be shaken out so that it is full of room air. The open end of the bag is placed loosely over the nose and mouth allowing free passage of air between face and bag. The patient should breathe freely within the bag. Rebreathing of the expired gases takes place thus raising the $PaCO_2$. After approximately six to eight breaths, the bag should be removed from the face and shaken out to refill it with fresh room air. The procedure should continue with regular shaking of the bag until the acute presenting symptoms subside or until the patient is capable of controlling the breathing pattern effectively. For safety reasons the rebreathing bag must only be used in the sitting or standing position and never in lying. Should the patient lose consciousness, the bag would fall away from the face and not remain in situ with the risk of asphyxia.

Rebreathing only raises the $PaCO_2$ during the procedure and, if the breathing pattern is not changed, it would fall back when rebreathing ceased. The purpose of the procedure is to raise the carbon dioxide sufficiently to enable conscious control of the breathing pattern.

An ordinary oxygen mask with large holes, as used for inhalation therapy, may be used for patients who are unable to control the breathing sufficiently at certain times or who, as a result of hyperventilation, are housebound and unable to do household and personal routines. The face mask may be worn for the duration of the task. The $PaCO_2$ is artificially raised by the rebreathing function of the mask. The vent holes are left open so that room air can be drawn in to maintain sufficient oxygen concentration.

The face mask may be the short-term therapy of choice for patients who are terminally ill and hyperventilate with anxiety.

It is unwise to use bags or masks too freely as some patients can become dependent on the aid and never learn to reorder the breathing cycle. They should only be used when the patient's personality and situation is understood and when all other avenues have been investigated.

Speech

Many patients report that speaking and singing stimulate the symptoms. Normal conversational speech occurs at the upper end of tidal flows and there is a delicate interplay between breathing and speaking. New patterns of the interrelationships of expiration, smoothness of speech and small inspirations at punctuation points need to be found and practised. It may be helpful to practise reading aloud and to listen to the new pattern of speech in order to re-educate the feed-back-loop.

Home programme

Therapy is directed towards re-educating the breathing pattern, not to breathing exercises. Practice sessions should be as many and for as long as possible. By using a practical approach, an acceptable programme must be worked out by the physiotherapist and the patient. At first it may only be possible to practise for 5 minutes a day, but three or four sessions of 20–30 minutes each is obviously more beneficial. Many patients find that as their lifestyle changes, more time can be made available for breathing control and relaxation sessions.

It is good to start the day with a period of conscious control of breathing. It is suggested that 10–15 minutes is spent in practice before rising in the morning. Travelling by bus or train is time well spent in conscious breathing control and relaxation. Car drivers can constructively use the time while waiting at traffic lights. Coffee, lunch and tea breaks could afford a few minutes of practice. Fifteen or 20 minutes should be put aside when returning home from work or shopping to relax and practise breathing control. It is worth spending this time after a working day to allow the body to equilibrate. The evening can be more enjoyable when not fighting symptoms. The last period of practice can be done having retired to bed using the favourite sleeping position.

Compensatory breath holding, intermittent breath holding and general physical and mental relaxation should become part of the normal day. People who have experienced hyperventilation syndrome are probably always at risk even after the presenting episode has been resolved. It would be judicious to remember to practise breathing control before aggravating situations such as flying, travelling to a high altitude, heat and periods of prolonged excitement or stress.

Exercise and fitness programmes

As a result of the disordered breathing pattern, many patients have been unable to exercise and have become unfit, thus compounding the problem. Guidance in a slowly graded exercise scheme can be helpful. It may need to start with very simple movements two or three times only. The progression must be carefully graded, and to err on the slow side is preferable to advancing too quickly. Impatience for progress may cause decline rather than improvement. Swimming is an excellent form of free exercise which encompasses general movement synchronized with breathing.

Group therapy

Some centres arrange self-help groups for exercise, relaxation and discussion. These sessions can be beneficial after an individual pattern of breathing control has been mastered and the patient is progressing with control in exercise. At a later stage, fitness training can be carried out in a group, although it should never be competitive. Each person should be following an individual programme.

These group sessions must be monitored carefully to ensure that they are not used for 'swapping symptoms'. With careful guidance they can help to give confidence.

CONCLUSION

Patience and perseverance of physiotherapist and patient is necessary for the long-term re-education of the breathing pattern, which aims at slowly increasing the resting $PaCO_2$ to more normal levels. The chosen pattern should eventually become the new, unconscious, habitual method of breathing. This chapter is related mainly to the description of this method of re-educating the manner of breathing. It does not discuss methods of associated relaxation techniques which may need to be part of the treatment.

Chronic habitual hyperventilators are often gifted and interesting people who are generally highly motivated and compliant towards treatment. A high proportion of sufferers are helped by a systematic, individual treatment programme and by an intelligent and sympathetic approach to the syndrome. The condition is a challenging one for the physiotherapist and the patient's improvement is pleasing.

Recently more recognition is being given to the syndrome and there is a concerted effort among some physicians and researchers to agree a more suitable diagnostic label for this breathing disorder. Breathing is a very complex mechanism which is affected by many stimuli and appears to have effects other than the exchange of gases (van Dixhoorn 1996). Some of the patients' symptoms may be attributed to various dysfunctional aspects of the breathing systems other than the variable or low levels of $PaCO_2$. There are many phenomena which are not yet understood and there are many areas inviting research. Work is currently in progress in a few centres which is offering a greater understanding of the physiological complexities and the interplay with responses to life events.

REFERENCES

Baker D M 1934 Sighing respiration as a symptom. Lancet 1: 174–177

Bass C, Gardner W N 1985 Respiratory and psychiatric abnormalities in chronic symptomatic hyperventilation. British Medical Journal 290: 1387–1390

Callaham M 1989 Hypoxic hazards of traditional paper bag rebreathing in hyperventilating patients. American Emergency Medicine 18(b): 622–628

Clark T J H, Cochrane G N 1970 Effect of personality on alveolar ventilation in patients with chronic airways obstruction. British Medical Journal 1: 273–275

Cowley D S, Roy-Byrne P P 1987 Hyperventilation and panic disorder. American Journal of Medicine 83: 929–937

Folgering H, Ruttern H, Rouman Y 1983 Beta-blockade in the hyperventilation syndrome. A retrospective assessment of symptoms and complaints. Respiration 44(1): 19–25

Freeman L J, Nixon P G F 1985 Chest pain and the hyperventilation syndrome: some etiological considerations. Postgraduate Medical Journal 61: 957–961

Gardner W N 1994 Diagnosis and organic causes of symptomatic hyperventilation. In: Timmons B H, Ley R (eds) Behavioural and psychological approaches to breathing disorders. Plenum Press, New York, ch 6. p 111

Gardner W N, Bass C 1989 Hyperventilation in clinical practice. British Journal of Hospital Medicine 41(1): 73–81

Glyn C J, Lloyd J W, Folkard S 1981 Ventilatory responses to intractable pain. Pain 11(2): 201–211

Hardonk H J, Beumer H M 1979 Hyperventilation syndrome. In: Vinken P J, Bruyn G W (eds) The handbook of clinical neurology. North Holland, Amsterdam, vol 38, pp 309–360

Kerr W J, Dalton J W, Gliebe P A 1937 Some physical phenomena associated with the anxiety states and their relation to hyperventilation. Annals of Internal Medicine 11: 961–962

Lum L C 1994 Hyperventilation syndromes: physiological considerations in clinical management. In: Timmons B H, Ley R (eds) Behavioural and psychological approaches to breathing disorders. Plenum Press, New York, ch 8, pp 118, 120

Macefield G, Burke D 1991 Parasthesia and tetany induced by voluntary hyperventilation. Brain 114: 527–540

Magarian G J 1982 Hyperventilation syndromes: infrequently recognised common expressions of anxiety and stress. Medicine 61(4): 219–236

Nixon P G F, Freeman L J 1988 The 'think test': a further technique to elicit hyperventilation. Journal of the Royal Society of Medicine 81: 277–279

Pilsbury D, Hibbert G A 1987 An ambulatory system for long term continuous monitoring of transcutaneous PCO_2. Clinical Respiratory Physiology 23: 9–13

van Dixhoorn J 1996 Hyperventilation and dysfunctional breathing. A presentation at the Third Annual Meeting of the International Society for the Advancement of Respiratory Psychophysiology (ISARP). University of Nijmegen

van Dixhoorn J, Duivenvoorden H J 1985 Efficacy of Nijmegen questionnaire in recognition of the hyperventilation syndrome. Journal of Psychosomatic Research 29(2): 199–206

van Doorn P, Colla P, Folgering H 1982 Control of end-tidal PCO_2 in the hyperventilation syndrome: effects of biofeedback and breathing instructions compared. Bulletin Europeen de Physiopathologie Respiratoire 18: 829–836

Vansteenkiste J, Rochette M, Demedts M 1991 Diagnostic tests of hyperventilation syndrome. European Respiratory Journal 4: 393–399

Wood P 1941 Da Costa's syndrome (or effort syndrome). British Medical Journal 1: 767–772, 805–811, 845–851

FURTHER READING

Bradley D 1994 Hyperventilation syndrome – a handbook for bad breathers. Kyle Kathie, London

Lum L C 1976 The syndrome of chronic hyperventilation. In: Hill O (ed) Modern trends in psychosomatic medicine. Butterworth, London, ch 11, pp 196–230

Tenny S M, Lamb T W 1965 Physiological consequences of hypoventilation and hyperventilation. Handbook of physiology. American Physiological Society, Bethesda Maryland, sect 3, vol 2, pp 979–1003

Timmons B H, Ley R 1994 (eds) Behavioural and psychological approaches to breathing disorders. Plenum Press, New York

MANCHESTER ROYAL INFIRMARY

SCHOOL OF PHYSIOTHERAPY

20

Bronchiectasis, primary ciliary dyskinesia and cystic fibrosis

Barbara A. Webber   Jennifer A. Pryor

BRONCHIECTASIS

'Bronchiectasis' is the term used for chronic dilatation of one or more bronchi (Cole 1995). This leads to impaired drainage of bronchial secretions, usually with persistent infection of the affected lobe or segment.

The cause of bronchiectasis may be congenital, for example primary ciliary dyskinesia, cystic fibrosis, sequestrated lung segments or bronchomalacia. Pertussis, measles, tuberculosis and pneumonia may also cause bronchiectasis, but with early medical intervention the incidence following these conditions has fallen. Bronchiectasis may complicate hypogammaglobulinaemia because of the patient's reduced capacity to resist bacterial infection. Other causes include allergic bronchopulmonary aspergillosis and obstruction of a bronchus by a tumour, mucus plug or an inhaled foreign body where persistent secondary infection in the distal airways leads to dilatation and distortion of the bronchi.

The bronchial wall damage with destruction of cartilage and alteration in the normal ciliated epithelium is a result of the inflammatory process. The bronchial circulation may show widespread anastomoses with varicosities and there is an increase in mucus-secreting glands.

Clinical features of bronchiectasis include cough, purulent sputum, wheeze, haemoptysis, breathlessness, chest pain, malaise, fever, weight loss, finger clubbing (rare in bronchiectasis unassociated with cystic fibrosis), crackles and wheezes over the affected areas, signs of consolidation and collapse with a superimposed infection and purulent rhinosinusitis including post-nasal drip.

There is a rare form of bronchiectasis known as 'dry' bronchiectasis which may be a consequence of pulmonary tuberculosis or a type where the patient has recurrent haemoptyses, but no infected secretions.

There are more specific signs and symptoms which occur with primary ciliary dyskinesia and cystic fibrosis which are discussed later in this chapter.

Investigations for bronchiectasis include:

- *Assessment* using subjective and objective findings as discussed in Chapter 1
- *The chest radiograph* may be normal but there may be signs of thickened bronchial walls (tramlining), crowding of vessels with loss of volume and cyst-like shadows with fluid levels
- *High-resolution computed tomography* is the imaging method of choice as a diagnostic tool in bronchiectasis (Smith & Flower 1996) and the invasive technique of bronchography is rarely used
- *Sputum specimens* for examination and culture to identify the microorganisms and their sensitivity to antibiotics, and for cytological examination to exclude malignant disease
- *Bronchoscopy* should be considered if a foreign body or tumour is suspected
- *Lung function tests*
- *Serum immunoglobulins* will detect patients with hypogammaglobulinaemia
- *Serum precipitins test* may help to identify allergic bronchopulmonary aspergillosis and would be carried out following positive skin tests to *Aspergillus*
- *Sweat test* to exclude cystic fibrosis
- *Nasomucociliary clearance test* and microscopic examination of the cilia to exclude cilial defects.

Medical management

Antibiotics are often required for infective exacerbations and are sometimes given long term

prophylactically. Bronchospasm is commonly present, needing bronchodilator therapy particularly before physiotherapy. Inhaled corticosteroids may reduce the need for bronchodilators and may have additional value in reducing the inflammation which is an important part of the pathogenesis of the disease.

Topical medication may be indicated for chronic mucopurulent rhinosinusitis and the recommended technique for inhaled, topical deposition of drugs is in the head-down and forward position to encourage entry of the drops to the ethmoid and maxillary sinuses (Wilson et al 1987).

A general practitioner may provide the patient with a prescription for an antibiotic which he can start immediately an infective episode occurs. Where there is an immunoglobulin deficiency, replacement therapy should be given in an attempt to prevent further lung damage.

Surgical resection would only be considered if the bronchiectasis is localized. In very severe widespread bronchiectasis with respiratory failure, lung transplantation may be considered.

The inhalation of recombinant human deoxyribonuclease (DNase) does not appear to improve ciliary transportability, spirometry, dyspnoea or quality of life in patients with bronchiectasis not associated with cystic fibrosis (Wills et al 1996).

Bronchography

The instillation of a radio-opaque medium is now rarely used as an investigative procedure, indeed contrast material for this purpose is no longer readily available. If it should be used for patients with probable bronchiectasis, physiotherapy would help to clear the airways before the bronchogram and to assist the clearance of the contrast medium immediately after.

Much of the contrast medium would either be expectorated spontaneously or absorbed from the peripheral airways into the bloodstream, but where the peripheral airways are blocked, as in bronchiectasis, physiotherapy can assist in the clearance of the medium.

It is important that patients have nothing to eat or drink for at least 3 hours after a bronchogram when the effect of the local anaesthetic will have worn off. If the procedure has been performed through the cricothyroid membrane, the patient should apply pressure over the cricothyroid cartilage during huffing or coughing for at least 6 hours to avoid the possibility of subcutaneous (surgical) emphysema.

Physiotherapy

Physiotherapy may help in the treatment of patients' problems of excess bronchial secretions, breathlessness, reduced exercise tolerance and chest wall pain of musculoskeletal origin.

Excess bronchial secretions

Following assessment the affected areas of the lung can be determined. It is important that the patient understands the pathology of the condition and the reasons for treatment. Clinically, effective physiotherapy will reduce the episodes of superimposed infection and may help to minimize further lung damage.

The active cycle of breathing techniques in gravity-assisted positions, as indicated on assessment, is used. Self-treatment is introduced with or without self-chest clapping accompanying the thoracic expansion exercises and self-chest compression may be combined with huffing (Fig. 20.1). It is likely that a minimum of 10 minutes in any one productive position will be necessary and the end-point of treatment must be recognized by self-assessment, that is two consecutive cycles where effective huffs are dry sounding and non-productive. The sitting position may be adequate for patients with minimal secretions.

Regular daily treatment is essential but the number of times in a day will vary among individuals and must be increased during episodes of superimposed infection. For many patients treatment once a day is sufficient. Some patients find their chest is 'dry' at the beginning of the day and it is important that the time for treatment is not only when their chest is productive, but also at a time that is compatible with their lifestyle. Compliance/adherence is also increased by agreeing a suitable home programme with the patient.

Patients using gravity-assisted positions for the lower and middle zones may find a full length postural drainage frame (Fig. 20.2) comfortable and convenient for treatment.

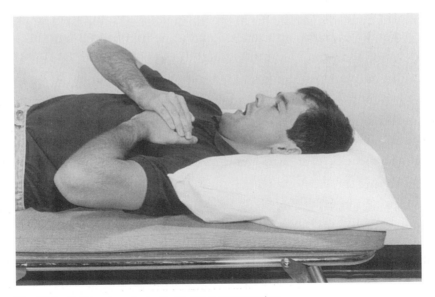

Fig. 20.1 Self-treatment – huff with chest compression.

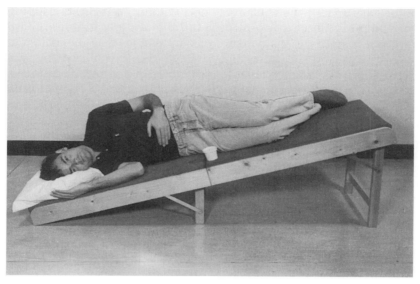

Fig. 20.2 Postural drainage frame.

Elderly or frail patients may benefit from assistance, by a relative or other carer, with chest clapping and shaking during the thoracic expansion exercises. Careful instruction needs to be given by a physiotherapist.

It is important that the physiotherapy techniques and positions for treatment are reassessed at intervals. Currie et al (1986) recommended a regular review. Most patients should be reassessed within 3 months of initial instruction and at least annually thereafter.

Acute exacerbation of infection. Patients may be admitted to hospital with an acute exacerbation of their chest infection. The patient will probably be expectorating an increased amount of more purulent sputum and may be febrile, dehydrated and breathless. Haemoptysis is not uncommon and pleuritic chest pain may be present. The most severely affected may be in respiratory failure.

It is likely that mechanical adjuncts will be required in addition to the active cycle of breathing techniques to assist in the clearance of excess bronchial secretions. A nebulized bronchodilator and/or humidification before treatment may help in the mobilization of tenacious secretions.

Intermittent positive pressure breathing (IPPB)

could help both in the clearance of secretions and in the relief of the work of breathing. There are patients who many years ago received the more radical treatment of resection of more than one lobe and by the time they reach middle age they have very poor respiratory reserve. A superimposed infection in these patients may precipitate respiratory failure. Modified positioning, for example side lying or high side lying, combined with IPPB may be an effective form of treatment in minimizing the effort of clearing secretions (p. 169).

Following resection of lung tissue the anatomy of the bronchial tree may alter and the traditional positions for drainage of segments of the remaining lobes may be unsuitable. The physiotherapist should try varying positions until the optimal ones are found.

The presence of blood streaking in the sputum is not a contraindication to physiotherapy and treatment should be continued. If there is frank haemoptysis physiotherapy should be temporarily discontinued, but resumed as soon as the sputum is only mildly bloodstained to avoid retention of old blood and mucus. Before discharge from hospital it is important that the patient is able to take the responsibility for his treatment and is confident with the positions and techniques required to continue regularly at home. If a bronchodilator has been prescribed, this would be given before treatment and a few patients with bronchiectasis may be prescribed nebulized antibiotic drugs which should be inhaled after clearance of secretions. If a patient is on the waiting list for lung transplantation, a preoperative rehabilitation programme should be established and postoperative treatment would be as outlined in Chapter 16.

Breathlessness

Some patients with bronchiectasis also demonstrate a degree of bronchospasm and will benefit from the inhalation of a bronchodilator before physiotherapy to clear secretions. Instruction in the use of an appropriate device for drug delivery is important.

It is the minority of patients with bronchiectasis who complain of breathlessness, and for these patients the rest positions to relieve breathlessness, and breathing control while walking and stair climbing should be included in the treatment programme.

Reduced exercise tolerance

Exercise should be encouraged to improve general physical fitness. It will also assist the mobilization of bronchial secretions. Patients with severe bronchiectasis may benefit from a group pulmonary rehabilitation programme (see Ch. 14).

Chest wall pain of musculoskeletal origin

See pages 192–203.

Evaluation of physiotherapy

Effective treatment will be recognized by a decrease in quantity of sputum, possible decrease in purulence of sputum, absence of fever, improvements in spirometry, a reduction in breathlessness, an increase in exercise tolerance and a reduction or absence of chest wall pain.

Improvements in oxygen saturation and blood gas tensions may also be apparent.

PRIMARY CILIARY DYSKINESIA

Primary ciliary dyskinesia (PCD) is an autosomal recessive inherited condition with a frequency of between 1 in 15 000 and 1 in 30 000 (Cole 1995). It affects the cilia, resulting in recurrent infections in the nose, ears, sinuses and lungs, and abnormalities in sperm motility may cause infertility in males.

Kartagener (1933) described the triad of bronchiectasis, dextrocardia and situs inversus. These patients were later found to have abnormalities of the cilia, but cases of ciliary abnormality without dextrocardia or situs inversus were later identified. The condition then became known as 'immotile cilia syndrome', but with the discovery of a range of cilial abnormalities both in beat frequency and ultrastructure and the knowledge that not all abnormal cilia are completely immotile, the term 'primary ciliary dyskinesia' was adopted (Greenstone et al 1988).

Pneumonia may be the presenting feature in infants, but the early signs in children may be a loose cough, runny nose and recurrent upper and lower respiratory tract infections with or without wheeze. Frequently the child has hearing problems associated with secretory otitis media (glue ear).

Specific investigations which would clarify the diagnosis of PCD include the nasal mucociliary clearance test (Stanley et al 1984), photometric determination of ciliary beat frequency (Rutland & Cole 1980) and electron micrographic analysis. A sweat test will exclude the diagnosis of cystic fibrosis.

Medical management

Early diagnosis is important as early treatment may minimize lung damage. Antibiotic therapy may be indicated for upper and lower respiratory tract infections. The insertion of grommets may be necessary to control the accumulation of fluid in the middle ear, but limited use is recommended as complications are common.

Occasionally hearing aids may be required. Nasal douching may help to keep the nose clear.

Physiotherapy

Daily physiotherapy if introduced at the time of diagnosis becomes a way of life for the child. It is important that parents detect signs of infection early: a child may be lethargic, 'off colour' and feel abnormally hot. Physiotherapy should be increased during infective episodes and parents must understand that it is not only antibiotics which will cope with an infection.

Owing to the cilial defect, secretions are most likely to collect in the dependent areas: the lower lobes and often the middle lobe and lingula. The middle lobe which may be situated on the left side, owing to situs inversus, is more commonly affected than the lingula. The goal of treatment should be to assist clearance of secretions from the dependent parts of the lungs using gravity-assisted positions and the active cycle of breathing techniques. Even if the chest is dry sounding and non-productive the parents should be shown the positions for the middle lobe (Fig. 20.3), lingula and lateral segments of the lower lobes, and encouraged to use these positions for drainage daily. A child should be encouraged to blow his nose regularly.

Huffing games can be introduced from the age of 2 years and by the age of 8 or 9 years the child can begin to do some of the treatment himself and gradually become independent. Sports and other active exercises should be encouraged. Even with grommets in place children can enjoy swimming (Pringle 1992).

Very occasionally, nasopharyngeal suction may be indicated in the infant when it is impossible to clear nasal and bronchial secretions by any other means.

Regular assessment of techniques, remotivation of the patient and support for the parents are important aspects of physiotherapy. It is probable that chronic lung damage will be minimized if physiotherapy is continued on a regular basis.

Evaluation of physiotherapy

In the young patient with primary ciliary dyskinesia effective treatment in the stable condition will be recognized by the presence of only minimal coughing on exertion. During an infective episode signs and symptoms of effective treatment include a reduction in shortness of breath and coughing, and a reduction in wheeze and fever if either or both had been present.

In addition in the older patient, a constant

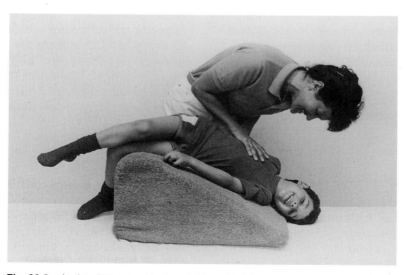

Fig. 20.3 Assisted treatment for the right middle lobe.

volume of sputum would be expectorated while stable, and during an episode of infection an increased volume of expectorated sputum should decrease with effective treatment.

CYSTIC FIBROSIS

Cystic fibrosis is the most frequent cause of suppurative lung disease in Caucasian children and young adults and is characterized by chronic pulmonary disease, pancreatic insufficiency and increased concentrations of electrolytes in the sweat (Høiby & Koch 1990).

Cystic fibrosis is an autosomal recessive condition most commonly found in Caucasian populations with a carrier rate of 1 in 25 and the disease occurring in approximately 1 in 2500 live births (Cystic Fibrosis Trust, British Paediatric Association, British Thoracic Society 1996). Carriers of the cystic fibrosis gene show no signs of cystic fibrosis, but if both parents carry the abnormal gene each child born has a theoretical 1 in 4 chance of inheriting the condition.

When the condition was first described by Anderson (1938) life expectancy was less than 2 years, but with increased recognition of the disease especially in its milder forms and improved treatment the median age of survival is approximately 31 years (Shale 1997a). Cohort survival graphs indicate an improvement in survival with time in the UK in all age groups (Dodge et al 1993). If the trend of improved survival continues it is likely that many of the patients born in the 1990s will live well into their 50s (P A Lewis, personal communication, 1997).

Diagnosis can be made by measuring the amount of sodium in the sweat and a concentration of more than 70 mmol/l is diagnostic of cystic fibrosis (di Sant'Agnese & Davis 1979)

The cystic fibrosis defect lies on chromosome 7 and the gene was identified in 1989 (Rommens et al 1989). Genes are made from the chemical deoxyribonucleic acid (DNA) and some pieces of DNA code for protein. The faulty gene in cystic fibrosis codes for the transmembrane conductance regulator (CFTR). The abnormality in this protein leads to changes in ion transport (McBride 1990) producing changes in the nature of the mucous and serous secretions produced by the exocrine glands and cells of the respiratory system and digestive tract.

Ion transport in human airways is dominated by the absorption of sodium ions from the mucosal surface (Alton et al 1992) and this is associated with the movement of water into the epithelial cells. It is also thought that chloride ions pass from the epithelial cells into the airway lumen taking water with them. The balance between the movement of sodium and chloride probably determines the volume and composition of airway surface liquid and this will affect mucociliary clearance (Alton et al 1992).

In cystic fibrosis there is a reduction in chloride secretion from the epithelial cells of the respiratory mucosa. This results in excess absorption of sodium and increased movement of fluid from the lumen of the airway into the cells reducing the airway surface liquid (mucous layer), increasing the viscosity of mucus and impairing mucociliary clearance.

The lungs in people with cystic fibrosis are structurally normal at birth (Reid & de Haller 1967), but studies have demonstrated evidence of inflammation and infection in infants and children with cystic fibrosis (Birrer et al 1994, Khan et al 1995) and in asymptomatic adults with normal lung function (Konstan et al 1994). Infection stimulates further mucus secretion and a generalized obstructive, suppurative cycle is set up. Repeated infections cause bronchiolitis, mucus impaction and cyst formation eventually leading to bronchiectasis and fibrosis (Fig. 20.4). The cycle of infection and inflammation impairs ciliary function and reduces mucus clearance. As the pulmonary disease progresses chronic hypoxia leads to pulmonary hypertension and cor pulmonale. The majority of patients die as a result of respiratory failure often associated with cor pulmonale.

There is a broad spectrum of presenting signs and symptoms in cystic fibrosis and this may be a reflection of the many gene variants. Over 400 mutations have been identified (Shale 1997b). Many patients are diagnosed early in life with signs and symptoms related either to the respiratory or gastrointestinal systems.

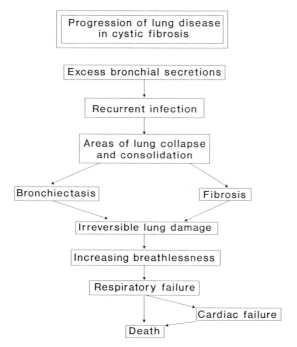

Fig. 20.4 Progression of lung disease in cystic fibrosis.

Screening may be undertaken if there is a known family history of cystic fibrosis and these tests are becoming more reliable (Super et al 1994). Neonatal screening is available and although it may positively influence long-term outcome (Ranieri et al 1994) it has not yet been widely accepted.

In the neonate, meconium ileus is the most common presenting feature occurring in about 10–15% of cases (Park & Grand 1981). Signs of intestinal obstruction may occur within 48 hours of birth. The infant fails to pass meconium after birth because the bowel is obstructed by sticky inspissated intestinal contents, but in milder cases there may only be delay in the passing of meconium. Three or 4 weeks after birth a sweat test should be performed in infants with meconium ileus to clarify the diagnosis, as this condition can occur in infants who do not have cystic fibrosis.

Another common presenting sign in infants and young children is a voracious appetite and failure to thrive due to malabsorption from the alimentary tract. Gastro-oesophageal reflux is a problem in some patients.

Abnormalities in ion transport in the pancreas lead to inflammation and later to fibrosis of the acinar portion of the gland and to hyposecretion of the major digestive enzymes secreted by the pancreas. The presenting symptom is steatorrhoea, the passing of characteristically fatty and offensive stools. Pancreatic steatorrhoea is often accompanied by abdominal discomfort and distension. In some patients steatorrhoea is not a presenting feature or may be mild.

The complication of diabetes mellitus in the older patient may possibly result from progressive fibrosis of the pancreas and is thought to be associated with a decline in the patient's clinical condition (Lanng et al 1992). Another feature occurring in adults is liver damage which starts as focal biliary cirrhosis and may in a few patients progress to portal hypertension and occasionally hepatic failure.

Meconium ileus equivalent (MIE) is a form of small intestinal obstruction occurring in some adults with cystic fibrosis. It causes abdominal distension and discomfort, vomiting and constipation, and should not be confused with appendicitis.

Most women with cystic fibrosis have normal or near normal fertility, but puberty may be delayed. Most males are subfertile because of developmental defects of the vas deferens, epididymis and seminal vesicles. Possible methods of reproduction may be discussed with the specialist.

Approximately one-third of adult patients with cystic fibrosis develop rheumatic symptoms (Bourke et al 1987). The two most common forms are an episodic and recurrent arthritis and hypertrophic pulmonary osteoarthropathy. They are characterized by joint pain, tenderness, swelling and limitation of movement, usually symmetrical and affecting particularly the knees, ankles and wrists (Johnson & Knox 1994).

The respiratory signs and symptoms vary. Some patients may be asymptomatic for many years, others may have a dry cough and later a persistent cough with purulent sputum. The respiratory pathogens most commonly isolated in 1990 were *Pseudomonas aeruginosa* (61%), *Staphylococcus aureus* (28.3%), *Haemophilus in-*

fluenzae (8.9%) and *Pseudomonas cepacia* (now known as *Burkholderia cepacia*) (3.2%) (FitzSimmons 1993). *Staphylococcus aureus* used to be the most frequently isolated organism, but it is now only in patients of less than 1 year of age in which this is the case (FitzSimmons 1993). Colonization with *Burkholderia cepacia* appears to be associated with deterioration in respiratory function, and a worse prognosis when a patient is colonized with both *Burkholderia cepacia* and *Pseudomonas aeruginosa* (Muhdi et al 1996). Mucus hypersecretion, impaired mucociliary clearance and inflammation create an environment in which bacteria will thrive. In patients with cystic fibrosis there is in addition a marked attraction between *Pseudomonas aeruginosa* and the airways (Smith 1994).

Haemoptysis is common and usually mild, although episodes of frank haemoptysis may occur. A wheeze is sometimes present, and patients may be breathless on exertion. With increasing breathlessness appetite becomes poor and the patient loses weight. Chest pain may be associated with an exacerbation of a bronchopulmonary infection, a pneumothorax or musculoskeletal dysfunction. Most patients develop finger clubbing and with more severe disease may become cyanosed.

The chest radiograph is usually normal at birth but an early change is bronchial wall thickening, particularly in the upper zones. As the disease progresses, overinflation of the lungs may occur with ill-defined nodular shadows, numerous ring and parallel line shadows indicating bronchial wall thickening and bronchiectasis (Fig. 2.20, p. 48). Crackles and wheezes may be heard on auscultation. Some patients develop nasal polyps; these may grow rapidly and are frequently recurrent. They may be related to chronic sinus infection.

Pulmonary function tests initially show signs of obstruction, but with advanced disease a restrictive pattern may be superimposed on the obstructive defect and a diffusion abnormality will also become apparent. Pulmonary function measurements (FEV$_1$, PaO$_2$, PaCO$_2$) have been shown to be predictors of mortality (Kerem et al 1992). As the disease progresses ventilation/perfusion imbalance occurs leading to hypoxaemia, pulmonary hypertension and cardiac failure.

Asthma is as common in patients with cystic fibrosis as it is among the normal population. Many cystic fibrosis patients have a positive skin test to *Aspergillus fumigatus*. This is often seen in the sputum (up to 57% of patients), but allergic bronchopulmonary aspergillosis (ABPA) is less common occurring in approximately 11% of patients (Nelson et al 1979, Brueton et al 1980). ABPA is recognized by recurrent wheezing, deteriorating chest symptoms and fleeting fluffy shadows on the chest radiograph.

Investigations for cystic fibrosis are similar to those for bronchiectasis, but may also include pancreatic function studies, tests for faecal fat, examination of the liver, spleen and gall bladder, and screening for diabetes mellitus.

Medical management

There is a wide range of antibiotics used in the treatment of cystic fibrosis and both the choice of drug and method of delivery vary. Early treatment is more effective (Valerius et al 1991) and the aim is to eradicate the organism. Sometimes control of infection is the best that can be achieved.

Intravenous antibiotics are frequently used for acute exacerbations of infection, but opinions differ as to the regular use of intravenous antibiotics for example 3-monthly. Treatment usually needs to continue for at least 10 days and can be evaluated by monitoring respiratory function and oxygen saturation (Hodson 1996). Nebulized antibiotics (Webb & Dodd 1997) have been shown to be effective in the treatment of *Pseudomonas aeruginosa* and this has been highlighted in the meta-analyses by Touw et al (1995) and Mukhopadhyay et al (1996). Antibiotics are usually inhaled twice daily and should follow physiotherapy for airway clearance.

Patients needing frequent or prolonged antipseudomonal treatment may require implantable intravenous access devices as thromboses may occur when long-term access is via peripheral veins. Selected patients use these devices at home (Stead et al 1987, Shale 1997b).

Segregation of patients colonized with *Burkholderia cepacia* from other patients with cystic fibrosis appears to limit spread of the organism (Muhdi et al 1996). Health professionals must pay particular attention to hygiene and washing their hands thoroughly between patients. This is essential when treating patients with *Burkholderia cepacia* as there is evidence of transmission from patient to patient (LiPuma et al 1990). Contamination of nebulizers is common and patients must be given instruction in the cleaning and care of nebulizer equipment. To minimize contamination the cleaning and drying of this equipment after use is essential (Hutchinson et al 1996).

Some patients benefit from the inhalation of bronchodilator drugs. Steroids may be indicated if asthma or allergic bronchopulmonary aspergillosis complicate cystic fibrosis. The use of aerosol steroids to improve airflow obstruction in the long-term management of cystic fibrosis is under investigation.

As a consequence of lung infection there are large quantities of DNA from the destruction of inflammatory cells, e.g. neutrophils. The inhalation of recombinant human deoxyribonuclease (DNase/Dornase alpha) acts on the DNA in the purulent lung secretions (Range & Knox 1995). It has been shown to improve lung function (Shah et al 1995), reduce viscoelasticity of the mucus (Shah et al 1996) and decrease exacerbations of bronchopulmonary infection (Fuchs et al 1994). Occasionally alteration in voice and episodes of pharyngitis may be experienced, but these are usually minor and transient (Hodson & Shah 1995).

Normal saline (0.9%) or hypertonic saline (3–7%) inhaled before physiotherapy may assist in clearance of secretions (Pavia et al 1978, Eng et al 1996).There is little evidence to support the use of other mucolytic agents such as acetylcysteine (Parvolex). They should be used with caution as bronchospasm may be induced. Acetylcysteine is, however, of benefit either orally or by enema in the treatment of meconium ileus equivalent (Hodson et al 1976).

In cystic fibrosis a high energy intake is needed as a result of malabsorption and the increased metabolic requirements during infection. The dietary energy intake should exceed the normal daily recommendation to sustain and maintain adequate weight, muscle bulk and function (Poole 1995). Supplements of fat-soluble vitamins and vitamin K are usually necessary in addition to pancreatic enzymes which should be taken with all meals and snacks.

When nasal obstruction by polyps is incomplete a corticosteroid nasal spray may be tried. Complete obstruction is unusual and polypectomy may be indicated.

Haemoptysis will usually stop spontaneously, but if bleeding is severe and prolonged, embolization of the bronchial artery to the affected lobe would be considered (Fairfax et al 1980, Cohen 1992).

Pneumothorax can occur spontaneously in the older patient. It may absorb without treatment, but if it persists or increases in size an intercostal drain will probably be inserted. Surgical intervention is withheld if possible, as transplantation may be more difficult if considered in the future. If necessary oversewing of the bleb and a localized surgical pleurodesis may be performed.

Heart–lung and lung transplantation (Ch. 16, p. 413) have been successfully carried out in patients with end-stage lung disease but there is a critical shortage of donor organs. Non-invasive positive pressure ventilation may be indicated for some patients on the waiting list for transplantation (Hodson et al 1991).

In end-stage cystic fibrosis, right ventricular failure is treated using diuretics and long-term oxygen therapy. To allay anxiety and to reduce breathlessness morphine or one of its derivatives is a useful treatment.

Gene therapy aims to correct the underlying pathophysiological defect through the transfer of genes. The gene is transferred in a 'carrier'. Liposomes and adenovirus have been used, but difficulties have been experienced. The adenovirus can stimulate an inflammatory response and the liposome is not as efficient as a 'carrier' (du Bois 1995). Theoretically the transfer of sufficient normal copies of the CFTR gene to sufficient numbers of affected cells should result in the production of enough normal protein to reduce the clinical manifestations of cystic fibrosis (Stern & Geddes 1994). There is considerable research in progress which may lead to effective gene therapy in the future.

Home treatment

In many countries the emphasis on treatment is moving from hospital to home. The benefits for patients of treatment at home include less disruption to school, work and family life while avoiding isolation from friends and family that hospitalization incurs.

For the newly diagnosed or newly referred patient a home visit by a member of the specialist team (usually the clinical nurse specialist) provides an opportunity for advice, education and support for the patient and family, as necessary. Domiciliary physiotherapy services are sometimes available and can provide the opportunity for discussion and demonstration of physiotherapy techniques in the home, an opportunity for a more effective assessment of the necessity and appropriateness of equipment and the possibility of specialist physiotherapy during terminal care. There is also evidence of improved compliance with treatment and a reduction in the stress of coping with the disease (Rogers & Goodchild 1996).

Many patients awaiting heart–lung transplantation can be cared for at home with a clinical nurse specialist visiting to provide assessment and to identify the needs for changes in treatment to maintain their optimal health status. It may be appropriate for a patient to either receive a course of intravenous antibiotics at home or to continue a course which has been started in hospital. This has been facilitated by developments in technology, for example the small, portable, prefilled antibiotic infusion devices (Bramwell et al 1995).

Physiotherapy

It is the knowledge of the condition and understanding of the treatment for cystic fibrosis which influence patient compliance and treatment outcomes (Conway et al 1996). The presenting problems of each patient will vary, and will fluctuate from a chronic stable state to an acute changing state. An exacerbation of a bronchopulmonary infection will produce changes which can be detected by accurate assessment of the signs and symptoms.

Physiotherapy may help in the treatment of patients' problems of excess bronchial secretions, reduced exercise tolerance, breathlessness and chest wall stiffness and pain of musculoskeletal origin. Arthropathy, unstable diabetes and the abdominal pain of meconium ileus equivalent are examples of medical problems which will affect the physiotherapist's treatment plan.

Excess bronchial secretions

With cystic fibrosis, bronchial secretions may be minimal or copious. The infant at the time of diagnosis may be asymptomatic, but there is evidence of inflammation and infection in the lungs. Most paediatricians recommend introducing physiotherapy at this time in an attempt to delay the destructive process of infection and fibrosis. If physiotherapy becomes an accepted part of life, compliance will probably be better than if physiotherapy is introduced at a later stage. A close bonding usually develops between the parents and the child. It is important that both parents are involved and that the siblings are included in the care of the affected child so that they do not feel left out.

In the infant, in the absence of specific radiological signs, drainage of the apical segments of the upper lobes is included as the infant will spend much of his time lying down. The position is sitting upright on the parent's lap with the head and shoulders supported (Fig. 20.5). Other recommended positions are lying on each side with the chest tilted downwards, the infant supported on the parent's lap and thighs (lateral segments of the lower lobes (Fig. 20.6)). By rolling the infant slightly backwards towards the supine position the right middle lobe and lingula can be drained.

The techniques of positioning, chest clapping and chest vibrations will assist the mobilization of secretions and stimulate coughing. For the

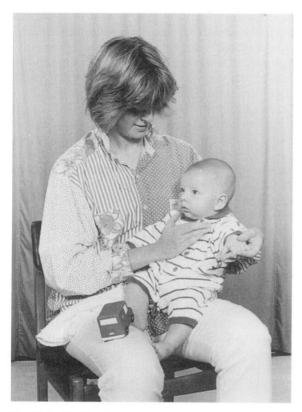

Fig. 20.5 Position for treatment of the apical segments of the upper lobes.

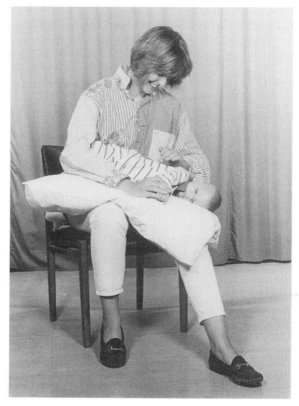

Fig. 20.6 Position for treatment of the lateral segment of the right lower lobe.

infant, chest clapping is performed using the first three fingers of one hand with the middle finger slightly elevated and should always be done over a layer of clothing. Treatment should be undertaken before feeds and probably for 5–10 minutes twice a day, for example sitting up and then positioning the infant for the lower lobe and middle zone of either the right or left lung, the other side being treated during the second session of the day.

Infants with cystic fibrosis have a higher incidence of gastro-oesophageal reflux (GOR), but there is conflicting evidence as to whether this is exacerbated by positioning with physiotherapy, especially the head-down position (Phillips 1996, Button et al 1997, Taylor & Threlfall 1997). Owing to the effect of gravity in the tipped position, intra-abdominal pressure will be at its lowest and there will be an increase in intra-

thoracic pressure. This together with an increase in diaphragmatic activity may enhance the competence of the oesophageal sphincter (Sindel et al 1989). When an increase in GOR is suspected the effect of positioning must be assessed. Anti-reflux medication may be prescribed.

When the child begins to walk the apical segments can be omitted from treatment, but it is then important to include the anterior segments of the upper lobes. The posterior segments of the upper lobes will probably be drained while the child is leaning forward playing with his toys.

If an infant or child has specific radiological signs, chest clapping in the appropriate gravity-assisted positions (p. 151) should be used. Treatments may need to be more frequent and, if tolerated, of slightly longer duration.

Treatment even at a young age should be fun.

The young child can be bounced up and down on his parent's knees and another exercise which is fun for the family is 'wheelbarrows' (Fig. 20.7). Laughing will also stimulate coughing and the minitrampoline can be introduced (Fig. 20.8).

From the age of 2 years, 'huffing' games can be started, for example blowing pieces of cotton wool or tissue using a tube in the mouth. The whole family can be involved in these games (Fig. 20.9). From 2–3 years of age the child can be encouraged to take deep breaths during the periods of chest clapping, but this should be for no more than three or four breaths before pausing for a period of breathing control. This is the introduction of the active cycle of breathing techniques (p. 140). At this stage if the head-down position is indicated the child can lie over a wedge of foam (Fig. 20.10) or pillows.

Infants and small children swallow their bronchial secretions, but as soon as possible expecto-

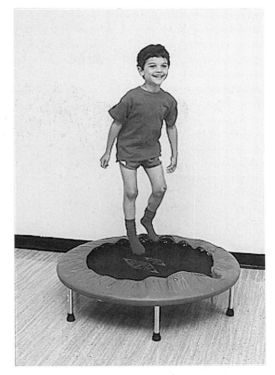

Fig. 20.8 Exercise on the minitrampoline.

ration should be encouraged. Nasopharyngeal suction should only be used if it is essential to obtain a sputum specimen or if the infant is distressed by the secretions. Learning to blow the nose is important to keep the upper airways clear.

By the age of 8 or 9 years the child can begin to do some of the treatment himself and gradually learn to be independent of his parents for periods of time. This will give his parents confidence that he will be able to continue his treatment when away from home staying with friends. For the adolescent a tipping frame supporting the whole body (Fig. 20.2) will be more comfortable and more appropriate than a wedge of foam.

Most adolescents prefer to take responsibility for their own physiotherapy, but assistance with treatment is often appropriate during an exacerbation of infection and for patients who are too frail to manage on their own. Sometimes patients have a preference for assistance.

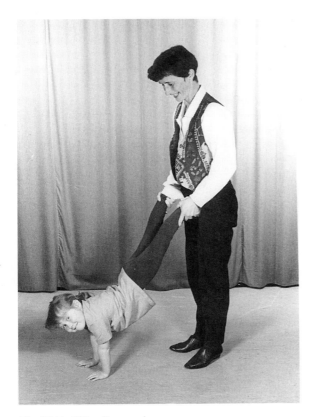

Fig. 20.7 'Wheelbarrows'.

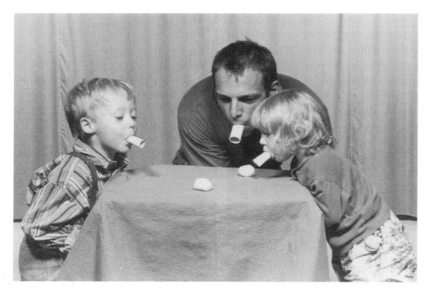

Fig. 20.9 Huffing games.

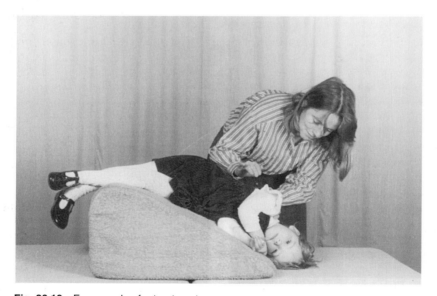

Fig. 20.10 Foam wedge for treatment.

Many patients with cystic fibrosis have a marked degree of airflow obstruction and to clear secretions effectively, sufficiently long periods of breathing control need to be emphasized. Paroxysms of coughing are exhausting and in-effective. They can be minimized by adapting the length of the huff and using breathing control. When control is gained, one or two huffs combined with breathing control will be more effective than coughing in the clearance of secretions.

The physiotherapist should be involved with

the changes in techniques from infancy to adulthood. Assessment and reassessment of the patient's condition are essential for the necessary changes in treatment to be recognized and recommended.

The frequency and duration of treatment will vary. When secretions are minimal, treatment once a day may be sufficient but additionally some form of exercise should be encouraged. Many patients will require treatment two or three times a day, but the programme should be realistic and allow for other normal activities. If a session is required in the middle of the day, this can probably be done in a sitting position at school, college or work.

Treatment is usually more effective if no more than three positions are used, as a minimum of 10 minutes in any one productive position is recommended. Although the cause is unknown, the upper lobes are frequently the most severely affected (Tomashefski et al 1986) and it is important to consider the anterior and posterior segments of the upper lobes when assessing the patient and planning treatment.

On occasions devices such as positive expiratory pressure (PEP) (p. 156), the Flutter (p. 157) or mechanical oscillators and percussors (p. 158) may increase adherence to treatment. Autogenic drainage (p. 155) is widely used in some countries. These regimens have been developed in different parts of the world to provide a means of treatment that does not require assistance and thereby improves patient compliance. Many of these regimens now include the forced expiration technique from the active cycle of breathing techniques and this has increased the effectiveness of these regimens.

In some parts of the world patients are given the opportunity to try each device and select their preferred treatment. In countries where even small costs are significant the active cycle of breathing techniques should be recommended as it is an effective regimen requiring no equipment.

Inhalation of drugs. Bronchodilator drugs may be prescribed and these should be inhaled before treatment to clear secretions. In some patients the airflow obstruction is partially reversible with bronchodilators. Another possible effect of β-adrenergic drugs is an increase in cilial action (Wood et al 1975) and this may improve mucociliary clearance.

Normal saline (0.9%) or hypertonic saline (3–7%) (Pavia et al 1978, Eng et al 1996) may be inhaled before physiotherapy to assist in clearance of secretions. If hypertonic saline is used a test dose should be given with recordings of PEF or FEV_1 before and 5 minutes after inhalation to identify any increase in airflow obstruction.

The optimal time for administration of Pulmozyme (DNase) in relation to physiotherapy has not yet been adequately studied and needs to be assessed for each individual. Some patients benefit most by inhaling it about 30 minutes before physiotherapy for airway clearance. Others find it takes several hours to reach a maximal effect and take it after one physiotherapy session with the result that the next session is more productive.

Pulmozyme should be aerolized on its own as it requires isotonic conditions and a neutral pH for maximal activity. On theoretical grounds, sufficient time (probably at least 30 minutes) should be allowed to elapse between the inhalation of Pulmozyme and other drugs, e.g. antibiotics, which may be either acidic or alkaline, to ensure maximum benefit from the drugs.

Mucolytic agents, for example acetylcysteine (Parvolex), reduce mucus viscosity. They should be used with caution as bronchospasm may be induced.

Aerosol antibiotics (p. 180) should be inhaled after secretions have been cleared. Spirometry is necessary before and after the initial dose to detect any increase in airflow obstruction. If this should occur the effect is usually minimized by the inhalation of a bronchodilator before treatment.

Acute exacerbation of a bronchopulmonary infection. Signs of an acute exacerbation include an increase in the volume and purulence of sputum, breathlessness, fever, a deterioration in lung function, possible pleuritic chest pain and a reduction in exercise tolerance.

An increase in the duration and frequency of physiotherapy treatments will be indicated and the patient will require assistance with chest clapping, shaking (Fig. 20.11) and compression. The pauses for breathing control may need to be lengthened and treatment should be discontinued before the patient becomes too tired. It may not be possible to reach the 'end-point' (p. 465) of treatment at this stage. There are such wide variations in pathology, and signs and symptoms, that for the inexperienced physiotherapist it is very difficult to know when to discontinue a treatment session. As a guide, a treatment session may range from about 20–45 minutes.

If oxygen therapy has been prescribed this should be continued throughout treatment. When secretions are very tenacious humidification should be considered, either continuously with oxygen therapy or for 10–15 minutes before physiotherapy (p. 188).

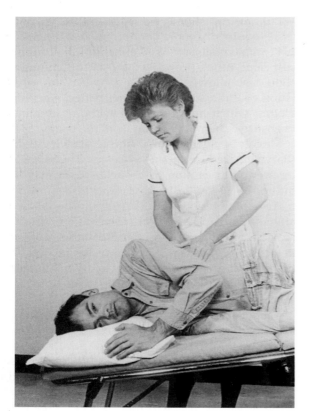

Fig. 20.11 Assisted treatment.

Intermittent positive pressure breathing (IPPB) may be indicated to reduce the work of breathing and assist in the clearance of secretions. If the patient has had a recent pneumothorax or a history of recurrent pneumothoraces IPPB is probably contraindicated.

Non-invasive positive pressure ventilation (NIPPV) (p. 106) may be used to improve ventilation and the physiotherapist may be involved in introducing the patient to the ventilator. By adjustment of the settings it is possible to continue NIPPV while carrying out physiotherapy, but it may be more appropriate to disconnect the patient from NIPPV and to use an airway clearance technique alone or an IPPB device with a mouthpiece.

Maintenance/increase in exercise tolerance

Exercise should play an important part in the management of cystic fibrosis through all stages of the disease to improve general physical fitness and muscle strength. It has been shown to improve cardiopulmonary fitness and muscle endurance (Orenstein et al 1981), to reduce breathlessness (O'Neill et al 1987) and to improve self-esteem and promote a feeling of well-being (Stanghelle et al 1988). Exercise increases mucociliary clearance, but it is less effective in the clearance of bronchial secretions than the active cycle of breathing techniques (Salh et al 1989).

From the time of diagnosis, exercise should be an integral part of the management. The family should be encouraged to take up some form of exercise that they will all enjoy. Children should take part in normal school games when possible and adults should be encouraged to take some form of enjoyable exercise regularly. In the winter months when outdoor sports may not be appropriate a stationary bicycle (Fig. 20.12) is often useful to provide a progressive exercise programme.

Exercise capacity can be assessed and monitored by measuring maximum oxygen uptake ($\dot{V}O_2$max) using a bicycle ergometer test. A progressive exercise programme should be based on a workload to achieve 50–60% of $\dot{V}O_2$max. If formal exercise testing is not available, 50%

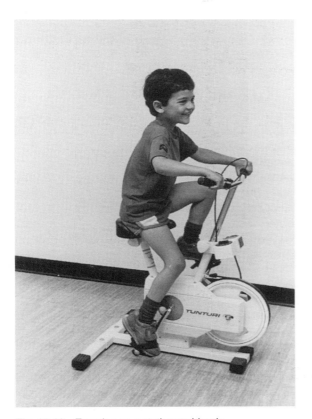

Fig. 20.12 Exercise on a stationary bicycle.

of peak work capacity (PWC) can be used as the starting point for exercise (Dodd 1991).

The PWC (in watts (W)) can be calculated using a bicycle ergometer. The patient starts cycling at a low wattage, for example 10–25 W (judged by fitness levels and disease severity) and this is increased by 10–25 W each minute until the patient can cycle no further. In patients with cystic fibrosis the limiting factor to exercise may be either breathlessness or muscle fatigue (Moorcroft et al 1996). The workload reached in this test approximates the PWC. Oxygen saturation and heart rate should be monitored. Many of these patients will tolerate a low oxygen saturation (SaO_2).

In patients with advanced pulmonary disease who desaturate during exercise, supplemental oxygen has been shown to increase exercise tolerance and aerobic capacity, and it can reduce

exercise-related arterial oxygen desaturation (Marcus et al 1992). The long-term effects of oxygen desaturation and therefore the place of oxygen therapy in chronic pulmonary disease remains controversial (Coates 1992).

Posture and trunk mobility exercises should be encouraged to try to maintain flexibility of the thoracic cage. Exercise programmes should combine endurance exercises for aerobic fitness and muscle strengthening exercises.

Exercise should be discontinued if a patient develops a fever as his metabolic requirements will be increased during this period. However, if confined to bed muscle strengthening exercises are important.

A patient who has exercise-induced asthma should remember to inhale his bronchodilator before starting exercise. When exercising a patient who has a small pneumothorax, or following a recent pneumothorax or haemoptysis, the physiotherapist should monitor the signs and symptoms during an exercise session.

In the occasional patient with osteoarthropathy exercise may be contraindicated during a period of acute joint involvement. The patient with diabetes should maintain an adequate sugar level during increased physical activity and a sweet drink or biscuit before exercise may be all that is required. Salt depletion may occur if exercising in hot weather or when in a hot climate, and salt supplements may be needed.

Some patients exercise after postural drainage, either because they are too breathless to exercise until they have cleared their secretions or because they find it more socially acceptable to be coughing less while participating in social sports. Other patients prefer to exercise before physiotherapy. Bilton et al (1992) could find no objective difference in sputum expectoration when exercise either preceded or followed physiotherapy.

Breathlessness

The use of breathing control while walking up stairs and hills should be introduced when breathlessness on exertion becomes noticeable. An irritable cough at night or breathlessness

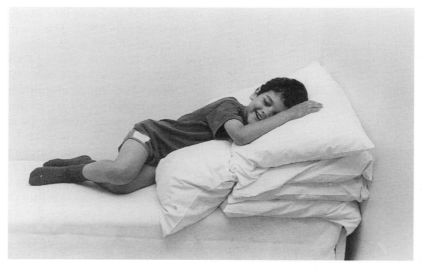

Fig. 20.13 High side lying position for breathlessness.

may be minimized by the use of the high side lying position (Fig. 20.13) and other rest positions are often of value to reduce breathlessness.

Chest wall stiffness and pain of musculoskeletal origin

Alterations in chest wall mechanics probably develop as a consequence of an increase in the work of breathing and hyperinflation of the chest leading to a shortening of the accessory muscles of respiration. Manual therapy techniques may increase thoracic mobility (p. 192) in patients with cystic fibrosis and may improve lung function (Vibekk 1991).

Complications of cystic fibrosis

Haemoptysis. Blood streaking of sputum is a frequent occurrence in patients with cystic fibrosis and there is no indication to alter the physiotherapy regimen. In cases of frank haemoptysis it is appropriate to discontinue physiotherapy temporarily until the bleeding begins to settle. Positioning may need to be modified and chest clapping withheld, but it is important to restart treatment as soon as possible to avoid

the accumulation of old blood in the airways and retention of sputum.

If severe haemoptysis persists a fibreoptic bronchoscopy may be undertaken to identify the bleeding point and embolization of the bronchial artery may be carried out (Cohen 1992). Following embolization, physiotherapy should be resumed without delay.

Pneumothorax. A small pneumothorax is not a contraindication to chest physiotherapy, but if during treatment the patient becomes more breathless or complains of chest pain the doctor should be notified immediately as it is possible that the pneumothorax could have increased in size.

A larger pneumothorax will require an intercostal drain and physiotherapy should be withheld until the drain has been inserted. Analgesia will probably be required before treatment and the patient's usual physiotherapy regimen should be continued, but chest clapping may be unnecessary and may cause discomfort.

If the air leak persists and surgical intervention is undertaken, it is essential that physiotherapy is restarted as soon as the patient is awake postoperatively. Adequate analgesia and humidification will assist the clearance of secretions.

Allergic bronchopulmonary aspergillosis. In

addition to the purulent secretions of cystic fibrosis there is mucus plugging caused by allergic bronchopulmonary aspergillosis (ABPA). Wheezing is also common. Treatment should include nebulized bronchodilators. Intermittent positive pressure breathing may be indicated.

Implantable venous access devices. These devices allow many patients to have intravenous antibiotic therapy at home, but it must be remembered that physiotherapy should also be increased during an exacerbation of a bronchopulmonary infection. Chest clapping over the site of the implanted device is uncomfortable and should be avoided, but all other techniques can be used.

Pregnancy. Pregnancy is not a complication in itself, but in the later stages of pregnancy the respiratory system is compromised and lung function will be reduced. Gravity-assisted positions will need to be modified and side lying or high side lying may be the positions of choice for physiotherapy.

The reduction in lung function continues for some time after the birth, especially if the patient has had an anaesthetic and caesarean section. Intensive physiotherapy is important throughout this stage.

Transplantation. The physiotherapist should be involved both before and after heart–lung or lung transplantation. Before transplantation the patient's exercise ability will be very limited but an exercise programme should be undertaken to optimize muscle strength and cardiovascular function. Postoperatively an extensive rehabilitation programme is essential to gain maximum benefit and improved quality of life (Ch. 16, p. 413).

Following heart–lung or double lung transplantation the lungs are denervated below the tracheal anastomosis with loss of all pulmonary innervation except postganglionic efferent nerves (Hathaway et al 1991). With the loss of the cough reflex and impaired mucociliary clearance, early recognition of signs of a chest infection is particularly important to minimize granulation tissue formation in the region of the large airway anastomoses, and pooling of secretions in the transplanted lung which may lead to bronchiec-

tasis (Madden & Hodson 1995). It is therefore often recommended that a short session of physiotherapy for airway clearance be continued on a daily basis, and increased as necessary during periods of chest infection.

Terminal care. The physiotherapist has an important role in the life of patients with cystic fibrosis and it is inappropriate to withdraw support in the terminal stages even though physiotherapy may no longer be effective. Assistance can be given with positioning the breathless patient to make him as comfortable as possible. Occasionally IPPB can be used to assist the clearance of secretions from the upper airways, but care must be taken to use it only as a part of physiotherapy treatment and not as a form of pseudo-ventilation.

The active cycle of breathing techniques is modified and will probably consist of encouraging a few deep breaths, long periods of breathing control and supported huffing either in high side lying or sitting leaning forward. The expectoration of one or two plugs of sputum can be a great relief to the patient. Nasotracheal suction is not indicated as it would serve no useful purpose at this stage. Morphine or one of its derivatives will help to relieve anxiety and breathlessness.

Evaluation of physiotherapy

In the patient in a stable condition, the daily weight or volume of sputum expectorated should remain approximately constant with effective physiotherapy and medical management. During an acute exacerbation effective treatment would be indicated by a reduction in sputum.

Appetite will return and weight will be gained as fever subsides and breathlessness is reduced.

Lung function including arterial blood gases and oxygen saturation are other indicators of improvement in response to treatment of an acute exacerbation. In long-term studies measurements of lung function must be viewed carefully as most of these will increase as the child grows older and decrease with progression of the disease.

Other measures include breathlessness, exercise capacity and endurance, chest wall pain and quality of life. Activities of daily living and absenteeism from school or work can also be used as indicators.

Continuity of care

Continuous assessment and reassessment of patients with cystic fibrosis is essential for effective management. The patient's needs will change as he progresses from infancy through school, college, university and work, but the emphasis is on leading as normal a life as possible while making time to include regular physiotherapy. Visits to schools to support individual patients and to increase the awareness and knowledge of the teachers is beneficial (Dyer & Morais 1996). Children should be encouraged to attend normal schools.

It is the knowledge and understanding of the condition and the effects of physiotherapy which will influence patient compliance through these stages (Passero et al 1981, Hames et al 1991). It is important to elicit and understand the patients' views and beliefs when negotiating a treatment programme (Carr et al 1996). Parents and patients should be involved in the planning of home treatment and realistic programmes can then be established.

Although the majority of parents and, when he is older, the patient himself can take the responsibility for physiotherapy treatments, it is essential that there is a regular review of the techniques by a physiotherapist. This also provides an opportunity to update the techniques and to discuss any problems. There are times when the parents or patient are unable to cope effectively on their own and the need for assistance during these periods should be recognized and help should be arranged.

If the patient is treated at both a local hospital and a specialist cystic fibrosis unit, communication between physiotherapists is essential to avoid confusion about treatment.

The physiotherapist must remember that she is a part of a multidisciplinary team and must be aware of the roles of the other members. Good communication within the team is essential. Members of the team may experience considerable stress from long-term involvement with patients with a chronic progressive illness. Coping with this stress can be helped by the team members recognizing each other's needs and providing the necessary support.

In caring for the patient with cystic fibrosis the physical care is important, but the psychological effects on both the family and the patient must also be considered. Many countries have cystic fibrosis associations which offer encouragement and support for patients and their families. In spite of the frequently high demands of treatment, most patients with cystic fibrosis are leading fulfilling lives and many adults are in full time employment (Walters et al 1993).

REFERENCES

Alton E, Caplen N, Geddes D, Williamson R 1992 New treatments for cystic fibrosis. British Medical Bulletin 48: 785–804

Anderson D H 1938 Cystic fibrosis of the pancreas and its relation to celiac disease: clinical and pathological study. American Journal of Disease in Childhood 56: 344–399

Bilton D, Dodd M E, Abbot J V, Webb A K 1992 The benefits of exercise combined with physiotherapy in the treatment of adults with cystic fibrosis. Respiratory Medicine 86: 507–511

Birrer P, McElvaney N G, Rüdeberg A et al 1994 Protease–antiprotease imbalance in the lungs of children with cystic fibrosis. American Journal of Respiratory and Critical Care Medicine 150: 207–213

Bourke S, Rooney M, Fitzgerald M, Bresnihan B 1987 Episodic arthropathy in adult cystic fibrosis. Quarterly

Journal of Medicine, New Series 64(244): 651–659

Bramwell E C, Halpin D M G, Duncan-Skingle F, Hodson M E, Geddes D M 1995 Home treatment of patients with cystic fibrosis using the 'Intermate': the first year's experience. Journal of Advanced Nursing 22: 1063–1067

Brueton M J, Ormerod L P, Shah K J, Anderson C M 1980 Allergic bronchopulmonary aspergillosis complicating cystic fibrosis in childhood. Archives of Disease in Childhood 55: 348–353

Button B M, Heine R G, Catto-Smith A G, Phelan P D, Olinsky A 1997 Postural drainage and gastro-oesophageal reflux in infants with cystic fibrosis. Archives of Disease in Childhood 76: 148–150

Carr L, Smith R E, Pryor J A, Partridge C 1996 Cystic fibrosis patients' views and beliefs about chest clearance and exercise – a pilot study. Physiotherapy 82: 621–627

Coates A L 1992 Oxygen therapy, exercise, and cystic fibrosis. Chest 101: 2–4

Cohen A M 1992 Hemoptysis: role of angiography and embolization. Pediatric Pulmonology Suppl 8: 85–86

Cole P 1995 Bronchiectasis. In: Brewis R A L, Corrin B, Geddes D M, Gibson G J (eds) Respiratory medicine, 2nd edn. Saunders, London, vol 2, ch 39

Conway S P, Pond M N, Watson A, Hamnett T 1996 Knowledge of adult patients with cystic fibrosis about their illness. Thorax 51: 34–38

Currie D, Munro C, Gaskell D, Cole P J 1986 Practice, problems and compliance with postural drainage: a survey of chronic sputum producers. British Journal of Diseases of the Chest 80: 249–253

Cystic Fibrosis Trust, British Paediatric Association, British Thoracic Society 1996 Clinical guidelines for cystic fibrosis care. Royal College of Physicians of London

di Sant'Agnese P A, Davis P B 1979 Cystic fibrosis in adults. American Journal of Medicine 66: 121–132

Dodd M E 1991 Exercise in cystic fibrosis adults. In: Pryor J A (ed) Respiratory care. Churchill Livingstone, Edinburgh, pp 27–50

Dodge J A, Morison S, Lewis P A et al 1993 Cystic fibrosis in the United Kingdom, 1968–1988: incidence, population and survival. Paediatric and Perinatal Epidemiology 7: 157–166

du Bois R M 1995 Respiratory medicine – recent advances. British Medical Journal 310: 1594–1597

Dyer J, Morais J A 1996 Supporting children with cystic fibrosis in school. Professional Nurse 11: 518–520

Eng P A, Morton J, Douglass J A, Riedler J, Wilson J, Robertson C F 1996 Short-term efficacy of ultrasonically nebulized hypertonic saline in cystic fibrosis. Pediatric Pulmonology 21: 77–83

Fairfax A J, Ball J, Batten J C, Heard B E 1980 A pathological study following bronchial artery embolization for haemoptysis in cystic fibrosis. British Journal of Diseases of the Chest 74: 345–352

FitzSimmons S C 1993 The changing epidemiology of cystic fibrosis. Journal of Pediatrics 122: 1–9

Fuchs H J, Borowitz D S, Christiansen D H et al 1994 Effect of aerolized recombinant human DNase on exacerbations of respiratory symptoms and on pulmonary function in patients with cystic fibrosis. New England Journal of Medicine 331: 637–642

Greenstone M, Rutman A, Dewar I, Mckay I, Cole P J 1988 Primary ciliary dyskinesia: cytological and clinical features. Quarterly Journal of Medicine, New Series 67(253): 405–430

Hames A, Beesley J, Nelson R 1991 Cystic fibrosis: what do patients know and what else would they like to know? Respiratory Medicine 85: 389–392

Hathaway T, Higenbottam T, Lowry R, Wallwork J 1991 Pulmonary reflexes after human heart–lung transplantation. Respiratory Medicine 85(suppl A): 17–21

Hodson M E 1996 Principles of antibiotic management. In: Issues in cystic fibrosis: antibiotic therapy. Report of a meeting held at Royal College of Pathologists November 1996 (Zeneca), 6–14

Hodson M E, Shah P L 1995 DNase trials in cystic fibrosis. European Respiratory Journal 8: 1786–1791

Hodson M E, Mearns M B, Batten J C, 1976 Meconium ileus equivalent in adults with cystic fibrosis of pancreas: a report of six cases. British Medical Journal 2: 790–791

Hodson M E, Madden B P, Steven M H et al 1991 Non-invasive mechanical ventilation for cystic fibrosis patients – a potential bridge to transplantation. European Respiratory Journal 4: 524–527

Høiby N, Koch C 1990 *Pseudomonas aeruginosa* infection in cystic fibrosis and its management. Thorax 45: 881–884

Hutchinson G R, Parker S, Pryor J A et al 1996 Home-nebulizers: a potential primary source of *Burkholderia cepacia* and other colistin-resistant, gram-negative bacteria in patients with cystic fibrosis. Journal of Clinical Microbiology 34: 584–587

Johnson S, Knox A J 1994 Arthropathy in cystic fibrosis. Respiratory Medicine 88: 567–570

Kartagener M 1933 Zur Pathogenese der Bronchiektasien. Beitrage zur Klinik der Tuberkulose 83: 489–501

Kerem E, Reisman J, Corey M, Canny G J, Levison H 1992 Prediction of mortality in patients with cystic fibrosis. New England Journal of Medicine 326: 1187–1191

Khan T Z, Wagener J S, Bost T, Martinez J, Accurso F J, Riches D W H 1995 Early pulmonary inflammation in infants with cystic fibrosis. American Journal of Respiratory and Critical Care Medicine 151: 1075–1082

Konstan M W, Hilliard K A, Norvell T M, Berger M 1994 Bronchoalveolar lavage findings in cystic fibrosis patients with stable, clinically mild lung disease suggest ongoing infection and inflammation. American Journal of Respiratory and Critical Care Medicine 150: 448–454

Lanng S, Thorsteinsson B, Nerup J, Koch C 1992 Influence of the development of diabetes mellitus on clinical status in patients with cystic fibrosis. European Journal of Paediatrics 151: 684–687

LiPuma J J, Dasen S E, Nielson D W, Stern R C, Stull T L 1990 Person-to-person transmission of *Pseudomonas cepacia* between patients with cystic fibrosis. Lancet 336: 1094–1096

McBride G 1990 More progress in cystic fibrosis. British Medical Journal 301: 627

Madden B P, Hodson M E 1995 Rehabilitation considerations for the lung transplant patient. In: Bach J R (ed) Pulmonary rehabilitation. Hanley & Belfus, Philadelphia, ch 15, pp 193–202

Marcus C L, Bader D, Stabile M W et al 1992 Supplemental oxygen and exercise performance in patients with cystic fibrosis with severe pulmonary disease. Chest 101: 52–57

Moorcroft A J, Dodd M E, Howarth C, Webb A K 1996 Muscular fatigue, ventilation and perception of limitation at peak exercise in adults with cystic fibrosis. Pediatric Pulmonology Suppl 3: 306

Muhdi K, Edenborough F P, Gumery L, O'Hickey S, Smith E G, Smith D L, Stableforth D E 1996 Outcome for patients colonised with *Burkholderia cepacia* in a Birmingham adult cystic fibrosis clinic and the end of an epidemic. Thorax 51: 374–377

Mukhopadhyay S, Singh M, Cater J I, Ogston S, Franklin M, Olver R E 1996 Nebulised antipseudomonal antibiotic therapy in cystic fibrosis: a meta-analysis of benefits and risks. Thorax 51: 364–368

Nelson L A, Callerame M L, Schwartz R H 1979 Aspergillosis and atopy in cystic fibrosis. American Review of Respiratory Disease 120: 863–873

O'Neill P, Dodd M, Phillips B et al 1987 Regular exercise and reduction of breathlessness in patients with cystic fibrosis. British Journal of Diseases of the Chest 81: 62–69

Orenstein D M, Franklin B A, Doershuk C F et al 1981

Exercise conditioning and cardiopulmonary fitness in cystic fibrosis. Chest 80: 392–398

Park R W, Grand R J 1981 Gastrointestinal manifestations of cystic fibrosis: a review. Gastroenterology 81: 1143–1161

Passero M A, Remor B, Salomon J 1981 Patient-reported compliance with cystic fibrosis therapy. Clinical Pediatrics 20: 264–268

Pavia D, Thomson M L, Clarke S W 1978 Enhanced clearance of secretions from the human lung after the administration of hypertonic saline aerosol. American Review of Respiratory Disease 117: 199–203

Phillips G 1996 To tip or not to tip? Physiotherapy Research International 1: 1–6

Poole S 1995 Dietary treatment of cystic fibrosis. In: Hodson M E, Geddes D M (eds) Cystic fibrosis. Chapman & Hall, London, ch 15, pp 383–395

Pringle M B 1992 Swimming and grommets. British Medical Journal 304: 198

Range S P, Knox A J 1995 rhDNase in cystic fibrosis. Thorax 50: 321–322

Ranieri E, Lewis B D, Gerace R L et al 1994 Neonatal screening for cystic fibrosis using immunoreactive trypsinogen and direct gene analysis: four years' experience. British Medical Journal 308: 1469–1472

Reid L, de Haller R 1967 The bronchial mucous glands – their hypertrophy and changes in intracellular mucus. Bibliotheca Pedriatica 86: 195–200

Rogers D, Goodchild M C 1996 Role of a domiciliary physiotherapist in the treatment of children with cystic fibrosis. Physiotherapy 82: 396–402

Rommens J M, Iannuzzi M C, Kerem B et al 1989 Identification of the cystic fibrosis gene: chromosome walking and jumping. Science 245: 1059–1065

Rutland J, Cole P J 1980 Non-invasive sampling of nasal cilia for measurement of beat frequency and study of ultrastructure. Lancet ii: 564–565

Salh W, Bilton D, Dodd M, Webb A K 1989 Effect of exercise and physiotherapy in aiding sputum expectoration in adults with cystic fibrosis. Thorax 44: 1006–1008

Shah P L, Scott S F, Fuchs H J, Geddes D M, Hodson M E 1995 Medium term treatment of stable stage cystic fibrosis with recombinant human DNase I. Thorax 50: 333–338

Shah P L, Scott S F, Knight R A, Marriott C, Ranasinha C, Hodson M E 1996 In vivo effects of recombinant human DNase I on sputum in patients with cystic fibrosis. Thorax 51: 119–125

Shale D J 1997a Predicting survival in cystic fibrosis. Thorax 52: 309

Shale D J 1997b Commentary. Thorax 52: 95–96

Sindel B D, Maisels M J, Ballantine T V N 1989 Gastroesophageal reflux to the proximal esophagus in infants with bronchopulmonary dysplasia. American Journal of Disease in Childhood 143: 1103–1106

Smith A L 1994 *Pseudomonas aeruginosa* infections in cystic fibrosis: epidemiology and biologic mechanisms. New Insights into Cystic Fibrosis (University of Washington School of Medicine) 2(2): 1–5

Smith I E, Flower C D R 1996 Review article: imaging in bronchiectasis. British Journal of Radiology 69: 589–593

Stanghelle J K, Winnem M, Roaldsen K et al 1988 Young patients with cystic fibrosis: attitude toward physical activity and influence on physical fitness and spirometric values of a 2-week training course. International Journal of Sports Medicine 9: 25–31

Stanley P, MacWilliam L, Greenstone M, Mackay I S, Cole P J 1984 Efficacy of a saccharin test for screening to detect abnormal mucociliary clearance. British Journal of Diseases of the Chest 78: 62–65

Stead R J, Davidson T I, Duncan F R, Hodson M E, Batten J C 1987 Use of a totally implantable system for venous access in cystic fibrosis. Thorax 42: 149–150

Stern M, Geddes D 1994 Gene therapy for cystic fibrosis. Respiratory Disease in Practice Winter: 18–23

Super M, Schwarz M J, Malone G, Roberts T, Haworth A, Dermody G 1994 Active cascade testing for carriers of cystic fibrosis gene. British Medical Journal 308: 1462–1468

Taylor C J, Threlfall D 1997 Postural drainage techniques and gastro-oesophageal reflux in cystic fibrosis. Lancet 349: 1567–1568

Tomashefski J F, Bruce M, Goldberg H I, Dearborn D G 1986 Regional distribution of macroscopic lung disease in cystic fibrosis. American Review of Respiratory Disease 133: 535–540

Touw D J, Brimicombe R W, Hodson M E, Heijerman H G M, Bakker W 1995 Inhalation of antibiotics in cystic fibrosis. European Respiratory Journal 8: 1594–1604

Valerius N H, Koch C, Høiby N 1991 Prevention of chronic *Pseudomonas aeruginosa* colonisation in cystic fibrosis by early treatment. Lancet 338: 725–726

Vibekk P 1991 Chest mobilization and respiratory function. In: Pryor J A (ed) Respiratory care. Churchill Livingstone, Edinburgh, pp 103–119

Walters S, Britton J, Hodson M E 1993 Demographic and social characteristics of adults with cystic fibrosis in the United Kingdom. British Medical Journal 306: 549–552

Webb A K, Dodd M E 1997 Nebulised antibiotics for adults with cystic fibrosis. Thorax 52(suppl 2): S69–S71

Wills P J, Wodehouse T, Corkery K, Mallon K, Wilson R, Cole P J 1996 Short-term recombinant human DNase in bronchiectasis. American Journal of Respiratory and Critical Care Medicine 154: 413–417

Wilson R, Sykes D A, Chan K L, Cole P J, Mackay I S 1987 Effect of head position on the efficacy of topical treatment of chronic mucopurulent rhinosinusitis. Thorax 42: 631–632

Wood R E, Wanner A, Hirsch J, Farrell P M 1975 Tracheal mucociliary transport in patients with cystic fibrosis and its stimulation by terbutaline. American Review of Respiratory Disease 11: 733–738

FURTHER READING

Brewis R A L, Corrin B, Geddes D M, Gibson G J (eds) 1995 Respiratory medicine, 2nd edn. Saunders, London, vols 1, 2

Dinwiddie R 1997 The diagnosis and management of paediatric respiratory disease, 2nd edn. Churchill Livingstone, Edinburgh

Hodson M E, Geddes D M (eds) 1995 Cystic fibrosis. Chapman & Hall, London

21

Immunosuppression or deficiency

Denise Hills

INTRODUCTION

The ability of an individual to remain healthy requires the cooperation and interaction of a very sensitive series of components, all designated to protect the host. Undifferentiated stem cells (originating from bone marrow) specialize into two major defence systems. These are the cellular and the humoral immune systems.

The cellular immune system

Cell-mediated immunity is made up of T lymphocytes (T cells) which are derived from the thymus and then migrate to the lymph nodes and spleen. When stimulated, some of these cells migrate via the bloodstream into affected tissue where they interact with foreign material. The key to the cell-mediated immune system is the CD4 positive lymphocyte (T-helper cell), one of the T lymphocytes (Weir 1977). T-helper cells process foreign antigen presented to them by macrophages and stimulate the appropriate cytotoxic cell lines (killer cells, CD8 cells) and B lymphocytes (B cells) to mount a response against all foreign cells or viruses with the same antigen make-up. These cells attack foreign material, both individually and in conjunction with macrophages (phagocytic cells). Phagocytic cells are either fixed in tissues, for example in the spleen, bone marrow, lung, liver (reticuloendothelial system), or in the circulation, that is the monocytes and polymorphonuclear neutrophils. This system helps to guard primarily against viral,

485

fungal and protozoal invasion as a first line of defence, along with circulating humoral factors.

The humoral system

The humoral immune system consists of B lymphocytes which produce immunoglobulins (antibodies), i.e. IgG, IgA, IgM, IgD and IgE. These immunoglobulins, found in serum, tissue fluids and secretions, develop an affinity for foreign (non-self) proteins during primary infection and they retain this affinity during subsequent infections. The immunoglobulin pool is made up of approximately 75% IgG (found in vascular and intervascular spaces), 15% IgA (in saliva, tears, colostrum, intestinal and bronchial secretions) and 10% IgM (in intravascular spaces). The remainder is made up of IgD found on the surface of B lymphocytes, and IgE on the membrane of mast cells where it interacts with allergens in allergic individuals.

Should any aspect of the complex host immune system be deficient or suppressed, the response elicited to a particular infective agent may be ineffective, leaving the host open to overwhelming and possibly life-threatening infection.

Classification of immune deficient states

There are many different congenital immunodeficiency syndromes in existence, usually rare and of little clinical importance to the physiotherapist. More frequently, the physiotherapist in a general hospital will be involved with patients suffering from immunodeficiency or suppression secondary to malignancies, immunosuppressive drugs, organ transplantation (see Ch. 16), chronic disease and, increasingly, human immunodeficiency virus (HIV) infection. However, of greater importance is the understanding of the overall type of deficiency, cellular, humoral or mixed, which in each case may be associated with certain patterns of infection (Table 21.1).

Infective agents

The immunosuppressed or deficient individual may be infected by a range of organisms varying from the more common pathogens, for example *Haemophilus influenzae*, to opportunistic infections which are only pathogenic in the presence of severe immune dysfunction, of which *Pneumocystis carinii* is an example (Table 21.2). Cell-mediated defects leave the host susceptible to infection from viruses, fungi, mycobacteria and protozoa, in contrast to humoral system defects, which are associated with infection by bacteria. Mixed defects will show the complete range of susceptibility, causing a complex clinical situation.

Presenting problems

The severity and extent of the presenting problems will depend on the type of defect from which the patient suffers. In the Swiss-type agammaglobulinaemia, for example, survival is rarely beyond the second year of life owing to overwhelming viral and bacterial infection. The most frequently affected site in immunosuppressed or deficient states is the respiratory tract, with sinusitis and pulmonary infections often recurrent and persistent. Bronchiectasis is a common complication of repeated pulmonary infections; however, abscess and cavity formation, empyemas and pleural effusions may occur.

Otitis media is a frequent complication and skin infections can also be present (bacterial or viral).

Gastrointestinal infections and resultant malabsorption may cause generalized weakness and emaciation. Mobility may be affected by septic arthritis and osteomyelitis, secondary to bacterial infection.

The neurological system does not escape susceptibility, and problems include meningitis, encephalitis and mental deterioration, peripheral nerve lesions, myelopathy, neuropathy, space-occupying lesions and demyelinating diseases.

The result is that the physiotherapist is often faced with a patient who has multiple, complex problems presenting separately or concurrently. This complexity is highlighted by the acquired immune deficiency syndrome (AIDS) patient, for example, who, as the immune deficiency increases (reflected by decreasing CD4 lympho-

Table 21.1   Immunodeficiency states with major types of immune defect

Immunodeficient state	Immune defect	Site*
Congenital		
Swiss-type agammaglobulinaemia (AGGA)	Immature stem cells	M
Bruton-type AGGA	Immature B cells	H
DiGeorge syndrome	Immature T cells	C
Immunodeficiency with ataxia telangiectasia	Immature T cells	C
Wiskott–Aldrich syndrome	Inability to respond to polysaccharide antigens	H
Partial defects, e.g. types I, III, V and VI dysimmunoglobulinaemia	Altered antibody levels	H
Infections		
HIV/AIDS	T-helper cell destruction	C
Leishmaniasis, malaria	Organism suppresses stem cell function	M
Malignancies		
Lymphomasarcoma		
Hodgkin's disease	Defective T cells and defective B cell function	M
Chronic lymphocytic leukaemia		
Iatrogenic		
Immunosuppressive drugs, e.g. corticosteroid and cytotoxic drugs		
Irradiation therapy	Suppressed T cell and B cell function	M
Organ transplants		
Splenectomy	Loss of phagocytic activity	M
Other		
Diabetes mellitus	Reduced neutrophil function	M
Uraemia	Reduced lymphocyte function	M
Malnutrition	Reduced T cell and phagocytic activity	C
Chronic disease	Reduced cell proliferation and response	M

* C, cellular immune defect; H, humoral immune defect; M, mixed defect.

Table 21.2   Common opportunistic pathogens with their main clinical features, found in immunocompromised patients

Pathogen	Characteristics
Bacteria	
Streptococcus pneumoniae	Pulmonary: lobar pneumonia, empyema Meningitis Septic arthritis Pericarditis Septicaemia Otitis media Sinusitis
Staphylococcus aureus	Bronchopneumonia Abscess formation Osteomyelitis Endocarditis Septic arthritis Skin infection
Streptococcus pyogenes	Consolidation with or without pleural disease Septicaemia
Klebsiella pneumoniae	Bronchopneumonia with or without abscess, possible septicaemia
Pseudomonas aeruginosa	Common nosocomial infection, e.g. burns, skin sites, central lines, focal with or without septicaemia
Haemophilus influenzae	Bronchopulmonary disease Sinusitis Otitis media Septic arthritis

Table 21.2 (contd)

Pathogen	Characteristics
Legionella pneumophila	Interstitial pneumonia
Escherichia coli	Colitis with or without septicaemia
Salmonella	Colitis – not self-limiting
Fungi	
Candida albicans	Dermatological Oral, oesophageal, bronchial in AIDS Disseminated infections in neutropenic patients
Cryptococcus neoformans	Interstitial pneumonitis with haematological spread to meninges, liver, spleen Localized at a site as cryptococcoma
Aspergillus fumigatus	Necrotizing bronchopneumonia Intracavitary fungal growth Invasive spread to tissues Generalized dissemination
Histoplasma capsulatum	Dermatological Disseminated Pulmonary with or without cavitation
Nocardia asteroides	Pulmonary: solitary or widespread consolidation Disseminated to brain Dermatological
Mycobacteria	
Mycobacterium tuberculosis	Pneumonitis Systemic
Atypical mycobacteria e.g. *Mycobacterium avium intracellulare*	Low-grade disseminated infection pulmonary
Viruses	
Cytomegalovirus	Pneumonitis with patchy diffuse infiltrates Enteritis Chorioretinitis
Herpes simplex/herpes zoster	Dermatological Pulmonary Neurological
Protozoa	
Pneumocystis carinii	Diffuse interstitial pneumonia
Toxoplasma gondii	Disseminated disease Interstitial pneumonitis Cerebral abscess, encephalopathy, meningoencephalitis

cyte cell numbers) shows progressive and fairly unpredictable presentations of increasingly severe infections covering all body systems. This can be a challenge for the medical staff, who need to diagnose each infection and instigate specific treatment regimens to combat each infection to maximal effect.

PHYSIOTHERAPY

The problems a physiotherapist may encounter in this group of patients are many and varied, offering a challenge not only in the short-term problem solving, but also in the achievement of long-term goals which may be very complex. Frequent communication with the multidisciplinary team is essential to coordinate appropriate treatment objectives.

The physiotherapist should make a detailed assessment of the patient to identify physiotherapy problems and to plan the treatment programme. Accurate documentation will assist in the long-term management of this group of patients, allowing trends to be recognized. The physiotherapist must also be aware of the patient's social situation, occupation, hobbies and functional needs. Treatment goals should then be agreed with the patient. The treatment of physiotherapy problems caused by immuno-suppression or deficiencies in children must be modified appropriately.

The following are some of the problems the physiotherapist may find on examination and be required to deal with in patients with immuno-suppression or deficiency.

Respiratory problems

In immune deficiency states the respiratory system is the most frequently affected site.

Breathlessness

The degree of breathlessness may vary from breathlessness on exertion to that occurring even at rest, dependent on the extent of the pathology.

The main causes include hypoxaemia, pleural effusions, pneumothorax and pneumonia. *Pneumocystis carinii* pneumonia (PCP) is a major life threatening infection in AIDS patients which causes progressive severe hypoxaemia and breathlessness (Fig. 21.1).

Positioning can be used to optimize ventilation and perfusion. The pattern of breathing control should be encouraged and the use of rest positions, for example high side lying and forward lean sitting.

When hypoxaemia is a major cause of the breathlessness, oxygen therapy is likely to be used. If a venturi system is not used, or a high oxygen concentration is necessary (e.g. 60% and above), high humidity should be considered.

The medical management may include the use of continuous positive airway pressure (CPAP) via a full face mask or nasal mask at approximately 5–10 cmH$_2$O if patients have not responded to oxygen therapy alone. CPAP has been demonstrated to increase the PaO_2 and decrease breathlessness in AIDS patients with severe PCP (Kesten & Rebuck 1988, Miller &

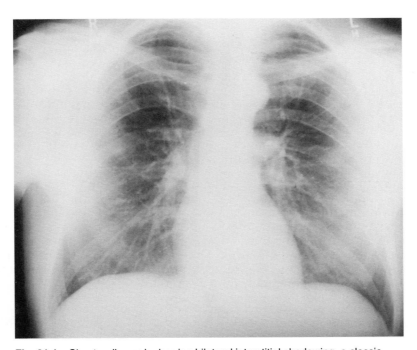

Fig. 21.1 Chest radiograph showing bilateral interstitial shadowing, a classic indication of PCP.

Mitchell 1990, Boix et al 1995), but patients need to be monitored closely.

Patients with suspected PCP who suffer from progressive breathlessness, hypoxaemia and a dry cough may be referred for sputum induction to assist in the diagnosis. Sputum induction involves the nebulization of hypertonic saline (3–5%) inhaled from an ultrasonic nebulizer (Fig. 21.2) or efficient jet nebulizer. The mode of action of the hypertonic saline is unclear. Several studies (Bigby et al 1986, Leigh et al 1989) advocate the use of strict protocols to avoid contamination of the sample. The patient may be requested to be 'nil by mouth' overnight, and thorough brushing of the teeth, tongue and gums with rinsing the mouth using large quantities of water or normal saline is important to clear oral debris. The nebulized hypertonic saline should be inhaled for up to 20 minutes, during which time the patient is encouraged to huff and cough until an adequate sample is obtained. Occasionally a sample may be unobtainable.

The sensitivity of sputum induction using an ultrasonic nebulizer ranges from 28 to 94.7%

depending on the availability of diagnostic techniques such as immunofluorescence or polymerase chain reaction (PCR) testing (Bigby et al 1986, Leigh et al 1989, Miller et al 1991, Lipschik et al 1992). However, there is the possibility of serious side-effects such as the rapid development of life-threatening pleural effusion if a small effusion is already present (Nelson et al 1990). Other adverse effects include breathlessness, nausea and bronchoconstriction (Miller et al 1991). If there is a negative response from sputum induction, fibreoptic bronchoscopy would probably be undertaken. The higher sensitivity of the procedure of bronchoscopy and its minimal side-effects have led to its preferred use in some centres (Miller et al 1990). The physiotherapist must be aware that a small proportion of HIV-infected patients undergoing investigation for PCP will in fact have pulmonary tuberculosis and appropriate precautions need to be used (Klein & Motyl 1993).

Excess secretions

This problem is usually caused by a bacterial

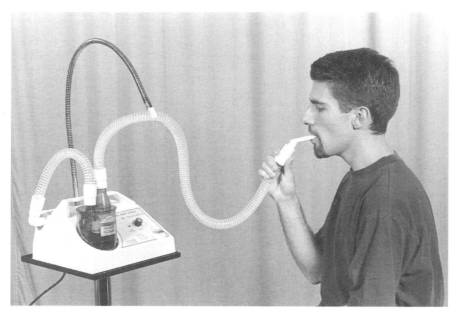

Fig. 21.2 An induced sputum procedure using the Devilbiss Ultra-neb 2000 ultrasonic nebulizer.

chest infection or pneumonia. The use of the airway clearance techniques, possibly including positioning, vibrations and chest clapping will help to clear excess secretions. The patient should be encouraged to continue these breathing techniques as necessary to maintain a clear chest.

Pain

Chest pain may occur in association with pneumonia (pleurisy) or as a result of a chest drain in situ for the treatment of a pneumothorax or pleural effusion. Chest pain may result in a shallow, rapid breathing pattern. Adequate analgesia is essential to allow the patient to breathe more normally and to facilitate the use of breathing techniques. This will reduce the possibility of subsegmental lung collapse and secretion retention as a secondary complication.

Prophylaxis and education

In all immunosuppressed or deficient patients a heightened awareness of developing infection is an asset. Patients can be taught to recognize signs of respiratory infection, giving them the opportunity not only to report early for medical treatment, but also allowing them to begin self-treatment, for example their breathing exercises, at an early stage. It is useful for patients who develop frequent, recurrent pulmonary infections to be taught airway clearance techniques which they can carry out themselves and to have these techniques reviewed at regular intervals to ensure effectiveness. Patients with bronchiectasis should be encouraged to continue their breathing exercises daily to help prevent further infections.

One aspect of care in which the physiotherapist may become involved is that of supervising or administering nebulized pentamidine isethionate to HIV/AIDS patients to prevent the occurrence of PCP. This treatment modality is sometimes used in patients unable to tolerate co-trimoxazole prophylaxis (Bozzette et al 1995). Pentamidine persists within the lung for long periods of time (Conte & Golden 1988) and therefore dose intervals of 2–4 weeks are appropriate (Leoung et al 1990, Smith et al 1991). The technique involves the administration of a solution of pentamidine dissolved in sterile water, delivered to the patient via an efficient nebulizer and exhalation system (Smaldone et al 1991). In practice, the nebulizer should produce a particle size of 2–5 μm (maximizing deposition to the alveolar region of the lungs). The exhalation of droplets into the room should be prevented by using a one-way valve system and wide-bore tubing out of the window, or an exhalation filter. The efficacy and benefits of this form of prophylaxis have been documented (Smith et al 1991). Side-effects are nearly always minimal and local. These may include bronchospasm, increased salivation, cough, unpleasant taste, nausea and a sore throat. The use of a nebulized bronchodilator before the nebulized pentamidine may help to keep the bronchospasm to a minimum (Smith et al 1988). This treatment can be administered as an outpatient procedure, or the patient may be taught to carry out the treatment at home.

Musculoskeletal problems

Pain

Joint and bone pain occur with osteomyelitis and septic arthritis and in these instances contractures could occur as a result of badly positioned limbs, particularly during periods of bed rest. Correct positioning is essential to maintain joint range and muscle extensibility. Joint splinting may be necessary during acute episodes for comfort and to decrease the likelihood of contractures. Ice packs applied to the affected area may help to decrease the pain.

Severe Kaposi's sarcoma lesions on the lower limbs in AIDS patients may result in extensive oedema and pain. Patients are inclined to draw their legs up into the flexed position, providing the ideal posture for the development of hip and knee flexion contractures. Advice and explanation on elevation, circulatory exercises and the use of lymphoedema massage or intermittent compression therapy via pumps may be of some value to help decrease oedema and pain.

This should be combined with compression in the form of an elastic lymphoedema stocking to help prevent recurrence of the oedema (Badger 1987) and daily passive/active exercise and stretches must also be included in the treatment programme. Techniques such as transcutaneous electrical nerve stimulation (TENS) may also be of use in the management of pain associated with the above conditions or HIV neuropathies.

Wasting and weakness

Malabsorption is a frequent complication of gastrointestinal infections, chemotherapy or malnutrition. The resultant wasting and weakness can be extremely debilitating, not only in the acute presentation but also as a chronic illness. This will have an effect on physiotherapy regimens as the patient's overall level of tolerance of a physical treatment may be lowered. It is necessary to allow for lethargy and fatigue and to include a generalized exercise programme in the treatment sessions to help build up muscle bulk and strength. Supervised exercise programmes, as well as showing expected improvements in cardiovascular fitness, do not appear to adversely affect the immune system and in one small study of HIV-infected individuals actually improved CD4 counts (Keyes et al 1989). The exercise programme should be progressive, and continual reassessment is necessary to evaluate the correct amount and variety of exercise needed. Imaginative use of equipment both on the ward and in a physiotherapy gymnasium will help to capture and maintain the patient's interest. Advice on on-going exercises and local facilities, for example swimming pools, to continue appropriate levels of activity following discharge is important to reinforce independence and self-care.

Altered tone and coordination

Neurological manifestations of immunosuppression or deficiency are many and varied and may not always fit a predictable pattern. The physiotherapist must treat problems such as spasticity, flaccidity and ataxia as they affect each individual. The techniques the physiotherapist may use are many and varied, but the overall goal should be one of maximal functional gain to achieve the best possible quality of life for each individual.

Mobility

Mobility is affected not only by weakness, wasting and neurological problems, but also by other complications such as joint contractures. During any episode of immobility it is essential to include the use of passive movements, active-assisted, active or resisted exercises and stretches for the joints and muscles. Where contractures already exist, the use of serial splinting and hold–relax proprioceptive neuromuscular facilitation techniques may help to regain some range of movement in combination with strengthening exercises.

Assessment and provision of mobility aids is an important part of achieving and maintaining functional independence and safety.

Where mobility is limited by breathlessness on exertion, for example in severe bronchiectasis or acute PCP, patients can be taught breathing control while walking and stair climbing.

Psychological problems

Physiotherapy students rarely receive tuition in counselling patients with chronic illness and terminal disease (see Chs 9 and 18). It is important to develop these skills to give the physiotherapist a better understanding and ability to deal more effectively and confidently with the complex emotions and reactions displayed by patients. The psychological support that can be provided by offering adequate time and using effective listening skills, can be invaluable to the patient and very rewarding to the physiotherapist.

Immunosuppressed or deficient patients who are suffering from HIV/AIDS may require more support than other groups as they may feel socially rejected and have guilt attached to their illness. This isolation may be compounded by estrangement from their family if they are homosexual or intravenous drug users. It is useful for physiotherapists to be aware of appropriate organizations that are available for patients to contact for help or advice.

INFECTION CONTROL

Some infections seen in immunodeficient patients can be contracted by other patients or hospital staff. Every hospital should have a policy or document on infection control with reference to the prevention of transmission of HIV, bacterial infections, TB and hepatitis B. Protocols for infection control must be known and adhered to by the physiotherapist. The philosophy and clinical application of universal

precautions for infection control is one of the most effective in protecting staff from transmission by 'unknown' carriers of HIV and the hepatitis B virus, and it also addresses the issue of confidentiality. The aim is to treat every patient equally and without prejudice (Mullen et al 1989).

CONCLUSION

Immunosuppressed or deficient patients form a challenging group for the physiotherapist. The patients' problems are often complex, but accurate assessment and effective treatment procedures can lead to exciting and rewarding improvements in their quality of life.

REFERENCES

Badger C 1987 Lymphoedema: management of patients with advanced cancer. Professional Nurse (January): 100–102

Bigby T D, Margolskee D, Curtis J L et al 1986 The usefulness of induced sputum in the diagnosis of *Pneumocystis carinii* pneumonia in patients with the acquired immunodeficiency syndrome. American Review of Respiratory Disease 133: 515–518

Boix J H, Miguel V, Arnar O et al 1995 Airway continuous positive pressure in acute respiratory failure caused by *Pneumocystis carinii* pneumonia [Spanish]. Revista Clinica Espanola 195: 69–73

Bozzette S A, Finkelstein D M, Spector S A et al 1995 A randomized trial of three antipneumocystis agents in patients with advanced human immunodeficiency virus infection. New England Journal of Medicine 332: 693–699

Conte J E, Golden J A 1988 Concentrations of aerosolized pentamidine in bronchoalveolar lavage in patients with AIDS. Journal of Infectious Diseases 157(5): 985–989

Kesten S, Rebuck A S 1988 Nasal continuous positive airway pressure in *Pneumocystis carinii* pneumonia. Lancet (17 Dec): 1414–1415

Keyes C, Rodgers P, Wolbert J et al 1989 Effect of cardiovascular conditioning in HIV infection (abstract). International Conference on AIDS

Klein R S, Motyl M 1993 Frequency of pulmonary tuberculosis in patients undergoing sputum induction for diagnosis of suspected *Pneumocystis carinii* pneumonia. AIDS 7: 1351–1355

Leigh T R, Hume C, Gazzard B et al 1989 Sputum induction for diagnosis of *Pneumocystis carinii* pneumonia. Lancet (22 July): 205–206

Leoung G S, Feigal D W, Montgomery A B et al 1990 Aerosolized pentamidine for prophylaxis against *Pneumocystis carinii* pneumonia. New England Journal of Medicine 323: 769–775

Lipschik G Y, Gill V J, Lundgren J D et al 1992 Improved diagnosis of *Pneumocystis carinii* infection by polymerase chain reaction on induced sputum and blood. Lancet 340: 203–206

Miller R F, Mitchell D M 1990 Management of respiratory failure in patients with the acquired immune deficiency syndrome and *Pneumocystis carinii* pneumonia. Thorax 45: 140–146

Miller R F, Semple S J 1991 Continuous positive airway pressure ventilation for respiratory failure associated with *Pneumocystis carinii* pneumonia. Respiratory Medicine 85: 133–138

Miller R F, Semple S J G, Kocjan G 1990 Difficulties with sputum induction for diagnosis of *Pneumocystis carinii* pneumonia. Lancet 335: 112

Miller R F, Kocjan G, Buckland J et al 1991 Sputum induction for the diagnosis of pulmonary disease in HIV positive patients. Journal of Infection 23: 5–15

Mullen R J, Baker E L, Bell D M et al 1989 Guidelines for prevention of transmission of human immunodeficiency virus and hepatitis B virus to health-care workers and public-safety workers. Morbidity and Mortality Weekly Report 38(suppl 6): 1–37

Nelson M, Bower M, Smith D et al 1990 Life-threatening complication of sputum induction. Lancet 335: 112–113

Smaldone G C, Vinciguerra C, Marchese J 1991 Detection of inhaled pentamidine in health care workers. New England Journal of Medicine 325(12): 891–892

Smith D E, Herd D A, Gazzard B G 1988 Reversible bronchoconstriction with nebulised pentamidine. Lancet ii: 905

Smith D E, Hills D A, Harman C et al 1991 Nebulized pentamidine for the prevention of *Pneumocystis carinii* pneumonia in AIDS patients: experience of 173 patients and a review of the literature. Quarterly Journal of Medicine 79(291): 619–629

Weir D 1977 Immunology – an outline for students of medicine and biology, 4th edn. Churchill Livingstone, Edinburgh, ch 4, pp 79–81

FURTHER READING

Braunwald E, Isselbacher K J, Petersdorf R G et al (eds) 1987 Harrison's principles of internal medicine, 11th edn. McGraw-Hill, New York, part 3, sections 1–9
Hughes W T 1977 Infections in the compromised host. Advances in Internal Medicine 22: 73–96

Pratt R 1991 AIDS, a strategy for nursing care, 3rd edn. Edward Arnold, London
Weir D 1977 Immunology — an outline for students of medicine and biology, 4th edn. Churchill Livingstone, Edinburgh

Normal values and abbreviations

NORMAL VALUES

	Heart rate (beats/min)	Respiratory rate (breaths/min)	Blood pressure (mmHg)
Pre-term infants	120–140	40–60	70/40
Full-term infants	100–140	30–40	80/40
1–4 years	80–120	25–30	100/65
Adults	50–100	12–16	95/60–140/90

Conversion tables

0.133 kPa = 1.0 mmHg		$pH = 9 - \log[H^+]$ where $[H^+]$ is in nmol/l	
kPa	mmHg	pH	$[H^+]$
1	7.5	7.52	30
2	15.0	7.45	35
4	30	7.40	40
6	45	7.35	45
8	60	7.30	50
10	75	7.26	55
12	90	7.22	60
14	105	7.19	65

Arterial blood

pH	7.35–7.45 $[H^+]$ 45–35 nmol/l
PaO_2	10.7–13.3 kPa (80–100 mmHg)
$PaCO_2$	4.7–6.0 kPa (35–45 mmHg)
HCO_3^-	22–26 mmol/l
Base excess	−2 to +2

Venous blood

pH	7.31–7.41 $[H^+]$ 46–38 nmol/l
PO_2	5.0–5.6 kPa (37–42 mmHg)
PCO_2	5.6–6.7 kPa (42–50 mmHg)

Ventilation/perfusion

Alveolar–arterial oxygen gradient A–aPO_2:
Breathing air   0.7–2.7 kPa (5–20 mmHg)
Breathing 100%   3.3–8.6 kPa (25–65 mmHg)
oxygen

Pressures

		mmHg	kPa
Right atrial (RA) pressure	Mean	−1 to +7	−0.13 to 0.93
Right ventricular (RV) pressure	Systolic	15–25	2.0–3.3
	Diastolic	0–8	0–1.0
Pulmonary artery (PA) pressure	Systolic	15–25	2.0–3.3
	Diastolic	8–15	1.0–2.0
	Mean	10–20	1.3–2.7
Pulmonary capillary wedge pressure (PCWP)	Mean	6–15	0.8–2.0
Central venous pressure (CVP)		3–15 cmH$_2$O	
Intracranial pressure (ICP)		< 10 mmHg (< 1.3 kPa)	
Peak inspiratory mouth pressure (*Pi*Max)	Male	103–124 cmH$_2$O (age dependent)	
	Female	65–87 cmH$_2$O (age dependent)	
Peak expiratory mouth pressure (*Pe*Max)	Male	185–233 cmH$_2$O (age dependent)	
	Female	128–152 cmH$_2$O (age dependent)	

Blood chemistry

Albumin	37–53 g/l
Calcium (Ca^{2+})	2.25–2.65 mmol/l
Creatinine	60–120 µmol/l
Glucose	4–6 mmol/l
Potassium (K$^+$)	3.4–5.0 mmol/l
Sodium (Na$^+$)	134–140 mmol/l
Urea	2.5–6.5 mmol/l
Haemoglobin (Hb)	14.0–18.0 g/100 ml (men)
	11.5–15.5 g/100 ml (women)
Platelets	150–400 × 10^9/l
White blood cell count (WBC)	4–11 × 10^9/l
Urine output	1 ml/kg/h

ABBREVIATIONS

A–aDO$_2$	alveolar–arterial oxygen gradient
A–aPO_2	alveolar–arterial oxygen gradient
ABPA	allergic bronchopulmonary aspergillosis
ADH	antidiuretic hormone
ADL	activities of daily living
AF	atrial fibrillation
AIDS	acquired immune deficiency syndrome
AMBER	advanced multiple beam equalization radiography
AP	anteroposterior
APACHE	acute physiology and chronic health evaluation
ARDS	acute respiratory distress syndrome
ARDS	adult respiratory distress syndrome
ARF	acute renal failure
ASD	atrial septal defect
ATN	acute tubular necrosis
ATPS	ambient temperature and pressure saturated
AVAS	absolute visual analogue scale
AVSD	atrioventricular septal defect
BiPAP	bilevel positive airway pressure
BIPAP	bilevel positive airway pressure
BIVAD	biventricular device
BMI	body mass index
BP	blood pressure
BPD	bronchopulmonary dysplasia
BPF	bronchopleural fistula
bpm	beats per minute
BSA	body surface area
BTPS	body temperature and pressure saturated
Ca^{2+}	calcium
CABG	coronary artery bypass graft
CABGS	coronary artery bypass graft surgery
CAD	coronary artery disease
CAL	chronic airflow limitation
CAVG	coronary artery vein graft
CBF	cerebral blood flow
CF	cystic fibrosis
CFA	cryptogenic fibrosing alveolitis
CFTR	cystic fibrosis transmembrane conductance regulator

CK	creatine kinase
CLD	chronic lung disease
cm	centimetre
CMV	controlled mandatory ventilation
CMV	cytomegalovirus
CO	cardiac output
CO_2	carbon dioxide
COAD	chronic obstructive airways disease
CPAP	continuous positive airway pressure
CPP	cerebral perfusion pressure
CRF	chronic renal failure
CRP	conditioning rehabilitation programme
CSF	cerebrospinal fluid
CT	computed tomography
CV	closing volume
CVP	central venous pressure
DH	drug history
DIC	disseminated intravascular coagulopathy
dl	decilitre
DLCO	diffusing capacity for carbon monoxide
DNA	deoxyribonucleic acid
DVT	deep vein thrombosis
EBV	Epstein–Barr virus
$ECCO_2R$	extracorporeal carbon dioxide removal
ECG	electrocardiograph
ECMO	extracorporeal membrane oxygenation
EEG	electroencephalogram
EIA	exercise-induced asthma
EOG	electro-oculogram
EPP	equal pressure point
ERV	expiratory reserve volume
$ETCO_2$	end-tidal carbon dioxide
ETT	endotracheal tube
FEF_{50}	forced expiratory flow at 50% of forced vital capacity
FEF_{75}	forced expiratory flow at 75% of forced vital capacity
FET	forced expiration technique
FEV_1	forced expiratory volume in 1 second
FG	French gauge
FH	family history

FHF	fulminant hepatic failure
FiO_2	fractional inspired oxygen concentration
FRC	functional residual capacity
ft	feet
FVC	forced vital capacity
g	gram
g/dl	gram per decilitre
GCS	Glasgow coma scale
GOR	gastro-oesophageal reflux
GPB	glossopharyngeal breathing
GTN	glyceryl trinitrate
h	hour
H^+	hydrogen ion
$[H^+]$	hydrogen ion concentration
H_2O	water
Hb	haemoglobin
HCO_3^-	bicarbonate
Hct	haematocrit
HD	haemodialysis
HDU	high dependency unit
HFJV	high-frequency jet ventilation
HFO	high-frequency oscillation
HFPPV	high-frequency positive pressure ventilation
HIV	human immunodeficiency virus
HLA	human leucocyte antigen
HLT	heart–lung transplantation
HME	heat and moisture exchanger
HPC	history of presenting condition
HR	heart rate
Hz	hertz
IABP	intra-aortic balloon pump
ICC	intercostal catheter
ICP	intracranial pressure
ICU	intensive care unit
Ig	immunoglobulin
IHD	ischaemic heart disease
IMV	intermittent mandatory ventilation
in	inches
INR	international normalized ratio
IPPB	intermittent positive pressure breathing
IPPV	intermittent positive pressure ventilation

IPS	inspiratory pressure support
IV	intravenous
IVH	intraventricular haemorrhage
IVOX	intravenacaval oxygenation
JVP	jugular venous pressure
K^+	potassium
KCO	coefficient of gas transfer
kg	kilogram
kJ	kilojoule
kPa	kilopascal
kVp	kilovoltage
l	litre
LAP	left atrial pressure
LED	light-emitting diode
LTOT	long-term oxygen therapy
LVAD	left ventricular assist device
LVF	left ventricular failure
LVRS	lung volume reduction surgery
m	metre
μm	micrometre (10^{-6} m)
μs	microsecond
MAP	mean arterial pressure
MCH	mean corpuscular haemoglobin
MCV	mean corpuscular volume
MDI	metered-dose inhaler
MEF_{50}	maximal expiratory flow at 50% of forced vital capacity
MEF_{75}	maximal expiratory flow at 75% of forced vital capacity
METs	metabolic equivalents
MHz	megahertz
MI	myocardial infarction
MIE	meconium ileus equivalent
min	minute
ml	millilitre
mm	millimetre
MMAD	mass median aerodynamic diameter
mmHg	millimetres of mercury
mmol	millimole
MRI	magnetic resonance imaging
MRSA	methicillin-resistant *Staphylococcus aureus*
ms	millisecond
MVV	maximum voluntary ventilation

n	number
Na^+	sodium
NEPV	negative extrathoracic pressure ventilation
NICU	neonatal intensive care unit
NIPPV	non-invasive intermittent positive pressure ventilation
nm	nanometre
nmol	nanomole
NO	nitric oxide
NPV	negative pressure ventilation
NSAID	non-steroidal anti-inflammatory drug
O_2	oxygen
OB	obliterative bronchiolitis
OHFO	oral high-frequency oscillation
OLT	orthotopic liver transplantation
PA	posteroanterior
PA	pulmonary artery
$PaCO_2$	partial pressure of carbon dioxide in alveolar gas
$PaCO_2$	partial pressure of carbon dioxide in arterial blood
PaO_2	partial pressure of oxygen in alveolar gas
PaO_2	partial pressure of oxygen in arterial blood
PAP	pulmonary artery pressure
PAWP	pulmonary artery wedge pressure
PCA	patient-controlled analgesia
PCD	primary ciliary dyskinesia
PCIRV	pressure-controlled inverse ratio ventilation
PCP	*Pneumocystis carinii* pneumonia
PCPAP	periodic continuous positive airway pressure
PCV	packed cell volume
PCWP	pulmonary capillary wedge pressure
PD	peritoneal dialysis
PD	postural drainage
PDA	patient ductus arteriosus
Pdi	transdiaphragmatic pressure
PE	pulmonary embolus
PEEP	positive end-expiratory pressure
PEF	peak expiratory flow

PEFR	peak expiratory flow rate	SG_{AW}	specific airway conductance
*Pe*Max	peak expiratory mouth pressure	SH	social history
PEP	positive expiratory pressure	SIMV	synchronized intermittent
pH	hydrogen ion concentration		mandatory ventilation
PIE	pulmonary interstitial emphysema	SOB	shortness of breath
PIF	peak inspiratory flow	SpO_2	nocturnal arterial oxygen saturation
PIFR	peak inspiratory flow rate	SVC	superior vena cava
*Pi*Max	peak inspiratory mouth pressure	SVO_2	mixed venous oxygen saturation
PIP	peak inspiratory pressure	SVR	systemic vascular resistance
PMH	previous medical history		
PN	percussion note	$TcCO_2$	transcutaneous carbon dioxide
PND	paroxysmal nocturnal dyspnoea	TcO_2	transcutaneous oxygen
POMR	problem oriented medical record	TED	thromboembolic deterrent
PTB	pulmonary tuberculosis	TENS	transcutaneous electrical nerve
PTCA	percutaneous transluminal coronary		stimulation
	angioplasty	TGA	transposition of the great arteries
$P_{TC}CO_2$	transcutaneous carbon dioxide	TLC	total lung capacity
	tension	TLCO	transfer factor in lung of carbon
PTFE	polytetrafluoroethylene		monoxide
PTT	partial thromboplastin time	TV	tidal volume
PVC	polyvinyl chloride		
PVH	periventricular haemorrhage	UAS	upper abdominal surgery
PVL	periventricular leucomalacia		
PVR	pulmonary vascular resistance	$\dot{V}$	ventilation
PWC	peak work capacity	$\dot{V}_A$	alveolar ventilation/alveolar volume
		VAD	ventricular assist device
$\dot{Q}$	blood flow	VAS	visual analogue scale
QOL	quality of life	VC	vital capacity
		V_D	dead-space ventilation
RAP	right atrial pressure	$\dot{V}_E$	minute ventilation
R_{AW}	airway resistance	VF	ventricular fibrillation
RBC	red blood cell	VF	vocal fremitus
RDS	respiratory distress syndrome	$\dot{V}O_2$	oxygen consumption
REM	rapid eye movement sleep	$\dot{V}O_2$max	maximum oxygen uptake
ROP	retinopathy of prematurity	$\dot{V}/\dot{Q}$	ventilation/perfusion ratio
RPE	rating of perceived exertion	VR	vocal resonance
RSV	respiratory syncytial virus	VRE	vancomycin-resistant enterococcus
RTA	road traffic accident	VSD	ventricular septal defect
RV	residual volume	V_T	tidal volume
RVF	right ventricular failure		
		W	watt
s	second	WBC	white blood count
SA	sinoatrial	WCC	white cell count
SaO_2	arterial oxygen saturation	WOB	work of breathing

Index